www.harcourt-international.com

Bringing you products from all Harcourt Health Sciences companies including Baillière Tindall, Churchill Livingstone, Mosby and W.B. Saunders

- ▶ **Browse** for latest information on new books, journals and electronic products

- ▶ **Search** for information on over 20 000 published titles with full product information including tables of contents and sample chapters

- ▶ **Keep up to date** with our extensive publishing programme in your field by registering with **eAlert** or requesting postal updates

- ▶ **Secure online ordering** with prompt delivery, as well as full contact details to order by phone, fax or post

- ▶ **News** of special features and promotions

If you are based in the following countries, please visit the country-specific site to receive full details of product availability and local ordering information

USA: www.harcourthealth.com

Canada: www.harcourtcanada.com

Australia: www.harcourt.com.au

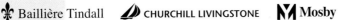 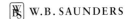
Baillière Tindall   CHURCHILL LIVINGSTONE   Mosby   W.B. SAUNDERS

Gynaecological Nursing

For Churchill Livingstone:

Publishing Manager, Health Professions: Inta Ozols
Head of Project Management: Ewan Halley
Project Development Manager: Katrina Mather
Designer: George Ajayi

Gynaecological Nursing

A Practical Guide

Edited by

Elizabeth Gangar RN RMT FPCert
Formerly Research Sister, Menopause Clinic, Queen Charlotte's & Chelsea Hospital,
London, UK

Foreword by

Vicki Allanach RN RM FETC DMS
Adviser in Midwifery and Women's Health, Royal College of Nursing, London, UK

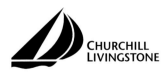

CHURCHILL
LIVINGSTONE

EDINBURGH LONDON NEW YORK PHILADELPHIA ST LOUIS SYDNEY TORONTO 2001

CHURCHILL LIVINGSTONE
An imprint of Harcourt Publishers Limited

First published 2001

ISBN 0 443 06202 1

British Library Cataloguing in Publication Data
A catalogue record for this book is available from the British Library

Library of Congress Cataloging in Publication Data
A catalog record for this book is available from the Library of
Congress

Note
Medical knowledge is constantly changing. As new information
becomes available, changes in treatment, procedures, equipment and
the use of drugs become necessary. The editor, contributors and the
publishers have taken care to ensure that the information given in this
text is accurate and up to date. However, readers are strongly advised
to confirm that the information, especially with regard to drug usage,
complies with the latest legislation and standards of practice.

The
publisher's
policy is to use
**paper manufactured
from sustainable forests**

Printed in China

Contents

A colour plate section can be found between
pages **182** and **183**.

Contributors

Kate Anders RGN, BSc, ENB 134 Nephro/
Urology
Urogynaecology Nurse Specialist,
Urogynaecology Unit, King's College Hospital,
London, UK

Margaret Barron SRN
Research Nurse, Princess Anne Hospital,
Southampton, UK

Janet Brockie SRN DipN
Menopause Office, Women's Centre, John
Radcliffe Hospital, Oxford, UK

Sandra Brown RGN Certificate in Health
Promotion ENB 931
Senior Nurse – Surgery, University Hospitals of
Leicester, Leicester General Hospital, Leicester,
UK

Jacky Cotton RGN RM MHS
Operational Nurse Manager – Gynaecology,
Birmingham Women's Hospital, Edgbaston,
Birmingham, UK

Sarah Creighton MD MRCOG
Consultant Obstetrician and Gynaecologist,
Department of Obstetrics and Gynaecology,
University College London Hospital, London,
UK

Elizabeth Gangar RN RMT FPCert
Formerly, Research Sister, Menopause Clinic,
Queen Charlotte's & Chelsea Hospital, London,
UK

Joy Hall MSc (Human sexuality), BEd (Hons),
RGN, Dip Nursing (Lon) RNT RCNT
Senior Lecturer, University of Central England,
Faculty of Health and Community Care,
Edgbaston, Birmingham, UK

Karen Handscomb BSc (Hons) RGN
Senior Clinical Nurse Specialist, Gynaecological
Oncology, Royal Marsden NHS Trust, London,
UK

Hilary Hollis BSc (Hons) Nursing Studies, MSc
Nursing Studies, PG (Dip) Nurse Education,
ENB 237 Oncological Nursing
Senior Nurse Clinical Trials,
Royal Marsden Hospital, London, UK

Cathryn Hughes RGN MSc
Gynaecological Oncology Nurse Specialist,
St Mary's Hospital, London, UK

Christina McGlynn RGN
Senior Sister, Ambrose King Centre and Barts
Sexual Health Centre, Royal London Hospitals
Trust, London, UK

Lindsey Mitchem MSc RGN
Tutor, Department of Nursing & Health Studies,
The Waikato Polytechnic, Hamilton,
New Zealand

Terri Morgan RGN RM
Clinical Nurse Specialist, Reproductive
Medicine, Department of Reproductive
Medicine, Mayday University Hospital, Surrey,
UK

Rosemary Nicholl RGN
Senior Staff Nurse, Ward 30, Leicester General
Hospital, Leicester, UK

Vera Rogers SRN
Formerly, Clinical Nurse Specialist, The Pelvic
Pain Clinic, Northwick Park and St Mark's NHS
Trust, Middlesex, UK

Kathy Suffling RGN RM
Clinical Nurse Specialist, Menopause Office,
Women's Centre, John Radcliffe Hospital,
Oxford, UK

Alison Sutton RGN PG (Dip)
HIV Liaison Nurse, Guest Hospital, Dudley,
West Midlands, UK

Hazel Watson MSc RGN
Lecturer (Clinical), European Institute of Health
and Medical Sciences, University of Surrey,
Guildford, Surrey, UK

Barbara Walters MSc RN RM PDN RCNT RNT
Dip N(Lon) Dip N Ed(Lon) ENB 901
Lecturer, Women's Health Pathway Leader, City
University, St Bartholomew's School of Nursing
and Midwifery, London, UK

Angela Whitton RGN ENB225 (Gynaecology)
Miscarriage Nurse Specialist, University
Hospitals of Coventry and Warwickshire,
Coventry, UK

Foreword

Evidence over recent years has demonstrated that nurses have a crucial role within the health care team and that patients value the care that nurses can give. Nursing care also helps patients to get better quicker and patients may feel more at ease with a nurse who often acts as their advocate. There is also evidence to show that nursing care gives good value for money.

Gender is an important determinant in health and women not only have particular health needs because of their complex reproductive system, they also have a need for fertility, contraceptive and sexual health advice, pregnancy and gynaecological care and treatment. In addition to all of this, women are affected both negatively and positively by social factors and generally they have higher expectations of the national health service. Against this complex background, gynaecological nurses are developing their role.

Gynaecological nurses have been encouraged to develop their skills and many nurses throughout the United Kingdom are leading exciting initiatives such as nurse led pre-operative assessment clinics, miscarriage and early pregnancy units, menopause clinics and colposcopy. Nurses work closely with their patient/client group involving them in their care as they know that patients who have control over their treatment fare better, feel more satisfied and ultimately cost less to treat. Gynaecological nurses are no exception to this. The intimate nature of gynaecological problems and diseases can be embarrassing, distressing and frightening for women. The nurse is in a unique position to assess and plan the woman's care taking into account the different aspects of her individual life which may be affected, and then provide appropriate support and care. The gynaecological nurse who is able to give continuity and women centred care can often be a source of reassurance for these women and therefore the nurses role should not be underestimated.

The Royal College of Nursing Gynaecological Nursing Forum is committed to the development of high standards of nursing care and supports nurses in their endeavours to achieve this. It is therefore very pleasing to introduce this practical guide *Gynaecological Nursing* which is written by nurses and doctors all of whom are women themselves and have expertise and knowledge in specific areas of experiences and practice. This applies particularly to the case studies which are helpful in highlighting examples of real life scenarios which chart the management and interventions in specific gynaecological diseases and disorders and demonstrate the crucial role that nurses have in the continuum of care.

This book will be an invaluable resource for nurses who are just beginning a career in gynaecology and equally for nurses who are already actively engaged within this speciality and want to consolidate and expand their knowledge and nursing practice. This book will also enable nurses to offer greater choices to women.

As technology and medical advances progress and the general public have increasing access to information about their own health there is a crucial need for all nurses to ensure that their knowledge base is sound and that their practice is evidence based. Gynaecological problems and women's health initiatives present some interesting and challenging opportunities for gynaecological nurses and this comprehensive text should provide an excellent working guide for nurses and enable them to achieve the best care for women.

London 2001   Vicki Allanach

Preface

Nursing is undergoing rapid changes with the advent of Nurse Specialists, Nurse Practitioners and Nursing Consultants and the government has made clear its intentions of expanding the role and responsibility of nurses in the NHS. Just as nursing is changing, medical technology is moving ever forward with resulting alterations in practice and the introduction of new techniques.

As nurses, we need to be aware of these changes and advances and maintain our knowledge base not only for patient care but as a requirement for re-validation and professional development which is now mandatory. For patients to feel confident about the information and care we provide and to maintain their trust, we need to be able to provide sound accurate and consistent information.

This book is designed to provide that information in a comprehensive, practical way giving thorough coverage of medical advances but using a sensitive holistic approach based on the requirements of nursing practice. It covers diseases and disorders which are unique to, or are more common in, women. Starting with problems which occur in the early reproductive years such as disorders of puberty, infertility, recurrent miscarriage and ectopic pregnancy, it continues through the reproductive years covering the minefield of endocrine disorders, causes of pelvic pain and malignancy. Finally, it looks at the late and post menopausal years covering aspects of uterine displacement, disorders of micturition and the climacteric. It concludes with a section on gynaecological surgery looking at the pre-operative assessment and post operative complications in common gynaecological procedures and operations.

It provides clinically focused, helpful information for nurses by nurses and doctors from around the country who have been chosen because of their expertise and knowledge in their individual field. I feel that we have produced a professional reference book which presents clinical and practical issues, management and education in many aspects of gynaecological nursing.

Surrey 2001   Elizabeth Gangar

1

Anatomy and physiology of the female reproductive system

Elizabeth Gangar

The purpose of this chapter is to refresh our memories and help us to understand the problems which can occur in the female.

THE FEMALE REPRODUCTIVE TRACT

The female reproductive tract (Fig. 1.1) is divided into two: the external genital organs and the internal genital organs.

The external genitalia

The external female genital organs (genitalia) are known collectively as the vulva and consist of the labia majora and labia minora, the clitoris, the hymen, the vestibule and the perineum (Fig. 1.2).

The labia majora

The two large folds of skin that form the boundary of the vulva are known as the labia majora. The inner aspects are smooth and contain a number of sweat and sebaceous glands while the outer aspects, after puberty, are covered with hair.

The labia minora

These are the two smaller folds of skin, situated within the labia majora, that contain a few sweat and sebaceous glands; they enclose an area called the vestibule. They attach anteriorly to the under surface of the clitoris – the area known as the frenulum – and posteriorly to form the fourchette.

The clitoris

This is a small, sensitive structure containing erectile tissue corresponding to the male penis.

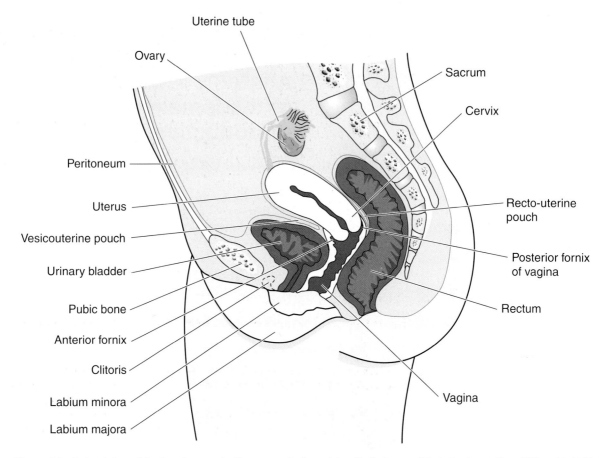

Figure 1.1 Lateral view of the female reproductive organs in the pelvis with their associated structures. From Wilson K, 1981 Foundation of Anatomy and Physiology 5e, Churchill Livingstone, Edinburgh.

The hymen

The thin layer of mucous membrane partially occluding the vaginal opening is called the hymen. Occasionally, the hymen completely covers the vaginal orifice and surgery is required to allow the passage of menstrual flow. This condition is known as an imperforate hymen and the accumulation of blood in the vagina is termed 'haematocolpos'. Very occasionally, the hymen is thick and fibrous and may need surgical treatment to allow penetrative intercourse (see Chapter 2).

The vestibule

The vestibule can be visualized when the labia minora are separated. Situated within the vestibule are: the external orifice of the urethra, two Skene's ducts, the vaginal orifice or introitus, and the two Bartholin's ducts. The Bartholin's glands secrete mucus, which keeps the external genitalia moist. If one or both glands become blocked, the secretions are unable to drain down the duct and the gland becomes acutely painful and swollen. Infected abscesses need to be incised and drained and antibiotics prescribed. If there is persistent cyst formation, then marsupialization is required.

The perineum

The triangular area that lies between the fourchette and the anus is known as the perineum. It gives attachment to the muscles of the pelvic floor and its function is to assist with the process of defecation and to act as a support for the genital tract. Trauma of this area,

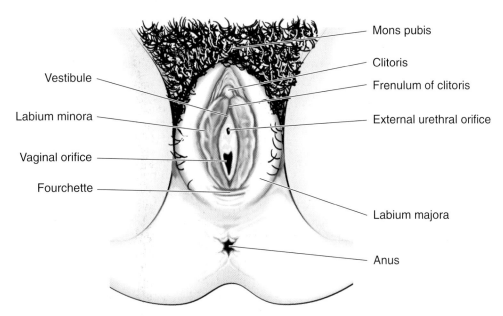

Mons pubis

Clitoris

Frenulum of clitoris

External urethral orifice

Vestibule

Labium minora

Vaginal orifice

Fourchette

Labium majora

Anus

Figure 1.2   The female external genitalia. From Wilson K, 1981 Foundation of Anatomy and Physiology 5e, Churchill Livingstone, Edinburgh.

such as during childbirth, can give rise to disorders of micturition, defecation and prolapse of the pelvic organs.

The internal genitalia

The internal genitalia of the female lie in the pelvic cavity and consist of the vagina, the uterus, the cervix, two fallopian tubes and two ovaries (see Plate 1).

The vagina

The vagina connects the vulva to the uterus and runs upwards and backwards into the pelvis. It is a fibromuscular structure. The walls lie closely together in folds and have the potential for separating and forming a tube to allow for sexual intercourse and childbirth. The anterior, posterior and two lateral fornices (named according to their position) are formed where the cervix protrudes into the vagina. The mucosa of the vagina, under the influence of oestrogen, contains a large amount of glycogen. Upon decomposition, this glycogen produces lactic acid, which creates a low pH and acid balance that inhibits bacterial growth and yeast and prevents infection; the acidity is also harmful to sperm. Semen (which is naturally alkaline) neutralizes this acidity to ensure sur-

vival of the sperm. The vagina can become susceptible to infection if the acidity balance is interfered with, such as during the postmenopausal years when oestrogen production is decreased (see Chapter 16) or when antibiotics are taken, which kill off the lactic acid-producing lactobacilli.

The uterus

The uterus is a hollow, muscular, pear-shaped organ that lies in the pelvis between the bladder and the rectum in an anteverted, anteflexed position. It is divided into three areas: (i) the fundus, which is the dome-shaped part of the uterus; (ii) the body, which is the main part of the uterus; and (iii) the cervix. The walls of the uterus are composed of three layers of tissue: (i) the serosa, or outer covering of peritoneum; (ii) the myometrium, or middle layer of smooth muscle fibres; and (iii) the endometrium, the epithelial lining. The structure of the endometrium varies with the menstrual cycle and the endometrium is largely shed during menstruation.

   Uterine support. The uterus is supported in the pelvic cavity by the round ligaments, which maintain it in the position of anteversion and anteflexion. However, in some women this position is not maintained and retroversion may be normal or caused by disease such as endometriosis or adhesion formation (see Chapter 17). The broad ligaments are folds of peritoneum draped over the uterus and fallopian tubes and attached to the sides of the pelvis. The cardinal ligaments, pubocervical ligaments and uterosacral ligaments give support to the cervix and uterus. Overstretching of these ligaments will result in prolapse of the uterus (see Chapter 17).

The cervix

The lower third of the uterus is the cervix, occasionally referred to as the neck of the uterus. It runs from the internal os, protrudes into the vagina and opens at the external os. The vaginal portion of the cervix (ectocervix) is lined with stratified squamous epithelium. It is replenished by basal cell proliferation during reproductive life and is glycogen-laden due to oestrogen stimulation. During the postmenopausal years this epithelium undergoes atrophy, with thinning and loss of glycogen. The endocervical canal is lined with columnar epithelium. The area where the endocervical columnar epithelium meets the ectocervical stratified squamous epithelium is referred to as the squamocolumnar junction (SCJ). This is not a fixed area and is important in the understanding of abnormal cell formation and their treatment (see Chapter 13). Under the influence of oestrogen, such as during puberty and pregnancy, the endocervical epithelium comes to lie on the ectocervix, moving the SCJ outwards. The visible red columnar epithelium is known as an erosion or ectopy. During the menopause the cervix tends to shrink and the SCJ moves up the endocervical canal and is difficult to visualize.

The fallopian tubes

The uterine or fallopian tubes lie on either side of the uterus, extending from the cornua. Each tube is approximately 3 mm diameter and about 10 cm long, ending at a dilated, trumpet-like portion. This end of the tube has finger-like projections, called fimbriae, which surround the orifice and collect the ovum. The lining of the tube consists of ciliated epithelium to aid the passage of the ovum from the ovary to the uterus. Fertilization of the ovum usually takes place in the fallopian tube and the slow, peristaltic movement of the cilia gives the fertilized ovum time to develop and prepare for implantation in the uterus. Implantation that occurs outside the uterine cavity is referred to as an ectopic pregnancy. The fertilized ovum may float freely in the pelvic cavity and implantation may occur on the pelvic viscera. More commonly, the fertilized ovum fails to descend to the uterus and implants in the fallopian tube, a type of pregnancy known as a tubal ectopic (see Chapter 5).

The ovaries

The ovaries are the female sex organs. They are situated near the fimbrial ends of the fallopian tubes and are attached to the posterior layer of the broad ligament by a band of peritoneum. The ovaries are smooth, dull, white and solid prior to puberty. Following puberty, the ovaries enlarge and develop an irregular surface; they become smaller and inactive again following the menopause. The ovaries are made up of two parts: (i) the medulla, the centre of the organ; and (ii) the cortex, which consists of connective tissue or stroma. It is in this stroma that the graafian follicles are embedded. These follicles each contain an ovum at different stages of development; only one of these will mature during each menstrual cycle. The ovaries are part of the endocrine system, which produces the female hormones, oestrogen and progesterone, and a small amount of testosterone. The hormones are produced in response to stimulation by the gonadotrophins secreted by the anterior pituitary gland (Fig. 1.3).

THE MENSTRUAL CYCLE

The menstrual cycle is a sequence of physiological changes that occur approximately every 28 days from puberty to the menopause (Fig. 1.4). The changes occur under the influence of the hormones produced by the ovaries, which, in turn, respond to stimulation by gonadotrophins produced by the anterior lobe of the pituitary gland. The menstrual cycle is divided into three phases:

1. The proliferative phase – the follicle stimulating hormone (FSH) produced by the anterior lobe of the pituitary gland stimulates the growth of an ovarian follicle. The follicle produces oestrogen, which stimulates the rapid growth and thickening (proliferation) of the endometrium. As the follicle reaches maturity and ruptures (ovulation) the production of oestrogen ceases and the proliferative phase ends.
2. The secretory phase – after ovulation, the ovarian follicle remnant is stimulated by luteinizing hormone, also from the anterior pituitary, to develop the corpus luteum; this produces progesterone. Progesterone stimulates the endometrium to produce a watery mucus to aid the passage of

Normal-Premenopausal

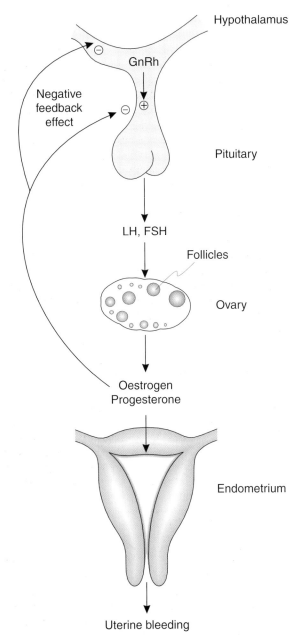

Figure 1.3 Negative feedback of the endocrine system in the normal premenopausal female.

sperm through the uterus to the fallopian tubes ready for fertilization. If fertilization does not occur, the menstrual phase begins.

3. The menstrual phase – if the ovum is not fertilized, the anterior pituitary stops producing luteinizing hormone and preparation for pregnancy ceases. The withdrawal of the luteinizing hormone causes degeneration of the corpus luteum and progesterone production decreases. The endometrium breaks down and menstruation begins. As the progesterone level falls it stimulates the negative feedback effect shown in Figure 1.4, and the anterior pituitary once again prepares for pregnancy by releasing follicle stimulating hormone at the start of the next cycle.

The changes in hormone balance that occur during the menstrual cycle inevitably cause changes throughout the body, in particular premenstrual syndrome, as discussed in Chapter 7.

THE LOWER URINARY TRACT

Strictly speaking the lower urinary tract is not part of the female genital tract. However, many conditions that send women to their general practitioners, and subsequently to the Gynaecology Department, are connected to both the female genital tract and/or the lower urinary tract.

The lower urinary tract consists of the bladder and urethra, with supporting ligaments and muscles.

The bladder

The bladder is a hollow, muscular organ situated in the pelvis. It lies posterior to the symphysis pubis, anterior to the vagina and inferior to the uterus. It is freely mobile and held in position by folds of peritoneum. The shape of the bladder varies – when empty it looks like a deflated balloon, when full it becomes pear-shaped and rises into the abdominal cavity. Its function is to act as a reservoir to store urine; it expels urine only when required to do so.

At the base of the bladder is a small triangular area known as the trigone. Entering obliquely at each upper angle of this triangle are the ureters; the urethra leaves the bladder at the third angle of the triangle. The surface mucosa of the trigone is typically smooth compared with the transitional epithelium of the rest of the bladder. Transitional epithelium can stretch and is enhanced by folds in the mucosa (rugae), which are visible when the bladder is empty. The muscle layer of the bladder is made up of three layers: (i) inner longitudinal fibres; (ii) middle circular fibres; and (iii) outer longitudinal fibres. Collectively, these are known as

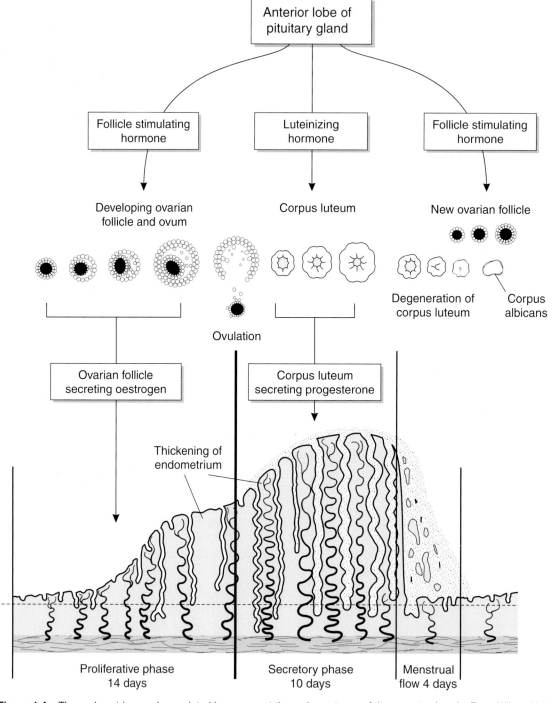

Figure 1.4 The endometrium and associated hormones at the various stages of the menstrual cycle. From Wilson K, 1981 Foundation of Anatomy and Physiology 5e, Churchill Livingstone, Edinburgh.

the detrusor muscle – the muscle that contracts during micturition. In the area around the opening to the urethra, circular fibres form an internal sphincter muscle and, below this, the external sphincter. Dislocation of this sphincter due to childbirth, ageing and menopause is the underlying cause of stress incontinence. Incontinence operations are intended to restore correct anatomical position of the bladder neck.

Bladder support. The bladder is supported by: (i) two lateral ligaments from the side walls of the bladder to the side walls of the pelvis; (ii) two pubo-vesical ligaments from the neck of the bladder to the symphysis pubis; and (iii) the urachus, which extends from the apex of the bladder to the umbilicus.

The urethra

The urethra is a small tube, 4–5 cm long, which leads from the base of the bladder to the urethral orifice in the vestibule of the vulva. The lower half of the urethra consists of stratified epithelium, the submucous folds of which provide a watertight seal for maintaining continence. It is important to note that these sub-mucous folds are oestrogen sensitive. Oestrogen deficiency can therefore affect the urethra, causing possible problems of incontinence, recurrent cystitis, etc. (see Chapters 16 and 18).

THE PELVIC FLOOR

The pelvic floor is a collective term for the layers of muscles that are stretched like a hammock from the pubic bone to the bottom of the backbone. These firm, supportive muscles help to hold the bladder, uterus and bowel in place; they also close off the urethral opening and anus. These muscles are kept firm and slightly tense to stop leakage of urine and faeces. When micturition and defecation occurs the muscles relax and tighten again afterwards to restore control. The pelvic floor muscles can become weak and sag due to childbirth, lack of exercise, hormonal effects and the ageing process. When they become weak, control over micturition and defecation can become poor and leakage and incontinence can occur (see Chapter 18).

Micturition

The sensation of a full bladder is conveyed to the brain by sensory sympathetic nerves. When the amount of urine in the bladder exceeds 300–400 ml (the average bladder capacity is >500 ml), receptors in the bladder wall transmit impulses to the spinal cord, initiating a conscious desire to expel urine. Then, at a suitable time, sympathetic nerves relax the internal sphincter, parasympathetic nerves (under voluntary cerebral control) cause the detrusor muscles to contract, the external sphincter relaxes and micturition takes place.

A lack of voluntary control occurs in infants, who void whenever the bladder is sufficiently distended to arouse a reflex stimulus. Continence occurs in children when they are taught to recognize the desire to void through 'potty training'. The involuntary urge to micturate or incontinence (i.e. urgency, urge incontinence) in adults may occur due to injury to the spinal nerves controlling the bladder, disease of the bladder and emotional stress, but most often is idiopathic (see Chapter 18).

2

Disorders of puberty and congenital malformations of the genital tract

Sarah Creighton

Gynaecological problems in children and adolescents are often poorly understood and poorly dealt with. Paediatricians and paediatric nurses are often mystified by disorders of the genital tract. Conversely, nurses and doctors working in the field of gynaecology are often unfamiliar with the specialized skills needed for dealing with young children and adolescents. This group of patients has special gynaecological needs and cannot just be treated as small versions of adults.

This chapter focuses on some of the gynaecological problems experienced by young children and adolescents. It covers the basic and common problems that may be found in any gynaecology clinic or ward, as well as the rarer aspects of intersex disorders.

NORMAL PUBERTY

Puberty is characterized by the development of secondary sexual characteristics and, eventually, the ability to reproduce. The endocrine changes leading to puberty are complex, starting in the fetus and continuing as a spectrum through childhood. In fetal life, the hypothalamic–pituitary axis is fully developed and the number of germ cells is maximum. There is evidence that ovarian maturation occurs throughout childhood (Stanhope et al 1985). At about 6–8 years of age, the adrenal cortex begins to secrete 17-keto steroids in response to adrenocorticotrophic hormone. This is called the adrenarche and may result in scanty pubic hair development and a minor growth spurt. Throughout puberty there is secretion of nocturnal pulsatile gonadotrophins (luteinizing hormone (LH) and follicle stimulating hormone (FSH)) and the amplitude of these pulses gradually increases (Boyar et al 1972). The mechanism of how gonadotrophin releasing hormone (GnRH) controls the secretion of the gonadotrophins is as yet unknown. As the secretion of gonadotrophins increases, so the ovary becomes stimulated to secrete

Table 2.1 Modified Tanner Staging

Stage	Age range (years)	Breast	Pubic hair
1	Prepubertal	Elevation of nipple only	None
2	9–13	Breast bud begins to grow beneath areola	Sparse, long, pigmented hair along labia
3	10–14	Further enlargement of breast and areola in same contour	Sparse, coarse, curlier hair over mons
4	11–15	Areola and nipple elevated above breast contour	Abundant adult-type hair mainly limited to mons
5	12–17	Recession of areola to contour of breast	Hair of adult type and distribution

the androgens and oestrogens responsible for development of the sexual characteristics.

The first sign of puberty in girls is characteristically breast development. Other changes include development of pubic hair, enlargement of the labia, enlarging of the hips due to widening of the pelvic inlet and fat deposition, and menstruation. Pubertal development was classified into stages by Marshall and Tanner (1970) and a modified description of these stages is given in Table 2.1.

The average age of puberty has been decreasing since about 1850 in the western world, with an average age of 12–13 years for the onset of menstruation at the time of writing (1999/2000). The reason for this may be better socioeconomic conditions and general health. Moderate obesity is associated with an earlier onset of puberty.

DISORDERS OF PUBERTY

Precocious puberty

Precocious puberty is defined as the onset of puberty before the age of 8 years in girls and 9 years in boys. It is more common in girls than boys and can occur at any age. Ovulation can take place and pregnancies have been described in children under the age of 10 (Dewhurst 1984).

Causes

True precocious puberty means activation of the hypothalamic–pituitary gonadal axis, which is gonadotrophin dependent. Pseudoprecocious puberty is independent of gonadotrophins and can be due to other conditions (Box 2.1).

True precocious puberty can be idiopathic or due to central nervous tumours such as gliomas or hamartomas; in rare circumstances it can be familial (Rangasami and Grant 1992). Pseudoprecocious puberty can be due to oestrogen-secreting ovarian

---

Box 2.1 Causes of precocious puberty

True precocious puberty (gonadotrophin-dependent)	Idiopathic Secondary to CNS tumours and other CNS disorders Primary hypothyroidism
Pseudoprecocious puberty (gonadotrophin-independent)	Tumours secreting gonadotrophin sex steroids, e.g. ovarian, adrenal Testoxicosis (in boys) McCune–Albright syndrome Premature thelarch

---

tumours such as granulosa cell tumours. The McCune–Albright syndrome is a cause of pseudoprecocious puberty and is characterized by café-au-lait spots, fibrous dysplasia and cysts of the long bones and skull; it is much more common in girls than boys.

Investigation

A full history and examination is essential. In true precocious puberty, the normal pubertal sequence of events occurs but in pseudoprecocious puberty these events may be out of sequence, e.g. vaginal bleeding before breast development.

Investigations may include bone age estimation and ultrasound scan of the ovaries. Hormonal investigations include thyroid function tests and baseline measurements of gonadotrophin levels. The nocturnal pulsatility of LH should be measured and the LH response to a bolus dose of GnRH assessed. In true precocious puberty, the gonadotrophin response resembles that seen in normal puberty.

Treatment

The major problem resulting from precocious puberty is premature skeletal maturation resulting in short stature. Other concerns are largely psychosocial, relating to the patient's and her parents/guardian's distress about the physical manifestations of precocious puberty.

If a specific cause is found, such as a central nervous system or ovarian tumour, then the cause must be treated appropriately. If the cause is idiopathic, the treatment of choice since the mid-1980s has been with GnRH analogues. Prior to this, cyproterone acetate and medroxyprogesterone acetate were used, although there was no clear evidence of a beneficial effect on final height. GnRH analogues act initially to stimulate pituitary function but then quickly downregulate it, leading to decreased LH and FSH secretion. The effects are all reversible and there is recent evidence that final height is improved by treatment (Oerter et al 1991). The future prospects for the child are good, with no evidence that the GnRH analogues interfere with future reproductive function.

Delayed puberty

Delayed puberty occurs when there are no signs of pubertal development by the age of 14 years; menstruation should start before the age of 16 years. In some cases of primary amenorrhoea there are no secondary sexual characteristics and sometimes there is normal development except for menstruation. The latter group will be discussed.

Causes of delayed puberty

There are many causes of delayed puberty and, for ease of understanding, these can be put into three groups:

- girls with short stature
- girls who are underweight
- girls with normal or excessive height and weight.

Examples in each group are given in Table 2.2 but there are many other rarer causes beyond the scope of this text.

Investigation

A careful history and detailed examination should give valuable pointers as to the presence of some of the conditions given above. With constitutional delay a similar history may be obtained from sisters or mother. In a patient with Turner's syndrome there are typical abnormalities including short stature, webbed neck and wide carrying angle. Special investigations may

Table 2.2   Causes of delayed puberty

Stature	Examples
Short stature	Chronic childhood illness
	Turner's syndrome (XO karyotype)
	Hypothalamic or pituitary lesion
	Hypothyroid
Underweight	Anorexia nervosa
	Malnutrition
	Excessive exercise
	Psychiatric problems
	Chronic illness
Normal height and weight or obese	Constitutional delay
	XY gonadal dysgenesis
	Pituitary tumour
	Kallman's syndrome
	Hypothyroidism
	Premature ovarian failure
	Polycystic ovarian syndrome

include chromosomal studies, serum gonadotrophins, thyroid function, radiology of the skull and bone age.

Treatment

The treatments vary depending on the underlying condition identified. With a diagnosis of constitutional delay, reassurance may be all that is necessary. However, if the girl is becoming anxious about her lack of development then induction of puberty should be considered. Successful treatment of anorexia resulting in weight gain will allow onset of normal pubertal development. Kallman's syndrome is rare and comprises hypogonadotrophic hypogonadism associated with anosmia (failure of LHRH production). This can be treated with gonadotrophins and/or pulsatile LHRH and pubertal development, and successful pregnancies have been described in women with this condition. The latter types of treatment should be carried out in units with specialized expertise in the treatment and monitoring of these rare conditions. It is essential that the patient understands that, although induction of puberty is the starting point, she will need to continue on her oestrogen long term to prevent chronic problems including osteoporosis, atherosclerosis and cardiovascular disease. Once puberty is reached, long-term treatment is best achieved with either the oral contraceptive pill or hormone replacement therapy. HRT is preferable as it provides continuous oestrogen whereas the contraceptive pill provides oestrogen for only three weeks out of four. However, the pill is free on prescription while HRT is not. The pill may also be more acceptable to a young girl than HRT, which her mother or grandmother may take.

COMMON ADOLESCENT GYNAECOLOGICAL PROBLEMS

Menorrhagia

The first few periods following the onset of menstruation are usually anovulatory. This means they are often irregular and heavy due to unopposed oestrogen stimulation of the endometrium. This can cause considerable distress and can be severe enough to cause anaemia in some cases. Polycystic ovarian syndrome can cause irregular periods and, although these are more commonly light, they may sometimes be heavy. Clotting abnormalities are rare but it has been reported that up to 20% of girls admitted to hospital with excessive menstruation have a coagulopathy (Claessens and Cowell 1981). The patient may give a history of excessive bleeding after other procedures such as dental extractions or there may be a family history such as von Willebrand's disease. Other causes, such as platelet disorders and leukaemia, must be borne in mind.

Investigation

A menstrual history, including the number of pads or tampons used, will give an idea of the problem. If the girl is already sexually active then it is important to exclude pregnancy-related causes for heavy vaginal bleeding. A sexual history should be taken in the absence of the parent if possible. Physical examination is usually normal and should be done in the presence of the parent or guardian. Features of polycystic ovarian syndrome, such as poor skin and hirsutism, may be difficult to separate from other normal pubertal changes. A vaginal examination is never indicated in a girl who is not sexually active. Rectal examinations are sometimes suggested as an alternative but are usually unhelpful, as well as painful and embarrassing.

Haemoglobin should be checked for anaemia and, if indicated, a coagulation screen should be done. Ultrasound scans may be helpful and, although they are almost always normal, the characteristic appearance of polycystic ovaries or a congenital abnormality such as a double uterus may occasionally be seen. It is almost never necessary to perform dilation and curettage or hysteroscopy.

Treatment

If all investigations are normal, the girl and her parents should be reassured. First-line treatment is antiprosta-

glandins or tranexamic acid taken during the period. Antiprostaglandins, such as mefanamic acid 500 mg q.d.s., reduce blood flow and also help with associated pain. There are few side-effects although gastro-intestinal disturbance is not uncommon. The advantage is that treatment is taken only during the first few days of bleeding and that the frequency of menstruation is not altered. Unfortunately, mefanamic acid is not always effective. Tranexamic acid has been show to be more effective than mefanamic acid in studies on adult women, although these studies have not included adolescents. Again, side-effects are few, although they include dizziness and diarrhoea. The treatment dose is usually 1 g q.d.s. and is needed only during the periods. If these regimes are not effective, or if the periods are very irregular, cyclical progestogens or the oral contraceptive pill are indicated. A common progestogen regime is oral dydrogesterone 10 mg daily from day 10 to day 25 of the cycle. Treatment is usually continued for 3 to 6 months. If this is unhelpful, or if contraception is required, a combined oral contraceptive pill is very effective.

The hope is that treatment is temporary whilst the pituitary–ovarian axis matures and establishes a more normal pattern. Unfortunately, there is no good, long-term outcome data on the future menstrual patterns of these girls. There is some evidence to suggest that, the longer the problem lasts, the more likely it is that problems will continue into adult life (Southam and Richart 1966) and effective treatment at an early stage would therefore seem sensible.

Dysmenorrhoea

Primary dysmenorrhoea is severe pain starting on the first day of menstruation. It may be associated with nausea and vomiting and can result in days lost from school. The pain is associated with ovulatory cycles and so often the first few periods are pain free until ovulation is established. The cause is not yet fully understood but prostaglandins have an important role to play (Ylorkala & Dawood 1978). Psychological factors can be important, particularly if the symptoms are refractory to treatment.

Investigation

A careful history should confirm the diagnosis and external examination should be normal. If the pain is atypical then an ultrasound scan may be useful; if the history is clear, an ultrasound scan is not indicated. If the symptoms are refractory to treatment, a laparo-

---

Case study 2.1: Nicola

Nicola was referred to the outpatient department by her GP with heavy, irregular and painful periods. She was 15 years old and attended the clinic with her mother. Her periods had started 18 months previously and had always been difficult. She bled for up to 14 days and had a period every 4 to 8 weeks. The first 2 days were very heavy requiring double 'super' sanitary towels day and night. Nicola missed 2 days of school with every period. She was unable to manage the heavy flow while at school and had been very upset by several accidents when she soaked through her school uniform in class. She had never been sexually active and had no other significant medical history. There was no significant family history and in particular no history of bleeding disorders.

On examination, Nicola was of normal height and weight for her age. She did not look anaemic or unwell and had secondary sexual development that was appropriate for her age. Abdominal palpation was normal and a vaginal examination was not performed. She was investigated with a full blood count and a pelvic ultrasound scan. The full blood count gave a haemoglobin of 10.5 g/dl and the picture was of an iron deficiency anaemia. A pelvic ultrasound scan was normal. In view of Nicola's distressing symptoms and anaemia, treatment was recommended.

Nicola was initially commenced on medroxy-progesterone 5 mg twice daily from days 15 to 26 of her cycle. She was also given ferrous sulphate 200 mg daily. She was asked to keep a menstrual calendar and to return in 3 months. On her return the periods were not greatly improved. They had become more regular and predictable. and were slightly shorter. The first 2 days were still very heavy and still required time off school. Nicola was then swapped over to the combined oral contraceptive pill Microgynon 30. This involved careful discussion with Nicola's mother, who was worried about someone so young being 'on the pill'. She did agree that with the severity of Nicola's symptoms it was worth trying. Nicola was therefore reviewed again after 3 months of Microgynon. Both Nicola and her mother were very pleased with the results. By the end of the second cycle her periods were noticeably shorter and lighter. They were completely regular and she had not missed any schooling. She had experienced some breast tenderness and slight nausea during the first packet of pills but these side-effects had completely resolved subsequently.

The plan was therefore for Nicola to continue on the pill for 6 months under GP follow-up. She was keen at that time to stop and see if her symptoms resolved. She was reassured by the fact that if her periods continued to be difficult, an effective treatment had been identified, which she could restart if necessary.

---

scopy can be performed. This is usually normal although endometriosis may be found occasionally. In very rare cases there may be a congenital uterine abnormality with an obstructed segment of the genital tract (see Plate 2). There is no place for a dilation and curettage, although this was recommended in the past, and there is no evidence that cervical stenosis has any role to play. Whilst it is true that symptoms may resolve after childbearing, this is not very consoling information to a girl in her early teens with severe period pain.

Treatment

If no abnormality is found, simple reassurance and explanation is essential; these symptoms are often self-limiting. First-line treatments involve the use of prostaglandin synthetase inhibitors such as mefenamic acid 500 mg t.d.s.; these are successful in most cases. If unsuccessful, then the combined oral contraceptive pill is also effective in producing light, regular and less painful cycles. If these treatments are unhelpful and a laparoscopy is normal, it is worth considering involving a psychologist.

Teenage contraception

The age at which young women are beginning sexual activity is decreasing worldwide. Although young women have the same physical requirements for effective contraception and protection against sexually transmitted disease as adults, their access to these facilities is often limited. The risks of early intercourse are given in Box 2.2.

Box 2.2 Risks of early age of first intercourse	
Infection	Sexually transmitted, e.g. gonorrhoea and chlamydia Chronic pelvic inflammatory disease Later tubal infertility
Cervical abnormalities	Abnormal smears requiring colposcopy and treatment Increased risk of cervical cancer in later life
Pregnancy	Increased abortion including surgical risks, risks of retained products, infection and bleeding, emotional sequelae Increased teenage pregnancy

Only half of sexually active teenagers use contraception (Bowie & Ford 1989). As one of the major reasons for this is fear of parental discovery of the fact that they are sexually active, it is essential that family planning services are easy to access and confidential. Discussion about contraception must be non-judgemental and empathetic. Explanations of different methods must be explicit and visual models are very helpful. Leaflets may sound a good idea but many adolescents would be reluctant to take these home in case of discovery. Facilities for pregnancy testing should also be available, as should sympathetic counselling on the options available if an unplanned pregnancy occurs. Vaginal examinations, especially the use of speculums for cervical smears, are very frightening. These do not need to be done at the first clinic visit; it is not harmful to defer them until the girl has been sexually active for several months. Hopefully, by this time she will have built up a rapport with her clinic nurse or doctor and will find the process less frightening. The importance of safe sex in preventing sexually transmitted diseases including HIV must be explained in simple and explicit terms.

Legal implications

Sexual intercourse before the age of consent is illegal in the UK. However, prosecution is unlikely to occur if both partners are of a similar age. Past ethical and legal concerns about prescribing contraception to girls under 16 were clarified by the famous Gillick case, in 1985. This case was brought against the then Department of Health and Social Services (DHSS) by Mrs Victoria Gillick, who sought to establish that it was unlawful to give young people under the age of 16 contraceptive advice or treatment without their parent's consent. The House of Lords ruled against her. Clearly, many young girls seeking contraceptive advice will begin or continue to have sexual activity with or without contraception. Currently, doctors are allowed to prescribe contraceptives to girls under 16 without parental knowledge within the guidelines set out in the Department of Health Memorandum of Guidance (DHSS HC(FP)86). The girl should be encouraged to inform her parents but must have assurance at all times of confidentiality.

Choice of contraception

Condoms These are usually the easiest to obtain and thus the most widely used. They provide protection against sexually transmitted disease as well as preg-nancy. Unfortunately, many young people report difficulties in using condoms. This may be because condoms are used by the male partner, who is even less likely to attend a family planning clinic than his female partner and may not know the correct way to use them. Explicit teaching with visual aids is essential and, if possible, directed towards young men. The female condom is also available now but is expensive and looks unappealing.

Oral contraception

The combined pill This is very popular as it is simple to use and very reliable if used well. Other benefits such as lighter and more regular periods also make it more attractive. It offers no protection against sexually transmitted infection and use of a condom in addition should be encouraged; the 'double dutch' method. Side-effects and risks are the same as for adult patients and there is no evidence of any detrimental effects on pubertal or bone development. Clear instructions must be given on when to start it and the importance of remembering. Breakthrough bleeding can occur and is most commonly due to missed pills.

Progesterone only pill This pill is much less reliable and more dependent on accurate pill taking than the combined pill. It is therefore not usually suitable in this group of patients.

Emergency contraception Young women must be made aware of the availability of emergency contraception. The most common method involves administering combined pills containing 100 µg oestradiol in two doses 12 hours apart. This must be commenced within 72 hours of intercourse. Insertion of an IUCD within 5 days is also effective postcoital contraception. Care must be taken to check that the girl is not already pregnant from contraceptive failure in the months preceding.

DepoProvera Long-acting hormonal methods such as DepoProvera can be very suitable for some adolescents. The injection needs only to be given every 3 months and this can make secrecy easier. There is less dependence on memory and so less scope for contraceptive failure compared with the contraceptive pill. The main problem with this method is the effects on the menstrual cycle, which include irregular periods and often amenorrhoea with prolonged use. However, with regular follow-up and reassurance these side-effects may be acceptable. There are no long-term health implications with this method. Fertility return may be delayed but this is less likely to be a problem to an adolescent.

Intrauterine contraceptive devices (IUCD) The IUCD is usually unsuitable for adolescents. They are at higher

---

Case study 2.2: Jane

Jane was a self-referral to the Casualty department with severe abdominal pain. She was aged 14 and had been brought to the hospital by her parents. She had a 6-hour history of severe abdominal pain causing her to vomit. She was initially referred to the surgical team as a possible appendicitis. On examination, however, they found a 16-week-sized acutely tender pelvic mass and referred her to the on-call gynaecology team.

On further questioning it became apparent that the pain had happened before, although never as severely. The pain had occurred at monthly intervals for approximately the last 6 months. Jane had not yet started her periods. She denied any previous sexual activity although she did have a steady boyfriend. She was otherwise in good health.

On examination Jane was very distressed and in pain. Gentle palpation of her abdomen did confirm a 16-week-sized tender mass arising from the pelvis. Parting of the labia and external inspection of the genitalia revealed a blue mass distending the vagina.

A diagnosis of imperforate hymen was made based on the history of cyclical pain and amenorrhoea. This was confirmed by ultrasound scan, which also excluded pregnancy as a diagnosis.

Jane was admitted and placed on the emergency theatre list for that day. At operation, examination under anaesthetic did reveal an imperforate hymen. This was incised and 500 ml of old blood was drained. Jane remained in hospital overnight. Her symptoms were relieved immediately and she had minimal vaginal loss. On discussion with her named nurse once her parents had gone home, Jane did reveal that she had actually been sexually active and was worried about pregnancy. Jane was reassured that her hospital admission was not related to sexual activity but that it was an important issue to tackle. Jane was encouraged to tell her mother and, after discussion and reassurance, she agreed. This was in fact done during her admission. Jane was discharged after 48 hours. She was advised that she should not have intercourse for 6 weeks to allow healing after surgery.

Jane was reviewed for follow-up. She had made a good recovery and had had a normal period subsequently. She and her mother were happy to discuss contraception and it was finally agreed that Jane would start the combined oral contraceptive pill. Safe sex and the need for barrier methods of contraception were discussed. Longer-term follow-up was arranged for Jane at the family planning clinic at her GP surgery.

---

risk of sexually transmitted infection and an IUCD may exacerbate the risk of pelvic inflammatory disease. This will be detrimental to future fertility. In addition, as this group are very fertile, the failure rate may be higher.

Primary amenorrhoea

Primary amenorrhoea is defined as never having had menstruation. To understand the underlying cause it is helpful to classify this further into amenorrhoea in the absence or presence of secondary sexual characteristics. Primary amenorrhoea in the absence of secondary sexual characteristics has been discussed above (see Delayed puberty). Primary amenorrhoea in the presence of normal secondary sexual characteristics is most commonly due to an anatomical defect such as the absence of uterus or vagina.

Imperforate vagina

This is the most common anatomical cause of primary amenorrhoea. The obstruction can be at any level in the vagina but is most commonly found in the lower third at the level of the hymen. Pubertal development is initially normal and secondary sexual characteristics develop. The events leading up to menstruation occur but escape of the menstrual blood is obstructed. The usual presentation is with cyclical abdominal pain and the diagnosis can be suspected from this history. If diagnosis is delayed the patient may present with a pelvic and abdominal mass as a result of a **haematocolpos** and a **haematometra**. If the pelvic mass is very large it can even cause urinary retention.

Investigation Cyclical pain will point to the diagnosis and a pelvic mass may be palpable. If the obstruction is low, gentle parting of the labia may reveal a blue bulging membrane. An ultrasound scan will be helpful in confirming a haematometria and haematocolpos.

Treatment An examination under general anaesthetic will allow confirmation of the diagnosis. The membrane can then be excised and the blood released. As long as enough of the membrane is excised to prevent it resealing, no further reconstructive vaginal surgery is required. There is some evidence that these girls may have an increased chance of endometriosis, which may be related to the length of time the obstruction was present (San Filippo et al 1986).

Absence of the uterus

The Rokitansky–Kuster–Hauser–Mayer syndrome is the absence of uterus and vagina in a girl with otherwise normal development. The ovaries develop normally and so there are normal secondary sexual characteristics. Examination of the genital area will reveal normal labia and a normal hymen with a central dimple. The patient will be infertile and will never menstruate.

Investigation An ultrasound scan will confirm an absent uterus and the presence of ovaries; a hormonal profile will be normal. A **karyotype** will also show a normal female XX pattern and it is important to do this to exclude other more complex abnormalities.

Treatment The only treatment available is geared towards producing a vagina of sufficient capacity to allow sexual intercourse. This is often successfully done with the use of vaginal dilators. Major reconstructive surgery is sometimes, but not often, necessary. Psychological input is important as these girls must cope with the realization that they are infertile. As their ovaries are normal, current assisted conception techniques allow the possibility of ovum retrieval for a surrogate pregnancy. However, this option is currently fraught with financial and emotional pitfalls and is not easy to recommend.

Intersex states

The physical features determining the sex of an individual are the genotype (genetic material or karyotype), the internal and external sexual organs, the gonads and the secondary sexual characteristics, which appear at puberty. Intersex states are due to a defect in the normal process of sexual maturation in the fetus, which results in abnormalities of internal or external genitalia. They are usually classified into three groups:

- male pseudohermaphroditism
- female pseudohermaphroditism
- true hermaphroditism.

Male pseudohermaphroditism

In this condition there is failure of **virilization** of a genetic male (XY karyotype). The appearances of the external genitalia can vary ranging from a small penis with **hypospadias** through ambiguous appearance to a normal female appearance. This condition is rare and is most commonly due to androgen insensitivity and 5-alpha reductase deficiency.

Androgen insensitivity (previously known as testicular feminization syndrome). In complete androgen insensitivity, there is resistance of the developing external genitalia to androgens. This means that although the fetus has a male karyotype and has testes, the external genitalia do not respond to testosterone and so the external appearance is female; a penis and a scrotum do not develop. However, the internal genitalia are male, with testes and no uterus or ovaries. The vagina develops but usually only the lower third, leaving a short, blind-ending vagina. Breast development is normal and there may be scanty pubic hair.

The baby appears as a normal female at birth and through childhood. Presentation may be during childhood with palpable gonads (testes) in the groins or as inguinal hernias. If this does not happen then the girl will present with primary amenorrhoea.

As the condition is X-linked recessive the diagnosis may be made after a sister is found to be affected.

Androgen insensitivity can also be partial where there is some response of external genitalia to androgens. The external genital appearances at birth are often ambiguous and the diagnosis may be made sooner for this reason.

5-Alpha reductase deficiency. This is a very rare autosomal recessive condition. As above, there is failure of the developing fetus to respond to androgens so the fetus has female external genitalia. This failure is due to an absence of the enzyme 5-alpha reductase, which is necessary to convert testosterone to its active form in the fetus. However, virilization at puberty requires only testosterone, and not the enzyme, and so at puberty there is striking virilization. This includes marked clitoral enlargement (see Plate 3), hirsutism, deepening of the voice and male psychosexual virilization.

Investigation depends to some extent on the mode of presentation. All children will need a karyotype performing. An ultrasound will confirm absent female internal genitalia. Complex genetic studies can identify a genetic problem in some families.

Treatment is complicated. These children have been brought up as girls and should in most cases remain in that gender. Counselling is crucial and should be done by an expert in these disorders. The child and her parents will have many concerns about gender and sexual identity. She must also come to terms with infertility. The current view is that girls with androgen insensitivity and related disorders should be made aware of their diagnosis and its implications for future general and sexual health. The relaying of the diagnosis must be done very gently and may take several consultations. In the past, the diagnosis was often deliberately concealed, leading to terrible confusion among the patients who knew something was wrong but not what it was.

The testes do have an increased risk of malignancy and must be removed either at laparotomy or laparoscopically, depending on their position. Other surgical procedures depend on the presentation. If the girl has normal external genitalia then external surgery is unnecessary. If there is clitoral enlargement then a surgical clitoral reduction is necessary. The vagina is usually short and most patients will require at least the use of vaginal dilators. Occasionally patients will already be sexually active and have unknowingly performed their own vaginal dilation through initiating and continuing intercourse. If dilators are unsuccessful then major surgery is indicated. In all cases where surgery is required this should be done in a centre used to dealing with these unusual cases to ensure the best possible surgical outcome. After gonadectomy, oestrogen supplements are essential to maintain female development and prevent osteoporosis.

Vaginal dilators have good success rates and should be the treatment of first choice. They avoid the risks of major surgery and can give excellent results. Motivation is key and this should be stressed to the patient. There is no right time to start using dilators but the girl is often most motivated in her mid to late teens when sexual relationships are being considered. Many girls are keen to start treatment before going away to college or embarking on a career after leaving school.

Various types of dilators are available. The Amielle dilators shown in Plate 4 seem to be the most acceptable to the patients when compared to other types on offer. The patient should be shown the dilators and taught how to use them by a nurse or doctor familiar with their use. The consultation should be unhurried and in relaxed surroundings. The girl may prefer to be seen alone or with a family member such as her mother. She should be given an opportunity to insert the smallest dilator under supervision if the wishes. She should be asked to gently insert it into the vagina as far as is comfortable. The dilator should be left in place for half an hour three times a week in the first instance. This must be done as part of a routine and the girl should be encouraged to use a set time, e.g. while watching a TV series. Once she is confident with the insertion, she should be encouraged to insert the dilator a little further each time it is used and to gradually work her way up through the sizes. If regular penetrative sexual intercourse becomes established then the dilators can be discontinued as intercourse itself will maintain the vaginal capacity. In a few cases the girl is already in a stable sexual relationship and her partner can be involved in use of the dilators.

Surgical **vaginoplasty** is an option if vaginal dilators fail. There is no single ideal surgical option and many approaches have been tried. The simplest operation is a Williams vulvovaginoplasty, which involves making a pouch in the perineum. A U-shaped incision is made from the level of the urethra down to the perineum anterior to the anus. The inner skin edges are sutured together, as are the two outer skin edges. This leaves a tunnel adequate for intercourse. The advantages are that this is not major surgery and that vaginal dilators are not required to keep the pouch open. However, the perineum does look very abnormal and the angle of the new vagina is very posterior compared with the normal angle. For these reasons this technique is becoming less popular.

Another option is a McIndoe vaginoplasty (McIndoe and Bannister 1938), which involves making a space for the vagina by blunt dissection between the urethra and rectum. The vagina is then lined with skin taken from a split skin graft on the patient's thigh. A vaginal mould must be left in place for up to 3 months and after that the patient will need to use vaginal dilators. Although good results have been reported with this technique, there are disadvantages. The surgery is major and an ugly scar is left at the donor site. The skin graft can contract down and dilators must be used regularly unless the patient is having regular sexual intercourse. The vagina is very dry and lubrication must be used during intercourse.

The most complex technique is to use a section of bowel to line the vaginal space instead of a split skin graft. Ileum, caecum and sigmoid colon have all been used in various modifications of the surgery. The advantage is that the problem of contraction is not seen and a good length and capacity vagina can be achieved. This procedure does, however, require major surgery by a surgeon experienced in bowel surgery. The mucosa can prolapse through the vaginal entrance giving an ugly stoma. Vaginal mucus production can be inconvenient although it may reduce over time.

Female pseudohermaphroditism

This occurs when a genetically female fetus is exposed to excessive circulating androgen in utero. While the karyotype and internal genitalia are female, the external genitalia become virilized. The excess androgens can come from the mother or from the fetus. The most common cause of this is congenital adrenal hyperplasia. Other causes are rarer and are given in Box 2.3.

Congenital adrenal hyperplasia

This affects 1 in 12 000 births and is an autosomal recessive inheritance. It is due to an enzyme defect in

---

Box 2.3 Causes of virilization of female fetus

Congenital adrenal hyperplasia

Maternal androgen-secreting tumour, e.g.
  arrheoblastoma, placental luteoma

Androgen drugs administered to the mother, e.g.
  Danazol, progestogens

---

the synthesis of cortisol. Low cortisol levels stimulate overproduction of adrenocorticotrophic hormone (ACTH) leading to adrenal hyperplasia and excess androgen production. The most common defect is 21-hydroxylase deficiency but other abnormalities cause the same picture. In over half of the children affected by this disorder, there is a serious salt losing problem. This is due to a deficiency in aldosterone secretion and can be life-threatening if not detected and treated.

Diagnosis The female baby will present at birth with ambiguous genitalia (see Plate 5). The clitoris is enlarged and resembles a phallus and the urethral opening can be anywhere along the phallus. The labia are usually fused and the skin of the labia is very rugose and scrotal. If the baby is a salt loser this will present in the first 2 weeks of life with vomiting, diarrhoea, weight loss and poor feeding. Diagnosis is confirmed by high levels of plasma 17-hydroxy-progesterone. Although the details of diagnosis and treatment are beyond the scope of a gynaecological textbook, the main aims are to correct the electrolyte imbalance by replacement of glucocorticoids and mineralocorticoids. This treatment is lifelong and the child must have specialist follow-up. Regardless of the degree of virilization, the child must be brought up in the female role as they have female genotype as well as normal ovaries and are potentially fertile.

Surgical treatment Surgical correction of the genital virilization is usually necessary. The appearance causing most concern to the parents will be the large clitoris. This can cause such concern that they are unhappy for anyone else, e.g. grandparents or nanny, to change nappies or be in charge of the baby. A clitoral reduction is usually performed at about 1 year of age. This is thought to be the best time as the baby has grown enough to make surgery practical but has not yet become aware of their own genitals and differences with peers. There is controversy as to the right time to perform a vaginoplasty. Most paediatric surgeons would separate the fused labial folds and perform a minor vaginoplasty at the same time as performing the clitoral reduction.

In adolescence it is highly likely that further surgery to the lower vagina will be necessary to allow tampon use and eventually intercourse. Surgery is best deferred until after puberty as the vaginal skin is then fully oestrogenized and most suitable for operating on. After puberty the girl is usually admitted for an examination under anaesthesia. This will allow careful assessment about the need for further genital surgery and the extent of surgery required. This decision cannot be made in the outpatient department and a full assessment without general anaesthetic will be uncomfortable and embarrassing for the girl. If further surgery is indicated, the timing thereafter depends upon the wishes of the individual girl. Most are keen to proceed with surgery soon and certainly would prefer to have it done before beginning any sexual relationships. As surgery is only usually necessary to the lower third of the vagina this can often be achieved with relatively simple procedures such as vaginal flaps and does not usually require the more complex types of vaginoplasty described earlier.

Long-term outlook. In terms of general health, this is good, although regular specialist follow-up is essential. In terms of gynaecological wellbeing there is little long-term follow-up data. As these girls have a normal upper genital tract and ovaries they are fertile. Puberty may be delayed if steroid control of their congenital adrenal hyperplasia is poor. Menstrual irregularity can occur for the same reason. If control is good then pregnancy can be achieved. Pregnancy is more likely in non-salt losers than in salt losers. There may be other factors involved in infertility apart from poor steroid control. Poor sexual function may be due to psychosexual concerns as well as to poor surgical results (Mulaikal et al 1987).

If pregnancy is achieved there is a risk of inheritance by the fetus. Prenatal diagnosis has been available for some time via a chorion villus sample or amniocentesis (Forest et al 1981). This is suitable where the mother herself has congenital adrenal hyperplasia or where a sibling has been diagnosed. There is evidence that administration of steroids to the mother will prevent virilization, although there are associated risks to the mother of high dose steroid administration throughout pregnancy.

True hermaphroditism

This rare condition occurs when the child has both ovarian and testicular tissue present. The karyotype is most commonly female (46, XX) but can be a mosaic or rarely a normal male 46, XY karyotype. The tissue may be ovarian on one side and testicular on the other or combined as an ovotestis. Presentation can vary but is usually with ambiguous genitalia, although other presentations such as breast development in a child thought to be male can occur. Internal anatomy can also vary and both male and female structures can be present to varying degrees. These children are usually assigned to the female gender and the testicular tissue needs to be removed because of the risks of malignancy.

CONCLUSION

Paediatric and adolescent gynaecology is only now being recognized as an area that requires specialized nursing and medical input. Some of the very rare conditions described in this chapter will be looked after in dedicated units, which are used to the care of these unusual cases. However, the more common problems, such as menstrual difficulties and contraceptive dilemmas, will appear in both general practice and hospital-based gynaecology clinics. It is important to have a clear understanding of any medical disorder and also not to underestimate the impact of psychological, sexual and family pressures in this particular group of patients. Only by careful consideration of all of these factors can we care for these children and young women as they deserve.

GLOSSARY

Haematocolpos: retained blood in the vagina
Haematometra: an accumulation of blood (or menstrual fluid) in the uterus
Hypospadias: a congenital malformation of the male urethra. Divided into two groups:
a) penile – when the terminal urethral orifice opens at any point along the posterior shaft of the penis
b) perineal – when the orifice opens on the perineum and may give rise to problems of sexual differentiation

Karyotype: creation of an orderly array of chromosomes, usually derived from the study of cultured cells. Usually done for diagnostic purposes in the detection of chromosomal abnormalities
Virilization: the appearances of secondary male characteristics in the female
Vaginoplasty: formation and construction of a vagina

REFERENCES

Bowie C, Ford N 1989 Sexual behaviour of young people and the risk of HIV infection. Journal of Epidemiology and Community Health 43:61–65
Boyar F, Finkelstein J, Roffenwarg H, et al 1972 Synchronization of augmented secretion of luteinizing hormone secretion with sleep during puberty. New England Journal of Medicine 287:2521
Claessens EA, Cowell CA 1981 Acute adolescent menorrhagia. American Journal of Obstetrics and Gynecology 39:277–280
Dewhurst J 1984 Female puberty and its abnormalities. Current reviews in Obstetrics and Gynaecology 9:91–119
Forest MG, Betuel H, Couillin P, Boue A 1981 Prenatal diagnosis of congenital adrenal hyperplasia due to 21-hydroxylase deficiency by steroid analysis in the amniotic fluid of mid-pregnancy; comparison with HLA typing in 17 pregnancies at risk for CAH. Prenatal Diagnosis 1:197
McIndoe AH, Bannister JB 1938 An operation for the cure of congenital absence of the vagina. Journal of Obstetrics and Gynaecology of the British Commonwealth 45:490–494
Marshall WA, Tanner JM 1970 Variations in the pattern of pubertal changes in girls. Archives of Diseases in Childhood 44:291–303

Mulaikal RM, Migeon CJ, Rock JA 1987 Fertility rates in female patients with congenital adrenal hyperplasia due to 21-hydroxylase deficiency. New England Journal of Medicine 316:178
Oerter KE, Manasco P, Barnes KM, Jones J, Hill S, Cutler GB 1991 Adult height in precocious puberty after long term treatment with deslorelin. Journal of Clinical Endocrinology and Metabolism 73:1235–1240
Rangasami JJ, Grant DB 1992 Familial precocious puberty in girls. Journal of the Royal Society of Medicine 85:497–498
San Filippo JS, Wakim NG, Schiker KN, Yussman MA 1986 Endometriosis in association with uterine anomaly. American Journal of Obstetrics and Gynecology 154:39–43
Southam AL, Richart RM 1966 The prognosis for adolescents with menstrual disorders. Adolescent and Pediatric Gynecology 2:157–159
Stanhope R, Adams J, Jacobs HS, Brook CGD 1985 Ovarian ultrasound assessment in normal children, idiopathic precocious puberty and during low dose 2. Pulsatile GnRH therapy of hypogonadotrophic hypogonadism. Archives of Diseases in Childhood 60:116–119
Ylorkala O, Dawood MY 1978 New concepts in dysmenorrhoea. American Journal of Obstetrics and Gynecology 130:833

FURTHER READING

Short overview
Garden AS (ed) 1997 Paediatric and Adolescent Gynaecology: Minisymposium. The Diplomate 4(3), Parthenon Press

Textbooks
Edmonds DK 1989 Practical Paediatric and Adolescent Gynaecology, 2nd edn. Butterworths, London
Garden AS 1998 Paediatric and Adolescent Gynaecology. Arnold, London

USEFUL ADDRESSES

Androgen Insensitivity Syndrome (AIS) Support Group
P O Box 269, Banbury, Oxon
email: orchids @ talk21.com
website: http://www.medhelp.org/www/ais
British Association for Counselling
1 Regent's Place, Rugby CV21 2PJ
Tel: 01788 578328
National Association of Young People's Counselling and Advisory Services
Magazine Business Centre
11 Newmarket, Leicester LE1 5SS
Tel: 01162 558763
Specialist Paediatric and Adolescent Gynaecology Clinics are run at:

Great Ormond Street and/or University College Hospital (depending on age and problem) by Miss Sarah Creighton, Consultant Gynaecologist
Address: Department of Obstetrics and Gynaecology, University College London Hospitals, Obstetric Hospital, Huntley Street, London WC1E 6AU
Tel: 020 7380 9566
Fax: 020 7380 9754
Queen Charlotte's Hospital by Mr Keith Edmunds, Consultant Gynaecologist
Address: Department of Obstetrics and Gynaecology, Queen Charlotte's and Chelsea Hospital, Goldhawk Road, London W6
Tel: 020 8383 1111

3

Subfertility/infertility

Terri Morgan

It is estimated that one in six couples seek specialist help to conceive at some stage in their lives (Greenhall & Vessey 1990, Templeton et al 1991). This demand is not necessarily indicative of an increased incidence, but more of a rise in the uptake of specialist medical care, which consequently reflects the need for expansion and progression.

The rapid advances in reproductive technology have heralded much controversy and publicity. From the birth of the first 'test tube' baby in 1978 through to the suggested use of eggs from aborted fetuses, an octuplet pregnancy and the birth of a child to a 60-year-old mother, there have been accusations that doctors extend their practice beyond accepted ethical boundaries. This extremely delicate and complex issue raises questions as to the moral and ethical implications of reproductive medicine.

Infertility provokes unique individual responses, which depend upon the sociological, cultural, religious and personal values held. Universal to all, however, is the knowledge that infertility is traditionally shrouded in stigma, partly as a result of controversial issues but often due to the 'inadequacy' and 'unnaturalness' that the disorder portrays.

It is the resultant psychological morbidity that should justify and enhance the need for a greater understanding of the specific dynamics of fertility care – the process of self-help and the availability of adequate management and treatment.

DEFINITION

The working definition of infertility that is generally applied is infertility:

…is the inability to achieve spontaneous conception following one year of unprotected intercourse.

The term 'infertility' refers to an absolute inability to conceive spontaneously; 'subfertility' indicates a reduction in the ability to conceive spontaneously. However, as a result of the wide use of the term 'infertility', it has come to be known by the same definition as subfertility, although many nurses and clinicians now share the view that the latter is less stigmatizing and reflects the potential for change and improvement in fertility status.

There are two classes of infertility:

1. *Primary infertility* – whereby no previous pregnancy has occurred.
2. *Secondary infertility* – where a previous pregnancy has occurred, irrespective of its outcome.

CAUSES OF SUBFERTILITY

The process of conception relies upon:

- ovulation and spermatogenesis (production of sperm)
- patent fallopian tubes – to allow uptake of ova and passage along the tubes to a site where fertilization can take place
- patent and functional epididymis, vas deferens, seminal vesicles and urethra – to allow maturation and transportation of sperm
- appropriately timed intercourse to deliver ejaculated sperm
- normal cervix and optimal timing for cervical mucus production and receptivity
- adequate sperm count and motility to penetrate cervical mucus and reach the tubes
- normal uterine and endometrial function to allow implantation of embryo.

Failure at any of the above stages can lead to subfertility. Table 3.1 shows the relative frequency of the different causes of subfertility.

It is important to note that a significant proportion of couples present with more that one reason for sub-

Table 3.1 Relative frequencies of the different causes of subfertility. (From Hull et al 1985, with permission.)

Cause	Relative frequency (%)
Unexplained	28
Sperm defects/dysfunction	24
Other male infertility	2
Annovulation	21
Tubal damage	14
Endometriosis	6
Coital failure	6
Cervical mucus defects/dysfunction	3
Others	11

fertility (as is reflected in the total percentages in Table 3.1) and effective management can be initiated only when both partners have been investigated appropriately.

MANAGEMENT OF SUBFERTILITY

The investigative procedures, often referred to as the 'fertility work-up', can be initiated in the primary healthcare setting. This is often where the couple first present and any tests performed here will expedite the investigative process when specialist referral is instigated.

The appropriate assessment of *both* partners is paramount. It should be remembered that there are two unique individuals within each relationship and that they are not necessarily accustomed to the discussion and revelation of their most intimate sexual encounters. Some couples do not share past events, such as previous pregnancies and their outcomes, sexually transmitted diseases, etc. and are reluctant to divulge what may be pertinent clinical information. This can often be overcome, however, during the inadvertent separation of the couple (i.e. for the physical examination) when information may be sought, although it is often volunteered.

History

General information regarding age, occupation, social and medical history is needed. Particular attention should be paid to the duration of infertility, frequency and timing of intercourse and any coital difficulties experienced. This will alert the practitioner to potential causative factors such as infrequent and inappropriate coital timing, possible psychosexual dysfunction or occupations that incur shift patterns or involve periods of separation that will disrupt sexual activity. Occasionally, the male partner may work with toxic chemicals or may be found to be taking certain medications that impair spermatogenesis. Cigarette smoking should be discouraged as it can be toxic to oocytes, increase the morphological abnormalities of sperm and cause an increased risk of miscarriage.

Female history

Menstrual cycle Note should be made of average cycle length and cyclic variations. Enquiries as to whether the woman is aware of mid-cycle pelvic discomfort (mittleschmerz), cervical mucus changes or has premenstrual symptoms can aid assessment of menstrual function.

Obstetric history Previous pregnancies, whether spontaneous or resulting from treatment, and their outcome should be detailed. Whether the pregnancy was achieved with the current partner or from a previous relationship should also be noted.

Previous surgery Particular attention is paid to pelvic surgery, as this could indicate pelvic adhesions or possible tubal damage.

Contraceptive history Note is made of the type of contraceptive devices that have been used and when they were stopped (it has been known for a female to present with infertility whilst still taking the oral contraceptive pill!). Previous use of the intrauterine contraceptive device (IUCD) is linked to pelvic inflammatory disease (PID), which in turn can lead to tubal damage. It is accepted that IUCD use is thought to increase the risk of developing clinical PID.

Sexually transmitted disease Any previous infections and their treatments should be documented because of their strong association with tubal damage.

Sexual activity This is a delicate subject to broach with some couples and is often responded to with trepidation when they await the possible verdict on their sexual function. It is commonly found that couples concentrate their sexual activity to the magical 'day 14', which is of little use for any cycle length that varies from 28 days. This is an ideal opportunity to explore and correct any misconceptions. Direct questioning about any coital difficulties or sexual dysfunction may indicate the need for psychosexual therapy. Any evidence of dyspareunia should be noted as this is often associated with endometriosis.

Galactorrhoea The presence of this may indicate hyperprolactinaemia and should be explored further.

Exercise Excessive exercise can cause hypothalamic disruption and lead to oligomenorrhoea or amenorrhoea. Advice should therefore be given accordingly.

Alcohol intake The weekly intake should be documented and should not exceed 14 units per week (Health Education Authority 1994), although a lower limit is advisable when preparing for pregnancy. Alcoholism can lead to amenorrhoea and ovulation disorders, as well as seriously affecting general health.

Family history It is often worth noting familial disorders for reference. Some inherited conditions can present with infertility.

Weight The body mass index (BMI) should be calculated (weight in kilograms divided by height in metres squared). The normal range is 20–25 kg/m^2. Underweight women become amenorrheic and anovulatory and weight gain may be the simple solution to their subfertility. Obese women should be referred to a dietician for professional advice and many fertility clinics will defer treatment until weight loss is attempted or achieved.

Male history

Answers to general health and lifestyle questions should be explored and appropriate advice and rationale given as previously mentioned.

Medical history Chronic conditions must be documented because of the possible association with infertility, for example, diabetes, which is associated with retrograde ejaculation. Pyrexial illness (e.g. streptococcal infection) could cause temporary azoospermia and any occurrence within the past 6 months is relevant when interpreting the results of a semen analysis.

Any problems with testicular descent in childhood, mumps, **orchitis** or testicular trauma should be noted. The history or presence of varicoceles is an important finding because of the association with impaired seminal parameters.

Previous pregnancies Enquiries are made as to any previous pregnancies the male partner has fathered and whether any difficulties were experienced prior to conception.

Previous surgery Knowledge of pelvic or genital tract surgery is of paramount importance, as complications affecting fertility could have developed. For example, surgical obstruction of the vas deferens may have occurred during childhood surgery for an inguinal hernia, or retrograde ejaculation may be a consequence of surgery on the lower urinary tract.

Sexual activity General enquiries as with the female. Any physical problems such as impotence or premature ejaculation should be ruled out and patients should be referred appropriately.

Sexually transmitted diseases All previous infections and their treatment are noted as STDs are known to increase the risk of blocked sperm ducts and the development of antisperm antibodies.

Alcohol intake The weekly intake should be documented and should not exceed 20 units per week, as alcohol can have a marked effect on spermatogenesis. Advice must be given to cut down or stop altogether; however, improvement may not be noticed for over 3 months.

Family history Some chromosomal conditions affect fertility. Cystic fibrosis is an example, and one of its presenting anomalies is a congenital bilateral absence of the vas deferens. Apart from the obvious problem for those who are trying to conceive, there are also the genetic implications for the couples' offspring.

Counselling and genetic screening should be explored before undergoing any treatment.

Examination

A general physical and pelvic examination is carried out on the woman alongside a genital examination of the man (some units will not examine the male unless indicated). Female examination includes:

- height, weight and estimation of body mass index
- observation for signs of endocrine disorders – acne, hursutism (e.g. polycystic ovarian syndrome). Palpation of the thyroid gland and general observation for signs of hyper/hypothyroidism
- breast examination, to assess for signs of galactorrhoea
- abdominal examination noting previous surgical scars and abdominal tenderness
- pelvic examination to detect the presence of adnexal masses, tenderness and nodules in the vagina and pouch of Douglas, which may be suggestive of endometriosis. Mixed or reduced mobility of the pelvic organs may indicate adhesions
- cervical smears and endocervical swabs for microscopy and chlamydia are often taken routinely.

Examination of the male (at this stage) will include:

- estimation of testicular size – using an orchidometer
- exclusion of testicular masses or varicoceles.

General investigations

Fertility investigations are complex. A significant proportion of general investigations can be performed at the primary healthcare level, whilst more specific investigations can be performed only at specialist centres. Table 3.2 summarizes the general investigations of subfertility.

Hormone profile

See Table 3.3 for a guide to the normal values.

Table 3.3 Hormone profile – normal values

Hormone	Normal value
Follicle stimulating hormone (FSH)	1–10 iu/l
Luteinizing hormone (LH)	1–10 iu/l
Thyroid stimulating hormone (TSH)	0.5–5.9 μm/l
Prolactin	0–360 μm/l
Luteal phase progesterone	>30 nmol/l

Follicle stimulating hormone levels. Serum levels of follicle stimulating hormone (FSH) are used as an indicator of ovarian function. It is generally found that levels above 20 iu/l on more than one occasion signify premature ovarian failure, whereas levels of 11–20 iu/l indicate that the ovaries are failing and are unlikely to respond to stimulation with gonadotrophins (especially if >15 iu/l). This is likely to come as a great shock as perimenopausal women may continue to menstruate and acceptance may take time and require counselling.

Luteinizing hormone levels. Elevated levels of luteinizing hormone (LH) in the presence of elevated FSH levels indicate premature ovarian failure.

Polycystic ovarian syndrome (PCOS) will manifest a rise in LH levels in the presence of a normal FSH level.

Low levels of LH and FSH (< 2 iu/l) indicate pituitary dysfunction, e.g. hypogonadotrophic hypogonadism.

The mid-cycle rise in LH (the LH surge) can be detected in blood or urine and is a normal physiological occurrence that triggers ovulation.

Thyroid stimulating hormone levels. Thyroid dysfunction can have a notable effect on fertility and women may present with infertility caused by thyroid disease. Elevated levels of thyroid stimulating hormone (TSH) suggest hypothyroidism and a suppressed level can point to hyperthyroidism, although estimations of free T3 and T4 will aid diagnosis.

Prolactin levels. Raised serum prolactin levels must be repeated and, if significantly raised, referral to an endocrinologist should be initiated. Hypothyroidism is associated with a rise in serum prolactin levels although a more sinister cause may be apparent, such as a pituitary adenoma, which is diagnosed through

Table 3.2 Summary of the general investigations of subfertility

Investigation	Hormones monitored
1. Hormone profile	• Follicle stimulating hormone (FSH)
Stage – early follicular phase, day 2–5 of cycle	• Luteinizing hormone (LH) • Thyroid stimulating hormone (TSH) • Prolactin levels
Stage – luteal phase, approximately 7 days before the onset of the next period	• Progesterone
2. Rubella status	
3. Semen analysis	

computerized tomography (CT) scanning or magnetic resonance imaging (MRI) scanning.

Prolactin levels can be elevated by stress and can vary daily.

Progesterone levels. Ovulation is often determined by a rise in the serum progesterone levels (> 30 mmol/l) in the luteal phase of the cycle. The correct timing for performance of the test is approximately 7 days before the next period. Therefore, in a 28-day cycle it would be day 21 and in a 34-day cycle, day 27.

Testosterone levels. These are often checked when PCOS is suspected as a significantly raised level can assist confirmation of diagnosis.

Rubella status

Rubella status is routinely established because of the known risks to the developing fetus during the first trimester. It is unwise to rely on evidence of vaccination alone and immunization is recommended if the antibody titre is low or absent. Advice is given to avoid pregnancy for 1 month following vaccination.

Semen analysis

Table 3.4 represents the criteria applied for interpretation of semen parameters. The generalized use of the World Health Organization guidelines ensures standardization and consistency between units.

The amount of samples required for analysis differs between units, but is usually either two samples, 4 weeks apart or one sample that is repeated if abnormal. Samples are produced through masturbation following 3 days abstinence.

The investigations described above can be carried out within the primary healthcare setting and will indeed speed up the process of diagnosis. The following procedures come under the umbrella of the specialist centre.

Table 3.4 WHO criteria for semen parameters

Standard tests	Normal values
Volume	≥2.0 ml or more
pH	7.2–8.0
Sperm concentration	≥20 million sperm/ml
Total sperm count	≥40 million sperm per ejaculate
Motility	≥50% with forward progression
	≥25% with rapid progression within 60 minutes of ejaculation
Morphology	≥30% with normal forms
White blood cells	<1 million/ml
Immunobead test	Fewer than 20% with adherent particles
MAR test	Fewer than 10% with adherent particles

Source: WHO 1992.

Specific investigations

Cycle monitoring

Many of the baseline investigations can be combined and observed within a 1-month cycle. Table 3.5 shows the average timing (subject to cycle length) and type of procedures currently assessed.

Ultrasound scans Although ultrasound scans were traditionally performed transabdominally, this has been superseded by the advent of transvaginal sonography (TVS). This approach has the advantage of more accurate and precise views of the pelvic organs and is performed without the need for a full bladder.

Serial ultrasound scanning allows assessment of the uterus and detection of congenital abnormalities, for example, bicornuate uterus. Other potential concerns such as fibroids or endometrial polyps can be detected at the same time. The ovaries are assessed for size and morphology and polycystic or multifollicular ovaries are clearly visible. Ovarian cysts are excluded or confirmed and clarification of type is often possible.

Table 3.5 Cycle monitoring

Average day of cycle	Procedure	Rationale
Day 2–5	Hormone profile	Baseline assessment of uterine and ovarian
	Ultrasound scan	morphology
Day 8–10	Ultrasound scan	Follicular tracking
	Monitor urine for LH surge	Predict ovulation and accurately time coitus/PCT
Day 10–14	Postcoital test	Assessment of sperm/mucus interaction and survival
Day 20–25	Ultrasound scan	Detection of ovulation/corpus luteum
	Serum progesterone	Hormonal evidence of ovulation

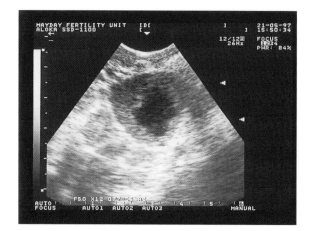

Figure 3.1 Corpus luteum-luteal phase of cycle.

Although fallopian tubes of normal appearance are not visible through ultrasound, it is possible to identify hydrosalpinges.

Around mid-cycle the growth of the dominant follicle is monitored (follicular tracking) to allow accurate prediction of ovulation and prompt testing for the LH surge. Towards the end of the cycle a further scan is performed to look for evidence of ovulation in the form of a collapsed follicle or corpus luteum (Fig. 3.1).

Transvaginal scanning has a vital role in the monitoring of cycles stimulated with exogenous gonadotrophins. It allows adequate observation of follicular response, minimizes the risk of ovarian hyperstimulation syndrome (OHSS) and ensures accurate timing of insemination.

Postcoital test

The postcoital test (PCT) is usually conducted in specialist fertility units, although it may easily be incorporated into the investigations carried out within the primary healthcare setting.

The test is performed immediately prior to ovulation when the cervical mucus, under the influence of oestrogen, becomes thin and most readily penetrated by sperm. The couple are instructed to have intercourse on the day of detection of the LH surge and attend the clinic/GP surgery within 6 to 18 hours. The woman is advised not to bathe or douche, although she may have a wash or shower. A small amount of mucus is retrieved from the cervical canal and examined under a microscope, where the characteristics are assessed and a positive or negative result is given.

The purpose of this test is to confirm adequate coital technique, assess the state and receptivity of the cervical mucus and observe the number and behaviour of the sperm within the sample.

The PCT is, however, highly controversial. In a recent review of the literature specific to current practice (Morgan, unpublished work, 1997), many discrepancies were uncovered that cast doubt upon the value of PCT as practised by some.

In a large quantitative study, Oei et al (1995) noted that the PCT was performed in 92% of the responding major teaching hospitals in western Europe, but

Table 3.6 The characteristics assessed during the postcoital test

Characteristic	Excellent findings Positive result	Poor findings Negative result
Cervical mucus		
Volume – collected	0.3 ml or more	0 ml
Consistency	Watery, minimally viscous preovulatory	Thick, viscous, premenstrual mucus
Ferning	Tertiary and quarternary stem ferning	No crystallization
Spinnbarkeit – length of cervical mucus thread when stretched.	9 cm or more	0–4 cm
Cellularity – estimated no. of leucocytes and other cells in cervical mucus	0 cells per hpf	>20 cells per hpf
Sperm		
Number of sperm	>20 sperm per hpf Highly debated!	<3 sperm per hpf
Motility – type of movement displayed	Rapid progressive motility	Immotile or non-progressive

hpf, high power field
Source: WHO 1992

remarked that there was an overwhelming lack of uniformity and standardization for performance, assessment and subsequent action taken.

The development of standard reporting criteria covering all parameters of the PCT can be adopted by GPs/clinics to facilitate accurate results. The WHO (1992) guidelines laid out in the laboratory manual for the examination of human semen and sperm–cervical mucus interaction is the most widely used at present and can easily be implemented. All practitioners involved in fertility investigations can then be cognisant to the characteristics responsible, and the meaning of a positive or negative test (Table 3.6).

Nevertheless, fertility patients often find the PCT one of the most psychologically traumatic investigative procedures. Boivin et al (1992) remark that the reason why the test is associated with sexual difficulties and trauma is that couples are obliged to engage in sex regardless of their level of sexual desire and that they must do so with the knowledge that the clinician will grade (indirectly) the outcome of their sexual performance.

Tests for tubal patency

Laparoscopy and dye test. Laparoscopic inspection of the pelvic organs is often the first-line management option and is complemented by the ability to assess tubal patency. Methylene blue dye is injected transcervically and the fimbrial ends of the fallopian tubes are observed for free spill of dye. In addition to this, the presence of endometriosis or adhesions are revealed. Minor adhesiolysis may be performed at the time of diagnostic laparoscopy but more complicated adhesions are managed at a later stage by laparotomy.

The procedure is usually performed in day surgery units allowing discharge home the same day.

Hysterosalpingography. This is an additional means of assessing tubal patency. The procedure is performed after the menses have ceased and prior to ovulation to ensure the woman is not pregnant. Patients are advised to use a barrier form of contraception in the month leading up to the hysterosalpingogram (HSG).

The procedure involves the injection of contrast medium into the cervical canal. The fallopian tubes are monitored through X-ray imaging for free spill into the peritoneum. The procedure has the advantage of not requiring a general anaesthetic and is useful in the investigation of obese patients. It is often employed as an adjunct when laparoscopic findings are negative or inconclusive and has the added ability to outline abnormalities within the uterine cavity that are not possible with laparoscopy alone. It is not possible, however, to detect peritubal adhesions, which may affect the function of the fimbrial end of the tube with respect to oocyte pick-up.

Caution is necessary where a history of PID is noted and, in severe cases, laparoscopy is favoured. Prophylactic antibiotics are administered if there are any concerns. The process can be uncomfortable for the patient (especially if tubal damage exists) and oral analgesia is recommended 30–45 min prior to the procedure.

Hysterosalpingo-contrast sonography (HyCoSy). This is similar to the HSG. Visualization is through ultrasound with the use of an echogenic contrast medium or saline to outline the uterine cavity and determine tubal patency. This technique can be performed in an outpatient setting. Adopting a selective criterion for use (e.g. no suspicion of tubal damage) has the advantage of expediting the fertility work-up. Any evidence of tubal blockage or uncertain findings must be reassessed through follow-up laparoscopy or HSG.

Uterine assessment

Hysteroscopy. Now commonly performed at the time of diagnostic laparoscopy, hysteroscopy permits systematic inspection of the uterine cavity and canal. Diagnosis of interuterine lesions such as endometrial hyperplasia, malignancy, polyps, submucus fibroids, uterine congenital anomalies and intrauterine adhesions are possible.

Treatment

Following the investigative process the couple return for a follow-up consultation to discuss the findings and explore options. In the percentage of patients where a problem exists a treatment plan can be formulated. Involvement of the couple during the decision-making process is extremely valuable and has the fundamental benefit of curtailing feelings of loss of control. For the couple there are far more issues surrounding the agreement to treatment such as religion, culture and financial position.

The appropriate options are explored. The benefits of medical or surgical intervention should be outlined and supported by facts with respect to resumption of fertility and spontaneous pregnancy. More dynamic treatments with the aid of assisted reproductive technologies may be indicated and occasionally a combination of both is necessary.

The specialist fertility nurse is an invaluable source here, not only to interpret medical terminology and clarify implications, but also to help the couple recognize their feelings and establish their personal limitations regarding treatment.

Regular medical review of the couple is paramount as, if conception is not achieved within a given time, further progressive options involving more advanced (and usually more invasive) techniques can be considered and initiated.

Occasionally couples feel pressurized to continue with treatment or wish to consider alternative pathways such as adoption or remaining childless. Professional counselling can provide the support and guidance these couples need to facilitate this transition. Each fertility unit will have access to appropriately trained counsellors.

Coexisting medical or gynaecological disorders

Paramount to the successful treatment of those women who present with infertility is the adequate management of coexisting medical or gynaecological problems.

Case study: Sue

Sue and Neil presented with secondary infertility of 3 years, having previously conceived spontaneously without difficulty. No obvious cause was identified on routine history taking and examination. Baseline investigations were performed and the initial semen analysis from Neil proved to have a low count, although this was found to be normal on subsequent testing. Routine cycle monitoring to include a hormone profile was undertaken by Sue and revealed a TSH level of less than 0.1, with a free T3 level of 12.2 pmol/l (ref range = 4.6–9.2 pmol/l). No obvious symptoms referable to her thyroid dysfunction were evident.

Review by the endocrinologist concluded that although she was clinically euthyroid, the biochemical results indicate thyrotoxicosis and warranted treatment. Thionamide therapy was commenced, however an adverse reaction was experienced and medication had to be discontinued.

Following lengthy discussions with Sue and her family it was felt that in view of her desire to conceive the quickest way of achieving permanent euthyroidism would be through the performance of a total thyroidectomy, which she underwent later that year. Postoperative recovery was uneventful and she was commenced on thyroxin replacement of 200 μg per day, anticipating no further thyroid problems. Within 5 months of surgery Sue conceived spontaneously. The pregnancy progressed normally and resulted in the birth of a live male infant.

Thyroid disease. Anovulation can result from hyperthyroidism or hypothyroidism, however, spontaneous conception is usually possible once the woman is rendered euthyroid. Hypothyroidism can also be an associative factor of hyperprolactinaemia.

Fibroids. Fibroids are thought to affect fertility only if they distort the uterine cavity or block the cornual region of the fallopian tube. An altered uterine cavity may impede implantation or later development of pregnancy. In this situation, medical treatment with a gonadotrophin-releasing hormone anologue (e.g. Zoladex) is used to decrease the size and vascularity of the fibroid prior to surgical removal (myomectomy).

Endometriosis. The aetiology, diagnosis and treatment of endometriosis are covered extensively in Chapter 11, however, the following information is with reference to the effect on fertility.

The link with endometriosis and subfertility is widely recognized, although the precise relationship between the two conditions remains unclear. Vessey et al (1993) notes that 18% of woman with proven fertility will reveal signs of endometriosis during laparoscopic assessment of the pelvis.

Endometriosis is associated with pelvic pain and a deciding factor in management may be the degree of the predominant symptom, i.e. pain or infertility. Many clinicians advocate treatment based on the degree of endometriosis present. This is confirmed through direct visualization, as symptoms alone do not always correlate with laparoscopic findings and some patients who present with infertility are asymptomatic with regards to endometriosis.

Severe endometriosis can affect fertility by distorting pelvic anatomy as a result of extensive adhesion formation and endometriotic ovarian cysts. The effect of mild endometrial deposits remains uncertain although the resulting dyspareunia may play a part.

Medical management will postpone the possibility of conception and may not be a desirable option for some. However, it is recommended by others as an interim prior to assisted conception.

Surgical treatment of endometriosis has the benefit of restoring pelvic anatomy and therefore increasing the chances of spontaneous conception. If a pregnancy has not resulted within 6 to 12 months, **in vitro fertilization** (IVF) is recommended. Fertility treatment in mild to moderate cases of endometriosis initially involves ovulation induction with or without intrauterine insemination (IUI)/**gamete** intrafallopian transfer (GIFT). If this is not deemed suitable (perhaps because of age and/or sperm dysfunction) or is unsuccessful, the couple will be advised to undergo IVF.

ANOVULATORY INFERTILITY

Correction of the underlying disorder is implicit to the management of annovulation. Balen and Jacobs (1997) state that this should lead to cumulative conception rates that approach those expected for the patient's age.

Hypothalamic–pituitary causes

Hyperprolactinaemia

Hyperprolactinaemia is the most common pituitary reason for amenorrhoea (Balen 1997). Management should be monitored by a clinical endocrinologist in conjunction with the gynaecologist and methods of treatment are detailed in Chapter 6.

If, however, cycle function (ovulation) does not return in the presence of normal serum prolactin levels, then ovulation induction should be considered.

Hypogonadotrophic hypogonadism

This refers to the condition whereby insufficient amounts of the gonadotrophins FSH and LH are secreted to stimulate the ovary. The cause may be a congenital absence of luteinizing hormone releasing hormone (LHRH), which is normally released in pulses from the hypothalamus and stimulates the pituitary to secrete LH and FSH. As those affected would not have reached the menarche, this condition is likely to have been detected prior to presentation for fertility treatment.

Diagnosis is made through serum FSH/LH levels alongside serum oestradiol (E2) levels, all of which would be low. The uterus and ovaries would appear abnormally small on ultrasound. Management is dictated by the cause.

If there is a reduction in LHRH release, treatment by pulsatile LHRH therapy is indicated.

Weight-related amenorrhoea

Weight-related anovulation can be caused by starvation (voluntary or involuntary), illness and exercise, which results in disruption of gonadotrophic secretion (see Chapter 6).

A normal body mass index (BMI) should be encouraged and this may be the only treatment necessary to ensure resumption of menstrual function. Professional support must be available and any indication of eating disorders should be managed in collaboration with a psychiatrist.

Ovarian causes

Polycystic ovarian syndrome

This condition and its management is covered separately in Chapter 8.

Premature ovarian failure

Premature ovarian failure (POF), is defined as the cessation of periods combined with raised gonadotrophin levels prior to the age of 40 years. Aetiology is multifocal and includes chromosomal abnormalities (e.g. Turner's syndrome), ovarian destruction from radiotherapy or chemotherapy, infection and previous surgery.

Treatment to restore ovarian function is not usually successful as the ovaries are unlikely to respond to exogenous gonadotrophins. However, pregnancy may be possible in perimenopausal women prior to the absolute cessation of periods. Recommendation is normally given to the use of donated oocytes as part of an IVF programme to overcome this problem.

TUBAL DAMAGE

The predominant cause of tubal damage is primarily chlamydial and gonoccocal sexually transmitted pelvic infections. Tubal factors account for approximately 14% of known cases of subfertility. Physiological function of the fallopian tubes is impaired by adhesions that can distort their anatomy.

Treatment options are either tubal surgery or IVF and the choice of management is influenced by age, degree of pathology, previous attempt at repair and other contributory factors for subfertility. All points must be considered to ensure that the most appropriate treatment is carried out.

Age is of particular concern and evidence exists to support the fact that fecundity declines markedly in women over the age of 38 years. For these women surgery may not be a realistic option and, the greater the extent of tubal damage, the lower the chance of spontaneous conception. Concern is also placed around the risk of ectopic pregnancy, which would be slightly higher than the general population.

Tubal microsurgery is an area requiring expertise and access may be limited to specialist units, even though this is the advocated method for restoration of tubal function and is noted to be superior to conventional surgical techniques (ESHRE Capri Workshop 1996). Various methods are available including salpingostomy, fimbrioplasty, salpingolysis and tubal anastomosis (commonly employed for reversal of sterilization).

Hull (1992) stresses the importance of selectivity based on location and extent of damage. Coexisting pelvic disease should also be considered as factors influencing outcome.

Other parameters of fertility investigation should be within normal limits and if suboptimal factors present then IVF would be indicated, as treatment with essentially no chance of success would be futile.

If a pregnancy has not been achieved within a given time (usually 1 year) following surgery then IVF is normally considered.

UNEXPLAINED INFERTILITY

This is often not a true diagnostic label but a term to describe a group of people for whom no cause for infertility has yet been found. The accuracy of the title is difficult to assess as centres differ in the amount of investigation performed before this description is reached and many fertility specialists adopt the term 'undiagnosed infertility' to reflect the potential for location of cause. Hull (1992) remarks that couples with unexplained infertility of less than 3 years have so far been 'unlucky' but goes on to say that in cases of more than 3 years duration, natural conception is an unrealistic hope.

Management strategies differ between units and are influenced by age and duration of infertility. Clomiphene citrate therapy is often used before progression to IUI, GIFT or IVF. Some centres advocate that one cycle of IVF be undertaken initially as this can double as a diagnostic tool with regard to knowledge of sperm/egg interaction and fertilization capacity.

It is important to remember that this is a desperate position emotionally. Frustration and anguish can often be overwhelming when conception fails to occur in the presence of 'supposed' normality.

MALE INFERTILITY

Male infertility can be due to an abnormality of the semen or a problem with its delivery to the female genital tract (Hirsh 1997).

The exact aetiology of sperm dysfunction is often unknown and correction of the cause is therefore problematic. The solution is usually that the disorder is 'overcome' with the use of assisted reproductive technologies (ART).

Diagnosis may also be hindered by the subjective nature and criteria applied for interpretation of semen parameters. Furthermore, individual semen samples are not necessarily static and a single specimen may not be an accurate representation of the general quality of the sperm, which is the reason that some units automatically analyse a second sample.

Although general guidelines for analysis are available (e.g. WHO 1992) they do not indicate the fertilizing capacity of the sperm in vitro, although this situation may improve with the advent of computer assisted sperm analysis (CASA). Its use in assessment of sperm count, motility and morphological parameters may have considerable advantages in terms of speed and reduction of inter–intra observer variation (Thornton and Fischel 1995) However, research into its true value is ongoing and debated (Barratt 1996).

Physical and psychosexual concerns will have been established by this point and referral made to the appropriate bodies.

The management of specific male disorders and investigations will be conducted in conjunction with a clinical andrologist (reproductive urologist); some larger units will have an andrologist working within the fertility team.

Further investigations are dependent upon the findings at semen analysis.

Azoospermia

Azoospermia is defined as the absence of sperm in the ejaculate. The causes can be identified at any of the following levels of the male reproductive physiology.

Hypogonadotrophism

There are reduced testosterone levels with low or normal FSH and LH. Treatment consists of prolonged use of hMG and human chorionic gonadotrophin (hCG).

Failure of spermatogenesis

Common causes include chromosomal abnormalities (e.g. Klinefelter's syndrome), spermatogenic arrest, testicular atrophy and Sertoli-only syndrome.

Treatment is difficult, although surgical sperm extraction combined with intracytoplasmic sperm injection; ICSI, see p. 32) may be successful in some cases.

Obstruction

Assessment is through semen analysis, vasography and hormone profiles. In selected cases treatment is surgical. Common causes of obstruction are detailed below.

Bilateral congenital absence of the vas deferens. The role of the vas deferens is to transport seminal fluid from the testes to the seminal vesicles. Congenital absence occurs in 1:1000 men and in 20% of men with obstructive azoospermia (Hirsch 1997).

This condition is associated with cystic fibrosis and genetic screening and counselling may be indicated prior to treatment.

If normal spermatogenesis is found then sperm can be extracted from the epididymis and used in conjunction with assisted reproductive technologies.

Vasectomy. Although an obvious cause, increasing numbers of couples are presenting for postvasectomy treatment of infertility.

There are two options: (i) surgical reversal; or (ii) sperm retrieval and assisted conception.

Surgical reversal has the benefit of allowing spontaneous conception (in the presence of normal female fertility). However, the success of surgery declines with time (usually over 5 years) and epididymal obstruction may occur rendering the male azoospermic once more.

Assisted conception combining intracytoplasmic sperm injection (ICSI) using retrieved sperm has major implications for the woman as she would have to undergo IVF treatment. There may also be financial restrictions as this option is expensive.

A recent study by Parlovich and Schlegel (1997) concluded that the most effective single intervention in terms of cost and pregnancy rate is microsurgical vasectomy reversal.

Ejaculatory failure

Associated neurological disorders are treated accordingly. If psychosexual problems are identified, specialist counselling may help. Postcoital examination of urine may reveal retrograde ejaculation.

Oligospermia

Oligospermia is defined as a sperm count lower that 20 million/ml. If the count falls below 10 million/ml it is described as severe oligospermia.

Causes are often idiopathic and circumnavigated with assisted conception. Other associated conditions are retrograde ejaculation, varicocele and infection.

Retrograde ejaculation

In this condition little or no semen is present at ejaculation, instead the sperm are ejaculated into the bladder. This is confirmed by the presence of sperm in the urine. It may be a result of nerve damage from injury, surgery or infection.

The postorgasmic urine can be collected and the sperm recovered and prepared as for IUI. Alternatively, antegrade ejaculation may be achieved during intercourse with a very full bladder.

Varicocele

The link between infertility and the presence of a varicocele is highly debated, although a rise in scrotal temperature may play a part.

Management varies between specialists and some consider that surgery holds no improvement to male infertility. However, the results of a recent WHO trial (1996) concludes that the varicocele is an important cause of male infertility.

Infection

The presence of infection is detected by a significantly raised white cell count on semen analysis. Treatment should be commenced with doxycycline 100 mg/day for approximately 4 weeks. Infection is known to reduce the fertilizing capacity of sperm and sexually transmitted infections can result in permanent damage.

Antisperm antibodies

Antisperm antibodies (ASAB) are found in blood, serum and cervical mucus. The condition is characterized by the agglutination (clumping together) of sperm, and is suggestive of an immunological cause of subfertility. ASAB are thought to develop in men when the blood–testes barrier is breached as a result of obstruction or injury to the reproductive ducts, e.g. after vasectomy, testicular trauma and infection. Antibodies impair sperm motility, which in turn could affect fertilization.

Treatment is through careful laboratory preparation of sperm combined with IUI, although in cases of severe ASAB, in vitro fertilization and/or ICSI is indicated.

ASSISTED REPRODUCTIVE TECHNIQUES

Treatment options for severe male factor infertility

Until 1992 treatment options for severe male factor infertility were limited. IVF is restrictive in so far as it requires a minimum sperm count of 500 000/ml, and anything below this meant that donor sperm was often recommended in order to achieve a pregnancy.

Since the introduction of gamete micromanipulation techniques, fertilization can be assisted and no longer requires large quantities of sperm, displaying specific motility. These techniques include:

- Partial zona dissection (PZD) – this involves the introduction of a glass needle into the zona pellucida (the outer shell of the oocyte) causing a breach through which the sperm can enter.
- Subzonal insemination (SUZI) – a process whereby sperm is injected beneath the zona pellucida.

However, these methods do not yield large quantities of embryos as fertilization rates do not exceed 20–25% of the micromanipulated oocytes (Van Steirteghem et al 1994), which therefore results in a reduced pregnancy and take-home baby rate.

Intracytoplasmic sperm injection (ICSI)

In 1992 a new treatment that was set to revolutionize the management of men with severely compromised semen parameters and change the outlook of repeated failed fertilization during conventional IVF was reported (Palermo et al 1992). The process, known as intracytoplasmic sperm injection (ICSI), involves the injection of a single sperm into the cytoplasm of an oocyte (Fig. 3.2). Successful fertilization is achieved in around 60% of oocytes undergoing microinjection, which results in a clinical pregnancy rate of approximately 30% (Van Steirtegham et al 1994).

By 1995 evidence was available regarding the use of surgically retrieved testicular sperm in conjunction with assisted reproductive technologies to achieve fertilization in patients with both obstructive and non-obstructive azoospermia (Devroey et al 1995).

At present there are a variety of methods employed for obtaining sperm, and their use in conjunction with ICSI (owing to the relatively few sperm required) is fast becoming part of routine treatment throughout the world.

Current methods of sperm retrieval are (Fig 3.3):

- Percutaneous epididymal sperm aspiration (PESA) – occasionally sperm can be aspirated directly from the epididymis with a very fine needle inserted through the skin of the scrotum. This is a simple procedure and can be performed under local anaesthetic.
- Microepididymal sperm aspiration (MESA) – this procedure is employed for the extraction of sperm directly from the epididymis using microsurgical techniques and is performed under general anaesthetic. It is often used when PESA is not possible or unsuccessful.
- Testicular sperm extraction (TESE) – if no sperm are present in the epididymis, as a result of either severe testicular sperm impairment or absence of the epididymis, a testicular biopsy is performed to extract the sperm directly from the testicular tissue.

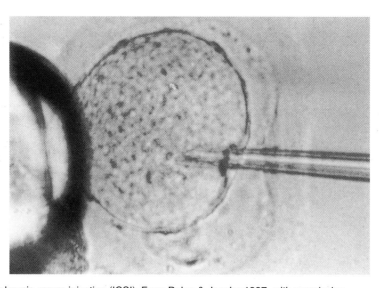

Figure 3.2   Intracytoplasmic sperm injection (ICSI). From Balen & Jacobs 1997, with permission

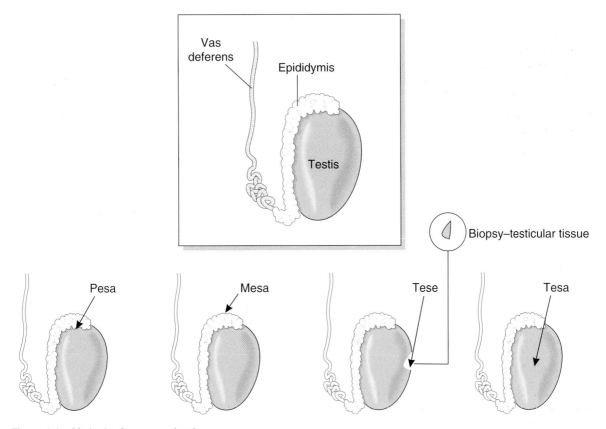

Figure 3.3   Methods of sperm retrieval.

● Testicular sperm aspiration (TESA) – indications are as in TESE but sperm recovery is achieved by inserting a needle directly into the testis through the skin.

In all the above methods surplus sperm may be cryopreserved for later use in subsequent cycles.

● Pentoxyphylline – this is a caffeine derivative used to enhance sperm motility. It is indicated for use with severe oligospermia, evidence of poor motility and previous poor fertilization rates, however its true role in fertilization is debated (Yovich et al 1990).

● Spermatids – Although a child conceived using this treatment was reported in 1995 (Fishel et al 1995), the use of spermatids (immature sperm cells) in conjunction with ICSI is not yet licensed in the UK. The HFEA remark that 'whilst technically possible, it has not yet been proven to be safe for both the intended child and the mother'. They also warn that

receiving this treatment in another country may expose the couple and their hoped for child to risk (HFEA 1997a).

Repercussions of micromanipulation techniques

The possibility of potential congenital abnormalities arising in children conceived with the use of ICSI and related micromanipulation techniques remains ongoing and under continued scrutiny. Initial data comes from Boudelle et al (1995), who conducted a comparative follow-up study of the first 130 children born after ICSI, alongside 130 children born through conventional IVF. No statistically significant differences were found between the two groups and no recognized instances of major abnormalities above that expected in the general population were apparent.

However, the rapid implementation of these techniques and the successful treatment of profound male factor indications (of which some arise from chromosomal anomalies) has led to concerns regarding the genetic risk inherent to the offspring (Baschat et al 1996, Martin 1996, The-Hung Bui & Wramsby 1996).

Boudelle et al (1996) pursued a more extensive follow-up study of 877 children born after ICSI and found that the incidence of major malformations was within an expected range comparable with previous results. The latest findings did reveal an increase in transmitted chromosomal aberrations, which led the authors to conclude that these observations must be completed by others and by collaborative efforts. It was recommended that patients be counselled about the available data, and the risk of transmitting fertility problems to their offspring.

This was supported by Baschet et al (1996), who stress that in view of the genetic implications, accurate diagnosis for male factor infertility should be established prior to treatment to allow prospective parents to make an informed choice regarding continuation of treatment.

Some units routinely conduct genetic screening on all patients requiring management with ICSI. As new information becomes available and genetic implications are confirmed, screening may become a mandatory requirement.

GENERAL TREATMENT OPTIONS USING ASSISTED REPRODUCTION

Ovulation induction

Oral – clomiphene citrate therapy

Clomiphene (clomid/serophene) is an antioestrogen that causes increased pituitary gonadotrophin release and ovarian stimulation. It works by preventing the normal negative feedback effect of oestrogen, which allows further endogenous FSH and LH secretion leading to folliculargenesis. Initial monitoring with serial ultrasound scans (USS) and endocrine/hormone profiles are indicated to assess response to treatment and detect increased folliculargenesis.

Complications and side-effects include:

- multiple pregnancy – (6% chance of twins)
- clomid cysts – these often resolve spontaneously but may require aspiration if they persist because of the predisposition to ovarian torsion (Fig. 3.4)
- blurring of vision – medication should be stopped if this occurs
- hot flushes

- abdominal distension and pain.

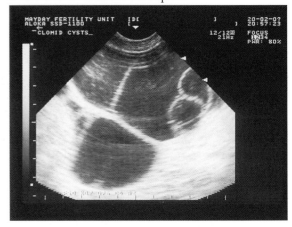

Figure 3.4 Ovarian cysts occuring during a cycle stimulated with Clomid.

Tamoxifen is sometimes substituted for clomiphene in those who experience unpleasant side-effects.

In 1994 a report by Rossing et al found an association between the use of clomiphene and ovarian cancer with more than 12 months continuous therapy. However, there is no evidence that clomiphene used for the recommended duration of 6 months increases the risk.

Treatment with clomiphene is occasionally initiated by the GP. This is not recommended where the cause of anovulation is uncertain or where adequate surveillance with USS is unavailable.

Parenteral – gonadotrophin therapy

The indications for parenteral gonadotrophin therapy are induction of ovulation in anovulatory women, failed response to clomiphene and in conjunction with intrauterine insemination (IUI).

Gonadotrophins are now available in several forms and include:

- *Human menopausal gonadotrophins (hMG)* – extracted from the urine of postmenopausal women and contains equal amounts of FSH and LH
- *Highly purified FSH* – which has little or no LH
- *Recombinant FSH* – this is a synthetic, pure FSH created through the utilization of molecular biology and is increasing in popularity between units.

Administration is by injection via the intramuscular or subcutaneous route.

Parenteral induction of ovulation (PIO)

Regimes to induce ovulation vary between centres and there is no 'correct' schedule for gonadotrophin therapy. Hormone levels, ovarian morphology and the nature of annovulatory dysfunction will define the parameters of therapy. Most regimes involve either daily injections or alternate day injections starting on day 2–3 of the cycle and continuing for approximately 7–14 days until follicular maturity is reached. The aim is to achieve up to three follicles of 17–20 mm in diameter. Administration of 5–10 000 iu of human chorionic gonadotrophin (hCG) will induce ovulation approximately 36 hours later, thus permitting insemination procedures or timed intercourse to be planned accordingly. If a greater number of follicles are found, hCG must be withheld and the couple advised to use contraception until the next period arrives because of the risk of multiple pregnancy and ovarian hyperstimulation syndrome (OHSS) (see p. 38).

Adequate monitoring with serial oestrodial levels and USS to assess follicular growth will enable the clinician to determine progress and accurately assess response to therapy. The couple should be aware of the need for continued monitoring and adequate instruction is crucial for the safe and successful outcome of treatment. The woman and her partner may wish to be taught how to administer injections, although some couples prefer the hospital or practice nurse/GP to give the drugs. Success rates for parenteral induction of ovulation (PIO) are difficult to assess, partly due to the variation in regimes, but also because of the underlying reason for performance. Unlike IVF there is no national data that considers the multitude of variables present, hence the limitation of unit comparison.

Intrauterine insemination (IUI)

Intrauterine insemination (IUI) is now often incorporated into PIO cycles and is indicated in the presence of mild sperm dysfunction, cervical mucus problems, unexplained infertility or functional abnormalities such as vaginismus, retrograde ejaculation or impotence.

The process involves the insemination of a prepared sample of sperm into the uterine cavity at the time of ovulation.

Preparation is achieved by 'washing' the sperm to remove the seminal plasma. This has a high concentration of prostaglandins that, if not removed, will cause painful uterine cramps following insemination. One of two techniques are usually employed to prepare the sperm. In the 'swim up' method the sperm is diluted in culture medium and centrifuged, followed by resuspension in the medium. This process is usually repeated and the sperm sample left to stand for 30–60 minutes. During this time the motile sperm can 'swim up' to the surface. The sperm recovered from the surface will contain a higher number of motile sperm with normal morphology. An alternative is the use of density gradients to separate the most morphologically normal and motile sperm. The cycle is stimulated with gonadotrophins (PIO) and is governed by the same criteria (maximum of three mature follicles) and surveillance guidelines. IUI can be achieved in a natural cycle although it is more successful when combined with PIO, probably due to the availability of more than one oocyte. This has led to pregnancy rates of 14% per cycle (Dodson and Haney 1991).

IUI is usually more accessible to couples owing to its relative inexpense, and is often available within district general hospitals. Absolute contraindications would be bilateral tubal damage and severe male factor infertility. Usually, three to six cycles are attempted before resorting to alternatives.

Gamete intrafallopian transfer (GIFT)

Gamete intrafallopian transfer (GIFT) is available to women who have at least one functional tube. Superovulation is achieved in the same way as IVF but the method and site of fertilization differ. Oocytes are retrieved either transvaginally under ultrasound direction or through laparoscopic aspiration. Up to three eggs, together with a small amount of medium containing prepared motile sperm, are transferred directly into the fallopian tubes laparoscopically.

Advantages of this method are that fertilization and early embryo development take place at their 'natural' site, which makes this technique acceptable to those who, for religious or moral reasons, find the 'creation of life' in vitro unacceptable.

The main disadvantage is that it does not indicate the fertilizing capacity of sperm and in cases of unexplained infertility or borderline male factor, where IUI has failed, IVF would be a more suitable treatment. Success rates are again subject to many variables but pregnancy rates of 26–36% per cycle have been reported by Hull (1992).

Zygote intrafallopian transfer (ZIFT) and tubal embryo transfer (TET)

These techniques are identical to GIFT in so far as superovulation regimes and oocyte retrieval.

However, fertilization is performed in vitro and the timing of return of the fertilised egg is variable.

In zygote intrafallopian transfer (ZIFT), the fertilized oocyte is transferred at the pronuclear stage (which will fuse to form the nucleus), usually 18–24 hours after insemination.

Tubal embryo transfer (TET) is performed approximately 48 hours after fertilization either by laparoscopy or retrograde transfallopian cannulation (whereby the cannula is passed through the fimbrial end and its contents deposited in the mid-ampulla region of the tube) or transcervical cannulation (passed up through the cervix) of the fallopian tube.

The main disadvantage of this treatment is that if oocytes are collected laparoscopically, two operative procedures may be required within 2 days. Nevertheless, attempted fertilization in vitro reveals valuable insight into sperm–egg interaction and fertilizing capability. Embryo development in vivo is regarded by some couples to be more acceptable. From a technical viewpoint, ZIFT/TET is of benefit when cervical transfer of embryos is difficult.

Rates for intrauterine pregnancy, ectopic and spontaneous abortions are within the same range as IVF and as yet no evidence of superiority regarding tubal or intrauterine transfer of gametes or embryos exists (Van den Eede 1995).

Direct intraperitoneal insemination (DIPI)

This procedure involves the injection of prepared sperm through the posterior vaginal wall into the peritoneal cavity, where it can be picked up by the fallopian tubes. Insemination is usually performed under ultrasound guidance and is often used by units where more advanced techniques are unavailable. The pooled data of published results shows a pregnancy rate of roughly 10% per cycle (Tan & Jacobs 1991).

IN VITRO FERTILIZATION (IVF)

Often thought of as the pinnacle of fertility treatments, in vitro fertilization (IVF) was initially devised to overcome the problem of tubal infertility. Modern application of this technique now circumvents almost all cases of infertility where other methods have failed.

The first live birth following IVF was achieved during a natural cycle but this approach was soon superseded by stimulated cycles, largely due to the greater yield of oocytes and embryos, which allowed multiple embryo transfer.

The process involves three main stages:

- superovulation
- oocyte retrieval
- embryo transfer.

Most centres will initiate treatment with a gonadotrophin releasing hormone (GnRH) agonist starting either in the follicular phase (day 1–2) or luteal phase (day 21).

Administration via nasal spray (e.g. Syneral) or subcutaneous injection (e.g. Buserelin) is continued for approximately 2 weeks. This causes pituitary desensitization ('downregulation') and leads to a reduction in endogenous FSH and LH rendering the ovaries quiescent. The advantage of using GnRH analogues is that it allows control of the stimulation regime, enabling timing of cycles and oocyte recovery. It also prevents an early surge of LH, which could cause ovulation or premature luteinization of follicles. Follicular recruitment is achieved by stimulation with gonadotrophins following regimes similar to PIO, although the dose is likely to be higher and continue for longer. The final trigger for maturation is given through s.c. or i.m. injection of hCG and oocyte retrieval is timed to occur 34–36 hours later.

A percentage of cycles may be cancelled prior to egg collection either because of a poor response (<4 mature follicles) or as a result of over response (>25 follicles) due to the risk of OHSS.

Oocyte retrieval is normally performed vaginally under ultrasound guidance, although some units perform the procedure laparoscopically. The transvaginal approach has the advantage of not requiring a general anaesthetic and is performed under sedation. Following aspiration of the follicles, the oocytes are recovered from the fluid by an embryologist. The sperm sample is produced through masturbation and then prepared through selection of the most motile and morphologically normal sperm. Insemination is usually performed 1–6 hours after oocyte recovery with the addition of around 100 000 sperm with each egg. Approximately 16–18 hours later the oocytes are examined to ensure that normal fertilization has occurred, as defined by the presence of two pronuclei. Occasionally all the eggs fail to fertilize, which is a devastating blow to the couple and in this situation ICSI would be indicated in a subsequent attempt.

Embryo transfer is performed 2–3 days after oocyte retrieval when the embryos have reached the four-cell stage of development. A small amount of culture medium is added to the embryos, which are replaced transvaginally into the uterus using a fine catheter. The number of embryos replaced is influenced by many factors, although the transfer of more than three embryos is prohibited by the Human Fertilization and Embryology Act (1990). Many centres routinely transfer two but in some instances the decision is purely academic as only one or two embryos may be available for transfer. Couples must be thoroughly counselled regarding the potential outcomes of a triple embryo transfer. Surplus embryos may be frozen (cryopreserved) for use in subsequent cycles, or donated, following adequate counselling because of the potential emotional repercussions.

Luteal support in the form or progesterone pessaries or injections is often advocated.

The ensuing fortnight is generally the most stressful as the couple wait to see if the treatment has been successful. This is governed by the onset of a period or a negative pregnancy test 2 weeks after embryo transfer.

Success rates vary between centres. The overall pregnancy rate in the UK per treatment started is

---

Case study: Celene

Celene and John are 24 and 26 years, respectively, and had previously achieved one pregnancy. This conception was ectopic and subsequently ruptured requiring a left salpingectomy.

Specialist help was sought after 2 years of unsuccessful attempts at pregnancy. Routine baseline investigations of hormone profile and semen analysis proved normal although laparoscopy and dye testing revealed irreparable tubal damage. IVF therefore was their only option.

Treatment was commenced 13 months later. Downregulation was achieved with a GnRH agonist in the form of a nasal spray, followed by daily injections of FSH.

The final ultrasound scan showed 11 follicles and serum oestrodial concentration was 8786 pmol/l. Transvaginal ultrasound directed oocyte retrieval was performed and nine eggs were collected.

Insemination took place approximately 5 hours later and the couple were told to ring the next day to establish how many eggs had fertilized. Quite unexpectedly fertilization failed to occur, even though egg quality was fair and sperm survival was excellent. It was decided that ICSI should be performed in any future cycle and this was attempted 5 months later.

Six eggs were collected and ICSI was performed on all of them. Five fertilized and two embryos of good quality were transferred. Following 2 weeks of progesterone supplements a subsequent pregnancy test proved positive. Transvaginal ultrasonography performed 4 weeks after embryo transfer revealed a single intrauterine pregnancy equivalent to 6 weeks gestation.

18.5% (between 1 January 1995 and 31 March 1996) (HFEA 1997b).

Transport/satellite IVF

IVF is becoming more accessible through the availability of transport IVF programmes. District general and private hospitals can provide an IVF service in conjunction with a specialist centre providing embryological laboratory expertise. In transport IVF, treatment up to and including egg collection is conducted at the local hospital and the male partner transports the follicular fluids to the central IVF unit, where the oocytes are recovered and fertilized. Embryo transfer is normally performed 2 days later at the central unit, although some centres transport the embryos back for replacement at the local unit.

Satellite IVF differs in so far as treatment is initiated at the local unit but care is transferred at the point of oocyte retrieval.

This adaptation restores the advantage of continuity of care and serves to limit the required time commitments that are often incurred when travelling to larger central units.

Cryopreservation

Supernumerary embryos resulting from IVF/GIFT cycles may be frozen for use in subsequent treatment cycles. This has the advantage of not requiring another egg collection and necessitates only minimal drug therapy to render the ovaries quiescent and prepare the endometrial environment for the replacement of embryos. Financial implications are also apparent as frozen embryo replacement cycles are often much cheaper than IVF, although a charge is made for the original storage of embryos. The disadvantage is that not all the embryos will survive the freeze–thaw process. Survival rates have been reported at between 45 and 80%, with embryo grade and cleavage stage at the time of freezing being good prognostic factors for the determination of freeze–thaw survival (Karlstrom et al 1997).

The HFEA details overall pregnancy rates from frozen embryo replacement cycles as 14% (HFEA 1997b).

Oocyte donation

The use of donated eggs for women with ovarian failure and certain genetic disorders is now widely established, although demand far exceeds supply. This is primarily due to the fact that the donor has to go through the same ovarian stimulation/egg retrieval process as that required by IVF. Many well-intentioned women who make enquiries are often unable to justify or set aside the time or commitment necessary for this. Some units have recruitment incentives that allow the potential recipients to divert waiting lists if they provide a donor in return. Donors are usually anonymous to the recipient because of the possible emotional and social repercussions.

The HFEA sets a minimum donor age of 18 years and a maximum limit of 35 years because of the increased risk of chromosomal abnormalities.

Complications of treatment

Ovarian hyperstimulation syndrome (OHSS)

Ovarian hyperstimulation syndrome (OHSS) is one of the most serious complications of ovulation induction and ovarian stimulation for IVF. Its development warrants prompt management to prevent rapid deterioration. OHSS is graded according to severity and classified as shown in Table 3.7.

Mild cases are managed at home and are concerned with relief of symptoms. The woman must be alerted to the fact that a more severe state may occur and should be issued with an advice sheet regarding the symptoms of OHSS and what to do if any arise.

Moderate to severe cases require hospitalization to correct fluid balance and provide pain relief. Paracentesis may be necessary if breathing becomes laboured.

Severe OHSS is life-threatening and adequate management within an intensive care unit is essential.

PCOS is a risk factor for the potential manifestation of OHSS and pretreatment identification of the syndrome will allow drug dosage to be tailored accordingly. Surveillance of follicular growth by USS and E2 estimations are imperative as it is on the basis of these findings that the woman is deemed at risk. OHSS is triggered by the administration of hCG and should be withheld in women who are considered to be in danger of its subsequent development.

Although abandoning the cycle appears to be the best safeguard, this is generally difficult for the couple to accept because of the emotional, financial and social commitments they have made. Two further courses of action may be considered or undertaken. First, the hCG may be administered (often at a lower dose) and oocyte retrieval carried out as previously planned. All resulting embryos are then cryopreserved to be replaced at a later stage. Pregnancy will increase the chance of OHSS occurring owing to the high levels of circulating hCG.

Alternatively, intravenous albumin may be administered prophylactically following egg collection. Both actions have been compared by Shaker et al (1996), who conclude that the two appeared equally as effective in the prevention of OHSS.

Multiple pregnancy

Stassen at al (1995) remark that the ultimate goal of infertility treatment is a singleton pregnancy and the birth of a healthy child. This statement underpins a poignant message that is sometimes sacrificed during the pursuit of infertility management. Multiple pregnancy is a common factor associated with assisted reproduction and its profound effect is encapsulated by Price (1992) who notes that when making arrangements to overcome the biological problem of infertility it seems that little thought has been given to the social and emotional aspects of possibly having many children at once, which will render the familiar, unfamiliar and the normal, abnormal.

In cases where high order (four or more) multiple pregnancy occurs the couple will be offered the chance to undergo selective fetal reduction. The aim here is to enhance the chance of survival of some of the fetuses by the sacrifice of others. The decision is fraught with emotional, moral and religious implications and for some is not an option. The procedure is usually performed in the first trimester and has an associated rate of pregnancy loss of 8–9% in experienced centres (Balen & Jacobs 1997).

The ruling in the Human Fertilization and Embryology Act (1990) on the maximum number of embryos/gametes permitted to be replaced in the

Table 3.7 OHSS grading

Degree of severity	Clinical manifestations
Mild	Weight gain, abdominal distension and discomfort, ovarian enlargement
Moderate	Nausea, vomiting, distension, pain, dyspnoea and ultrasound evidence of ascities and ovarian enlargement
Severe	Pain, tense ascites, haemoconcentration, hypovolaemia, electrolyte disruption, oliguria, renal failure and ovarian enlargement (>12 cm in diameter)

uterus has served to minimize this risk, although in other countries with no such legislation, multiple pregnancies are commonplace.

Results The overall chance of a single pregnancy after transfer of three embryos is approximately 25–30%, while the chance of multiple pregnancy is 1–5%.

The take-home baby rate is 15–20% for each cycle with IVF and GIFT, while the relevant rate with ICSI is about 30% per cycle (Stirrat 1997).

Cumulative conception rates (CCR) This is defined by Tan & Jacobs (1991) as a statistical method of expressing the success rate of infertility treatment. It takes into account treatment success and failure as well as patients who discontinue treatment and also copes with different rates of follow-up.

THE HUMAN FERTILIZATION AND EMBRYOLOGY AUTHORITY

The advancing technologies of assisted conception and scientific medical research relating to human fertilization and embryology have been under debate and scrutiny for many years. This led to the 1990 Human Fertilization and Embryology Act, which recommended the establishment of a regulating authority.

The Human Fertilization and Embryology Authority (HFEA) assumed its full powers in 1991. Its principal tasks are to licence and monitor clinics that conduct IVF cycles, that use and store donated gametes, and that undertake embryo storage or research.

The authority consists of 21 members representing scientific, medical, nursing, social, legal, religious and lay public views. Their fundamental aims and objectives are to oversee, regulate and maintain unit responsibility in the treatment offered and research undertaken. In doing so they act as a safeguard to protect the wellbeing of patients, children, the general public and future generations.

The code of practice

The code of practice is, in essence, the manual for fertility units and sets out levels of service to which licensed centres must abide. It includes guidance on staffing, facilities, counselling, welfare of the child, information and standards of practice.

The code stipulates that consideration should be given to the welfare of the resulting child when assessment is made of the suitability of clients to receive treatment. Some units require the couple and/or their GP to complete questionnaires regarding previous history and suitability to receive treatment. It is hoped, however, that initial referral by GPs would not be made if concerns are evident.

Following acceptance for licensed practice, centres are inspected annually by a team who report to the licensing and fees committee. Licences can be suspended or revoked at any time if the unit does not comply with the regulations set out in the code of practice.

Provision of NHS treatment

In 1996 the College of Health undertook its fourth study of NHS funding of infertility services in the UK. A response rate of 82%, which covered approximately 90% of the UK population was received from the postal questionnaires enquiring into the purchasing arrangements and criteria.

The overall findings showed an increase of NHS funding for IVF of around 15% but this tended to be within areas that already funded IVF and not from those who were previous non-funders, indicating a sharp divide between authorities. The establishment of formal policies for infertility treatment are increasing although conceptualization and forward movement remains low key. Aspects of eligibility criteria appear to be more uniform although wide variations in detailed criteria exist, e.g. age limitations for IVF of 34–43 years and the continuation of some authorities to refuse funding if either partner within the couple has had a child.

Concerns are also present with regard to type of treatment accessible. For example, in areas where IVF is not funded but tubal surgery is available, situations could occur where women undergo tubal surgery when IVF is more appropriate.

They conclude by remarking that few authorities were able to provide information of funds allocated for infertility treatment, or divulge details of the numbers of fertility treatments they had funded (other than assisted conception). This consequently casts doubt on whether the limited funds the authorities have at their disposal are used effectively (College of Health 1996).

THE ROLE OF THE NURSE

The degree of participation nurses have within the field of reproductive medicine varies enormously. Ranging from brief encounters during outpatient visits or the short stay diagnostic procedures through to the specialist fertility nurses who coordinate and manage every aspect of fertility care. One factor common to all is the tremendous support that is gained from the nursing staff.

Nurses working within the primary healthcare setting (GP practice, family planning or well women clinics) are ideally placed to assist couples with the initial management of fertility problems. The provision of basic advice regarding lifestyle, health and frequency or timing of intercourse is sometimes all that is required to correct the situation. Careful listening and questioning can also prevent unnecessary investigations and inappropriate medical interventions.

In addition to the advice on health and lifestyle (detailed within the section on history taking) the instruction and promotion of fertility awareness is of extreme value. Many couples are unsure of the physiological events that occur each month and are usually guided by family/friends and filled with well intended (but sometimes wrong) advice. Infertility creates an overwhelming vulnerability and there is often reluctance to admit lack of understanding for fear of ridicule. This should be borne in mind and no assumptions made when formulating an action plan.

Table 3.8 outlines a programme of observations to detect normal physiological changes that will enable the woman to recognize and assess her period of fertility through retrospective analysis.

In general, the measures displayed are best used as a guide to assess the fertile period. It may take a few months to become familiar with the pattern but persistence is worthwhile and rewarding with regard to control. The couple should be deterred from concentrating intercourse solely to the day of LH surge and ovulation as valuable potentially fertile days may be missed.

Fertility nursing

The position of fertility specialist requires a number of skills and encompasses numerous roles such as nurse, advocate, counsellor and friend. The scope for extended practice is immense and not within the confines of this chapter. It is one of the less known areas of nursing but one that is constantly changing as technology and feasibility advances.

Recognition of this nursing role is increasing with the advent of the Fertility Nurses Group (subgroup of the RCN) and the establishment of the Assisted Conception Nursing Care course (ENB N40 – long course). At the time of writing, the development of a specialist diploma course in fertility nursing to incorporate the ENB N40 is underway.

Counselling

Couples experiencing difficulties in conceiving have particular needs and nurses from areas outside of specialist centres may be confronted with these. A unique set of anxieties present for each individual and these are influenced by society's views and their own religious and social standing. It is these values that are contemplated when attempting to balance their wish for a child against the methods that may need to be employed to achieve this.

The couple are continually reminded of their situation. Comments from others, however well intended, deliver striking reminders of their plight, shopping trips become a nightmare, the onset of periods

Table 3.8 Assessment of fertility

Observation	Rationale
Cycle length	Recorded from the first day of red loss until (but not including) the next period. This will allow identification of the luteal phase, which is the only static period and can aid the pinpointing of ovulation
Basal body temperature	Temperature recordings performed daily (early morning) A rise in temperature of approximately 0.2 degrees centigrade is detectable within 24 hours of ovulation A sustained rise for 3 days would indicate 48 hours post ovulation
Cervical mucus	Recorded at the end of the day, oestrogenized 'fertile' mucus will be thin and 'stretchy' when placed between the fingers Viscous, non-stretchy mucus signifies non-ovulatory/non-fertile period A watery discharge can indicate potential fertility
Mittelschmerz	Ovulation pain The presence of dull pain in the lower abdomen (often unilateral) lasting up to a few hours can indicate ovulation
Detection of the surge in luteinizing hormone (LH surge)	The LH surge triggers ovulation approximately 32–36 hours later Commercially available urine testing kits can be used to predict ovulation and time intercourse

reinforce another month's failure. Often, social/family events are avoided for fear of exposure to more pain.

Diagnosis of infertility disrupts natural, lifecycle events that have been assumed since childhood. Not a mother, not a grandmother and not able to continue the blood line. The resulting cascade of emotions is known to affect relationships and self-esteem (Hirsch & Hirsch 1989). The causes for infertility, especially if confined to one partner, can result in feelings of guilt and often lead to tension and lack of communication with each other.

The 'roller coaster' of highs and lows are often extreme, ranging from euphoria when hope is restored and plummeting to despair when a treatment fails. The continued subjection to these situations will inevitably take its toll and professional counselling should be offered to allow exploration of feelings and beliefs, either as a couple or separately, in order to understand their present circumstances so that they may rationalize, live more effectively and gain a clearer perspective.

Although nurses acquire and utilize a number of counselling skills, the implications of fertility treatment are long-lasting and extreme. Situations may present that are beyond the capabilities and time constraints of daily practice and it is here that input from a specialist counsellor should be sought.

The HFEA Code of Practice (1995) details three distinct types of counselling that should be available to couples receiving licensed treatments:

- Implications counselling, which concerns the implications of undertaking the proposed treatment with respect to themselves, their families and any children born as a result.
- Support counselling, which concerns the provision of emotional support throughout the duration of treatment and is of particular importance during times of heightened stress when a treatment has failed.
- Therapeutic counselling, which is concerned with helping the couple cope with the consequences of fertility treatment. The aim is to assist with the adjustment and acceptance of their position by helping them to resolve any conflicts that may exist.

Although the availability of counselling in licensed centres is mandatory, the acceptance of such is not. Counselling is viewed by some as an indication of failure or inability to cope and uptake may be dependent upon the way in which it is offered. Couples should never be pressurized to attend and it must be emphasized that counselling can be initiated at a later stage.

THE DECISION TO END TREATMENT

The decision to discontinue treatment is probably the most traumatic that the couple will have to face. Confronting the pain of childlessness is to some unbearable and can be the reason for the continued drive for active therapy. In cases of absolute infertility (e.g. ovarian failure) the result is final, but for those whose diagnosis is uncertain or minor, as in the case of unexplained infertility, a question mark will persist with regard to future **fecundity**. The possibility that the next cycle might be the one that works or the poor understanding of cumulative success rates will cast doubt upon the accuracy of a decision to give up.

The individual merit of each case is considered when dealing with the number of cycles offered and medical decisions will be influenced by the same factors that determine any successful outcome. By this stage most couples have undergone many years of investigation and treatment and a realistic view of chances must be presented to enable acceptance of their situation. It is often the medical team that will suggest a time to stop thus preventing the couple from initiating the final decision. Whether this is excepted or dismissed is a further issue.

There are, of course, couples who drop out at the point of IVF for various reasons but overall people who discontinue medical care do so because the process becomes too stressful, overwhelming, painful and expensive. At whatever stage treatment ends it is imperative that these couples have access to therapeutic counselling to ease the transition and provide the help and support needed to let go and move on to new pathways.

Adoption

Following the introduction of the oral contraceptive pill and the legal performance of abortions, very few babies are available for adoption in the UK. Frequently it is older children who are placed for adoption, with a high percentage coming through the care system.

The process of adoption is controlled through local social service departments or voluntary agencies. The procedure, which is subject to regional variations in accessibility and criteria, can take up to 2 years to complete. Unfortunately, many couples are unsuccessful.

None the less, adoptive parents continue to need support. They are likely to experience diverse emotions and may have unrealistic expectations of themselves as parents, which may be hampered by friends and relatives who perhaps do not agree with their decision to adopt. Networks of support do now exist that aim to bridge the postadoption problems and fears that may arise (see Useful Addresses, p. 44).

Surrogacy

As an alternative to adoption, surrogacy offers to some the chance of a child to which they are the biological parents. Although dependent on IVF the surrogate acts as an incubator to the developing baby, following successful implantation of embryos developed from the eggs and sperm of the intended parents. This type of arrangement is often referred to as 'host surrogacy'. A second form of surrogacy involves the artificial insemination of the intended father's sperm and will mean that any resulting children are genetically related to the surrogate.

Controversy engulfs surrogacy and 'bad press' has shaped public opinion, although reservations are justified when assessing the suitability of this course of action. This can be a hazardous pathway and the potential emotional repercussions must not be underestimated.

Nevertheless, Kim Cotton, the first UK surrogate mother and former chairperson of COTS (Childlessness Overcome Through Surrogacy) argues that this method should not be ignored if it is an alternative to childlessness. She further remarks that surrogacy is often ignored by society in favour of adoption but, as approximately 6000 couples are waiting to adopt with only 300 babies available, for many this is an unrealistic option (Cotton 1997).

The intervention of a third party (i.e. fertility centre) is not mandatory and many surrogacy arrangements are conducted privately and it is here that the concerns lie. It is imperative that all surrogates and their commissioning parents have access to professionals who can ensure full exploration of the implications before any agreements are undertaken.

CONCLUSION

Subfertility is relatively common, although the true incidence may be grossly underestimated. Early recognition of fertility disruption will permit prompt referral and initiation of interim baseline investigations.

The advances in reproductive technologies have allowed the circumnavigation of most causes of infertility, although caution must be maintained with the development of micromanipulation techniques and associated methods until long-term outcomes are known.

The long-lasting and profound impact of infertility can engulf all aspects of the individual's life. Driven by the overwhelming desire for a child the couple may become consumed by their situation. Adequate support and guidance, with access to professional counsellors, is imperative to minimize the potential psychological morbidity.

Levels of nurse involvement vary between settings but of particular value is the education of couples with regard to fertility awareness, which can prevent unnecessary referral and inappropriate investigation.

The social stigma shrouding infertility is beginning to shift but general awareness of reproductive technologies remains tarnished by the bad press it continues to receive. The demand for assisted conception will increase as more people, whether part of a traditional couple or as single individuals, present for treatment. It is therefore paramount that nurses working within the field of women's health become aware of the issues surrounding and factors involved in fertility care.

GLOSSARY

Fecundity: the ability to procreate
Gamete: collective term referring to the males' sperm or the females' eggs
In-vitro fertilization: fertilization performed outside of the body, usually in a glass dish

In-vivo: process occurring within the body
Orchitis: inflammation of the testis

REFERENCES

Balen AH 1997 Amenorrhoea and anovulation. In: Rainsbury PA and Viniker DA (eds). Practical guide to reproductive medicine. Parthenon Publishing, New York, ch 4, p 49–63

Balen A, Jacobs H 1997 Infertility in practice. Churchill Livingston, New York.

Barratt CLR 1996 Consensus workshop on advanced diagnostic andrology techniques. Excerpts on Human Reproduction. No 3:1–5

Baschat AA, Schwinger E, Diedrich K 1996 Assisted reproductive techniques – are we avoiding the genetic issues? Human Reproduction 11(5):926–928

Boivin J, Takefman JE, Brender W, Tulandi T 1992 The effects of female sexual response in coitus on early reproductive processes. Journal of Behavioural Medicine 15(5):509–517

Bouduelle M, Legein J, Derde M-P et al 1995 Comparative follow-up study of 130 children born after intracytoplasmic sperm injection and 130 children born after in vitro fertilisation. Human Reproduction 10:3327–3331

Bouduelle M, Wilikens A, Buysse A et al 1996 Prospective follow-up study of 877 children born after intracytoplasmic sperm injection (ICSI), with ejaculated epididymal and testicular spermatozoa and after replacement of cryopreserved embryos obtained after ICSI. Human Reproduction 11 (Suppl 4):131–155

College of Health 1996 Report of the fourth national survey of NHS funding of infertility services. College of Health, National infertility awareness campaign London.

Cotton K 1997 Labour of love. Nursing Times 93(11):38–39

Devroey P, Lui J, Nagy Z et al 1995 Pregnancies after testicular sperm extraction and intracytoplasmic sperm injection in non-obstructive azoospermia. Human Reproduction 10(6):1457–1460

Dodson W, Haney F 1991 Controlled ovarian hyperstimulation and intrauterine insemination for treatment of infertility. Fertility and Sterility 55:457–467

ESHRE Capri Workshop 1996 Guidelines to the prevalence, diagnosis, treatment and management of infertility. Excerpts on Human Reproduction No 4, Oxford University Press, Oxford.

Fischel S, Green S, Bishop M, et al 1995 Pregnancy after intracytoplasmic injection of spermatid. Lancet 345:1641–1642

Greenhall E, Vessey M 1990 The prevalence of subfertility: a review of the current confusion and a report of two new studies. Fertility and Sterility 54(6):978–983

Health Education Authority 1994 That's the Limit – A Guide to Sensible Drinking. Health Education Authority, London

Hirsch AM, Hirsch SM 1989 The long-term psychosocial effects of infertility. Journal of Obstetrics, Gynaecology and Neonatal Nursing 24(6):517–522

Hirsch AV 1997 A guide to the practice of andrology in the assisted conception unit. In: Rainsbury PA and Viniker DA (eds). Practical guide to reproductive medicine. Parthenon Publishing, New York, ch 11, pp. 179–213

Hull MGR, Glazener CMA, Kelly NJ, et al 1985 Population study of causes, treatment and outcome of infertility. British Medical Journal 291:1693–1697

Hull MGR 1992 Infertility treatment: relative effectiveness of conventional and assisted conception methods. Human Reproduction 7(6):785–796

Human Fertilisation and Embryology Authority (HFEA) 1995 Code of practice. HFEA, London

Human Fertilisation and Embryology Authority (HFEA) 1997a The patients' guide to DI and IVF clinics, 3rd edn. HFEA, London.

Human Fertilisation and Embryology Authority (HFEA) 1997b Sixth Annual Report. HFEA, London

Karlstrom PO, Bergh T, Forsberg AS, Sandkvist U, Wilkland M 1997 Prognostic factors for the success rate of embryo freezing. Human Reproduction 12(6):1263–1266

Martin R 1996 The risk of chromosomal abnormalities following ICSI. Human Reproduction 11(5):924–925

Oei SG, Keirse MJNC, Bloemenkamp KWM, Helmerhost FM 1995 European postcoital tests: opinions and practice. British Journal of Obstetrics and Gynaecology 102:621–624

Palermo G, Joris H, Devroey P, van Steirteghem AC 1992 Pregnancies after intracytoplasmic injection of a single spermatozoon into an oocyte. Lancet 340:17–18

Pavlovich CP, Schlegel PN 1997 Fertility options after vasectomy: a cost-effectiveness analysis. Fertility and Sterility 67(1):133–141

Price F 1992 In: Stacey M (ed) Changing human reproduction – social science perspectives. Sage Publications, London, p. 112

Rossing MA, Daling JR, Weiss NS, Moore DE, Self SG 1994 Ovarian tumors in a cohort of infertile women. New England Journal of Medicine 331:771–776

Shaker AG, Zosmer AZ, Dean N, Bekir J, Jacobs HS, Tan SL 1996 Comparison of intravenous albumin and transfer of fresh embryos with cryopreservation of all embryos for subsequent transfer in prevention of ovarian hyperstimulation syndrome. Fertility and Sterility 65(5):992–996

Staessen C, Nagy ZP, Lui J, Janssenswillen C, Camus M, Devroey P, van Steirteghem AC 1995 One years experience with elective transfer of two good quality embryos in the human in vitro fertilisation and intracytoplasmic sperm injection programmes. Human Reproduction 10:3305–3312

Stirrat GM 1997 Aids to obstetrics and gynaecology for the MRCOG, 4th edn. Churchill Livingstone, New York, p. 216

Tan SL, Jacobs H 1991 Infertility – your questions answered. McGraw-Hill, Singapore

Templeton A, Fraser C, Thompson B. 1991 Infertility – epidemiology and referral practice. Human Reproduction 6(10):1391–1394

The-Hung Bui, Wramsby H 1996 Micromanipulative assisted fertilisation – still clinical research. Human Reproduction 11(5):925–926

Thornton S, Fischel S 1995 Infertility in men. Infertility, Update Postgraduate Centre Series, Reed Healthcare Communications, pp. 48–53

Vessey MP, Villard-Macintosh L, Painter R 1993 Epidemiology of endometriosis in women attending family planning clinics. British Medical Journal 306:182–184

Van den Eede B 1995 Investigation and treatment of infertile couples: ESHRE guidelines for good clinical and laboratory practice. Human Reproduction 10(5):1246–1271

Van Steirteghem AC, Nagy P, Lui J et al 1994 Intracytoplasmic sperm injection – ICSI. Reproductive Medicine Review 3:199–207

World Health Organization 1992 WHO laboratory manual for the examination of human semen and sperm– cervical mucus interaction, 3rd edn. Cambridge University Press, Cambridge

World Health Organization 1996 WHO varicocele trial. British Journal of Urology 77 (Suppl 1):19

Yovich JM, Edirisinghe WR, Cummins JM, Yovich JL 1990 Influence of pentoxifylline in severe male factor infertility. Fertility and Sterility 53:715–722

USEFUL ADDRESSES

CHILD (The National Infertility Support Network)
Charter House, 43 St Leonards Road, Bexhill-on-Sea, East Sussex TN40 1JA

COTS (Childlessness Overcome Through Surrogacy)
Loandhu Cottage, Gruids, Lairg, Sutherland IV27 4EF

DI Network (Donor Insemination Support Group)
PO Box 256, Sheffield S3 7YX

Human Fertilization and Embryology Authority
Paxton House, 30 Artillery Lane, London E1 7LS

ISSUE (The National Fertility Association)
114 Lichfield Street, Walsall WS1 1SZ

Multiple Births Foundation
Queen Charlotte's & Chelsea Hospital, Goldhawk Road, London W6 0XG

Parent to Parent Information on Adoption Services
Lower Boddington, Daventry, Northants NN11 6YB

Post-Adoption Centre
5 Torriano Avenue, London NW5 2RZ

4

Sexually transmitted infections

Christina McGlynn

Sexually transmitted infections (STIs) affect a large proportion of the sexually active population, to a greater or lesser degree, at some time in their life. This could be a very minor 'infection' or could lead to a chronic gynaecological problem. Sex and STIs are subjects that many people would prefer to ignore, they remain taboo areas and it is therefore important for all workers involved in women's healthcare to understand the basics of sexual health and STIs. STIs can have a broad range of effects on women's lives. This chapter will look at some common STIs and their diagnosis and treatments. It will not cover *Chlamydia trachomatis* and pelvic inflammatory disease (PID), which are dealt with in Chapter 10.

When women attend a genitourinary medicine (GUM) sexual health clinic they will be offered a full sexual health screen. This will include looking at the external vulvovaginal area and enables a thorough check to eliminate the presence of any abnormal pathology, which might include genital warts, genital herpes, pubic lice, molluscum contagiosum and any breaks in the skin, redness or erythema. After this is completed a speculum examination will be performed to check for any internal abnormal pathology and allow for any swabs to be taken.

These will check for chlamydia, gonorrhoea, candidiasis (thrush) and a cervical smear test can be taken, if indicated. Specimens will be taken for Gram-staining looking for thrush, bacterial vaginosis (BV) and gonorrhoea, and a wet-preparation slide, which can be used to detect *Trichomonas vaginalis* (TV), will also be taken.

Diagnosing within a GUM/sexual health clinic can be performed in two ways. The initial diagnosis is made through microscopy, which is usually performed by nurses, although some clinics employ laboratory staff to do this. This is either on a wet-preparation or Gram-stained slide. The wet-preparation is a glass slide onto which approximately two drops of normal saline are mixed with vaginal discharge, covered and looked at through a microscope. This will be either on a dark field microscope or on low power. Gram-staining is a process whereby specimens are stained using a process to prepare the slides for oil immersion microscopy. The slide for Gram-staining will contain a sample from the vaginal walls, cervix, urethra and, in some cases, the rectum. The samples are then heat-dried and the slide is placed in methyl violet/crystal violet to stain any Gram-positive organisms (such as the spores and mycelia seen in thrush, or cocci). The slide is placed into iodine to fix the organisms in place and is then rinsed in acetone, which gets rid of any unwanted debris. Lastly, it is placed in saffronin/neutral red or carbol fuchsin, which stains the Gram-negative organisms (such as Gram-negative diplococci, which, if it is intracellular, is indicative of gonorrhoea). It is once again heat-dried and immersion oil is placed on the three samples before they are looked at through the microscope.

Usually, lactobacilli in the vagina produce lactic acid, which keeps the vaginal pH low and stops other organisms growing in the vagina; if they do grow, they can cause infections. There are many organisms present in normal vaginal flora, but in small numbers.

Vaginal discharge is a common reason for women presenting in a GUM or sexual health clinic. This may be physiological or pathological. Adler (1995) comments that 'vaginal discharge is a continuum, and as such the concept of normality does not exist'. Some women have very little discharge and others have a profuse discharge. It is important for women to be aware of their usual discharge to be able to determine what is abnormal. Physiologically, a degree of vaginal discharge is quite normal, helping to keep the vagina healthy. Vaginal secretions act as a lubricant during sexual intercourse, preventing friction and reducing soreness afterwards.

BACTERIAL VAGINOSIS

Definition

Bacterial vaginosis (BV) used to be known as *Gardnerella vaginalis*, which is now an outdated term. The history of BV has shown a change in name due to the complexities of the bacteria found and advances in the technology available to identify the bacteria.

BV is an overgrowth of naturally occurring bacteria found in the vagina. When the discharge from the vagina is looked at microscopically, after Gram-staining, a normal slide will contain epithelial cells and lactobacilli. If BV is present the slide will have a distinct lack of lactobacilli and an increase in numbers of other bacteria that are normally only present in small numbers.

Diagnosis

BV is one of the few infections that is diagnosed mainly through clinical features. The diagnosis is made by finding three out of the four criteria proposed by Amsel et al in 1983. These are:

1. homogenous, grey/white discharge
2. characteristic fishy smell when potassium hydroxide (KOH) 5–10% is added to the vaginal discharge, due to the release of amines, this is often referred to as the amines test or 'whiff' test
3. vaginal discharge with a pH of 4.5 and above
4. clue cells present on microscopy.

When the speculum is inserted there may be evidence of a homogenous, thin, grey/white discharge coating the vaginal walls.

The 'amine' test can be performed at various points: after the speculum is removed, using the discharge on the speculum; by placing a sample of vaginal discharge on a separate slide or by using the 'wet slide' specimen after examining it under the microscope.

As pH is one of the criteria used, it is important to know that the pH of water, water-based lubricants and blood is alkaline, i.e. the pH is greater than 7. So, if any of these are present they will alter the pH reading of the vaginal discharge.

Clue cells are epithelial cells that will appear to be granulated if the woman has BV (Gardner & Dukes 1955). Another way of describing their appearance is as 'salt and pepper' markings on the epithelial cells.

There is also the Nugent method of diagnosing BV (Nugent et al 1991); this method grades the vaginal flora on the Gram-stained slide and allows the person diagnosing to interpret the information in more detail; it does not rely solely on the presence of clue cells.

Treatment

The current first-line treatment for BV is metronidazole 400 mg twice a day for between 5 and 7 days; sometimes, a stat dose of 2 g metronidazole is given. Metronidazole is an antimicrobial drug that exerts selective activity against anaerobic bacteria by interfering with the activity of their DNA (Hopkins 1992). Lactobacilli are allowed to regrow when metronidazole is given, and this is essential for restoring the normal balance of vaginal flora. Metronidazole does have side-effects, which include darkening of the urine, especially with the 2 g stat dose; nausea and a metallic taste in the mouth; drowsiness and dizziness (Hopkins 1992). In addition, if patients drink any alcohol whilst taking metronidazole, and up to 24 hours after finishing, they can be profoundly sick. Turner and Richens (1978) recognized that metronidazole acts like disulfiram (antabuse) – a treatment for alcoholism. McGlynn (1996) emphasized the importance of explaining the side-effects of alcohol when giving metronidazole to patients.

Other treatments include clindamycin cream 2%, usually prescribed for 7 days. This is a 40 g tube with applicators and is inserted into the vagina each night. Women who are using condoms or a cap/diaphragm as their means of contraception should be told that clindamycin cream includes a mineral oil that weakens latex. They should therefore abstain from sexual intercourse for at least 72 hours after the treatment is finished. Some clinicians use chlorhexidine pessaries, ofloxacin 200 mg twice daily for 7 days or Aci-Jel, which contains acetic acid.

Patient education

Patients should be advised to avoid douching, as this disturbs the natural flora of the vagina. Tight clothing, strong detergents, bath oils and bubble baths, strong soaps and vaginal deodorants should be eliminated and some women may need to stop using tampons (McGlynn 1996). There has been research looking at male partners of women with recurrent BV, although treating male partners has not been shown to significantly reduce the number of recurrences. Dawson (1990) has stated that caution should be used in treating male partners as the suggestion is that BV is not sexually transmitted. However, research into this area is ongoing. Women who have sex with women appear to have a higher incidence of BV. In a study of women attending a lesbian sexual health clinic, Conway and Humphries (1994) state that 47% of women were found to have BV. Although many factors are involved in the aetiology, the role of transmission was unclear. Research is currently being undertaken to investigate the transmission of BV from woman to woman.

VULVOVAGINAL CANDIDIASIS

Definition

Vulvovaginal candidiasis is commonly known as thrush. It is usually caused by the fungus *Candida albi-*

Case study: Lily

Lily attended the sexual health clinic for a check-up; she presented with a history of a smelly, vaginal discharge. She attended with her partner, Chan. Three weeks prior to the attendance she had a miscarriage.

The doctor took an in depth sexual history. Lily had been in her first trimester when she miscarried and Chan felt that while he had been away she had been having an affair.

A full sexual health check-up was performed. This involved the doctor having a close look around Lily's vulva and labia, looking for any external signs of an STI, then a speculum examination to enable them to take swabs. The swabs taken were for candida, gonorrhoea, chlamydia and samples for microscopy to look for thrush, gonorrhoea, BV and TV.

After looking at the samples using the microscope an initial diagnosis of bacterial vaginosis (BV) was made. Lily and Chan had never heard of bacterial vaginosis, so the nurse spent a long time explaining to them in detail. Special attention was paid to explaining the link between BV and miscarriage. Also, the fact that it is not proven to be sexually transmitted. Lily was given a 1-week course of metronidazole 400 mg twice a day and advised of the side-effects. She was told to return the following week for the results and to have another examination to ensure the infection had been cleared up.

---

cans. Candida is not generally thought of as an STI, although sexual intercourse may lead to trauma causing damage to the vulval mucosa and allowing the candida to penetrate the deeper layers (Wooley 1994). One of the most common features in women with thrush is vulvovaginal pruritus, which is one of the main reasons women seek medical advice. The vulval itch combined with soreness often occurs with an increased vaginal discharge, which is often described as being like cottage cheese (Fagan 1996). It is usually thick and white and there is often oedema of the labia minora. The woman's genitalia can be excoriated due to scratching. It is important to check the urine for glucose, as thrush can often be a presentation of diabetes.

Diagnosis

Diagnosis is initially made through Gram-stain microscopy of the vaginal wall specimen and backed up with a culture sent to the laboratory. Traditionally, cultures are plated on Sabouraud's medium and incubated at 37°C for 48 hours; Stuart or Amies transport medium may be used when necessary.

Treatment

The most popular first-line treatment is clotrimazole. This is available as pessaries (500 mg single dose, 200 mg on three consecutive nights or 100 mg on six consecutive nights), topical cream 1% or vaginal cream 10%, with a 5 g applicator (which is inserted intravaginally at night for up to six consecutive nights). The pessaries and cream are now available over the counter in chemists without a prescription. Other treatments include econazole cream, 150 mg intravaginally; miconazole 1.2 g pessary, single dose; miconazole cream, 2% topically; nystatin, 100 000 unit pessaries inserted at night for 14–28 nights; fluconazole capsule, 150 mg stat dose and itraconazole, 200 mg capsules morning and evening for 1 day. The topical treatments can sometimes cause further irritation in the area if the patient is sensitive to them and, if this happens, the patient should be advised to stop using the treatment at once.

Patient information

Advice should be given to women to avoid wearing tights, leggings, lycra shorts and tight jeans or trousers and to wear cotton underwear to allow air to circulate and to reduce the risk of sweating and giving the candida a moist, hot environment in which to survive. Sanitary towels rather than tampons should be used when menstruating and panty liners for everyday use should be avoided, as should perfumed soaps, genital sprays, deodorants, bubble baths and disinfectants. The genital area should always be washed and wiped from front to back. If the patient is taking antibiotics, and has a history of thrush, she should be treated for thrush at the same time. She should be advised to make sure that her vagina is well lubricated during intercourse, to reduce trauma (Fagan 1996), and to ensure that her genital area is thoroughly dried after bathing or swimming. Partners should be checked and treated concurrently to avoid re-infection during sex.

TRICHOMONAS VAGINALIS
Definition

Trichomoniasis is caused by a **protozoan** pathogen *Trichomonas vaginalis* (TV). TV is a single-celled organism with four anterior flagellae and one posterior flagellum, which gives it the motility that is seen on microscopy. Trichomonads reproduce by binary fission

and feed by **phagocytosis**. The incubation period is usually between 3 and 21 days; Csonka (1990) has observed that it is commonly 7 days. Transmission is mainly sexual and male partners are rarely symptomatic, although they may suffer urethritis. Heine & McGregor (1993) state that the symptom women usually complain of is a vaginal discharge, often described as green/yellow, which appears frothy on examination. Many women also have pruritus and up to 50% complain of dyspareunia.

Diagnosis

A swab should be taken from the posterior vaginal fornix. Diagnosis is usually made from a wet-preparation slide for microscopy. This can be backed up by a culture media sent to the laboratory. Rein (1990) stated that there are various cultures used, the most popular being the Feinberg–Whittington medium, which is kept incubated for 48 hours and then examined daily for trichomonads for up to 7 days. TV can also be picked up when the laboratory is reporting the cervical smear results, as it can be Gram-stained, but it is difficult to differentiate TV from pus cells using this method.

Treatment

The current first-line treatment is metronidazole, either a 2 g stat dose or 400 mg twice daily for a week. Sexual partners should be treated stimultaneously otherwise the infection will be passed back and forth. Patients should be given the same advice regarding metronidazole as under BV. If TV is diagnosed within the first trimester of pregnancy, metronidazole should not be used as it is not licensed for use during pregnancy.

Patient information

Patients should be advised to avoid sexual intercourse whilst taking treatment and until they return to the clinic for a test of cure, to ensure the treatment was successful (Phillips 1996). As TV is often associated with other STIs, it is important that patients return to the clinic not only for the test of cure, as there are resistant strains, but also for their results and to ensure that no other infection was found on culture. Patients should not resume sexual intercourse until their partner has also been treated.

GONORRHOEA

Definition

Gonorrhoea is caused by the organism *Neisseria gonorrhoea*, which is a non-motile, non-spore forming Gram-negative diplococcus that characteristically grows in pairs. The gonococci attach to columnar epithelium and cause substantial mucosal cell damage in a short time; this is followed by a large **polymorphonuclear** leucocyte response, hence the profuse vaginal discharge that is characteristic of gonorrhoea. *Neisseria gonorrhoea* infects the mucosa of the genital tract, urinary tract, rectum, oropharynx, eye, epididymis and fallopian tubes.

Close physical contact with infected mucosa is required for transmission and the risk of infection from a single episode with an infected partner has been calculated at 60–90% for females and 20–50% for males (Sherrard & Bingham 1995). The higher rate for women is due to the vagina and cervix having a larger mucosal area than the male urethra. In women, urethritis and cervicitis, but not vaginitis, occur. Around 70% of cases in women are symptomless, although increased vaginal discharge, dysuria and frequency may result (Scott 1996a). Ascending infection from the cervix resulting in acute salpingitis occurs in 10% of cases and there is an increased risk of pelvic inflammatory disease (PID), chronic pelvic pain and ectopic pregnancy (Nicholas 1998). Bilateral salpingitis may lead to infertility. An infected woman may infect the eyes of her newborn baby at delivery, which is known as ophthalmia neonatorum, although this is fairly uncommon in the UK. The average incubation period is 3–7 days after exposure to the infection, although symptoms can be present from 1 to 14 days after exposure.

Many women and some men remain asymptomatic. Women may present with mucopurulent vaginal discharge, cervicitis, intermenstrual bleeding, severe menorrhagia, erythema and oedema of the cervix (this may bleed on contact with the swab) or dysuria.

Diagnosis

Diagnosis is made by reading Gram-stained specimens from the cervix and the urethra. The specimen shows Gram-negative intracellular diplococci, however, in women, positive microscopy is found in less than 50% of cases (Scott 1996a). The reasons for this could be that in women, gonococci are often present in single pairs only, rather than groups, making them much more difficult to identify and, if there is a concurrent infection, they could be obscured by the presence of many other organisms. A sample is sent to the laboratory, transported on selective medium such as modified New York City medium in a carbon-dioxide-enriched atmosphere.

Treatment

It is important that first-line treatment is given as a single dose to ensure patient compliance. The actual drug used will vary depending on factors such as local policies and resistance patterns. The World Health Organization (WHO, 1991) recommends the following single dose treatment:

- amoxycillin 3 g and probenicid 1 g, orally
- procaine benzylpenicillin 4.8 million units, i.m., with probenicid 1 g, orally (probenicid causes an increased and prolonged blood level of penicillin)
- ciprofloxacin 500 mg, orally
- ceftriaxone 250 mg, i.m.
- spectinomycin 2 g, i.m.

Drugs suitable for use in pregnancy include ampicillin, amoxycillin, ceftriaxone and spectinomycin.

Patient information

All patients diagnosed with gonorrhoea should be referred to the health adviser for contact tracing. They must be advised to refrain from having sexual intercourse until they have had a test of cure; some clinics do two tests. The National Standards for the Management of Gonorrhoea (1997) state that at least one follow-up test should be performed to establish the treatment has been successful; this is very important to ensure the strain was not penicillin- or multi-resistant. Advice regarding use of barrier methods of contraception should be promoted, as this has been shown to reduce transmission rates (Barlow 1977).

SYPHILIS

Definition

Syphilis is less common than the other STIs in the United Kingdom. It is important to treat syphilis as, untreated, it will become a chronic infection and is potentially fatal.

Syphilis is a bacterial infection, the causative organism is a spirochaete, *Treponema pallidum*. It is mainly

---

Case study: Sarah

Sarah attended the sexual health clinic complaining of pain when passing urine and abdominal pain. She had noticed that she had been bleeding, although her period wasn't due. It had been painful having sex with her partner. She had no other sexual partners, this was her first serious relationship and they had been together for 1 year. Her partner wasn't with her.

A full sexual health check-up was performed. The slides were looked at by the nurse and a diagnosis of gonorrhoea was made. Sarah was deeply shocked by this and burst into tears. The health advisor (HA) was informed and came to talk to her. The HA explained all about gonorrhoea, how it is transmitted and the incubation period (which averages 3–7 days after exposure). The implications were obvious to Sarah – that her partner had been having sex with someone else. This was a double shock for her; she spent a long time discussing this with the HA. The HA also issued Sarah with a contact slip for her sexual contact(s); in Sarah's case this was one contact slip. The information on this would be Sarah's clinic number (as all samples are sent to the laboratory with the patient's clinic number on and date of birth to ensure confidentiality), and the code used for the diagnosis. The codes are universal, so Sarah could take the contact slip to any sexual health clinic in the country and it would be understood.

Once she was feeling more in control, Sarah was given a stat dose of amoxycillin 3 g and probenicid 1 g. She was advised not to have sex until she returned for her test of cure and had been given the all clear.

---

sexually transmitted, but may also be passed vertically – from mother to the unborn child.

Diagnosis

The incubation period is usually 2–4 weeks, after which a painless genital ulcer (chancre) appears. The primary lesion resolves over 3–8 weeks and is followed 6–8 weeks later by secondary syphilis, characterized by a maculopapular rash, lymphadenopathy and mucosal ulcers. All mucosal lesions are potentially infectious and may recur the following year.

The diagnosis is suspected from the history and clinical signs. All genital sores should be investigated carefully to exclude syphilis. *T. pallidum* can be identified on microscopy of serous fluid from ulcers in primary and secondary syphilis, this is looked at using a dark ground microscope. Serological tests are the main way of diagnosing syphilis. The blood is screened using an ELISA method for detecting antitreponemal antibodies, with positive results being confirmed by the traditional Venereal Disease Research Laboratory

(VDRL), *Treponema pallidum* haemagglutination (TPHA) (or *Treponema pallidum* particle analysis (TPPA) and fluorescent *treponemal* antibody (FTA) tests (Scott 1996b). All new patients attending a sexual health clinic are offered a screen for syphilis. In the United Kingdom all pregnant women have a blood test for syphilis when they visit the antenatal clinic.

Primary stage syphilis

The primary stage is when one or more chancre(s) appear at the place where the bacterium entered the body. This can be anywhere on the body but is usually on the vulva, clitoris, urethra, cervix or penis and foreskin; they can also be found around the anus and mouth. The sore is very infectious and may take 2–6 weeks to heal.

Secondary stage syphilis

If the infection remains untreated the secondary stage may occur during the next 2 years. The symptoms include a non-itchy rash covering the whole body or appearing in patches, flat warty-looking growths on the vulva in women and around the anus in both sexes, a flu-like illness, a feeling of tiredness and loss of appetite, accompanied by swollen glands (this can last for weeks or months), white patches on the tongue or the roof of the mouth or patchy hair loss. When these symptoms are present syphilis is very infectious and may be sexually transmitted to a partner.

Latent stage syphilis

The latent stage occurs at any time after the first 2 years. During this time syphilis is rarely transmitted sexually. If left untreated the disease develops gradually, sometimes over many years. It is at the latent stage that syphilis can affect the heart, joints and possibly the nervous system.

Treatment

Treatment at any time during the first two stages of syphilis will cure the infection. If treatment is given during the latent stage the infection can be cured but any damage to the heart or nervous system may be irreversible.

The main treatment of choice for primary and secondary syphilis is benzathine penicillin 2.4 mega units i.m. daily for 10 to 21 days, with 500 mg of probenicid twice daily for the same time. The aim is to maintain a prolonged low concentration of penicillin in the blood.

Alternatively, doxycycline 100 mg twice daily for 15 to 28 days can be used. For treatment of latent syphilis the regime is the longer course. Patients must be informed that it is essential to complete the medical treatment in order to stop asymptomatic disease progression.

There are side-effects of treatment for syphilis using penicillin. The most common reaction is exacerbation of the flu-like symptoms and skin lesions. This is known as the Jarisch–Herxheimer reaction and occurs 3–12 h after the first injection and lasts 12–24 h. The reaction is most commonly seen in treatment of secondary syphilis but can occur in any stage. The patient can be reassured it will not happen with further treatment. In treatment of latent syphilis the reaction can be much more serious and the patient should be monitored closely following initial treatment.

Patient information

All patients must be seen by health advisers for contact tracing; it is important to get their contacts to attend. For primary and secondary syphilis the contacts from the previous 6 months must be traced and examined as soon as possible.

The patient must be advised that during untreated primary and secondary stages of the disease their saliva and vaginal and seminal secretions are infectious.

The follow-up will be according to the clinic protocol. The usual follow-up is 3, 6 and 12 months for early and congenital syphilis to ensure that serology tests (TPHA or TPPA) become negative or reach a very low titre and that there are no physical signs of infection. Secondary syphilis should also have a repeat test 2 years after treatment and anyone with latent syphilis should be followed-up for 5 years.

GENITAL WARTS (HPV)
Definition

Genital warts are caused by genitotropic strains of the human papilloma virus (HPV). Although the risk of HPV acquisition rises with the number of partners, it should be emphasized that prevalence in women with only one lifelong partner is as high as 20%. Transmission of HPV occurs by direct skin-to-skin contact. The incubation period for HPV is very variable and can be anywhere between 3 weeks and 9 months Schneider (1993). HPV enters through breaks in the skin and mucous membranes. The virus can be present in the body without ever causing any clinical symptoms Oriel (1990).

Diagnosis

The diagnosis is made by clinical observation. Application of 5% acetic acid may assist in the differential diagnosis by accentuating the surface appearance of the warts. If there is any doubt about diagnosis it should be resolved by biopsy.

Seventy-three genotypes of HPV have been identified (Bowman 1994), of which more than 30 types can affect the genital tract. Most types identified as genital warts are HPV6 and HPV11, which are associated with benign warts or mild dysplasia. Cervical intraepithelial neoplasia (CIN) has been linked particularly to HPV16 and HPV18 and is present in 80% of invasive squamous carcinomas of the cervix, vulva and penis.

Any part of the male and female genitalia can be affected, although it is more commonly seen on the moister areas and usually starts in areas that are more susceptible to trauma during sexual intercourse (Oriel 1990). Warts can be found around the anus or in the anal canal. When warts are seen around the anus it is important to perform a proctoscopy examination to check whether there are any inside. The cervical transformation zone is particularly important as this is the area where columnar epithelium undergoes a process of metaplasia, developing into squamous epithelium. This area of cellular change at the cervix is thought to make it more vulnerable to viral infection and to neoplastic change.

Treatment

There are various treatments for genital warts.

Podophyllin is a crude resin extract from the roots of different species of Berberidaceae, or may apple. It is generally available in 25% alcohol solution, although some clinics use 10%, 15% or 20%. Podophyllin is an antimitotic agent that acts by destroying keratinocytes and dermal cells and by injuring the microcirculation. Great care must be taken whilst applying podophyllin to the warts as it will cause irritation to the surrounding skin and mucous membrane. The smallest possible swab should be used to apply it. It is applied once to twice weekly by an experienced practitioner and the patient is advised that it should be washed off 4–6 h after application.

Podophyllotoxin is the main constituent of podophyllin. It can be given to the patient to use at home for self-administration. It comes in a solution 0.5% or cream 0.15% and is used twice daily for three sequential days, repeating up to three times at weekly intervals. Response rates at between 4 and 6 weeks are generally in the region of 60–80%, but subsequent lesions are common.

Podophyllin is not a uniform substance. The content of its active component, podophyllotoxin, varies between 2% and 10% and it is relatively unstable in solution (Murphy & Bloom 1991).

Podophyllin should not be used on women who are pregnant or if there is any chance they could become pregnant, as it is an antimitotic agent and has profound effects on tissues with rapid cell division, such as developing fetuses.

Cryotherapy is the treatment of choice for keratanized lesions. Ideally, liquid nitrogen is applied via a cryospray. The wart area is frozen then allowed to defrost before freezing again. This is usually repeated two to three times per visit, depending on protocol. Alternatively, a cryoprobe could be used. This is either nitrous oxide or carbon dioxide. The practitioner selects the appropriate size tip or probe to freeze a ball of lubricating gel, thereby freezing the wart. Enough gel is applied either to the wart itself or the tip of the probe, to ensure an ice ball around the wart. The protocol for the clinic should be followed but it is usual to freeze the wart for approximately 30 s, and then to defrost and repeat this two to three times.

Electrocautery is another treatment and is always performed by a doctor. This involves using a probe through which an electric current runs. The patient is earthed using an electrode plate, which makes the circuit complete, thus allowing the probe to burn away any warty tissue. The patient is given a local anaesthetic. A hand-held cautery can also be used to burn away the tissue. Hyfrecation is another treatment that uses electric current, again using local anaesthetic.

Trichloracetic acid (TCAA) is another solution that must be used with extreme caution and only by experienced practitioners. The TCAA must be applied only to the wart, it must not touch any healthy skin as it will cause a chemical burn to the area and possibly severe destruction of the surrounding tissue. This is a very effective treatment on hyperkeratanized warts.

Patient information

When patients are first diagnosed with genital warts it is important to give clear, concise information regarding the virus. The information about HPV/genital warts is constantly changing with the research that is being carried out and the guidelines regarding yearly and three-yearly smears have also changed. The advice now is that women remain on the 3-year programme unless abnormalities have been detected by the laboratory. The advice and follow-up will be determined by the clinical areas protocol. The woman will usually have had a colposcopy, either in the gynaecology department or the sexual health clinic.

It is important to inform the patient that, like any other virus, HPV will be present for the rest of their lives. The possibility of recurrence is partly dependent on the patient's own immune response. Stress and cigarette smoking will aid in reducing the immune response.

The use of condoms or barrier methods for safer sex is a debatable one. The wart virus is passed on via skin-to-skin contact and it is likely that the only time viral shedding occurs is when warts are present on the surface of the skin or epithelium (Oriel 1990). So, once the warts have been treated successfully, can the patient stop using condoms? Also, as the warts are not always visible, it may not be apparent that one of the partners has the virus. The warts may be flat or invisible on the skin surface, showing up only with acetic acid. Does this mean that partners should always use condoms?

Patients should be told that, currently, only the symptoms can be treated, not the cause. The treatments used are mostly destructive, therefore it is important to advise patients that they may experience discomfort or pain. As most people seek treatment of warts because they feel they are unsightly, the chosen treatment must be performed by an experienced practitioner as not only is it destructive to the warts but it will also destroy the surrounding healthy tissue, causing scarring, although this should go with time.

Patients should be told that several cofactors have been associated with HPV, which may promote its progression. These include the early onset of sexual activity, smoking, other STIs, multiple sexual partners, hormonal changes and poor nutrition.

GENITAL HERPES (HSV)

Definition

Genital herpes is caused by the herpes simplex virus (HSV). There are two types of this virus, either of which can effect the described parts of the body. Type I usually causes sores on the nose or mouth (and occasionally in the eyes), known as cold sores. Type II causes sores in the genital and anal area. Type I is now more commonly seen in the genital and anal area, perhaps because people are having oral sex more often.

As Scoular (1996) described, the classic presentation of primary genital herpes occurs 2–14 days after exposure and is characterized by bilateral genital **macules** and **papules**, followed by **vesicles, pustules, ulceration** and crusting.

The primary infection is likely to cause both men and women to have one or more of the signs and symptoms, such as an itching or tingling sensation in the genital or anal area, small fluid-filled blisters, pain when passing urine, a flu-like illness, backache, headache, swollen glands or fever. The blisters usually burst and leave small sores, which can be very painful. In time these dry out, scab over and heal. With the first infection they can take between 2 and 4 weeks to heal properly. At this time the virus is highly infectious. Recurrent infections are usually milder, the sores are fewer, smaller, less painful and heal more quickly, and there are no flu-like symptoms.

Although the most severe clinical disease is associated with primary genital herpetic infection, the majority of individuals with primary genital herpes can be asymptomatic or minimally symptomatic. They can present with minimal clinical features, such as genital cracks and fissures, mild balanitis or minor vulva lesions, which are easily overlooked.

Diagnosis

The diagnosis can be made on the clinical signs described above but this should always be confirmed with culture of a swab from a vesicle or ulcer, transported in appropriate transport medium to a laboratory with cell culture facilities.

Treatment

The treatment should include analgesia with local care of lesions. Accurate information and supportive counselling are essential elements of care. Antiviral treatments may be prescribed according to local protocol. There is good evidence for the effectiveness of antiviral treatment of initial episodes and suppressive therapy in patients with frequent and/or severe recurrences (Scoular 1996). There is conflicting evidence for the effectiveness of episodic treatment of recurrences and no evidence that suppressive therapy can prevent transmission.

Patient information

When suffering from herpes, patients should be advised to take pain killers, if they have any pain; keep the area as clean and dry as possible; wear loose clothing so air can get to the area; place an ice pack in a clean cloth or towel against the area; avoid sunbathing or using sunbeds; get plenty of rest. If it is difficult to pass urine it may help to try and do so in the bath. They should drink plenty of fluids to help neutralize the urine. If it is still difficult to pass urine they should be advised to contact their GP.

The blisters and sores are highly infectious and the virus can be passed to others by direct contact. The virus affects the areas where it enters the body. The advice given in the Health Education Authority (1997) leaflet is to reduce the risk of passing HSV on by avoiding kissing when either person has cold sores around the mouth, avoiding oral sex when either person has mouth or genital sores and avoiding any genital or anal contact, even with a condom or dental dam, when either person has genital sores. (A condom will only protect against herpes if it covers all the blisters. Herpes can also be transmitted by non-penetrative sex.) It is important not to share towels or face flannels and always to wash hands with soap after touching sores.

The virus is also present and can be shed prior to the blisters appearing. This makes it difficult to give exact advice to avoid sex because the patient may not have any signs or symptoms before the blisters appear. Asymptomatic shedding is a major health education/promotion issue.

Herpes and pregnancy

Herpes does not affect a woman's ability to become pregnant. If the primary infection occurs in the first 3 months of the pregnancy there is a small risk of miscarriage, however most women who have several episodes of herpes during pregnancy have a normal delivery. If the woman has herpes around the expected delivery date they may be advised to have a caesarean delivery to reduce the risk of infecting the baby.

SCABIES
Definition

Scabies is caused by a small mite, *Sarcoptes scabiei*, that spreads from person to person through close physical contact. The female mite is about twice the size (0.3 mm long) of the male and can just be seen by the naked eye as a black dot. Infestation occurs by close physical contact, not necessarily sexual. The symptoms are usually noticed 2–6 weeks after infestation. The patient complains of itching, which is often unbearable, intractable and worse at night when the body is warm. The symptoms are caused by the female burrowing into the uppermost layer of the skin (stratum corneum), laying eggs and defecating. The sites of itching and burrows bear no relation to the mode of transmission. Lesions may be found in the clefts of fingers and on the wrists and elbows as well as on the genitals.

Diagnosis

This is usually based on the clinical history and by physical examination and may be confirmed by finding the mite. A skin flake may be taken from one of the spots and examined under the microscope to look for evidence of mites.

Treatment

The usual treatment is with malathion 0.5% applied to all body surfaces, especially in between fingers and toes. It is not applied to the face and it is washed off after 24 h.

Patient information

Patients should be told to wash all clothing and bed linen after the treatment has been given. They should also be informed that the itching may persist for several weeks, despite successful treatment. Unless they know this, they may well think they have been reinfected and retreat themselves, running the risk of chemical dermatitis.

PUBIC LICE
Definition

Pediculosis pubis is caused by the pubic louse, *Phthirus pubis*, which is a different species from that causing head and body louse infestation. The insect is small and round (1–2 mm long) and has three sets of legs. The adult adheres not only to the pubic hair but also to other hairy areas (perineum, thighs, abdomen, axillas, eyebrows and eyelashes). It is a blood sucker. The female lays eggs at the base of the hairs and these usually hatch within 7 days. The adult louse is transferred from person to person during close physical contact. As lice do not leave the host, the condition is not spread by wearing or sleeping in infested clothing or sheets.

Diagnosis

This is usually based on clinical appearances alone. Bluish-grey macules occasionally occur on the abdomen, buttocks or thighs at the sites of bites. As the condition is usually acquired through sexual contact, a full sexual history and check-up is essential.

Treatment

The usual treatment is 0.5% malathion. This should be applied to all the hairy areas apart from the scalp. It should be left on for 24 h, after which the patients should wash it off. One application is usually sufficient but, if necessary, another application can be given within 7–10 days of the initial treatment.

Patient information

There is no need for patients to wash their clothes or bedclothes as the louse does not leave the host. Sexual partners should be seen and treated. Shaving of body hair is not necessary.

MOLLUSCUM CONTAGIOSUM
Definition

Molluscum contagiosum may be transmitted sexually but this is not the only route. It is a contagious viral condition that may be spread by close bodily contact, clothing or towels. The agent causing molluscum contagiosum is one of the pox viruses and has a variable incubation period of 2–12 weeks.

Diagnosis

Diagnosis is usually based on clinical appearance, as the virus cannot be grown successfully. The lesions are characteristic. The pearly white **umbilicated** papules appear in the genital area (penis, scrotum, vulva, perineum, abdomen and thighs). If transmission is not sexual they may also be found on any part of the body but particularly on the arms, face, eyelids and scalp.

Treatment

Cryotherapy is used to freeze the papules. Phenol can be used, applying it to the centre of the umbilicated core of the lesions with a sharpened orange stick.

Patient Information

Patients should be advised not to use other people's towels or to try-on other people's clothes, as these are vehicles for spreading molluscum contagiosum. They should avoid close physical contact until they are certain treatment has been successful.

CONCLUSION

Sexual health is a very important issue. As nurses it is our duty to have an understanding of sexual health and a clear idea of what an important part of the holistic care it comprises. Most adults will be in, or will have had, a sexual relationship, therefore when they access healthcare this will be an important aspect of their care. It is also important to recognize that people do not all have sex in the same way and with the opposite sex. Never use closed questions, allow women to feel comfortable and safe to express their sexual health needs without fear of judgement. If a woman discloses something about herself that you do not fully understand, ask someone to explain, never show surprise or disgust.

It is equally important for nurses to be aware of STIs and how they can manifest. This is very true in a gynaecological setting, as women's symptoms can be a reason for accessing the service. While women are being cared for in a gynaecological area, the healthcare professionals can also educate women about STIs and about the importance of having regular sexual health check-ups. This is the ideal time for health promotion and education about safer sex.

STIs are very common. Any woman having sexual intercourse without using a barrier method is at risk of acquiring an STI. Even with barrier methods, some STIs can be passed on. Having sex with another person can mean that you are also having sex with the other people they have had sex with, and with the people they have had sex with and it could go on and on. That is the reason we need to educate and promote sexual health check-ups. That is the reason, as nurses, we need to be aware and up to date with information about STIs and sexual health as a whole.

GLOSSARY

Macule: a discoloured spot, not raised above the skin's surface
Papule: a small, circumscribed elevation of the skin
Phagocytosis: the engulfment by phagocytes of foreign or other particles, or cells harmful to the body
Polymorphonuclear: having a many-shaped or lobulated nucleus, usually applied to the phagocytic neutrophil leucocytes (granulocytes) which constitute 70% of the total white blood cells

Protozoan: protozoa are the smallest and simplest creatures that can be called animals. They form a diverse group with the common characteristic that their bodies are not divided into separate functional units or cells
Pustule: a small, inflammatory swelling containing pus
Ulceration: an open sore in a body surface
Umbilicated: having a central depression
Vesicle: a small bladder, cell or hollow structure; a skin blister

REFERENCES

Adler MW (ed) 1995 ABC of sexually transmitted infections, 3rd edn. BMJ Publishing Group, London
Amsel R, Totten PA, Spiegel CA, Chen KCS, Eschenbach D, Holmes KK 1983 Non-specific vaginitis: diagnostic criteria and microbial and epidemiological associations. The American Journal of Medicine 74:14–22
Barlow D 1977 The condom and gonorrhoea. Lancet October 15:811–813
Bowman C 1994 Perspectives on HPV. British Journal of Sexual Medicine May/June:24–25
Conway M, Humphries E 1994 Bernhard Clinic, meeting the need in lesbian sexual health care. Nursing Times 90(32):40–41
Csonka GW 1990 Trichomonas vaginalis infestation. In: Csonka GW, Oates JK (eds) Sexually transmitted diseases – a textbook of genitourinary medicine. Baillière Tindall, London

Dawson S 1990 Bacterial vaginosis. In: Csonka GW, Oates JK (eds) Sexually transmitted diseases – a textbook of genitourinary medicine. Baillière Tindall, London
Fagan B 1996 Candidiasis. In: Sutton A, Payne S (eds) Genito-urinary medicine for nurses. Whurr Publishers Ltd, London
Gardner HL, Dukes CD 1955 Haemophilus Vaginalis Vaginitis, American Journal of Obstetrics and Gynaecology 69(5): 962–976
Health Education Authority 1997 Patient information leaflet, genital herpes (HSV)
Heine P, McGregor JA 1993 Trichomonas vaginalis: a re-emerging pathogen. Clinical Obstetrics & Gynaecology 36(1):137–144
Hopkins SJ 1992 Drugs and pharmacology for nurses, 11th edn. Churchill Livingstone, Edinburgh

McGlynn C 1996 Bacterial vaginosis. In: Sutton A, Payne S (eds) Genito-urinary medicine for nurses. Whurr Publishers Ltd, London

Murphy M, Bloom GD 1991 Podophyllin or podophyllotoxin as treatment for condylomata acuminata? Papillomavirus Report 2(4):87–89

Nicholas H 1998 Gonorrhoea: symptoms and treatment. Nursing Times 94(8): pp. 52–54

National Standards for the Managment of Gonorrhoea. In: The International Journal of STD + AIDS 1997 7:298–300

Nugent RP, Krohn MA, Hillier SL 1991 Reliability of diagnosing bacterial vaginosis is improved by a standardized method of Gram stain interpretation, Journal of Clinical Microbiology 29:297–301

Oriel D 1990 Genital human papilloma virus infections. In: Holmes KK, Mardh P-A, Sparling PF, Wiesner PJ (eds) Sexually transmitted diseases, 2nd edn. Churchill Livingstone, Edinburgh.

Phillips M 1996 Trichomoniasis. In: Sutton A, Payne S (eds) Genito-urinary medicine for nurses. Whurr Publishers Ltd, London

Rein MF 1990 Vulvovaginitis and cervicitis. In Bennett JE (ed) Principles and practice of infectious diseases, 3rd edn. Churchill Livingstone, New York

Schneider A 1993 Pathogenesis of genital HPV infection. Genito-urinary Medicine 69:165–173

Scott G 1996a Gonorrhoea. In: Prescriber guide: sexually transmitted diseases. A & M Publishing, Guildford

Scott G 1996b Syphilis. In: Prescriber guide: sexually transmitted diseases. A & M Publishing, Guildford

Scoular A 1996 Genital herpes. In: Prescriber guide: sexually transmitted diseases. A & M Publishing, Guildford

Sherrard JS, Bingham JS 1995 Gonorrhoea now. International Journal of STD & AIDS 6(3):162–166

Turner P, Richens A 1978 Clinical pharmacology, 3rd edn. Churchill Livingstone, Edinburgh

WHO 1991 In: The International Journal of STD + AIDS 1997 7:298–300

Wooley P 1994 Diagnosis and management of vaginal infections, Part 2. British Journal of Sexual Medicine, May/June:16–18

FURTHER READING

Adler MW (ed) 1995 ABC of sexually transmitted infections, 3rd edn. BMJ Publishing Group, London

Andrews G (ed) 1997 Women's sexual health. Baillière Tindall, London

Curtis H, Hoolaghan T, Jewitt C (eds) 1995 Sexual health promotion in general practice. Radcliffe Medical Press, Oxford

Knox H 1995 Sexplained, the uncensored guide to sexual health. Knox Publishing, London

Phillips A, Rakusen J 1989 The new our bodies, ourselves, a health book by women for women. Penguin, Harmondsworth

Savage J 1987 Nurses, gender and sexuality. Heinemann Nursing, London

Sutton A, Payne S (eds) 1996 Genito-urinary medicine for nurses. Whurr Publishers Ltd, London

USEFUL ADDRESSES

The Herpes Association
41 North Road, London N7 9DP
Tel: 020 7609 9061
Offers support to herpes sufferers and provides information sheets.
Health Education Authority
Hamilton House, Mabledon Place, London WC1H 9TX
Tel: 020 7383 3833

Provides a wide range of information for professionals, including leaflets and posters.
Women and Health
4 Carol Street, London NW1 0HU
Women's Health Concern
PO Box 1629, Earls Court, London W8

5

Early pregnancy disorders

Miscarriage and early pregnancy units
Angela Whitton
Ectopic pregnancy
Lindsey Mitchem
Termination of pregnancy
Rosemary Nicholl

MISCARRIAGE AND EARLY PREGNANCY UNITS

Women experiencing early pregnancy loss or undergoing a termination of pregnancy account for a significant percentage of patients cared for by gynaecological nurses or nurses involved in the area of women's health. In recent years there have been major developments in the management and treatment of these conditions. Greater emphasis is now placed on the psychological care of the women and their partners and the role of the nurse has played a major part in these changes and the care that is given.

SPONTANEOUS MISCARRIAGE
Definition and incidence

A miscarriage is defined as a pregnancy that ends spontaneously before 24 weeks gestation. The World Health Organization (WHO) defines miscarriage as the expulsion of an embryo or fetus weighing 500 g or less. This weight corresponds to approximately 22 weeks gestation. The terms miscarriage and abortion are synonymous. The latter term, often used by professionals to denote the spontaneous loss of a pregnancy, can cause unnecessary distress to a woman who only knows the term as meaning an induced legal termination of pregnancy, so if the term is used in her presence then it should always be clarified. A study group from the Royal College of Obstetricians and Gynaecologists (RCOG), considering problems in early pregnancy, recently recommended that the term abortion when used regarding early pregnancy loss

should be replaced. The changes in terminology that the group recommended are:
- spontaneous abortion should be replaced by spontaneous miscarriage

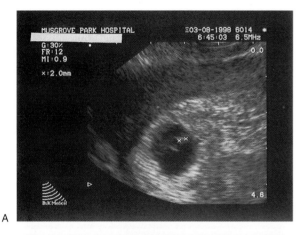

A

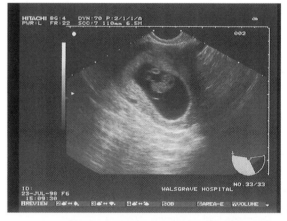

B

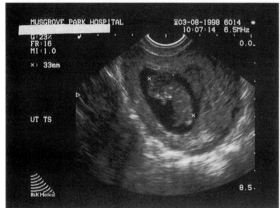

C

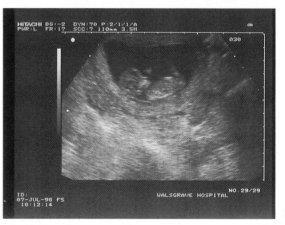

D

E

Figure 5.1 Pictures A–E show stages of early intrauterine fetal development 6–13 weeks
A/ 6 weeks gestation
B/ 8 weeks gestation with yolk sac clearly visible
C/ 10 weeks gestation
D/ 11 weeks gestation
E/ 13 weeks gestation

- missed abortion should be replaced by early fetal demise or missed miscarriage
- incomplete abortion should be replaced by incomplete miscarriage.

Approximately 20% of all pregnancies end in miscarriage, most in the first trimester, but this figure represents only the tip of the iceberg of reproductive loss; many more pregnancies are lost before pregnancy is diagnosed. The introduction of pregnancy test kits, which detect implantation before the first period is missed, suggests that the rate of subclinical pregnancy loss is 50–60%.

As many as 25% of women will experience a miscarriage at some stage during their reproductive years. Up to 50% of fertilized eggs will not implant in the uterus and 30% of those that do implant are lost before 7 weeks gestation (Girling & De Swiet 1996). Fig 5.1 shows the normal stages of fetal development from 6 weeks to 13 weeks gestation.

Types of miscarriage

There are several types of miscarriage, each with its distinctive pattern of presentation (Table 5.1). The diagnosis may not be clear until all the test results are available, and even then they may have to be repeated a week later to ensure a definite diagnosis. Any couple encountering such a wait require additional support and contact during this anxious time.

Threatened miscarriage

There are an estimated 700 000 threatened miscarriages in England and Wales each year, 50–75% of women experiencing them go on to full term with no increased risk of fetal abnormality (Allan 1995). However, once a fetal heart has been visualized, the risk of miscarriage is greatly reduced. In up to 98% of pregnancies that are threatening to miscarry, once a fetal heart has been visualized the pregnancy will proceed

Table 5.1 Presentation of different types of miscarriage

Type	Bleeding	Pain	Cervix	Uterus
Threatened	Slight Intermittent	None/mild	Closed	Enlarged Equal to dates
Inevitable	Heavy, often with clots	Cramping, intermittent period-like pains (uterine contractions)	Open	Enlarged
Incomplete	Heavy with clots and possible products of conception	As above	Open	May be smaller than gestational age
Complete	Previous heavy bleeding, patient presents with little bleeding or slight discharge	None, although will complain of severe abdominal cramps	Closed	Returned to non-pregnant size
Blighted ovum (anembryonic pregnancy)	Slight brownish loss	None	Closed	Smaller than gestational dates
Early fetal demise	Brownish discharge	Non-specific	Closed	Smaller than gestational dates
Hydatidiform mole	Brownish discharge	Non-specific	Closed	Larger than gestational dates, may palpate soft as no fetal parts
Septic	Heavy	Abdominal pain with pyrexia	Open/closed	Very tender on examination

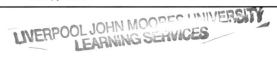

normally (Stabile et al 1987). The later the heart is seen beating, the lower the subsequent miscarriage rate.

When a woman presents with a threatened miscarriage she will complain of slight intermittent vaginal bleeding and/or mild abdominal pain after a spell of amenorrhoea. To make a diagnosis of threatened miscarriage it has to be confirmed that the woman is pregnant (as there are other causes of amenorrhoea), established that the bleeding is coming from inside the uterus (as there may be bleeding from a cervical erosion) and confirmed that any pain experienced is slight and the cervical os is closed.

On vaginal examination, fresh or altered blood may be found in the vagina, the cervix is closed and the uterus is enlarged to approximate gestational size. There is no evidence to suggest that a vaginal examination affects the outcome of the pregnancy but caution may be indicated in some cases.

In a threatened miscarriage there is bleeding into the choriodecidual space but this is not sufficient to kill the embryo. Some women bleed slightly at the time of the first missed period when the embryo is implanting into the endometrium, this is called an implantation haemorrhage. It may be difficult to distinguish this type of bleeding from a threatened miscarriage, but in the former the bleeding is slight, fresh and settles quickly.

There is no evidence to show that bedrest or refraining from intercourse improves the outcome of a threatened miscarriage, however, if a woman wishes to 'do something' then these measures can be suggested.

Inevitable miscarriage

A threatened miscarriage becomes inevitable when the bleeding becomes heavier and abdominal pains become rhythmic and strong as the uterus begins to contract. On examination the cervical os is dilated and products of conception (POC) may be felt. The process of miscarriage at this stage may be complete or incomplete. With an inevitable miscarriage there is always the risk of shock and haemorrhage and, as such, urgent medical treatment is normally required.

Unfortunately, once the cervix has begun to dilate there is no treatment available at present to prevent the miscarriage proceeding, so the main objective is to provide a quick and accurate diagnosis and provide treatment as necessary.

Complete miscarriage

A complete miscarriage is one in which all the POC have been expelled from the uterus. The woman may

---

Case study: Janet

Janet and Mark are in their mid thirties; Janet is presently 18 weeks pregnant with their first child. She contacts her midwife after experiencing a bright red vaginal loss for 3 hours with intermittent abdominal pain. Janet is admitted immediately to the gynaecology ward with a diagnosis of a threatened miscarriage. Mark accompanies her to the hospital; they are both extremely anxious on admission and require a lot of reassurance. On vaginal examination the cervical os is open and bleeding is heavy; it is sensitively explained to Janet and Mark that they will inevitably miscarry the baby within the next few hours. A suitably qualified nurse is allocated to care for Janet and Mark and she explains what they can expect. The miscarriage nurse (MN) for the unit is also involved in their care and offers support, advice and information.

Over the next 2 hours Janet's pain increases and she is given suitable analgesia; she spontaneously delivers the baby followed by the placenta, which is assessed as being complete. Janet and Mark are given the opportunity to see and hold the baby and photographs are taken. They spend several hours alone with their baby and eventually feel able to 'let go' and allow it to be taken to the mortuary.

The bleeding settles and the following day Janet is assessed as physically fit for discharge. Investigations into the cause of the miscarriage are discussed; Janet and Mark refuse a post-mortem but consent to other investigations as appropriate. Janet is prescribed medication to prevent her producing milk as she feels this will be a painful reminder. They are visited by the hospital chaplaincy to discuss the disposal of the baby. Information is given on what is available and Janet and Mark wish to have time to decide, so the chaplain will contact them at home.

The MN ensures that all documentation has been completed, a follow-up appointment is made and that suitable written information is offered. She also confirms that Janet and Mark are aware of the Baby Book of Remembrance, local support groups and have her contact number. Janet's GP and community midwife are informed of the outcome.

A week after discharge the MN makes contact. Janet and Mark are struggling to accept their loss; a home visit is arranged for the next day. Contact is maintained over the next 3 months between the MN and Janet and Mark until they feel able to cope; they are both aware they can ring again in the future.

---

complain of previous heavy bleeding associated with severe abdominal pain, both of which have subsequently settled. She may also claim that she has passed 'something', which, if saved for examination, will be found to be the whole of the conceptus.

On examination the cervical os is closed and the uterus is non-tender, firm and palpates smaller than gestational age as it returns to its non-pregnant size.

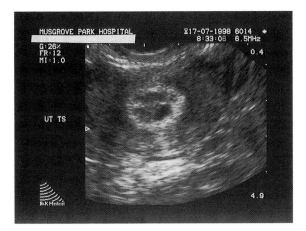

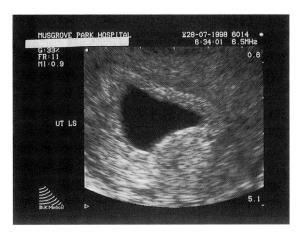

Figure 5.2   Retained products of conception; patient was 7 weeks pregnant by LMP.

Figure 5.3   Anembryonic pregnancy, mean sac diameter 20 mm, no fetal pole or yolk sac seen.

No treatment is necessary if a diagnosis of complete miscarriage is made. Any further bleeding should be light and settle within a few days, if not then further medical advice should be taken with the possibility of retained products of conception or infection to be investigated.

Incomplete miscarriage

As the name suggests, an incomplete miscarriage is one in which only part of the POC have been passed, usually the embryo, with the placenta being retained (Fig 5.2). Vaginal bleeding may be heavy, with painful uterine contractions. It is possible for a woman to bleed so severely that within a few hours her haemaglobin level drops to as low as 6 g/100 ml. In many cases intramuscular analgesia is required, with an antiemetic and possibly a blood transfusion. Surgery is often essential to stop the blood loss; once an evacuation of the uterus has been performed then bleeding settles immediately.

Blighted ovum (anembryonic pregnancy or early embryonic)

Also known as an anembryonic or early embryonic pregnancy, this occurs when the gestation sac develops in the absence of an embryo. Microscopic studies have shown that imperfect sperm are still able to fertilize a normal or defective ovum, which results in a blighted ovum. This is unable to develop or implant correctly and consequently the pregnancy results in a miscarriage.

The diagnosis is made by performing an ultrasound scan, often vaginally, which shows a gestation sac with a mean diameter of at least 20 mm and no evidence of an embryo or a yolk sac (Fig 5.3). This condition is commonly discovered at a routine early scan and therefore comes as a shock to the woman who has had no obvious signs that anything has gone wrong with the pregnancy. There is no urgency for treatment and if none is given then the woman will eventually spontaneously abort the sac. This condition is unlikely to reoccur in future pregnancies, so reassurance can be given to women with this diagnosis.

Missed miscarriage (early fetal demise)

A missed miscarriage occurs when there is retention of the fetus after death has occurred. On scan the **crown–rump length** (CRL) must be more than 6 mm on trans-vaginal scan to confirm that no fetal heart can be seen (Fig 5.4), any fetal pole below this measurement must be rescanned at least 1 week later to confirm the diagnosis, as per the recommendations following the Glamorgan Inquiry (Hately et al 1995).

If the embryo dies in the early weeks of pregnancy then bleeding occurs between the chorionic villi and the uterine wall, which can result in the formation of a carneous mole. If death occurs in the later stages of pregnancy, after about 18 weeks, then the dead fetus becomes mummified and is macerated by the time it is eventually passed; the gestation sac can be retained in the uterus for several weeks or months if left untreated. It is still unknown why the uterus does not expel the fetus at the time death occurs.

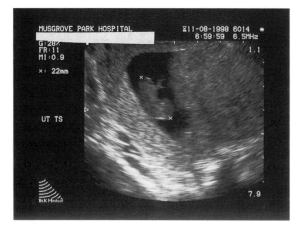

Figure 5.4 Fetal demise, CRL 22 mm, no fetal heart visible on scan.

The woman may notice a small amount of brown discharge for a couple of days between 8 and 12 weeks gestation. She may also complain that the signs and symptoms of pregnancy have disappeared or she may realize this in hindsight. On examination, the uterus feels smaller than gestational dates. The immunological test for pregnancy, which detects the presence of the hormone **human chorionic gonadatrophin (hCG)**, remains positive for as long as placental tissue survives; eventually all the trophoblastic tissue dies or is expelled and the test becomes negative.

Once the diagnosis of fetal demise has been made there is no urgency for treatment, spontaneous expulsion may occur without intervention, but many women feel distressed at the thought of carrying a dead fetus around. The treatment options are discussed later in this chapter. Early fetal demise and anembryonic pregnancy are possibly at opposite ends of the same spectrum (Girling & De Swiet 1996). On close examination of many pregnancies diagnosed as anembryonic, professionals think that an embryo is initially present but is absorbed after development stopped, whereas in a case of early fetal demise, death is diagnosed before reabsorption or miscarriage take place.

Hydatidiform mole (molar pregnancy)

Hydatidiform mole is an uncommon abnormal form of pregnancy where the trophoblastic tissue develops abnormally; over 90% of women who are diagnosed have no further trouble from it once it has been removed (Crawford & Pettit 1986). In the remainder,

Case study: Lisa

Lisa, who is 26 years old, presents to her GP with a 10-week history of amenorrhoea and complaining of abdominal pain and slight brown PV loss over the last 48 hours. This is her fourth pregnancy, she has two children aged two and four; she terminated her first pregnancy. The GP arranges an appointment in the local EPAU. On arrival a history is taken, ultrasound scan performed and bloods taken for FBC and blood group. The trans-vaginal scan shows an intrauterine gestation sac containing a fetus measuring 10 mm but no fetal heart, the cervix is closed; a diagnosis of fetal demise is confirmed by two qualified members of staff.

The scan results and possible treatment options are explained. Lisa is given the opportunity to go home and discuss it with her husband, but she chooses surgery. She feels that this is the best option for her as the thought of walking around with a dead baby inside for longer than necessary causes her great distress; she also has the opportunity to arrange childcare.

Arrangements are made for an EVAC to be performed on a routine operating list the next day. Suitable advice is given regarding preparation for theatre and what to do if the bleeding increases.

The operation is uneventful and the POC are sent to histology. Lisa recovers quickly and is soon ready for discharge home. She is given appropriate advice regarding bleeding, pain, resuming normal activities and future pregnancies; this is written as well as verbal. Contact numbers are given for counsellors and support groups.

A few days following discharge Lisa is contacted at home by a member of nursing staff to ensure that her and her family are coping. Lisa says she is feeling tearful, has lost her appetite and is having difficulty sleeping; she is reassured that this is normal. Lisa feels she has adequate support from family and friends, she has contacted the local support group and will be attending their next meeting as she feels it will help to talk to others who have experienced a similar loss.

treatment is vital to prevent further complications. If the abnormal tissue continues to proliferate then perforation of the uterus may occur, leading to severe haemorrhage. If this happens then an emergency hysterectomy has to be performed, with the resultant loss of fertility, otherwise the outcome is fatal. In about 3% of those patients diagnosed with a molar pregnancy the mole undergoes malignant changes resulting in choriocarcinoma.

Hydatidiform mole is a special form of chromosomal disorder in which abnormal proliferation of the trophoblast is followed by hydropic degeneration of the chorionic villi. In the case of a complete mole all the villi are involved and no fetus is present.

A partial mole contains a fetus/embryo that has three sets of chromosomes, they are more common than complete moles and usually mimic the appearance of an inevitable or complete miscarriage. As with other genetic abnormalities there is a higher incidence of molar pregnancies in conceptions that occur in women at both extremes of their childbearing years. The incidence in the UK is about 1 in 3000 pregnancies, but there are geographical variations across the world; in Asia the incidence is reported to be as high as 1 in 100 pregnancies. This may be due to their extended childbearing period.

The diagnosis of a hydatidiform mole is often made early in the pregnancy (Box 5.1), there may be some vaginal bleeding or the woman may visit her GP complaining of **hyperemesis gravidarum** as a result of the excessive amount of hCG excreted by the abnormal tissue. The molar tissue may abort spontaneously or it may be detected on ultrasound scan where it has a typical 'bunch of grapes' appearance.

Treatment is surgical evacuation and the specimen is sent for histological examination to confirm the diagnosis. As it is rare for most units to diagnose more than a handful of molar pregnancies each year it is national policy that follow-up is provided in three main centres: Charing Cross Hospital, London; Western Park Hospital, Sheffield; and Ninewells Hospital, Dundee. These centres follow the patient's progress by monitoring the levels of hCG in blood and urine samples taken at regular intervals (Box 5.2). These levels are measured as it has been found to be the most reliable method of determining how much trophoblastic tissue has been retained.

Choriocarcinoma is a curable form of cancer, the aim of the treatment when dealing with women of childbearing age is to eradicate all invasive tissue, thus pre-

---

Box 5.1 Diagnostic criteria for hydatidiform mole

- Uterus palpates larger than gestational dates in about 70% of cases.
- Uterus may feel soft if no fetal parts are felt. Fetal heart cannot be heard.
- Blood and urine hCG levels are raised. In normal pregnancy the levels peak between 60 and 90 days then fall.
- Hypertension and/or proteinuria in about 20% of cases. The larger the uterus the greater the possibility of this.
- Hyperthyroidism may occur but resolves following treatment of the mole.

Box 5.2 Patterns looked for in follow-up to molar pregnancy

- Very high levels 24 hours postsurgical evacuation of the uterus.
- Levels over 20 000 iu/litre of hCG 4 weeks postevacuation.

Both the above suggest residual molar tissue invading the uterus with the risk of severe haemorrhage or uterine perforation.

- Failure of hCG level to return to normal after 6 months.
- A rising hCG level or one that is not falling after 4 months.

Both the above suggest malignant changes.
(Source: Crawford & Pettit 1986).

---

venting neoplastic spread and haemorrhage whilst avoiding hysterectomy and the resultant loss of fertility. In the 1950s it was found that choriocarcinoma responded effectively to treatment with methotrexate, an antimetabolite of folic acid, which destroys rapidly dividing cells. If the disease is more extensive, then methotrexate is combined with other chemotherapeutic drugs. It is important to remember that women requiring such treatment are young, possibly with other children and may wish to have another child in the future, so there are many complex psychological and practical issues to address. On completion of the treatment more than 80% of women proceed to have a normal healthy pregnancy, although they are advised to avoid conceiving for at least a year as methotrexate remains in the body for several months and may cause genetic damage to the fetus. The issue of contraception during this time appears to evoke conflicting advice. Crawford & Pettit (1986) state that hormones taken by the patient following a molar pregnancy substantially increase the possibility of the need for treatment, therefore women should be advised to use a barrier method of contraception rather than the pill until their hCG levels have returned to normal. Alternatively, Llewellyn-Jones (1990) advises that patients may be prescribed oral contraceptives as there is no evidence that they cause residual disease to persist. There is no conclusive evidence available to confirm or contradict either opinion.

Septic miscarriage

A septic miscarriage normally arises as a complication of an incomplete miscarriage or a therapeutic abortion performed by an unskilled person or under non-sterile conditions. Septic miscarriage is becoming less common as more countries liberalize their laws on legal termination of pregnancy and there is a drastic reduction in the number of illegal abortions.

The woman presents with heavy vaginal bleeding accompanied by a pyrexia greater than 38°C and tachycardia. She may also complain of general malaise, abdominal pain and may have marked pelvic tenderness. The infection is mild in 80% of cases and localized to the decidua, but in 15% of cases it can spread to the myometrium and beyond. In the remaining 5% there is the risk of endotoxin shock and disseminating intravascular coagulation. The degree of pyrexia is not always related to the severity of the infection, although a pulse rate of higher than 120 beats per minute often indicates spread of the infection beyond the uterus.

The most common organisms involved in cases of septic miscarriage are *Escherichia coli* and other Gram-negative organisms that cause endotoxin shock. Initially, vaginal swabs are taken to isolate the organism and broad-spectrum antibiotic treatment commenced. Once the results of the culture and sensitivity are known then the treatment may be reviewed.

Most cases will require the uterus to be evacuated but, unless the bleeding is severe, this should be delayed for at least 12 hours to allow reasonable tissue levels of antibiotics to be achieved. However, in many cases the amount of bleeding is such that evacuation of the uterus cannot be deferred. Early evacuation reduces the risk of haemorrhage and removes necrotic tissue, which can act as a culture medium. In about 3–5% of all cases of septic abortion endotoxin shock occurs. This has a mortality rate of 30–50%.

Aetiology of sporadic miscarriage

The aetiology of sporadic miscarriage can be divided into various categories. Despite a long list of causative factors, in many cases the cause of a particular miscarriage is often indeterminable. Early miscarriages, up to 12 weeks gestation, occur mainly due to defects in the conceptus, after this time maternal factors become more common and the fetus can be born apparently normal but too immature to survive.

Chromosomal imbalance caused by the absence or duplication of genetic material possibly accounts for up to 60% of all sporadic miscarriages. However, this is probably an underestimate in light of recent improvements in tissue culture techniques (Wolf & Horger 1995). Numerical abnormalities (aneuploidies) are the most common genetic cause of spontaneous miscarriage and are either the presence of an extra chromosome (trisomy), or a missing chromosome (monosomy), resulting from segregation errors during cell division. Down's syndrome is an example of a trisomy, where there are three copies of chromosome number 21 instead of two, and Turner's syndrome is a monosomy, where there is only one X chromosome. Aneuploidies are sporadic and do not usually recur in subsequent pregnancies; parental chromosomes are usually normal. Chromosomal examination of the fetal tissue is performed only if the woman has a recurrent problem or it is specifically indicated, but estimates show that these abnormalities are incompatible with life. Unfortunately, increasing maternal age results in a greater risk of chromosomal abnormality and consequently an increased possibility of miscarriage.

The hormones involved in the continuation of pregnancy are oestrogen, progesterone and hCG but specifically it is the level of progesterone that appears to be of particular importance. Progesterone is secreted by the corpus luteum until about the 11th week of pregnancy, when the placenta is sufficiently developed to take over production of the hormone. One cause of sporadic miscarriage was thought to be when this change-over took place but more recent thinking believes that low levels of progesterone are as a result of the miscarriage rather than a cause. Consequently treatment with progesterone, once a pregnancy is established, is unlikely to avoid miscarriage. The possibility that its use is linked with an increased rate of congenital abnormalities has been suggested (Enkin et al 1995).

Diabetes and hyperthyroidism were previously associated with increased risks of spontaneous miscarriage, this is only the case if the problem remains undiagnosed or is not adequately controlled and is more likely to result in infertility than in miscarriage.

Viral infections in pregnancy are common and in the majority of cases there is no adverse effect on the pregnancy unless there is severe maternal illness. However, some viruses may cross the placenta and affect the fetus directly. These include listeria and toxoplasmosis, the former may be asymptomatic or may present as a mild flu-like illness associated with abdominal pain and diarrhoea, which can lead to late miscarriage, and the latter is contracted from cat faeces and can cause miscarriage only when the primary infection is acquired during pregnancy, thus pregnant women are advised to avoid contact with cat excreta. Other infections that can cause sporadic miscarriage include rubella, cytomegalovirus, genital herpes (first infection), parvovirus, severe influenza, malaria and any acute pyrexial illness or condition causing peritonitis.

Maternal age is thought to have some bearing on the risk of miscarriage, but only over the age of 35 years where there is an increased loss of both normal and abnormal fetuses. Between the ages of 35 and 39 years the risk increases to 21%, over the age of 42 years it increases to > 42% (Knudsen et al 1991).

There have been some positive links between cigarette smoking and miscarriage independent of maternal age or alcohol consumption (Kline et al 1980) and there is conflicting evidence on excessive alcohol consumption and an increased risk of miscarriage. The results of a National Lottery funded research project with the London School of Hygiene and Tropical Medicine on factors such as caffeine, alcohol, smoking, air travel, stress and occupation are eagerly awaited to hopefully give us more information as to possible causes of miscarriage. It has now been shown that the use of visual display units whilst pregnant does not increase the possibility of pregnancy loss (Parazzini et al 1993).

Women need to be reassured that the use of oral contraceptives or a previous uncomplicated termination of pregnancy does not confer any additional risk of miscarriage. Women who have previously undergone an abortion often feel very guilty and blame themselves if they subsequently miscarry a wanted pregnancy. These women require a lot of support and reassurance.

MANAGEMENT OF MISCARRIAGE

There are three possible methods of managing miscarriage; wherever possible a choice of treatment should be given to the patient unless surgery is necessary for a suspected ectopic pregnancy, to evacuate a molar pregnancy, if there is severe haemorrhage or where medical treatment is contraindicated.

Surgical management

Since the 1930s surgical evacuation of the uterus (ERPC or EVAC) under general anaesthetic has been the unquestionable treatment for first trimester miscarriage, in fact many women expect to go to theatre and are surprised when offered a choice. With this method there is the potential for surgical, anaesthetic, haemorrhagic or infective complications (Girling & De Swiet 1996) although it is the method of choice when bleeding is heavy. An opportunity is provided in theatre to obtain fetal tissue for further investigation and the whole procedure is dealt with in a limited time span, although there is often the disadvantage of a long wait for theatre time. A surgical evacuation involves the dilatation of the cervix and gentle removal of the contents of the uterus with a curette or a small suction catheter, it can be performed under local or spinal anaesthetic but most are performed under general anaesthetic.

Medical management

Over recent years, non-surgical methods of treating miscarriage have been investigated and in trials complete uterine evacuation has been achieved in 95% of early miscarriages (El-Refaey et al 1992, Henshaw et al 1993). Medical management involves a combination of the antiprogesterone mifepristone (RU486, Mifegyne) and a prostaglandin E, either vaginally (Gemeprost) or orally (Misoprostol, Cytotec). This form of management is less invasive and eliminates surgical and anaesthetic risks with possible financial savings to be made (Hughes et al 1996). The main drawback of this treatment is the duration, which can be up to 72 hours, and the fact that it is often difficult to obtain fetal tissue for further investigations.

The management of second trimester intrauterine death (IUD) and termination is usually medical as few units now have the surgical expertise to complete these procedures safely by dilatation and evacuation. The same combination of drugs are given which shorten the time taken to deliver the fetus without causing maternal side-effects (El-Refaey et al 1993, Hinshaw et al 1995).

Expectant management

Expectant or conservative management can be offered to women who are diagnosed with an inevitable or incomplete miscarriage. With the increased use of ultrasound in early pregnancy and the availability of sensitive hCG assays a diagnosis of miscarriage is now made at a stage when previously the diagnosis may have been 'late period' or 'abnormal bleeding'. As many of these episodes would previously have resolved spontaneously it can be assumed that most intervention is unnecessary. At the Fertility Institute of New Orleans all patients diagnosed with a non-viable pregnancy are offered expectant management with no known adverse outcome and weekly telephone contact until spontaneous miscarriage occurs (Dickey 1993).

With this method of management the woman goes home to miscarry. The drawbacks include the length of time the process can take, the psychological effects of carrying a 'dead baby' for days and possibly weeks, the inability to predict when miscarriage will actually take place, how much pain and bleeding will be experienced and the possibility that fetal tissue will not be obtained. It does, however, allow the woman to be in control of her own body and be involved in the process of miscarriage and for those women who are adamant that they do not want surgical or medical intervention it offers an alternative.

RECURRENT MISCARRIAGE

Definition and incidence

Recurrent miscarriage is defined as three or more consecutive spontaneous miscarriages. This can be subdivided into primary and secondary groups, primary consisting of those women who have miscarried all their previous pregnancies, and secondary consisting of those women who have had at least one successful pregnancy followed by at least three consecutive miscarriages (Stirrat 1990a). What has to be decided is whether there is a distinct clinical disorder or are these women the victims of chance? The frequency with which women miscarry three consecutive pregnancies if due to chance alone would be 0.3–0.4%, but the figure is nearer 1% suggesting that there may be a specific underlying cause.

Aetiology of recurrent miscarriage

Anatomical. Congenital abnormalities appear to contribute little to the incidence of recurrent miscarriages. Over 3% of women who carry a pregnancy to term have either a septate or bicornuate uterus (Simon et al 1991); this is a similar incidence to that found in the general population (Clifford et al 1994). One explanation for this is that the abnormal area of the uterus potentially has a reduced blood supply and is therefore unlikely to be the implantation site for every pregnancy.

Box 5.3 Causes of recurrent miscarriages

- Anatomical.
- Hormonal.
- Immunological.
- Hereditary thrombophilias.
- Genetic.
- Infection.
- Psychological.

In the past, treatment for congenital abnormalities was open surgical correction. This is now felt to be unsuitable, firstly because there is a lack of evidence that the abnormality is the sole cause of the miscarriages, and secondly because there is a high risk of postoperative infertility as a result of adhesion formation. The treatment of choice is now hysteroscopic resection of the septum, but even this requires further study as it is unclear whether any treatment is necessary unless infertility is also an issue.

A retroverted uterus is not a cause for recurrent miscarriage so if this is found on examination the woman can be reassured. However, the association of fibroids and miscarriage is an uncertain area, many women with fibroids become pregnant without any delays and experience an uncomplicated pregnancy, although in some women the presence of fibroids may enlarge the uterus and distort the uterine cavity to such an extent that they cause serious reproductive problems. If the woman is found to have a fibroid polyp then this can easily be removed during a routine dilatation and curettage (D and C). However, the decision to remove a submucous fibroid depends upon its size and position. It may be possible to resect the fibroid using a hysteroscope, other surgical alternatives require major abdominal surgery, which is more complex and can cause scar and adhesion formation resulting in infertility. Other methods of treatment are being developed, such as the embolization of fibroids, which may have fewer associated complications, but these are still in the early stages.

Cervical incompetence is a frequently quoted cause of recurrent second trimester miscarriage. Causes of cervical incompetence are thought to include congenital abnormality of the cervix, damage to the cervix following a difficult vaginal delivery and the use of excessive force or overdilatation of the cervix during a D and C or therapeutic abortion. Fortunately, with the development of more gentle surgical techniques and the introduction of prostaglandin pessaries for termination of pregnancy, the problem has greatly reduced.

A typical presentation is sudden rupture of membranes in the second trimester, followed by an often relatively painless delivery. It appears that the increasing weight of the fetus forces the cervical os to gape until the pregnancy can no longer be maintained. Diagnosis can be made before pregnancy by a hysterosalpingogram or the use of Hegar dilators to measure the internal os, or during pregnancy serial ultrasounds may show cervical shortening. All such available tests are imprecise, leading to an overdiagnosis of the condition. It is not present in over two-thirds of the cases in which it is diagnosed (Clifford et al 1994).

Treatment is normally the insertion of a purse-string suture around the cervix at the level of the internal os. This is performed over 14 weeks gestation under anaesthetic and the woman is advised to rest for the remainder of the pregnancy. Studies have shown that there is no real benefit gained from such surgery and so women in whom cervical incompetence is suspected should be referred to an obstetrician for an individual management plan.

Intrauterine adhesions, also known as synechiae, can cause the walls of the uterus to stick together. In its mild form this can prevent successful implantation, in more severe cases it can result in amenorrhoea. Intrauterine adhesions almost always follow a surgical procedure in the uterus such as a D and C, ERPC, termination of pregnancy or manual removal of the placenta.

Adhesions in the uterus are very common and, if left untreated, will usually resolve spontaneously. The traumatized uterine lining starts to regenerate and menstruation returns with no adverse consequences. If the problem continues then it is advisable for the woman to have the adhesions divided using a hysteroscope. Usually, the adhesions respond to treatment and do not cause long-term problems, thus women who have undergone several ERPCs can be reassured that this should have no bearing on their future fertility.

Diagnosis of anatomical abnormalities can be done with laparoscopy, hysteroscopy, hysterosalpingogram, ultrasound, magnetic resonance imaging (MRI) and computerized tomography (CT).

Hormonal. Hormonal explanations for recurrent miscarriage have always been attractive and studies into the treatment of infertility have shown that successful implantation and continuation of pregnancy depends partly on what happens in the first half of the menstrual cycle. In particular, high levels of luteinizing hormone (LH) have been associated with failure to conceive and a high incidence of miscarriage. Polycystic ovarian syndrome (PCOS) is the most common cause of high LH levels and can be found in up to 60% of women with recurrent miscarriage in comparison to 23% of women in the general population (Regan 1991). Trials conducted at St Mary's Hospital, London, assessed the effectiveness of pre-pregnancy pituitary suppression of LH secretion on the outcome of pregnancy in women with a history of recurrent miscarriage, PCOS and hypersecretion of LH. The conclusion was that there was no improvement and that the outcome without pituitary suppression was excellent. The trial also concluded that supportive care alone within the setting of a special-

ized clinic can result in a higher rate of successful pregnancy outcomes. It was suggested that further research should be directed at other endocrine factors that control implantation and that hypersecretion of LH is not a direct cause of miscarriage but a marker of some other endocrinopathy (Clifford et al 1996).

Some women may have a potentially remediable cause for the hypersecretion of LH, which may include suppression by gonadatrophin releasing agonists, ovarian diathermy or somatostatin (Prelevic et al 1990). Hamilton-Fairley et al (1992) showed an association between PCOS, obesity and miscarriage, and that women with a body mass index of $>25 \, kg/m^2$ were significantly more likely to miscarry than women with a normal body mass index. Thus it can be concluded that weight reduction is the single most important contribution a woman can make to improve the chances of a successful pregnancy.

Inadequate secretion of progesterone by the corpus luteum in the second half of the menstrual cycle and in early pregnancy has long been thought to be an important factor in recurrent miscarriage. Termed 'corpus luteum dysfunction' or 'luteal phase inadequacy' it is said to occur in between 23% and 80% of women with recurrent miscarriage (Fritz 1988), but there is no method to recognize luteal dysfunction in a woman who is already pregnant. As previously stated, it is now thought that low progesterone levels are a result of a failing pregnancy rather than a cause. Treatment of luteal dysfunction with progesterone or hCG, after conception, have failed to reduce the rate of miscarriage.

Immunological. A woman's ability to conceive, maintain and deliver a healthy baby are all affected by a complex web of immune factors. The fetus is a foreign body to the mother yet, in cases of a healthy pregnancy, it is not rejected. Both **autoimmune** and **alloimmune** causes of recurrent miscarriage have been possibly identified. In women of childbearing age systemic lupus erythematosis (SLE) is the most common autoimmune disorder and is associated with a high miscarriage rate as well as an increased risk of developing pre-eclampsia, growth retardation of the baby and placental abruption. It is now recognized that these problems are also associated with the presence of antiphospholipid antibodies (APA). Lupus anticoagulant (LA) and anticardiolipin antibody (ACA) are the two known antiphospholipid antibodies that are associated with recurrent pregnancy loss. Recurrent miscarriage in this group of patients is thought to occur as a result of thrombosis of placental vessels, which causes infarction and consequently fetal death (Out et al 1991), although there is also evidence to suggest that these antibodies can attack the cells of the placenta directly (Rote et al 1992).

The prevalence of APA in the general antenatal population is about 2%, compared with about 15% in women with recurrent miscarriage (Rai & Regan 1995). The successful pregnancy rate is only 10–15% in untreated women carrying APA and recurrent miscarriage is often how the condition first presents.

APA status cannot be determined on a single test as the levels of APA fluctuate over time. False negative results can be obtained due to incorrectly performed laboratory tests or as a consequence of the blood sample being taken using a tourniquet. The woman may have temporarily positive results caused by a virus or other infections so, in order for a definite diagnosis to be made, the woman must test positive for LA and/or ACA on at least two occasions at least 8 weeks apart.

Treatment of APA is now fairly standard, initially low-dose aspirin (75 mg daily) is started either pre-conceptially or at the first positive pregnancy test, combined with low molecular weight heparin when a fetal heart is detected on ultrasound. The rate of live births with this combination of drugs can be as high as 71% (Rai et al 1997). Caution must be taken when using heparin during pregnancy as it has been reported to cause a fall in the platelet count resulting in bleeding and, more seriously, osteoporosis (Shefras & Farquharson 1996), so women should be monitored carefully throughout their pregnancy.

The other possible immunological cause of recurrent miscarriage is an alloimmune response. Alloimmunity is the immune reaction that occurs between the tissues of different human beings, for example, an organ transplant. However carefully matched, the genetic makeup of the donor and recipient are not exactly the same, so drugs are used to suppress the alloimmune reaction. In pregnancy, the fetus is effectively a foreign transplant as it contains genetically different material than that of the mother, but it is not yet clearly understood why it is not immediately rejected by the mother's immune system. An alternative explanation is that some women have an immune deficiency that prevents them from mounting the appropriate protective response towards their fetus.

Treatment has been aimed at inducing the protective response that appears to be lacking in the alloimmune response to pregnancy. Research has included intervention with donor leucocytes, trophoblast or immunoglobulin and partner's leucocytes or seminal plasma (Stirrat 1990b). The current feeling is that immunotherapy does not have a role in the management of recurrent miscarriage at present, although further study and research into the subject continues.

Hereditary thrombophilias. Genetically determined thrombophilic defects have been the focus of much attention since the mid-1990s. These include deficiencies of antithrombin III, factor XII and of protein C and S, in addition to the more recently recognized activated protein C resistance (APCR) due to a single point mutation (factor V Leiden) in the factor V gene. APCR has a prevalence of 20% in women with second trimester miscarriages compared with 4% in the general population.

An association between inherited thrombophilic disorders and recurrent miscarriage is so recent that detailed studies are still required. However, it is likely that the most appropriate treatment is low-dose heparin and full anticoagulation may be necessary throughout the pregnancy.

Genetic. Although genetic abnormalities account for a large percentage of sporadic miscarriages, patients who suffer from recurrent losses tend to miscarry chromosomally normal pregnancies. However, in up to 4% of couples who suffer recurrent miscarriages one partner will carry a chromosomal abnormality. The most common of these is a reciprocal translocation in which a segment of one chromosome becomes attached to the broken end of another. Although the individual with a balanced translocation appears normal, when he or she produces eggs or sperm, some will be normal but others will inherit the abnormality. No longer is the abnormality balanced by the second normal chromosome in the pair, and as a result gametes frequently possess an unbalanced amount of chromosomal material (duplications and/or deficiencies). These imbalances are usually lethal to the developing embryo or fetus, resulting in miscarriage. Identification of these patients is essential so that they may be offered specialist genetic counselling and possible prenatal diagnosis in future pregnancies, via amniocentisis or chorionic villi sampling.

Infections. Most infections cause spontaneous miscarriage rather than recurrent losses. The exceptions to this rule include cytomegalovirus, which can be reactivated, and syphilis, which is now rarely seen. The human immunodeficiency virus (HIV) is an organism capable of causing recurrent miscarriage, although this theory still needs to be proved.

Currently under investigation is the role of vaginal infections in the aetiology of recurrent miscarriage, in particular the association of bacterial vaginosis and recurrent losses. Bacterial vaginosis is a condition where there is an overgrowth of anaerobic and other bacteria in the vagina with a corresponding decrease in the number of lactobacilli (Hay et al 1994). Bacterial vaginosis is diagnosed by Gram-staining of a vaginal smear.

A study conducted at Northwick Park Hospital concluded that 15% of pregnant women have abnormal vaginal flora in the form of bacterial vaginosis in early pregnancy and that these women have a five-fold increased risk of late miscarriage or preterm delivery (Hay et al 1994). Ralph et al (1999) looked at the influence of bacterial vaginosis on rates of conception and first trimester miscarriage in women undergoing in vitro fertilization. They concluded that bacterial vaginosis did not affect conception rate but did double the risk of miscarriage. As yet there is no evidence to suggest that treating bacterial vaginosis will alter this outcome, although further studies are anticipated.

Psychological. Many studies have examined the psychological effects of pregnancy loss but few have identified it as a cause of miscarriage. When investigating the effect of suppressing LH on the miscarriage rate, Clifford et al (1996) found that women in the control group who were given supportive care and no other treatment achieved excellent live birth rates. Other studies have noted the beneficial effect of 'tender loving care' on the outcome of pregnancy (Liddell et al 1991). So although there are great difficulties when trying to determine a psychological cause of miscarriage, it has been shown that supportive care in early pregnancy is the most important factor in determining the outcome in women with a history of unexplained recurrent miscarriage (Clifford et al 1995).

Investigations for recurrent miscarriage

Although most investigations for recurrent miscarriage are directed towards the woman it is important that both partners are seen together.

Initially, a full history should be taken including information on each miscarriage, any family history of pregnancy loss, problems with infertility or congenital abnormalities from either partner. This information provides the medical staff with an indication as to which investigations are appropriate. Table 5.2 shows the investigations that may be carried out for recurrent miscarriages. Most units operate a policy of investigating only after a third consecutive miscarriage, as the statistics show that even after two miscarriages there is still a higher chance of a successful pregnancy than that of a further pregnancy loss. However, some

Table 5.2 Investigations for recurrent miscarriages

Possible cause	Investigation
Anatomical	Hysterosalpingogram Hysteroscopy Vaginal ultrasound
Hormonal	Pelvic ultrasound Follicular phase LH levels and urinary LH excretion Endometrial biopsy
Immunological	Bloods for lupus anticoagulant and anticardiolipin antibodies (tests repeated at least 8 weeks apart)
Hereditary thrombophilias	Thrombophilia screen Antithrombin III Factor XII Protein C and protein S Activated protein C resistance (APCR)
Genetic	Peripheral blood karyotyping from both partners If possible, POC sent for cytogenetic investigations
Infection	Possible screening for bacterial vaginosis in early pregnancy
Psychological	No known investigation available

couples may warrant earlier investigation, such as those women over the age of 35 years who have experienced two consecutive losses and couples whose excessive concern over their miscarriage is interfering with their ability to perform the normal activities of daily living (Timbers & Fienberg 1997).

The first visit to the clinic should include a reassuring and realistic statement about the chances of a successful pregnancy. It may be that this is all that is required, and the fact that the problem has been taken seriously reassures the couple. It also has to be clearly stated at this stage that a 'cause' for the recurrent miscarriages may not be found, which may be more stressful for the couple.

A second appointment should be made when all the test results are available. If no apparent cause is found then reassurance for a successful pregnancy should again be given and the couple encouraged to try for another pregnancy when they both feel ready. In any subsequent pregnancy the woman must be seen early by an experienced obstetrician, preferably the one who investigated the recurrent miscarriages, the benefits of an early referral include the opportunity to choose the pattern of care they would like over the critical period and the availability of an ultrasound scan to show a developing pregnancy.

If the tests show a causative factor then appropriate treatment should be instigated either before or early in a subsequent pregnancy. The importance of psychological care and support for these couples should not be underestimated. If the pregnancy does unfortunately end in miscarriage then all attempts should be made to obtain fetal tissue for cytogenetic testing.

INFORMATION AND ADVICE FOLLOWING A MISCARRIAGE

Many women complain that they are given conflicting advice around the time they are miscarrying; this is as a result of many myths surrounding pregnancy loss. A typical example is when a woman presenting with a threatened miscarriage is advised to have bedrest, this in itself is not always appropriate and the benefits, if any, should be explained so that she is able to make an informed choice.

Following a miscarriage women need to be advised that they can expect some vaginal bleeding, which may last anything up to 2 weeks. If the bleeding becomes heavy or offensive then they need to seek medical advice either via their GP or the hospital, as it may indicate retained products of conception or an infection. They should be advised to use sanitary towels rather than tampons as the latter can pose a risk of infection, although tampons may be used for their next period. Women need to be aware of when to expect their next period, normally it is within 4 to 6 weeks of the miscarriage if they previously had a regular cycle. It is important to warn them that this period may be lighter or heavier than they would normally expect.

Depending on the gestation of the pregnancy there is the possibility of tender breasts and even the leakage of milk. This can be relieved by wearing a supportive bra, using a cold flannel and taking mild analgesia. If the problem persists or becomes a painful reminder of what has happened then further treatment can be sought from the GP.

Resuming sexual intercourse can be difficult for many couples. Physically, they should wait until the bleeding settles to allow the cervix to close thus reducing the risk of infection. Emotionally, it can take time before both partners are interested again so they will have to be patient and show love and understanding regarding how the other feels.

Many women experience fatigue and tiredness for several days following a miscarriage, so they should be advised to rest as much as possible. It is not unusual to take at least 2 weeks off work and GPs are willing to sign a sick leave certificate for as long as necessary. Returning to work is an individual decision, some women may feel the need to return swiftly as it provides the opportunity to escape their feelings, most women, however, need time to grieve for their loss and to feel strong again before facing the outside world. There is no right or wrong way, they must do whatever feels best for them.

Emotionally, it can surprise many couples how deeply an early pregnancy loss can affect them; there are obviously those who adjust quickly whereas others can be severely affected for several weeks even months. A range of feelings can be experienced including guilt, anger, resentment, despair, frustration, bitterness, emptiness, numbness and an acute sense of loss. Eventually the 'good' days will outnumber the 'bad', although there are times when the feelings will return such as an anniversary of the loss or the baby's due date. Some women release their feelings by crying a lot, others find it difficult to express themselves, many complain of a loss of appetite, difficulty sleeping and unpredictable outbursts usually aimed at their partner or close family. These are normal reactions to grief and given time and understanding the woman will return to 'normal'. In severe cases it may be appropriate to treat with antidepressants but this should be done in conjunction with counselling. Local support groups can provide an opportunity to talk about the miscarriage with other women and couples who have experienced a similar loss, which can be a great comfort, especially when family and friends feel they should have 'moved on' in the grieving process.

Men often find it difficult to express their feelings and try to be strong and supportive, which can be interpreted as being uncaring and unfeeling. It should be pointed out that this loss affects both partners and each will have their own way of coping so they need to be understanding and ensure they have the opportunity to communicate with each other.

Following a miscarriage one of the hardest things to do is tell people what has happened and it is often the man who has to perform this task. Meeting people after a miscarriage can be traumatic, some friends may be supportive and understanding while others appear not to care and may even avoid contact. This is often because they feel uncomfortable with death and are frightened to ask how the woman feels as they are unable to cope with her reactions.

All couples should be offered the opportunity to mark the loss of their baby and many hospitals and churches have a Book of Remembrance where a verse or message can be inscribed. It may be appropriate for a funeral to take place, which can allow the couple an opportunity to say goodbye and move on in the grieving process; every hospital will offer different services. If an identifiable fetus is passed then it is important that parents are given the option of seeing and holding the baby, spending time with the baby, taking photographs and obtaining momentos that will allow them to cope with their loss.

Many couples want information regarding future pregnancies, they should be advised that there is no fixed time they should wait before trying again – it is right when they feel ready – although it is a good idea that they wait until after the woman has her next period to allow her body to recover and to ensure accurate dating in the next pregnancy. Some health professionals advise waiting for three periods before trying again. There is no research to show that this results in a higher chance of a successful pregnancy and there is nothing to indicate an increased risk of miscarriage if the woman falls pregnant immediately. Every woman should be given positive information regarding future pregnancies, they have every chance of a successful pregnancy next time and there is no increased risk of miscarriage as a result of this pregnancy loss.

All women should be given advice regarding getting as fit as possible for future pregnancies, such as

---

Box 5.4 Foods rich in folic acid

- Green vegetables (broccoli, spinach, brussel sprouts and cauliflower).
- Yeast extract spread.
- Fortified breakfast cereals.
- Fortified and wholemeal bread.
- Nuts and chick peas.
- Citrus fruits (e.g. oranges).

---

stopping or cutting down smoking, eating a sensible diet and taking regular exercise. All women considering a pregnancy should be informed of the value of taking folic acid. In 1996 the government launched a £2.3 million publicity campaign to persuade women that taking folic acid for 3 months prior to conception and up to 12 weeks gestation can dramatically reduce their chances of giving birth to a baby with a neural tube defect, such as spina bifida or anencephaly. It is recommended by the Department of Health that women should take 0.4 mg of folic acid daily as well as eating foods rich in folic acid (Whyte 1995) as outlined in Box 5.4.

ACKNOWLEDGEMENTS

Thanks to Rachel Savage, Nurse Practitioner in Early Pregnancy Assessment, Taunton and Somerset NHS Trust, and Kathy Jackson, Staff Midwife, University Hospitals of Coventry & Warwickshire, for the time and effort involved in obtaining the ultrasound scan pictures.

ECTOPIC PREGNANCY

DEFINITION AND INCIDENCE

Although ectopic pregnancy refers to any pregnancy occurring outside the uterine cavity, this chapter concentrates mainly on tubal pregnancy, that is, those that are located within the fallopian tube (Fig 5.5). Ectopic pregnancy has been described as an unmitigated human reproductive catastrophe (De Cherney 1983). The effects of such a disaster have been widely studied across the world over the last few decades.

The first clear description of ectopic pregnancy was made in AD 936 by Abulcasis (Abul Qasim), a famous Arabic writer who studied surgical topics. It remained a potentially fatal condition until the late nineteenth

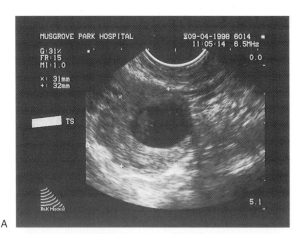

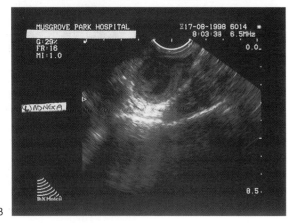

Figure 5.5 Tubal pregnancies
A/10 weeks gestation by LMP
B/7 weeks gestation by LMP

century when Lawson Tait described the first successful attempts to operate on patients with ruptured tubal ectopic pregnancy (Tait 1888, cited by Dimitry 1989). Since then, there have been many developments in the diagnostic techniques and clinical management of the condition, all of which have one common aim – to preserve maternal life and protect the woman's reproductive ability.

In the UK several studies have concluded that a rise in the incidence of ectopic pregnancy is apparent (Dimitry & Morcos 1990, Kok et al 1989). Indeed, Irvine et al (1994) identified an ectopic pregnancy rate of approximately one in 60 reported pregnancies, which is one of the highest rates reported worldwide.

There are, however, limitations in accurately identifying ectopic pregnancy rates. There has been some controversy over the denominator used in defining the incidence. This varies from the number of live births or the number of reported pregnancies to the total number of conceptions, including all abortions, spontaneous and therapeutic. These must be taken into account when reviewing the literature, as the denominator used may reflect differences in incidence rates. Another limitation to accuracy is the possibility that very early cases of ectopic pregnancy may be missed because they have resolved spontaneously with no intervention, even before pregnancy is suspected (Stabile 1996). It may be argued, however, that adverse effects on incidence rates can be attributed to the sophisticated diagnostic tests now widely available. Clinicians are now able to detect ectopic pregnancies earlier, many of which may have previously spontaneously resolved undetected.

In the UK ectopic pregnancy continues to be a cause of maternal death, resulting in seventeen deaths between 1985 and 1987 (Department of Health 1991). With this in mind, the need for knowledge and understanding of the factors affecting the incidence and the causes of the condition persists as an issue of paramount importance to clinicians and researchers alike.

RISK FACTORS

Risk factors for an ectopic pregnancy are as follows:

- sterilization
- previous pelvic surgery
- previous tubal surgery
- previous ectopic pregnancy
- pelvic inflammatory disease
- smoking
- infertility.

All women who are sexually active are at risk of developing an ectopic pregnancy, although in some the risk is increased by one or a combination of factors. Dimitry & Morcos (1990) suggest that changes in the reproductive behaviour of women, including the increased incidence of sexually transmitted diseases, changes in contraceptive patterns and family planning are contributing factors.

Intrauterine devices

The use of intrauterine devices (IUDs) was previously thought to have been a major determiner of ectopic pregnancy (Beral 1975), although it is not now accepted that it is a prime cause. Indeed, there is growing evidence that the IUD in situ reduces the risk of ectopic pregnancy (Wilson 1989).

Surgery

Previous pelvic surgery, including sterilization, is thought to be another contributing risk factor. Dimitry (1987) identified appendicectomy as an underlying cause due to the development of adhesions as a result of surgery performed in close proximity to the pelvic organs. Furthermore, De-Stephano et al (1982) found that sterilized women had a higher risk of ectopic pregnancy than if they had opted for barrier methods or oral contraception. As one in six pregnancies after tubal ligation is ectopic it may be suggested that the increase in the popularity of female sterilization may be contributing in part to the rise in incidence of tubal pregnancy. Similarly, advances in tubal surgery to correct tubal damage have also increased the risk of developing ectopic pregnancy (Winston 1980). This may be as a result of adhesion formation or scar tissue development within the fallopian tube. It is also accepted that women with a history of ectopic pregnancy have a higher risk of experiencing a second ectopic (Dimitry & Morcos 1990), especially if the fallopian tube is conserved or only partially removed.

Pelvic inflammatory disease

The evidence for pelvic inflammatory disease as a major risk factor is very strong. Many observers, for example Westrom et al (1981) and Brunham et al (1986) have suggested that tubal infections are mainly responsible for the increase in the incidence of ectopic pregnancy. This hypothesis is supported by the frequent finding of chronic salpingitis in treated cases.

Chronic salpingitis is often attributed to sexually transmitted disease and especially to *Chlamydia trachomatis*, a known major cause of tubal damage (Brunham et al 1986).

Smoking

Another fairly convincing and statistically significant association has been made between tobacco smoking and ectopic pregnancy in several studies (Levin et al 1982, Matsunga & Shiota 1980). It is thought that the pathophysiological effects of smoking on the immune system and the production of oestrogen are to blame, although it has been suggested that socioeconomic factors should also be considered. For example, Chow et al (1988) argue that women who smoke may be more likely to contract agents that cause tubal disease because of their choice of sexual partner, therefore increasing their risk of ectopic pregnancy.

Infertility

Women with a history of infertility are also at risk. The development of assisted reproduction techniques has meant that more patients with tubal damage have conceived. Not surprisingly, ectopic pregnancy is quite common following in vitro fertilization and embryo transfer (Cohen et al 1986).

DIAGNOSIS

The diagnosis of ectopic pregnancy is not straightforward. Stabile (1996) states that: 'ectopic pregnancy remains the great mimic of gynaecology; no other pelvic condition gives rise to more diagnostic errors.' Apart from the typical symptoms of pelvic pain and irregular vaginal bleeding, along with a positive high sensitivity pregnancy test and other signs of pregnancy that may or may not be present, the need for reliable and accurate diagnostic tools is evident. Toumivaara et al (1986, cited by Stabile 1996) suggest that on the basis of clinical features alone, only half of patients will be correctly diagnosed with the condition. In cases of ruptured ectopic pregnancy, symptoms may include shoulder-tip pain, distended abdomen due to intra-abdominal bleeding, and cardiopulmonary collapse.

Prompt diagnosis is important for several reasons. Most significantly, early screening is an important factor in reducing maternal deaths from ruptured ectopic pregnancy (Turnbull et al 1989). Diagnosis before tubal damage occurs has obvious physical and psychological benefits to the patient, the conservation of future fertility and reduction in the need for radical surgery being two of the most significant and the alleviation of patient anxiety another. It has been suggested, however, that early intervention may encourage overtreatment of ectopic pregnancies that might have otherwise resolved spontaneously (Stabile 1996). Screening should, therefore, be recommended to secure an accurate diagnosis before any intervention is decided, especially in women who are known to be at risk of tubal disease, are undergoing assisted reproduction programmes or in those who have a history of ectopic pregnancy.

hCG measurement

Measurement of human chorionic gonadotrophin (hCG) is the most commonly used biochemical test in the detection of pregnancy, hCG can be found in urine and blood and is relied upon to establish the normality or otherwise of the pregnancy. It is generally agreed that measurement of this hormone can be used as a sensitive marker for intra- and extrauterine **trophoblastic tissue** and that patients with ectopic pregnancy have lower hCG values that will either decline slowly, rise slowly or plateau. Furthermore, if the serum measurement of hCG is rising, the likelihood of ectopic pregnancy increases as the doubling time of the hormone increases (Stabile, 1996). In addition, Dimitry et al (1992) propose that a negative quantitative serum measurement almost always excludes the presence of ectopic pregnancy. The usefulness of the serial quantitative beta hCG test is enhanced when used in conjunction with clinical examination, although it has its limitations as a stand-alone test. It does not, for example, locate the pregnancy and it requires an interval of 48 hours between measurements. Two or three measurements may need to be taken before a provisional diagnosis may be made. During this time, anxiety levels of the patient may increase and symptoms, if present, may worsen. Several observers suggest that if this test is used in conjunction with other diagnostic tools, for example ultrasonography, it offers an accurate and reliable contribution to the diagnosis (Cacciatore et al 1990, Grudzinskas & Stabile 1993).

Ultrasonography and colour Doppler sonography

The role of ultrasonography as a diagnostic tool is to locate the suspected ectopic pregnancy. It may be per-

---

Case study: Rebecca

Rebecca is 36 years old with a history of infertility and a previous ectopic pregnancy 2 years ago, which resulted in a right partial salpingectomy. She presented to the EPAU at 6 weeks pregnant by last menstrual period (LMP) complaining of light vaginal spotting, a slightly raised temperature but no abdominal discomfort. An ultrasound scan showed an empty uterus, no obvious **adnexal** masses and normal ovaries.

Rebecca's hCG levels were measured and an appointment made for a second measurement 48 hours later. Rebecca was allowed home but given a contact number if she experienced any pain or had any other concerns. Her BhCG results were:
- 1st measurement: 850 units
- 2nd measurement: 1280 units.

Rebecca was recalled after the second result as the levels indicate the possibility of an ectopic pregnancy. She was admitted, prepared for a laparoscopy and told that this might need to proceed to surgery. She gave her permission for this.

The operation findings showed a 5-week tubal ectopic pregnancy on the right side at the site of the previous tubal anastamosis; the left tube and both ovaries appeared normal. A right salpingectomy was performed laparoscopically.

Postoperatively Rebecca had i.v. hydration, narcotic analgesia via a patient-controlled analgesia system (PCAS) and routine observations. She was discharged after 48 hours having been seen by the miscarriage nurse for the unit who will follow Rebecca up at home. Verbal and written information was given regarding ectopic pregnancies, future fertility and future pregnancies. Rebecca was also given contact numbers for the local support group and the miscarriage nurse.

---

formed abdominally or vaginally, although it has been argued that expert vaginal scanning provides better detail in identifying the pelvic organs and locating the implantation site of the pregnancy (Cacciatore et al 1989). However, even with transvaginal scanning, DeCrespigny (1988) found that an ectopic fetus is seen in only 20% of confirmed cases, suggesting that other sonographic features need to be identified to assist with the diagnosis. Another advantage of transvaginal scanning is that it does not require a full bladder, which is known to increase the patient's discomfort during the waiting time. It would be prudent to mention, however, that when abdominal pregnancy is suspected, vaginal scanning may not be effective in locating it and abdominal scanning is preferred.

Colour Doppler sonography, a relatively new method for diagnosing early tubal ectopic pregnancy, seeks to improve the speed and accuracy of diagnosis by analysing the flow of blood in the tubal arteries. Kirchler et al (1993) found an increase in tubal blood flow on the side that the ectopic pregnancy had implanted and concluded that this method enables the experienced clinician to locate and identify tubal pregnancy very quickly using a non-invasive and practical procedure.

It may be argued that repeated confirmation of the diagnosis by several means is important to the psychological wellbeing of the patient, who may be grieving for the potential loss of the pregnancy and who needs absolute reassurance that the pregnancy is non-viable. The production of protocols and guidelines in early pregnancy assessment units are a valuable means of enabling clinical presentations and diagnostic findings to be interpreted. If there are ambiguous results, the management of patients can be planned to monitor their condition safely whilst providing reassurance that no hasty intervention will be performed.

Surgical diagnosis

Invasive diagnostic tools play an important role in confirming the suspected presence of ectopic pregnancy and usually follow biochemical and sonographic tests. **Laparoscopy** (Plate 6) is considered to be the optimal invasive technique for diagnosing and excluding ectopic pregnancy, providing a positive diagnosis in over 90% of cases (Kim et al 1987). The risks to the patient are the need for a general anaesthetic and the potential complications of vascular, bowel and urinary tract trauma. The presence of adhesions may obscure the view, resulting in the need to proceed to laparotomy to locate the suspected ectopic pregnancy.

MANAGEMENT

As the diagnosis of ectopic pregnancy has become more sophisticated, so have the treatment options. These may be categorized into four groups:

- expectant management (non-medical and non-surgical methods)
- medical treatment
- conservative treatment (surgical techniques where the fallopian tube is conserved)
- radical surgical intervention.

Expectant management

In spite of the rising incidence of ectopic pregnancy, the rate of tubal rupture is declining (Pansky et al 1991). This is probably a result of the increasing ability to diagnose and treat the condition at an earlier stage, sometimes even before any symptoms are present. Over recent years, several authors have suggested that a changing clinical picture of ectopic pregnancy is emerging, allowing the development of new therapeutic techniques, one of them being expectant management.

There is growing evidence that, in some cases, ectopic pregnancy will resolve spontaneously, either by tubal abortion or resorption (Fernandez et al 1988, Ylostalo et al 1992). However, because of increasingly early diagnosis and intervention, the natural history of many ectopic pregnancies has been suppressed. Several studies have been conducted to examine the outcome of expectant management following confirmed diagnosis by laparoscopy and using strict protocols to monitor the progress of selected patients. Garcia et al (1987) suggest that asymptomatic patients with continually falling beta hCG levels probably have a non-viable gestation in the process of being reabsorbed and conclude that, under tightly controlled conditions, expectant management is appropriate. It is not clear how many patients might benefit from this type of management, although the avoidance of tubal surgery may be an attractive alternative to conventional methods of treatment.

The potential disadvantages to this method include the need for a longer period of surveillance and repeated visits to hospital. It has also been suggested that asymptomatic tubal pregnancies may result in tubal obstruction (Haney 1986, cited by Fernandez et al 1988), suggesting the need for hysterosalpingogram following this course of action to check tubal patency. Another disadvantage is the possibility that any intraperitoneal bleeding, not reabsorbed spontaneously, may cause peritoneal irritation and adhesion formation – with subsequent effects on fertility.

Medical treatment

Medical treatment of ectopic pregnancy has recently been introduced into clinical practice as an alternative to surgical management. It involves the administration of systemic or local drugs into the gestation sac, which is then left inside the fallopian tube to be absorbed. Drugs commonly used include:

- methotrexate
- potassium chloride
- mifepristone
- prostaglandin E2 and F2 alpha
- hyperosmolar glucose solution.

It is believed that as many as 25% of ectopic pregnancies may be suitable for this type of treatment (Stabile 1996).

Systemic chemotherapy (methotrexate) has been used to treat unruptured ectopic pregnancy since the 1980s. However, there is concern that this may expose patients to side-effects such as systemic toxicity, even when citrovorum is added to lessen the toxic effects. In view of this problem, local injection has been introduced to allow more accurate location of the drug and to reduce the volume needed for successful resolution (Kojima et al 1990).

Local injection of prostaglandins has also been used with successful results, although cardiovascular side-effects and abdominal discomfort have been recorded when higher doses are used (Egarter & Husslein 1988). More recently, it has been suggested that laparoscopic injection of hyperosmolar glucose solution is as effective as other methods and is without the side-effects (Lang et al 1992).

The advantages of using medical treatments are mainly the reduced need for tubal surgery. The subsequent fertility rate is high if there is no history of infertility and the recurrent ectopic rate is approximately 11% (Stabile 1996). However, selection criteria for medical treatment require that the tube is intact and that the pregnancy is less than 4 cm in diameter. Treatment failure is probable if a fetal pulse is seen on scan or if very high levels of hCG are present. Following treatment, it is important that all patients are monitored with serial hCG measurement, meaning further visits to hospital. If treatment is unsuccessful, surgery may be required to remove the ectopic pregnancy, exposing the patient to more risks. With this in mind it remains to be seen whether medical treatment carries advantages over conservative, surgical treatment.

Conservative treatment

Surgery continues to be the treatment of choice for many patients with ectopic pregnancy, although trends suggest that conservation of the fallopian tube is a major factor when deciding which treatment to opt for (Stabile 1996). Surgical techniques that conserve the tube include:

● linear salpingotomy
● **salpingostomy** (when the tube is left open to heal)
● fimbrial evacuation.

These procedures may be performed laparoscopically or by microsurgical laparotomy. Studies comparing laparoscopy and laparotomy have suggested that the economic advantages and more rapid recovery following laparoscopy, as well as the improved cosmetic result, outweigh those of laparotomy (Brumsted et al 1988). Nevertheless, if there is significant intra-abdominal bleeding or dense abdominal adhesions that may obscure the view, laparotomy is indicated. The major advantage of both these methods is that confirmation of the diagnosis and treatment can be performed during the same procedure.

Various methods are used to open the tube, including:

● **electrocautery**
● surgical instruments
● laser techniques.

Several observers have concluded that laser is the most effective method as it causes minimal trauma to the tube and provides active haemostasis with minimal adhesion formation postoperatively (Keckstein et al 1990; Paulson 1992). However, availability and personal preference seem to be the main indicators of which method is used as opposed to the actual performance of each tool.

Once the tube has been opened and the products of conception removed, the decision whether to close the tube (salpingotomy versus salpingostomy) is made. Closing the tube may aid haemostasis, although there is a difference in opinion whether consequent adhesion formation is greater following salpingotomy or salpingostomy. Stabile (1996) argues that, as the pregnancy does not usually lie inside the tubal lumen, carefully performed linear salpingotomy should not enter the cavity of the tube and, therefore, that it is unnecessary to close the incision to maintain tubal patency.

Fimbrial evacuation (milking out of the tube) provides an alternative method when the conceptus lies within the fimbrial region. A laparoscopic version, known as tubal aspiration, is sometimes used when a tubal abortion is already in progress and the products of conception are seen protruding through the distal tube opening. These methods have caused concern among observers because of the complications that may occur. Brosens et al (1984) identified problems such as tubal scarring with consequent adhesion formation, continued bleeding and persistent trophoblast. It is therefore recommended that great care is required when performing fimbrial evacuation and that the method should not be attempted on ectopic pregnancies that lie elsewhere in the tube.

Whichever conservative method is chosen, it must be stressed that the safe recovery of the patient should be the prime consideration. Saunders (1990) states that: 'conservatism should not be confused with complacency.'

Although it has been argued that conservative management should always be the first choice of treatment, the need for a more radical procedure may arise for a variety of reasons.

Radical surgical intervention

A radical procedure is indicated when the tube is irreparably damaged or if there is uncontrolled bleeding. It may also be considered in cases of repeat ectopic pregnancy in a tube that was previously treated conservatively or when fertility is no longer required. In patients that are undergoing assisted reproduction techniques, such as in vitro fertilization, radical surgery may be performed to improve ovarian access.

The main radical procedure used is salpingectomy, which may be partial or complete, usually performed at laparotomy. When the conceptus is smaller than 3 cm in diameter, however, laparoscopic salpingectomy may be successfully performed (Semm 1979). Cornual resection and/or oophorectomy may follow salpingectomy if the blood supply to the ovary is at risk, although every effort to conserve the ovary is usually made in case in vitro fertilization is subsequently indicated. In terms of future fertility, the condition of the unaffected tube is important and may influence the type of surgery chosen.

Whether radical surgery carries advantages or disadvantages to the patient depends on the history of each individual case. When performed as a life-saving technique, it carries obvious advantages, but for the woman who has lost her natural ability to conceive after bilateral salpingectomies, for example, the consequences of such radical surgery are severe. Physical recovery time may be reduced by advancing technology but for some women the emotional scars never heal.

FERTILITY AFTER ECTOPIC PREGNANCY

It is generally believed that reproductive performance after ectopic pregnancy is less successful, although other factors thought to influence prognosis rates should be considered, such as history of infertility, previous abdominal surgery and advancing age (Ory et al 1993). For example, Langer et al (1982) found that 80% of patients with a normal contralateral tube achieved a subsequent viable pregnancy following conservative surgery, compared with a 55% viable pregnancy rate in those with a damaged contralateral tube or periadnexal adhesions. Similarly, Sherman et al (1982) discovered that patients with a normal pelvis and no history of

---

> **Case study:** Aisha
>
> Aisha is 26 years old and presented to the local casualty department with acute left iliac fossa pain, which came on suddenly at work. She is known to be 7 weeks pregnant in her second pregnancy; she already has a son of 21 months. Aisha is transferred immediately to the gynaecology ward with a suspected ectopic pregnancy. On admission to the ward her observations are blood pressure 90/50 and pulse 128. She is complaining of shoulder-tip pain, nausea and light headedness. On examination her abdomen is extremely tender with rebound tenderness.
>
> Five minutes after her arrival Aisha suddenly collapses – blood pressure 70/40 and pulse 140 – a diagnosis of ruptured ectopic is made. i.v. access is gained, colloid fluids commenced and theatre arranged immediately.
>
> In theatre a laparotomy is performed, 2 litres of blood are found in the abdomen and a ruptured left cornual ectopic. A left salpingectomy is carried out with abdominal lavage. Postoperatively Aisha has i.v. hydration, analgesia via a PCAS, a urinary catheter and an abdominal drain. Routine observations of pulse, blood pressure and temperature remain within normal limits. On the first postoperative day the catheter and drain are removed, Aisha passes urine normally, light diet and fluids are commenced and by the second day the PCAS and i.v. fluids are discontinued.
>
> Ferrous sulphate 200 mg twice daily is commenced on the third day postoperatively as a routine check. FBC shows a haemaglobin level of 9.5 mg/100 ml. Aisha remains an inpatient for 5 days, during which she is seen by the miscarriage nurse and has an opportunity to discuss the events and ask questions regarding postoperative care, future fertility and her fears about getting pregnant again. She is given written information and contact numbers and is followed up after discharge by phone. Aisha receives support from her extended family and eventually returns to work 8 weeks after surgery.

---

infertility had an 85% subsequent intrauterine pregnancy rate following salpingotomy or salpingectomy. In a larger and more recent study, however, Gruft et al (1994) found no significant correlation between reproductive prognosis and parity, age, presence of adhesions in the contralateral tube or type of surgery performed.

Nevertheless, there is increasing evidence that of all the factors affecting future prognosis, a prior history of infertility is the most significant. Ory et al (1993) observed that patients with no history of infertility had a 68% term pregnancy rate following conservative or radical surgery. For patients with a history of infertility the rate was significantly lower, that is, 25% following conservative management and only 11% after radical surgery. This study suggests that, regardless of the procedure chosen, women with a prior history of infertility have a poor fertility prognosis and should perhaps be advised to consider alternatives, such as in vitro fertilization.

It would seem logical that unruptured tubal pregnancy is less likely to impede future fertility than if the tube were to rupture (Sherman et al 1982), whereby the argument for early diagnosis and prompt conservative treatment would be supported. The decision on whether to conserve the tube or not is usually related to the size of the gestation and it might be argued that a conservative procedure would be inadvisable if the contralateral tube is normal. In such circumstances, while subsequent fertility rates are comparable following radical and surgical procedures, the repeat ectopic pregnancy rate is thought to be higher following conservative treatment (Thorburn et al 1988). By removing the affected tube, however, the treatment options will be reduced should a further ectopic pregnancy occur in the other tube.

Reproductive performance following medical treatment of ectopic pregnancy has been little researched, although preliminary results appear promising. Stovall et al (1990) concluded that, following methotrexate and citrovorum factor treatment of unruptured ectopic pregnancy, reproductive performance is not impaired and that pregnancy rates are better than traditional conservative surgical methods and are comparable with laparoscopic salpingostomy.

Similarly, the long-term effects of expectant management on tubal performance are comparable to those of other treatments, with tubal patency on the affected side observed in 70–100% of patients following expectant management in comparison with 50–100% after medical and conservative surgical procedures (Fernandez et al 1988, Ylostalo et al 1992). Intrauterine and recurrent ectopic pregnancy rates are yet to be reliably compared, because studies of expectant management have been small and infrequent.

Fertility rates after different types of management are dependent on many factors, therefore making it difficult to suggest that one method of treatment is better or more successful than another. What is certain overall, however, is that the ability to go on to achieve a viable pregnancy has been greatly improved since the variety of treatment options has developed.

THE FUTURE

The diagnostic efficiency and techniques to treat ectopic pregnancy have been improving as technology grows and there is no reason to suggest that options will not continue to unfold. Current advances in the use of fibreoptic techniques, such as **falloposcopy**, are allowing ever more adventurous attempts to examine the tube 'from the inside', suggesting that even less traumatic diagnosis and more gentle treatment may develop. More recently, it has been suggested that relocating the ectopic pregnancy to the uterine cavity may be a worthwhile technique to explore, provided that certain prerequisites are addressed (Grudzinskas et al 1994). These include:

- efficient facilities for early diagnosis of ectopic pregnancy
- counselling for potential recruits
- on-call surgical and embryology teams
- accurate karyotyping techniques
- appropriate surgical technique for removal and relocation of the pregnancy.

It remains to be seen whether the idea will become a reality in the future: if successful, it will alter the present knowledge that every ectopic pregnancy is a doomed pregnancy and will offer at least a glimmer of hope to women affected by this condition.

EARLY PREGNANCY ASSESSMENT UNITS (EPAU)

Prior to the development of EPAUs most women with pain and/or bleeding in early pregnancy were admitted to the gynaecology ward as emergency admissions. Not only did this cause unnecessary distress and anxiety to the woman and her family, but she was often left for long periods of time waiting to see medical and nursing staff and for appropriate investigations to be arranged and results reviewed. Valuable bedspaces were taken up on a busy ward and there was not the opportunity to give the women the necessary emotional support. Most nurses would agree that the service offered was haphazard, disorganized and of poor quality.

Many units throughout the country now offer a 'one-stop' referral system; women with problems in early pregnancy are given an appointment time to attend a dedicated clinic often led by nurse practitioners. A history, examination, ultrasound scan, urine and blood tests are done immediately and a diagnosis reached quickly. The patient can then be discharged or treated as necessary and there is an opportunity to offer advice, support and counselling to those women who require it. Units such as these offer an improved quality of service and the women feel that they are a priority to the staff. Patients are spared the anxiety of unnecessary admission to hospital with the associated domestic problems (Bigrigg & Read 1991). The benefits of such a unit are felt by many departments, laboratories have a reduced number of on-call requests, out of hours work for junior doctors are decreased and obviously there is a reduced number of emergency admissions on the gynaecology ward.

Every unit will be managed differently in every hospital due to available resources and workload but the basic principle remains universal, the provision of an efficient service to women who experience problems in early pregnancy by offering a fast and accurate diagnosis, appropriate treatment with the availability of support, advice and follow-up.

THE ROLE OF THE NURSE IN EARLY PREGNANCY LOSS

Miscarriage is being increasingly recognized as a major and traumatic event in the lives of the women and their partners who experience it. This improved understanding is reflected in the care that couples receive and the role that the nurse plays.

There have been several studies into the psychological consequences of miscarriage and evidence suggests that many women experience intense emotional distress. Modern technology enables parents to bond with their baby very early in pregnancy and with it a possible range of names, a future and a personality. A heart beat can be seen on the screen as early as 8 weeks and a miniature baby can be recognized a couple of weeks later, which makes subsequent miscarriage all the harder to deal with.

The experience of miscarriage is unique, the intensity of the emotional response is not related to gestational age. A woman can be as distressed at 8 weeks as at 22 weeks. The extent of distress can sometimes be aggravated by poor medical care or the physical trauma. So it can be seen that while the physical care of the woman is important there is also a great need for psychological care. If a couple are given appropriate support and advice at the time of the pregnancy loss

they may be better able to deal with the long term consequences.

An important part of the nurse's role is to assess the woman's feelings, her perception of loss and the events surrounding the loss. Not all women and their partners experience the same intensity of pain and grief and what may be appropriate to offer one couple may be completely inappropriate for another. In cases of late miscarriage issues such as seeing and holding the baby, the taking of photographs, the opportunities for burial/cremation and the collecting of mementoes have to be addressed sensitively and at the appropriate moment. Most couples will be unaware of what is available so it is the role of the nurse to inform them.

More units are now appointing nurses to specifically deal with couples experiencing a miscarriage; they are able to provide continuity of care from clinic through treatment to discharge and follow-up. They are the contact point for women if they have any questions or problems; the nurse can provide relevant and accurate information on various aspects of miscarriage.

Many articles in the nursing press suggest that professionals are unable to provide the necessary support to couples who have suffered a pregnancy loss. Hopefully this situation is improving as more staff become aware of the important role they play.

CONCLUSION

The incidence, risk factors, diagnosis and management of pregnancy loss have been discussed. It is evident from the research to date that new knowledge and new hypotheses have continued to develop as interest in the subject has grown.

The contribution that nurses can make in helping patients, their partners and families to come to terms with the consequences of pregnancy loss is invaluable. Providing the right amount of information to enable them to make informed choices about their care, and offering them appropriate psychological support can aid both their physical and emotional recovery.

TERMINATION OF PREGNANCY

In 1996 in the United Kingdom nearly 200 000 pregnancies were terminated, with about 90% in the first 13 weeks of gestational age. Terminations of pregnancies are regulated by the 1967 Abortion Act (not applicable in Northern Ireland unless the woman's life is at risk) as amended by the Human Fertilization and Embryology Act 1990. This legislation allows pregnancies up to 24 weeks duration to be terminated if two doctors certify that:

- the continuation of the pregnancy would involve risk to the life of the pregnant woman greater than if the pregnancy were terminated
- the termination is deemed necessary to prevent any permanent injury to mental or physical health of the pregnant woman
- the pregnancy has *not* exceeded its 24th week and its continuation would involve risk greater than if the pregnancy were terminated to the physical or mental health of the pregnant woman
- the pregnancy has *not* exceeded its 24th week and its continuation would involve risk greater than if the pregnancy were terminated to the physical or mental health of any existing child(ren) of the pregnant woman
- there is a substantial risk that if the child were born it would suffer such physical or mental abnormalities as to be seriously disabled.

An exception to the two signatories is allowed in the case where a termination is required to save the life of the woman or to prevent injury to her physical or mental health – in this case only one doctor's signature is required.

The changes following the Human Fertilization and Embryology Act (1990) reduced the legal gestation of termination from 28 weeks to 24 weeks. It is illegal to perform a termination of pregnancy after 24 weeks unless there is a gross abnormality – in this case a termination can be carried out at any gestational age. Any treatment, either surgical or drug-induced, must be carried out in a National Health Hospital or a place approved by the Secretary of State for Health or Secretary of State for Scotland.

The practitioner terminating a pregnancy must complete the notification form HSA1 and send it to the Chief Medical Officer of the Department of Health or the Scottish Home and Health Department.

Box 5.5 The Royal College of Nursing's conscience clause

'The protection of the conscience clause is only given to those nurses who participate in any treatment The RCN advises that administering an abortifacient drug is participating in any treatment and a nurse who have a conscientious objection is not required by his or her employer to carry out this procedure except in an emergency when treatment is necessary to save the life or prevent grave permanent injury to the physical or mental health of the pregnant woman'.

Termination of pregnancy at any gestational age is undertaken for reasons that are deeply personal for the woman concerned. It can be distressing not only for the woman but also for the nursing and medical staff involved in her care. The later the termination the more likely problems are to arise. The Abortion Act (1967) does not contain a conscience clause, and the Royal College of Nursing has recognized this and drawn up guidelines (Box 5.5).

Terminations in the United Kingdom have now been legalized for more than 30 years, but women do not receive equality in the abortion services from the NHS. As with the conscience clause applying to nursing staff, the medical profession can also refrain from participation in a termination at any stage and this may be difficult for some women as the initial consultation may be with their GP, who may object to abortion. Besides this, the interpretation of the indicators is variable, depending on the individual medical practitioner. In some cases women have to consult one of the private or charitable agencies, but this is depends on financial considerations; it often involves travelling to the nearest clinic and possible accommodation charges.

UNPLANNED PREGNANCY

Every woman's experience is individual to her, and there will be a mixture of emotions related to the woman's individual circumstances and influenced by her personal and economic situation. It is often assumed that a woman with an unplanned pregnancy, or has 'brought this upon herself' or been unlucky or foolish. But some women have unplanned pregnancies even when using contraception – no method has a 100% guarantee. As health professionals, we must respond to the individual needs of the woman.

Confirmation of a pregnancy is normally the initial step. A consultation is usually prompted by a positive home pregnancy testing kit result or a chemist test, paid for by the woman herself. Discussing this result at an initial consultation may be the only opportunity that the woman has had to express her fears and anxieties about the pregnancy. It is the policy in some hospitals and clinics to repeat this test, regardless of the type of previous test and result. It is important that the woman is told about possible false positive results so that she understands why the test is being repeated. It is important that women understand what is happening, as many feel a sense of loss of control, although others may want to have their decisions made for them. It must be remembered it is the woman who has the final decision, as she is the one who has to live with the results of that decision, both in the short and long term. As professionals, nurses are there to aid help and support women in making their decision, without influencing them or making the decision for them. The process of decision making is an important one and it may be possible to offer another appointment, so that the issues can be explored further, at a time that is more acceptable to the woman and to the nursing staff. In some cases, further support may be needed, perhaps because the nurse feels unable to cope with the emotions expressed or because the nurse feels that a qualified counsellor may be a more appropriate person for the woman to talk to.

Referring the woman to an appropriate agency is a vital part of her care, not only initially but also in the long term, as research suggests that if a woman is not allowed to grieve following a termination she may be depressed, anxious or worried during subsequent pregnancies. It is vital that, throughout the process of decision making, it is the woman who makes the decisions and that she is encouraged to think about the options available to here:

- adoption
- continuing pregnancy
- termination.

Following a positive test it is important to explain the policy of the hospital or clinic the woman is attending in relation to time factors involved in receiving the results and the method in which they are given. Some hospitals have a 'walk-in service' with the results available in minutes whilst others may have to be sent outside the clinic for processing and can take several days. It is also the practice in some health authorities for a member of the medical profession to give the result, with an appointment required in some cases, whilst in others authorities the nurse may do this.

Information-giving enables the woman to decide if the particular facilities offered meet her individual needs. If they do not, it is important to give her information, at a local level if possible, about where she can meet her needs as far as possible, if not completely. National telephone numbers are available and give up-to-date information on what is available. It is vital that these, both written and verbal, are given to the woman before she leaves the clinic or hospital, so that she has means of contacting people who can help her, rather than leaving her wondering what to do next.

METHODS OF LEGAL TERMINATION

The referral system in each health authority is different but the principles remain the same. A woman may refer herself for a consultation and treatment to a charitable organization without GP consultation or she may see her GP and be referred within the local NHS service.

Each hospital has their own guidelines as to the gestational restrictions they are able to treat but most areas will discuss the needs, especially late termination, on an individual basis. Royal College of Gynaecology (RCOG) guidelines recommend that woman should be seen in a hospital environment within 5 days of referral, and can have the termination within 7 days of consultation. This is not always possible due to working constraints but, as stated previously, individual health authorities will have their own guidelines in place.

At a hospital outpatient consultation the woman is usually seen by a member of the medical profession who takes a medical and gynaecology history and also performs a vaginal examination. This consultation will include dates of the last menstrual cycle, contraception used and the outcomes of any previous pregnancies, including the method of delivery, as this needs to be taken into account when the decision as to whether cervical 'priming' is required is made. Some authorities have a specialist nurse/practitioner available to discuss what has been decided and to answer any questions the woman may have. In all although all health professional work under time restraints nurses may have more time the options with the woman. In some NHS hospitals, the nurse will continue the care of the woman throughout her stay and will be used as a point of contact for the woman. It has been recognized by some authorities that this a thought-provoking time for all concerned and this continuity of care enables the woman to discuss her fears and anxieties with one individual, building rapport and trust.

Once the consultation is complete, the woman will require investigations prior to admission for the termination. These will include:

- full Blood Count
- group and save
- **Rhesus group**
- rubella
- vaginal swabs including chlamydia
- ultrasound scan to confirm gestational age.

Following pregnancy confirmation, counselling and medical consultation, and after time taking to consider the choices available to her, the woman may decide to continue with the termination of the pregnancy. In whichever sector the woman decides to be treated, the method of termination is usually determined by the gestational age, although it may be restricted by the services a particular agency offers.

Terminations can be divided into two groups:

- early terminations – carried out before 12 weeks of **gestation**
- late terminations – performed from the 13th week of gestation up to the upper limit according to UK law of 24 weeks.

In all cases, it is important that vaginal swabs have been taken to exclude infection or, if not, that antibiotics are given prophalactively as pelvic inflammatory disease is a recognized complication and can lead to long-term sequelae of tubal infertility or ectopic pregnancy (see Box 5.7).

Early terminations

Most terminations are carried out before the 12th week of gestation by suction, dilatation and curettage (D&C), that is, they are surgical terminations.

Surgical Termination

This procedure is most commonly carried out as a day case. Some authorities offer a preassessment clinic appointment where the women can be assessed for suitably for the unit, as they usually have parameters to which to work. In rare cases, women may have to go to a 'main theatre' list and may require an overnight stay. This might happen if they had a high BMI ratio, or were asthmatic. A general anaesthetic is usually given, but in those cases not requiring a D&C (6–8 weeks gestation) the procedure may be done without an anaesthetic or with an anaesthetic block such as a paracervical block, in which lignocaine is injected into the cervix at 4, 8, and 12 o'clock. Some units 'prime' the cervix with Gemeprost prior to the procedure. Gemeprost (1 mg) is a vaginal **prostaglandin** pessary used to soften the cervix up to 3 h prior to surgery. The associated complications may include uterine pain, diarrhoea, flushing, chills or mild pyrexia, but referral to a drug formulary is advised if unsure.

In the theatre, the doctor will assess the uterus for size, shape and position by a bimanual examination. Once the cervix is visualized and immobilized the cervical canal is sounded for length and direction. In some cases the cervix may need to be dilated according to the gestational age. A small plastic tube is then inserted into the cervical canal and attached to a vacuum, which sucks out the contents. The contents are caught in the gauze trap so that they can be inspected. This is important to confirm that an intrauterine pregnancy has been evacuated. This sample is also sent to histology to avoid an ectopic pregnancy going unnoticed and also to ensure that the contents are not those of a molar pregnancy, which necessitates important follow-up care.

Many women experience some cramp-like pains initially, which will not persist for long. A mild analgesic may be required. The woman is observed for a few hours following this procedure and then allowed home, depending on her condition, with instructions and usually with a contact telephone number (See Box 5.5).

Medical termination

Since 1991 it has been possible for women to have a medical termination of pregnancy. This was developed and licenced for termination of pregnancy up to 63 days amenorrhoea and for second trimester pregnancy (13–20 weeks). It must be administered only in areas licenced under the Abortion Act 1967 and the amendments of 1990. Mifepristone (Mifegyne, also known as RU486) is given. This works by blocking the effect of progesterone, causing:

- detachment of the **embryo**
- increased contractibility of the myometrium
- ripening and opening of the cervix.

The treatment is not suitable for women with:

- suspected ectopic pregnancy
- chronic adrenal failure
- long-term corticosteroid therapy
- known allergy to mifepristone
- haemorrhagic disorders and who are being treated with anticoagulants.

It should not be given in conjunction with Gemeprost in smokers over 35 years of age and caution is also advised in women with asthma and chronic obstructive airways disease (COAD). The datasheet gives full details of all the precautions necessary.

The dosage of mifepistone varies: 200 mg (one tablet) or 600 mg (three tablets) are usual, followed 36–48 h later by either 1 mg of vaginal Gemeprost or 800 µgs of the orally active prostaglandin analogue Misoprostol, which is unlicensed. The alternative Misoprostol is used in some areas due to its reduced prostaglandin side-effects and low cost. It has been recommended in the RCOG Guidelines for Induced Abortions (July 1997). Investigations for this procedure as for those stated earlier in the chapter.

Women receiving a medical termination must attend on a specific day for the administration of mifepristone and be readmitted 2 days later as a day case. In the interim period she is able to continue normal activities. The woman has a 24-h contact telephone number for

---

Case study: Mary

Mary Smith is an 18-year-old student who is at present living with her parents in the Midlands. She is awaiting exam results and hoping to attend university in London.

She has been sexually active since the age of 16, and has been in her current relationship for 6 months. Mary has been using the combined oral contraceptive pill but, whilst on a weekend away with her boyfriend, complained of vomiting and diarrhoea. She did not realize about the need for extra protection during this time or the availability of emergency contraception.

She presented to her GP after having missed a period and also complaining of sickness. The GP took a urine sample during the consultation and carried out a pregnancy test, which came back as positive. Mary did not know what to do but the GP discussed the options available to her and gave her some information on the choices available should she continue with the pregnancy or decide to terminate the pregnancy. The GP made arrangements for her to return to the surgery in a weeks time. During the consultation they discussed her present relationship and also the reaction of her parents, as the GP felt they should be made aware of the pregnancy because Mary would need support, whatever her decision.

Mary has always been close to her mother and following her GP visit Mary confided in her mother. They discussed the options and felt that it was best not to tell her father at present until a decision had been made by Mary. Her father had recently been attending the hospital for tests as he had been complaining of pain in the chest. Mary and her mother decided not to put any more strain on her father at present.

During the next week Mary discussed the pregnancy with her boyfriend, who was also hoping to go to university. He felt that he could not give financial support and they were not sure what would happen to their relationship at the start of their university studies. He left the decision to Mary. Mary thought of nothing else over the next week and then returned to see her GP and asked for arrangements to be made for a termination. The GP contacted the local hospital and an out patient appointment was arranged for 10 days time. He completed as the first signatory on the Cert. A. Mary and her mother attended the hospital as planned. She was seen by the consultant on her own and they discussed the reason for her request. Mary explained, as she had done to her GP, the wish to continue with her studies.

The consultant asked about her medical and gynaecological history. He discussed her reasons for requesting a termination and agreed. He signed as the second signatory on the Cert. A. An internal examination was carried out, including swabs. Mary was given a prescription for antibiotics for prophylactic cover. The reason for this being that she had had several sexual relationships without using condoms, and was therefore at risk of pelvic inflammatory disease both pre- and postoperatively.

An ultrasound scan was performed to give an accurate gestational age so that a decision could be made regarding possible treatment. The scan showed an intrauterine gestational sac of 9#fr1/2> weeks. The option of a surgical termination was discussed, along with the possible effects.

Mary was introduced to the nurse at the preassessment clinic. They discussed the procedure in more depth. Contraception was talked about and Mary was given information leaflets given. Included was the use of condoms as a means to reduce infection risk. Routine bloods were taken including those for a rhesus group. A day case appointment was arranged. Mary and her mother attended on the given date and time.

Mary was seen again by the nurse who again discussed the procedure and answered any questions. Written consent was obtained by a member of the medical staff. The nurse prepared Mary for theatre and escorted her into the anaesthetic room. Immediately postoperatively the consultant completed the HSA1.

Following surgery, Mary was awake and orientated. Her blood pressure, pulse and vaginal loss were recorded. She was started on sips of water and fluids increased gradually. As this was tolerated a light diet was given. Mary was mobilized gently and passed urine.

Four hours postoperatively Mary was reviewed by a member of the medical staff. Her rhesus group was positive therefore anti-D was not required. Contraception was discussed. The oral contraceptive pill was dispensed and a pill teach given. A review appointment with the nurse was arranged for 6 weeks, verbal and written discharge advice, contact numbers and a GP letter was given. Mary was discharged home, escorted by her mother.

the interim period as she may experience some vaginal bleeding or abdominal cramps. It is important that the woman is told to avoid NSAIDs until the termination is complete, as these may reduce the efficacy of the treatment.

The woman returns to the treatment centre 36–48 hours later and the prostaglandin is administered. In the majority of cases the termination will occur within 4 h, but the woman must be observed for at least 6 h or until the bleeding or pain has diminished to an acceptable level.

If the termination has not been confirmed, the woman must be given specific instructions on who to contact in the event of any heavy bleeding and on the importance of attending for the follow-up appointment in 8–12 days to verify the expulsion, as she may pass the products at home. Verification is usually by ultrasound scan. If the pregnancy has continued then a surgical procedure may be carried out. It is important that the woman is aware that, if she decides to stop the treatment following the administration of mifepristone, that there is the risk of gross fetal abnormalities.

Late terminations

The main reason for a late termination is due to the delay in recognizing a pregnancy because the woman may:

- be frightened or embarrassed to seek help
- unawarene of where to seek help and advice
- have experienced slight bleeding in early pregnancy, which she assumed to be a normal period
- have assumed that a missed period could mean the beginning of the menopause.

After 12 weeks the procedure can become more difficult and an alternative method has to be decided upon by the gynaecologist to induce labour.

Surgical methods are available for the performance of a termination between 13 and 19 weeks gestation, but this varies between units. This procedure is normally carried out under a general anaesthetic, which is usually given after cervical preparation. A dilation and evacuation involves dilation of the cervix and removing the products of conception in pieces. The complications relating to this procedure may necessitate a blood transfusion or further surgery such as a hysterotomy.

Medical methods involve the use of mifepristone 600 mg orally followed 36–48 h later by vaginal prostaglandins every 3 h, with a maximum of five doses in 24 h. This method achieves a termination in 94% of cases within 24 hours. Some areas use intra-

---

> **Box 5.6** Complications associated with termination
>
> - Haemorrhage
> - Ongoing pregnancy
> - Hysterectomy
> - General anaesthetic
> - Perforation
> - Infection
> - Tubal damage
> - Incomplete termination
> - Psychological effects
> - Incompetent cervix
> - Rhesus Isoimmunisation

amniotic or oral preparations of prostaglandins as an alternative to the vaginal preparations. In terminations of greater than 20 weeks gestation it is important that there are no signs of life and this is usually achieved by injecting potassium chloride under the guidance of ultrasound in the cardiac cavity. These methods of termination can be a distressing experience for the woman as the labour is induced using the prostaglandins and she is usually offered analgesia such as Entonox, and in some areas an epidural. A general anaesthetic may be required to remove the placenta.

NURSING CARE

A termination of pregnancy at any stage is not without physical or mental complications, and therefore is a great dilemma for both the woman and the gynaecologist who will perform this (see Box 5.6).

All women need a clear explanation of the procedure and most importantly an understanding of what may occur. However, as many women may be feeling desperate to have the pregnancy terminated, the information may not absorbed and all verbal information must be allied with written advice. The nurse plays an important role throughout, as some women have no support or have told no-one they are pregnant and will require support throughout the procedure. If possible, it is advisable for the woman to have a trustworthy confidante throughout.

Following a surgical procedure the woman is nursed similarly to those who have had a D&C. In late terminations the woman requires more intensive nursing care as drug reactions can occur and she must be monitored closely for hypotension, tachycardia and vaginal loss. The woman experiencing labour requires support and care as for any labouring patient. Appropriate analgesia is important as the contractions may be distressing, this can range from oral to opiates. Once the contractions begin bed rest is recommended as progress may be difficult to assess and the woman usually receives little warning.

All products must be retained for examination by the doctor and pathologist. In most cases the placenta is retained and the **fetus** expelled. The cord should be clamped, cut and the fetus removed. A retained placenta can result in severe haemorrhage, and therefore vaginal loss – cumulative and immediate – should be monitored closely. Each unit has guidelines as to when a D&C should be scheduled if the placenta has not been expelled following medical intervention (usually 2 h). Infection can develop and signs of infection must be monitored every 4 h during the procedure. Following the expulsion or removal of the placenta the vaginal loss can be described by the woman as 'a heavy period'.

Most women are discharged within hours of aborting, or the next day. Whatever the case, clear instructions relating to their care must be given and contraception should be discussed. Contraception should ideally have been decided prior to this and, if appropriate, the chosen method given prior to discharge. If this is not possible, addresses and contact numbers of local family planning clinics should be given. Ovulation occurs as early as 18 days following a termination so a pregnancy is possible, although it is advisable that sexual intercourse should be avoided whilst bleeding due to an increased risk of infection.

DISCHARGE ADVICE

Most women undergoing a termination are discharged within hours or 1–2 days of the termination and it is important that clear, concise information is given so that they will understand their care in the few days that follow. They need to know that:

- they can resume normal activities as soon as possible, those following a general anaesthetic may do so more slowly
- vaginal bleeding may occur for up to 2 weeks and should decrease in amount
- sanitary towels, and not tampons, should be used for this bleed and during the next period to avoid any risk of infection
- some abdominal pain may occur, but should be relieved by simple analgesia at the stated dose and frequency
- they should contact their GP if they show any signs of fever, malaise or offensive vaginal discharge

- their next period should occur within the next 4–6 weeks and, in some cases, may be slightly heavier than normal. If this does not occur it may indicate an ongoing, extrauterine or a new pregnancy
- they should avoid sexual intercourse whilst bleeding, so as to reduce the risk of infection
- they must contact their GP or clinic if they are concerned about any unusual signs or symptoms
- they must return for follow-up care
- they can obtain help and support following discharge, and be given contact details.

Follow-up care

Follow-up care is an important factor in both the short and the long term. Individual areas have their own protocols, but a lot of women prefer to have this facility provided by the GP or family planning clinic, as they may not wish the return to the place were the termination took place and they prefer the familiar faces at the clinic. This is not true for some hospital environments, as the development of nurse specialist/practitioners gives a continuity of care within the hospital environment.

Follow-up care gives the woman the opportunity to discuss her physical and mental wellbeing, as no matter why she decided to have a termination she may suffer from feelings of doubt and guilt, which, as mentioned previously, can carry forward to future a pregnancy.

There is no ideal time to discuss contraception during the decision-making process, but for some women with an unwanted pregnancy this is a priority. It is important to understand what contraception was used and why it failed, or why no one method was used. Some methods may have been stopped due to misconceptions and it is an opportunity to give correct and accurate information, and details of where to obtain it at a local level. Some areas provide short-term contraception prior to discharge due to the possibility of ovulation with in 18 days postreatment. This gives immediate contraceptive cover in the short term and more leisurely discussions can then be carried out; these should include emergency contraception. If no contraception is required it is important to encourage the woman to have condoms available.

CONCLUSION

The request for a termination of pregnancy is a dilemma for the woman and also for all those professionals involved in her care. Using our skills as professionals we can help the woman to discuss her feelings and give her accurate and concise information relating to her request. We can also support her through this process, whatever the decision is, both in the short and the longer term. Fertility control is an important aspect of the health of women and however it develops there will always be unplanned pregnancies. It is essential that there is an abortion service that is easily accessible to all women, whatever their reasons for seeking it.

GLOSSARY

Adnexal: relating to the fallopian tubes and ovaries
Alloimmune: immunity against another person
Autoimmune: immunity against self
Crown–rump length (CRL): measurement of an embryo from head to bottom, used to accurately date a pregnancy in the early stages
Cytomegalovirus: a virus belonging to the same group as the herpes simplex virus. If contracted during pregnancy it may cause miscarriage or congenital abnormality
Electrocautery: searing heat treatment using electric current
Embryo: the stage of development from conceptus until the 8th week after fertilization
Falloposcopy: examination of the fallopian tube from the inside
Fetus: the developing pregnancy from the 9th week of pregnancy
Fibroid polyp: a fibroid attached to the endometrial lining by a stalk
Gestation: the period during which a fertilized egg develops into a baby that is ready to be delivered
Human chorionic gonadotrophin (hCG): hormone that is secreted from an early stage in pregnancy
Hyperemesis gravidarum: excessive vomiting in pregnancy
Hysterotomy: an incision of the womb, through either the abdominal wall or vagina
Laparoscopy: examination of the pelvic organs through a laparoscope

Listeria: a bacterial infection contracted from soft cheeses and raw meats which can lead to miscarriage
Parvovirus: a viral infection that can cause spontaneous miscarriage
Placental abruption: severe bleeding behind the placenta causing it to shear away from the uterine wall compromising the blood supply to the baby
Prostaglandin: one of a group of hormone-like substances with many actions, one of which is to cause uterine contractions
Rhesus group: a group of antigens that may or may not be present on the surface of the red blood cells. Certain antibodies in the serum react against the cells of the other
Salpingectomy: surgical removal of the fallopian tube
Salpingostomy: surgical procedure where the fallopian tube is left open to heal after cutting
Salpingotomy: surgical opening and closing of the fallopian tube
Submucous fibroid: a fibroid that protrudes into the uterine cavity
Toxoplasmosis: an infection transmitted by cat faeces which can cause miscarriage, stillbirth or damage to babies eyes and brain if contracted whilst pregnant
Trophoblastic tissue: tissue present in the early stages of embryonic development

REFERENCES

Allan A 1995 Types and causes of miscarriage. Modern Midwife 5(3):27–30
Beral V 1975 An epidemiological study of recent trends in ectopic pregnancy. British Journal of Obstetrics and Gynaecology 82:775–782
Bigrigg MA, Read MD 1991 Management of women referred to early pregnancy assessment unit: care and cost effectiveness. British Medical Journal 302:577–579
Brosens I, Gordts S, Vasquez G, Boeckx W 1984 Function retaining surgical management of ectopic pregnancy. European Journal of Obstetrics Gynaecology Reproductive Biology 18:395–402
Brumsted J, Kessler C, Gibson C, Nakajima S, Riddick DH, Gibson M 1988 A comparison of laparoscopy and laparotomy for the treatment of ectopic pregnancy. Obstetrics and Gynaecology 71(6):889–892
Brunham CB, Binns B, McDowell J, Paraskevas M 1986 Chlamydia trachomatis infection in women with ectopic pregnancy. Obstetrics and Gynaecology 67:722–726

Cacciatore B, Stenman UH, Ylostalo P 1989 Comparison of abdominal and vaginal sonography in suspected ectopic pregnancy. Obstetrics and Gynaecology 73:770–774
Cacciatore B, Stenman UH, Ylostalo P 1990 Diagnosis of ectopic pregnancy by vaginal ultrasound in combination with a discriminatory serum hCG level of 1000 IU/I (IRP). British Journal of Obstetrics and Gynaecology 97:904–908
Chow WH, Daling JR, Weiss NS, Voigt LF 1988 Maternal cigarette smoking and tubal pregnancy. Obstetrics and Gynaecology 71(2):167–170
Clifford K, Rai R, Watson H, Regan L 1994 An informative protocol for the investigation of recurrent miscarriage: experience of 500 consecutive cases. Human Reproduction 9:1328–1332
Clifford K, Rai R, Regan L 1995 Future pregnancy outcome in women with recurrent miscarriage (Abstract). Human Reproduction 10:19–20
Clifford K, Rai R, Watson H, Franks S, Regan L 1996 Does suppressing luteinising hormone secretion reduce the

miscarriage rate? Results from a randomised controlled trial. British Medical Journal 312:1508–1511

Cohen J, Mayux MJ, Guihard-Moscoto ML, Schwartz D 1986 In-vitro fertilisation and embryo transfer: a collaborative study of 1163 pregnancies on the incidence and risk factors of ectopic pregnancies. Human Reproduction 1:255–258

Crawford M, Pettit D 1986 Hydatidiform mole and choriocarcinoma. Nursing Times 82(49):38–39

DeCherney AH 1983 Ectopic pregnancy. In: Kase NG, Weingold AB (eds) Principles and practice of clinical gynaecology. New York, John Wiley, pp. 483–487

DeCrespigny L 1988 Early diagnosis of pregnancy failure with transvaginal ultrasound. American Journal of Obstetrics and Gynaecology 159:408–409

Department of Health 1991 Report on confidential enquiries into maternal deaths in the UK 1985–87. London, Her Majesty's Stationery Office

DeStephano F, Peterson HB, Layde PM, Robin GL 1982 Risk of ectopic pregnancy following tubal sterilisation. Obstetrics and Gynecology 60:326–330

Dickey R 1993 Patients' safe with expectant management. British Medical Journal 307:259

Dimitry ES 1987 Does previous appendicectomy predispose to ectopic pregnancy? – a retrospective case controlled study. Journal of Obstetrics and Gynaecology 7:221–224

Dimitry ES 1989 A ten year survey of 193 ectopic pregnancies. Journal of Obstetrics and Gynaecology 9(4):309–313

Dimitry ES, Morcos MY 1990 The increasing incidence of ectopic pregnancy: 193 cases in ten years in the Medway towns. Journal of Obstetrics and Gynaecology 10(3):181–185

Dimitry ES, Soussis I, Oskarsson RA, Winston RML 1992 The use of transvaginal ultrasound in the diagnosis of ectopic pregnancy. Journal of Obstetrics and Gynaecology 12(4):258–261

Egarter C, Husslein P 1987 Treatment of tubal pregnancy by prostaglandins. Lancet i:381–382

El-Refaey H, Hinshaw K, Henshaw RC, Smith N, Templeton AA 1992 Medical management of missed abortion and anembryonic pregnancy. British Medical Journal 305:1399

El-Refaey E, Hinshaw K, Templeton A 1993 The abortifacient effect of misoprostol in the second trimester. A randomised comparison with gemeprost in patients pre-treated with mifepristone (RU486). Human Reproduction 8:1744–1746

Enkin M, Keirse MJNC, Renfrew M, Neilson J 1995 Prevention of miscarriage. Cited in: Girling J, De Swiet M 1996 Miscarriage. Update November 394–410

Fernandez H, Rainhorn JD, Papiernik E, Bellet D, Frydman R 1988 Spontaneous resolution of ectopic pregnancy. Obstetrics and Gynaecology 71(2):171–174

Fritz MA 1988 Inadequate luteal function and recurrent abortion: Diagnosis and treatment of luteal phase deficiency. Seminar of Reproductive Endocrinology 6:129–143

Garcia AJ, Aubert JM, Sama J, Josimovich JB 1987 Expectant management of presumed ectopic pregnancy. Fertility and Sterility 48(3):395–400

Girling J, De Swiet M 1996 Miscarriage. Update November: 394–410

Grudzinskas JG, Stabile I 1993 Ectopic pregnancy: are biochemical tests at all useful? British Journal of Obstetrics and Gynaecology 100:510–511

Grudzinskas JG, Palomino M, Armstrong P, Lower A 1994 Relocation of ectopic pregnancy to the uterine cavity: a dream or a reality? British Journal of Obstetrics and Gynaecology 101:651–653

Gruft L, Bertola E, Luchini L, Azilonna C, Bigatti G, Parazzini F 1994 Determinants of reproductive prognosis after ectopic pregnancy. Human Reproduction 7:1333–1336

Hamilton-Fairley D, Kiddy D, Watson H, Peterson C, Franks S 1992 Association of moderate obesity with poor outcome in women with polycystic ovary syndrome treated with low dose gonadatrophin. British Journal of Obstetrics and Gynaecology 99:128–131

Hately W, Case J, Campbell S 1995 Establishing the death of an embryo by ultrasound – report of a public inquiry with recommendations. Ultrasound in Obstetrics and Gynaecology 5:353–357

Hay PE, Lamont RF, Taylor-Robinson D, Morgan DJ, Ison C, Pearson J 1994 Abnormal colonisation of the genital tract and subsequent preterm delivery and late miscarriage. British Medical Journal 308:295–298

Henshaw RC, Cooper K, El-Refaey H, Smith NC, Templeton AA 1993 The medical management of miscarriage: nonsurgical uterine evacuation of incomplete and inevitable spontaneous abortion. British Medical Journal 306:894–895

Hinshaw K, El-Refaey H, Rispin R, Templeton A 1995 Midtrimester termination for fetal abnormality: advantages of a new regimen using mifepristone and misoprostol. British Journal of Obstetrics and Gynaecology 102:559–560

Hughes J, Ryan M, Kinshaw K, Henshaw K, Rispin R, Templeton A 1996 The costs of treating miscarriage, a comparison of medical and surgical management. British Journal of Obstetrics and Gynaecology 103:1217–1221

Irvine LM, Hicks JL, Blair-Bell C, Setchell ME 1994 The incidence of ectopic pregnancy in the City and Hackney Health District of London 1990–1991. Journal of Obstetrics and Gynaecology 14(1):29–34

Keckstein J, Hepp S, Schneider V, Sasse V, Steiner R 1990 The contact Nd:YAG laser: a new technique for conservation of the fallopian tube in unruptured ectopic pregnancy. British Journal of Obstetrics and Gynaecology 97(4):352–356

Kim DS, Chung SR, Park MI, Kim YP 1987 Comparative review of diagnostic accuracy in tubal pregnancy: a 14 year survey of 1040 cases. Obstetrics and Gynaecology 70(4):547–554

Kirchler H, Seebacher S, Alge AA, Muller-Holzner E, Fessler S, Koller D 1993 Early diagnosis of tubal pregnancy: Changes in tubal blood flow evaluated by endovaginal colour Doppler sonography. Obstetrics and Gynaecology 82(4):561–565

Kline J, Shrout P, Stein ZA 1980 Drinking during pregnancy and spontaneous abortion. Lancet ii:76–80

Knudson UB, Hansen V, Juul S, Secher NJ 1991 Prognosis of a new pregnancy following spontaneous abortions. European Journal of Obstetric, Gynaecological and Reproductive Biology 39:31–36

Kojima E, Abe Y, Morita M, Ito M, Hirakawa S, Momose K 1990 The treatment of unruptured tubal pregnancy with intratubal methotrexate injection under laparoscopic control. Obstetrics and Gynaecology 75:723–725

Kok KP, Mahmood TA, Lees DAR 1989 A study of the incidence, the trend and the management of patients with ectopic pregnancies in the Scottish Highlands (1976–1987). Health Bulletin 47:295–303

Langer R, Bukovsky I, Herman A, Sherman D, Sadovski G, Caspi E 1982 Conservative surgery for tubal pregnancy. Fertility and Sterility 38:427–430

Lang PF, Tammussino K, Honigl W, Ralph G 1992 Treatment of unruptured tubal pregnancy by laparoscopic instillation of hyperosmolar glucose solution. American Journal of Obstetrics and Gynaecology 166(5):1378–1381

Levin AA, Schoenbaum SC, Stubblefield PG, Zimicki S, Monson RR, Ryan KJ 1982 Ectopic pregnancy and prior induced abortion. American Journal of Public Health 72:253–256

Liddell HS, Pattison NS, Zanderigo A 1991 Recurrent miscarriage – Outcome after supportive care in early pregnancy. Australia and New Zealand Journal of Obstetrics and Gynaecology 31:320–322

Llewellyn-Jones D 1990 Fundamentals of Obstetrics and Gynaecology, 5th edn. Faber and Faber, London, vol II, ch 2, p 208

Matsunga E, Shiota K 1980 Ectopic pregnancy and myoma uteri: teratogenic effects and maternal characteristics. Teratology 21:61–69

Ory SJ, Nnadi E, Herrmann R, O'Brien PS, Melton LJ 1993 Fertility after ectopic pregnancy. Fertility and Sterility 60:231–235

Out HJ, Bruinse HW, Derkson RHWM 1991 Antiphospholipid antibodies and pregnancy loss. Human Reproduction 6:889–897

Pansky M, Golan A, Bukovsky I, Caspi E 1991 Non-surgical management of tubal pregnancy. Necessity in view of the changing clinical appearance. American Journal of Obstetrics and Gynaecology 164:888–895

Parazzini F, Luchini L, La Vecchhia C, Crosignan PG 1993 Video display terminal use during pregnancy and reproductive outcome – a meta analysis. Journal of Epidemiology and Community Health 47:265–268

Paulson JD 1992 The use of carbon dioxide laser laparoscopy in the treatment of tubal ectopic pregnancies. American Journal of Obstetrics and Gynecology 167(2):382–386

Prevelic GM, Werzburger MI, Balint-Peric L, Nesic JS 1990 Inhibitory effect of sandostatin on secretion of luteinising hormone and ovarian steroids in polycystic ovary syndrome. The Lancet 336:900–903

Rai R, Regan L, Clifford K 1995 Antiphospholipid antibodies and beta 2 glycoprotein-1 in 500 women with recurrent miscarriage: results of a comprehensive screening approach. Human Reproduction 10:2001–2005

Rai R, Cohen H, Dave M, Regan L 1997 Randomised controlled trial of aspirin and aspirin plus heparin in pregnant women with recurrent miscarriage associated with phospholipid antibodies (or antiphospholipid antibodies). British Medical Journal 314:253–257

Ralph SG, Rutherford AJ, Wilson JD 1999 Influence of bacterial vaginosis on conception and miscarriage in the first trimester: cohort study. British Medical Journal 319:220–223

Regan L 1991 Recurrent miscarriage. British Medical Journal 302:543–544

Rote NS, Walter A, Lyden TW 1992 Antiphospholipid antibodies – lobsters or red herrings? American Journal of Reproductive Immunology 28:31–37

Saunders NJ 1990 Non-surgical treatment of ectopic pregnancy. British Journal of Obstetrics and Gynaecology 97(11):972–973

Semm K 1979 New methods of pelviscopy (gynaecologic laparoscopy) for myomectomy, ovariectomy, tubectomy and adnectomy. Endoscopy 11:85–89

Shefras J, Farquharson RG 1996 Bone density studies in pregnant women receiving heparin. European Journal of Obstetrics, Gynaecology and Reproductive Biology 65:171–174

Sherman D, Langer R, Sadovsky G, Bukovsky I, Caspi E 1982 Improved fertility following ectopic pregnancy. Fertility and Sterility 37:497–502

Simon C, Martinez L, Pardo F, Tortajada M, Pellicer A 1991 Müllerian defects in women with normal reproductive outcome. Fertility and Sterility 56:1192–1193

Stabile I, Cambell S, Grudzinskas JG 1987 Ultrasonic Assessment of complications during first trimester of pregnancy. Lancet ii:1237–1240

Stabile I 1996 Ectopic pregnancy: diagnosis and management. Cambridge University Press, Cambridge.

Stirrat GM 1990a Recurrent miscarriage I: definition and epidemiology. Lancet 336:673–675

Stirrat GM 1990b Recurrent miscarriage II: clinical associations, causes and management. Lancet 336:728–733

Stovall TG, Ling FW, Buster JE 1990 Reproductive performance after methotrexate treatment of ectopic pregnancy. American Journal of Obstetrics and Gynecology 162(6):1620–1624

Thorburn J, Philipson M, Lindblom B 1988 Fertility after ectopic pregnancy in relation to background factors and surgical treatment. Fertility and Sterility 49(4):595–601

Timbers KA, Feinberg RF 1997 Recurrent pregnancy loss: a review. Nurse Practitioner Forum 8:77–88

Turnbull A, Tindal VR, Beard RW, Robson G, Dawson IMP, Cloake EP, Ashley JSA, Botting A 1989 Report on confidential enquiries into maternal deaths in England and Wales 1982–1984, London. Her Majesty's Stationery Office, London, pp. 41–46

Westrom L, Bengtsson LPH, Mardh PA 1981 Incidence, trends and risks of ectopic pregnancy. British Journal of Obstetrics and Gynaecology 82:775–782

Whyte A 1995 Fortifying the pregnancy message. Health Visitor 68(10):397–398

Wilson JC 1989 A prospective New Zealand study of fertility after removal of copper intra uterine contraceptive devices for conception and because of complications: a four year study. American Journal of Obstetrics and Gynecology 160:391–396

Winston RML 1980 Microsurgery of the fallopian tube: from fantasy to reality. Fertility and Sterility 34:521

Wolf GC, Horger EO 3rd 1995 Indications for examination of spontaneous abortion specimens: A reassessment. American Journal of Obstetrics and Gynecology 173(5):1364–1368

Ylostalo P, Cacciatore B, Sjoberg J 1992 Expectant management of ectopic pregnancy. Obstetrics and Gynecology 80:345–348

FURTHER READING: MISCARRIAGE

Kohner N, Henley A 1995 When a baby dies. The experience of late miscarriage, stillbirth and neonatal death, 2nd edn. Pandora Press, London

Moulder C 1990 Miscarriage: women's experiences and needs. Pandora Press, London

Oakley A, McPherson A, Roberts H 1984 Miscarriage. Fontana William Collins & Sons, London

Regan L 1997 Miscarriage what every woman needs to know, 1st edn. A positive new approach. Bloomsbury Publishing plc, London

SANDS 1995 Pregnancy loss and the death of a baby. Guidelines for professionals. Stillbirth and Neonatal Death Society, London

Tschudin V 1991 Counselling skills for nurses, 3rd edn. Baillière Tindall, London

FURTHER READING: EARLY PREGNANCY ASSESSMENT UNITS

Child Bereavement Trust Information Pack
This information pack is for everyone, whether a parent or a professional, who is concerned about the emotional support available to grieving families after the death of a baby or child.

Death at birth – miscarriage, stillbirth, neonatal death and termination for abnormality
A two-part training video for healthcare professionals, with Trainer's Guide. Produced by Jenni Thomas and Bradbury Williams and available from the Child Bereavement Trust.

FURTHER READING: TERMINATION OF PREGNANCY

Chamberlain GVP 1995 Gynaecology by Ten Teachers, 16th edn. Arnold, London, pp. 208–212

Henshaw RC et al 1993 Comparison of medical abortion with surgical vacuum aspiration: women's preferences and acceptability of treatment. British Medical Journal 307:714–717

Hoechst Marion Roussel 1996 A guide to the use of Mifegyne in clinical practice.

Morgan D 1990 Blackstone's Guide to the Human Fertilisation and Embryology Act.

Ney PG 1987 Helping patients cope with pregnancy loss. Contempory Obstetrics/Gynaecology June: 117–130

Paterson C 1998 Induced abortion. Trends in Urology Gynaecology and Sexual Health, part 2. May/June: 36–41.

Royal College of Obstetricians and Gynaecologists 1997 Guidelines on Induced Abortion.

Royal College of Nursing 1992 Issues in nursing and health. Nurses and Abortion (11)

Termination of first trimester termination 1998 Drug and Therapeutics Bulletin 36 (2):13–15

USEFUL ADDRESSES

Abortion Anonymous
Tel: 020 7350 2229
Provides free counselling services

ARC (Antenatal Results and Choices) formerly known as SATFA (Support Around Termination For Abnormality)
73 Charlotte Street, London W1P 1LB
Helpline: 020 7631 0285
Admin: 020 7631 0280
Helping parents who discover that their unborn baby is abnormal

British Association for Counselling
1 Regent's Place, Rugby, CV21 2PJ
Tel: 01788 578328
Provides information on where to get counselling locally

British Victims of Abortion Helpline
Tel: 0845 6038501 (7 p.m.–10 p.m. 7 days per week)

Child Bereavement Trust
Harleyford Estate, Henley Road, Marlow, Buckinghamshire SL7 2DX
Tel/fax: 01628 488101
A charity that cares for bereaved families by offering training and support to the professional carer

Cruse Bereavement Care
126 Sheen Road, Richmond, Surrey TW9 1UR
Cruse Bereavement Line: 020 8332 7227
Provides a local contact for counselling

Foresight

28 The Paddock, Godalming, Surrey GU7 1XD
Tel: 01483 427839
Offers information and leaflets on promoting optimal
health in both parents prior to conception of a
child

LUPUS UK

1 Eastern Road, Romford, Essex RM1 3NH
Tel: 01708 731251
Fax: 01708 731252
Offers a full list of leaflets and publications on both lupus
and Hughes syndrome

Miscarriage Association

c/o Clayton Hospital, Northgate, Wakefield, West
Yorkshire WF1 3JS
Tel: 01924 200799
Fax: 01924 298834
Offers support, information and leaflets on all aspects of
miscarriage and ectopic pregnancy

SANDS (Stillbirth and Neonatal Death Society)

28 Portland Place, London W1N 4DE
Helpline: 020 7436 5881
Admin: 020 7436 7940
Offers support and information for parents whose baby is
born dead or dies soon after birth. Offers training for
professionals

Toxoplasmosis Trust (TTT)

61 Colier Street, London N1 9BE
Offers information on all aspects of toxoplasmosis from
primary prevention and follow-up to treatment of an
infected newborn

6

Menstrual disorders

Elizabeth Gangar

Disorders associated with the menstrual cycle are amongst the most common complaints seen in primary care. They also constitute a large part of the workload within the gynaecology outpatient department in hospital. In fact, menstrual disorders are the second most common cause of hospital referral (Coulter et al 1989).

Menstruation has long been a taboo subject with many myths associated with it. In many cultures it is considered unclean or sacred and even in our own society, until recent times, girls were encouraged not to take a bath or wash their hair during menstruation. As a result, menstruation is not a subject generally discussed. It is therefore often difficult for a woman to distinguish whether her cycle is normal or not. It is only when her menstrual pattern changes in such a way as to affect her quality of life, that she may seek help. Thus, 'menstrual disorders' can be highly subjective, which can make assessments and treatments difficult.

The purpose of this chapter is to look at the most common problems including amenorrhoea, **dysmenorrhea**, menorrhagia and postmenopausal bleeding.

AMENORRHOEA

Amenorrhoea is the absence or stopping of menstruation and is frequently divided into primary and secondary amenorrhoea.

Primary amenorrhoea is defined as no menstruation by the age of 14 accompanied by poor growth and the failure of the sex characteristics development, or when there is no menstruation by the age of 16 but where growth and sexual development is normal. Secondary amenorrhoea is defined as the absence of menstruation for 6 months in a woman who has previously menstruated.

Causes of amenorrhoea

There is considerable overlap between the causes of primary and secondary amenorrhoea (Box 6.1). It is important, therefore, that the above categories are not adhered to too rigidly. Primary amenorrhoea was covered in Chapter 2 and this chapter therefore concentrates on secondary amenorrhoea, which includes the following.

Weight loss

Amenorrhoea may occur when there is a loss of more than 10 kg in weight. For regular menstruation to be maintained, 17% of body weight needs to comprise fat (Frisch et al 1973). Amenorrhoea may occur in young women obsessed with their body image but may also occur in those who exercise strenuously, such as dancers. Oestrogen levels can be profoundly depressed to levels within the menopausal range. Normal menstruation usually returns when the weight increases. However, if there is prolonged amenorrhoea osteoporosis becomes a significant risk and hormone replacement therapy (HRT) should be considered.

Postoral contraceptive

The combined oestrogen/progestogen oral contraceptive pill does not predispose to amenorrhoea once the pill has been stopped. However, there are a small number of women who remain anovulatory after stopping the pill (Shearman 1986). These women appear to be those who had a tendency to irregular cycles prior to commencing the oral contraceptive, those who have lost a substantial amount of weight or who have undertaken a vigorous exercise programme whilst on the medication. Spontaneous menstruation usually occurs within 6 months of stopping the pill. However, it is important not to assume that it is an 'after effect' of the pill and other possible underlying causes should be excluded after 6 months of amenorrhoea. In the absence of any disease process, this type of amenorrhoea will respond well to ovulation induction with medications such as clomiphene if pregnancy is desired (see Chapter 3).

Following the use of the injectable contraceptives such as Depo-Provera, the resumption of menstruation may be delayed with transient infertility. The long-term consequences of a low oestradiol level and amenorrhoea with depot contraception, such as the possible effects on bone and the cardiovascular system, is controversial and continues to be researched and debated.

Polycystic ovarian syndrome

Polycystic ovarian syndrome (PCOS) is the presence of hyperandrogenism with chronic anovulation in women without a specific underlying disease of either the adrenal or pituitary gland (see Chapter 8).

Asherman's syndrome

Secondary amenorrhoea can occur due to the formation of uterine adhesions. This may occur following a

---

Box 6.1 Main causes of amenorrhoea

	Primary	**Overlap between both categories**	**Secondary**
Disorders of anatomy of vagina and/or uterus	Absent uterus and/or cryptomenorrhoea Testicular feminization syndrome	Vagina	Asherman's syndrome
Disorders of the hypothalamic–pituitary axis	Kallman's syndrome	Weight loss Hyperprolactinaemia Thyroid function defect	Postoral combined contraceptive
Disorders of the ovaries	Chromosomal abnormalities, e.g. Turner's syndrome Gonadal agenesis	Polycystic ovarian syndrome	Ovarian failure
Others		Pregnancy Emotional upset Strenuous exercise Radiotherapy Chemotherapy	

Case study: Debbie

Debbie, a 32-year-old woman, was referred by her GP to the gynaecology clinic with an 8-month history of amenorrhoea. A history revealed that the amenorrhoea stemmed from the birth of her second child 9 months earlier. Following an uneventful normal vaginal delivery, she had heavy vaginal bleeding for 2 weeks. On ultrasound scan, retained products of conception were observed and an evacuation of retained products of conception was performed. Since then she had not had any bleeding. Debbie had decided not to breastfeed her second child as she had problems feeding her first child. The amenorrhoea was not therefore due to hormonal suppression. Repeated pregnancy tests had been consistently negative.

Pelvic examination revealed an anteverted mobile uterus, which felt slightly enlarged and tender on palpation. After a long discussion, it was decided that a hysteroscopy was required with a possible diagnosis of Asherman's syndrome. At hysteroscopy, Asherman's syndrome was confirmed with the presence of multiple synechiae (intrauterine adhesions). These were divided laparoscopically and an intrauterine contraceptive device was inserted. The coil was inserted to keep the uterine walls apart and to prevent further adhesion formation. Ethinyloestradiol 30 μg to be taken daily was prescribed to rebuild the endometrium and to assist regeneration.

Postoperative recovery was uneventful and an appointment was made for 6 weeks later. At this appointment, Debbie reported that she had experienced no bleeding on the ethinyloestradiol and a progesterone, in the form of norethisterone 5 mg was prescribed. This was to be taken after 8 weeks of ethinyloestradiol to oppose the oestrogen and to induce a withdrawal bleed. A repeat appointment was made for 4 weeks' time.

At this visit Debbie was able to report that she had had a normal but slightly heavier period following the norethisterone. Pelvic examination revealed a normal, non-tender uterus. Debbie was prescribed the combined oral contraceptive, Marvelon, to maintain regular withdrawal bleeds and to ensure a healthy uterus. Debbie was instructed to continue with the Marvelon for a further 3 months at which time the coil would be removed.

Debbie was reviewed 3 months later when she reported that all was well and she had normal regular withdrawal bleeds on the Marvelon. The coil was therefore removed, which was an uneventful procedure. Debbie continued on the Marvelon for contraception under the care of the local Family Planning Clinic.

---

vigorous curettage where the endometrium has been destroyed or following a severe uterine infection. The most common example is following an evacuation for retained products of conception, especially if infection is present. To treat this problem, the adhesions first need to be divided hysteroscopically. On hysteroscopic examination multiple **synechiae** (adhesions) will be evident (see Plate 7). The insertion of an intrauterine contraceptive device is required to prevent reformation and the administration of an oral oestrogen such as ethinyl oestradiol for several weeks is required to rebuild the endometrium.

Ovarian failure

Ovarian failure is the presence of high levels of follicle stimulating hormone (FSH) and luteinizing hormone (LH) in conjunction with amenorrhoea, with or without other symptoms such as hot flushes and night sweats. Unfortunately, ovarian failure can occur at any age but prior to the age of 45 it is considered to be a premature menopause. There are three important factors to consider:

1. the emotional and psychological aspects
2. future fertility (see Chapter 3)
3. the increased risk of heart disease and osteoporosis (see Chapter 19).

Women who experience premature ovarian failure should be referred to a specialist clinic where the above issues may be addressed with the expertise that they require.

Hyperprolactinaemia

Excessive levels of prolactin in the blood due to the disruption of normal secretion of prolactin from the pituitary. These high levels of prolactin interfere with the menstrual cycle by suppressing normal pulsatile secretion of gonadotrophin releasing hormone (GnRH). Hyperprolactinaemia is most commonly and most importantly caused by prolactin-secreting tumours of the anterior pituitary. Other causes consist of:

- **idiopathic** (in 40% of cases)
- stress
- hypothyroidism
- endocrine side-effects of some drugs, i.e. metoclopramide, phenothiazines, cimetidine, haloperidol and methyldopa
- PCOS can be associated with a mild elevation of prolactin.

The clinical features of hyperprolactinaemia consist of amenorrhoea or **oligomenorrhoea**, breast enlargement and galactorrhoea. There is a significantly raised prolactin estimation, which should be repeated to avoid

Table 6.1 Laboratory findings in major causes of amenorrhoea

	FSH	LH	Prolactin	Testosterone	Karyotype
Hyperprolactinaemia	Normal	Normal	High	Normal	Normal
Premature menopause	Very high	High	Normal	Normal	Normal
Polycystic ovarian syndrome	Normal	Slightly raised	Normal or slightly raised	Slightly raised	Normal
'Hypothalamic'	Normal	Normal	Normal	Normal	Normal
Turner's syndrome	High	High	Normal	Normal	45, XO or mosaics
Testicular feminization	High	High	Normal	High	46, XY

From McPherson A (ed) 1993 Women's problems in general practice, 3rd edn. Oxford University Press, Oxford. With permission.

stress related elevations. In cases of marked or persistent elevations a computerized tomography (CT) scan of the pituitary gland is required. Where a patient complains of headaches or visual field disturbance, urgent investigations are necessary.

Management of hyperprolactinaemia

Medical. The treatments of choice are dopamine agonist drugs such as bromocriptine and newer preparations such as cabergoline and quinagoline. Quinagoline is longer-acting and can be taken on a once daily regimen and is therefore better tolerated. These will suppress the secretion of prolactin and correct the oestrogen deficiency. This will restore normal ovulation, therefore restoring menstruation and fertility. There is no contraindication to pregnancy although consultant care would be recommended. Bromocriptine will also reduce the size of most small tumours (known as microadenomas). These microadenomas tend to grow slowly and often regress spontaneously.

Surgical. Surgery and radiotherapy may be required in patients with large tumours (known as macroadenomas), particularly if there is visual field disturbance or severe headaches.

Investigations of amenorrhoea

The basic investigations consist of luteinizing hormone (LH), follicle stimulating hormone (FSH), oestradiol, serum prolactin levels, thyroid function, free testosterone (Table 6.1). Other less common tests to help establish the diagnosis would include a karyotype blood test where a chromosomal abnormality is likely on clinic examination, pelvic ultrasound scan and progesterone challenge test. The progesterone challenge test is performed in cases of amenorrhoea to check the endogenous oestrogen level. It consists of a progestogen, such as medroxy-progesterone or norethisterone, taken daily for approximately 10 days. The occurrence of a withdrawal bleed on completion of the course indicates that the endometrium is reactive and the outflow tract patent.

OLIGOMENORRHOEA

This is defined as the occurrence of menses on only five or fewer occasions in a year. The causes and management are as for secondary amenorrhoea.

DYSMENORRHOEA

Dysmenorrhoea, or painful periods, can be divided into primary or secondary. Primary dysmenorrhoea is a common problem affecting approximately 50% of young women. It is rarely associated with any pelvic pathology. The first few periods following **menarche** are irregular and anovulatory and are usually painless. Dysmenorrhoea becomes more common when a regular ovulatory pattern is established. A further discussion may be found in Chapter 2. It is a common complaint affecting most women at some stage of their life but many women never seek medical attention. They feel it is a trivial problem, despite causing significant distress and inconvenience.

Causes

An increased production of prostaglandins gives rise to uterine hypercontractility and hence painful contractions. The reason for the production of prostaglandins is unknown. Although considered a hormone, prostaglandins act locally via tissue fluid rather than travelling via the circulation. Most cells release prostaglandins as part of the inflammatory response (Box 6.2).

Box 6.2 Action of prostaglandins

- Stimulate smooth muscle in the uterine wall to contract.
- Increase the secretion of pepsin, mucus and hydrochloric acid in the stomach.
- Stimulate platelet aggregation and promote clot formation.
- Induce pain, inflammation and fever.

Symptoms

The symptoms of dysmenorrhoea include:

- lower abdominal colicky cramps
- pain occurring during the first 24–36 hours of menses
- backache
- occasional nausea, vomiting and diarrhoea
- occasional fainting and headaches.

Dysmenorrhoea is not usually associated with menorrhagia. Secondary dysmenorrhoea usually commences in adult life and is frequently associated with pelvic pathology such as endometriosis, adenomyosis, pelvic inflammatory disease and endometrial polyps, and less commonly with fibroids, the intrauterine contraceptive device and cervical stenosis. It frequently begins prior to the onset of the period and increases with intensity as the onset of period starts. This corresponds to a further surge of prostaglandin as endometrial shedding begins and the **myometrium** contracts, producing the most severe symptoms.

Investigations

Initially a full medical history to ascertain whether the symptoms are suggestive of primary or secondary dysmenorrhoea. A laparoscopy and/or hysteroscopy may be useful in making a diagnosis.

Treatment

This very much depends on the underlying cause. Once the correct diagnosis has been made the appropriate treatment may be introduced. Where there is no existing pathology the symptoms can be controlled by medical therapies such as the oral contraceptive or anti-inflammatory drugs. In women who require contraception, the oral combined contraceptive can be useful in controlling dysmenorrhoea. This can be used continuously by taking the pill without a break for three packets at a time, thus producing a withdrawal every three cycles. It inhibits ovulation, reduces menstrual flow and in turn reduces pain. Depo-Provera may also be used in severe cases of dysmenorrhoea to induce amenorrhoea but caution is required regarding the hypo-oestrogenic effects on the skeletal and cardiovascular systems.

Oral contraceptives may not be a suitable remedy for those who do not require or wish to use contraception. The non-steroidal anti-inflammatory drugs (NSAIDs) may be an acceptable alternative. These act by blocking the inflammatory response by inhibiting the release of an enzyme required in prostaglandin formation. The most common NSAID is aspirin. The advantages of aspirin are that it is easily accessible, well known and effective in controlling period pain. Its main disadvantage is its short half-life. It is metabolized rapidly and needs to be taken at regular intervals – every few hours – to remain effective. Gastrointestinal irritation with bleeding is associated with aspirin when taken in large doses and women should be aware of this. Mefenamic acid (Ponstan) is also useful. It is as effective as aspirin but is effective for longer (see p. 102). Anti-inflammatory drugs such as ibuprofen are also effective in the treatment of dysmenorrhoea.

As already mentioned, many women never seek medical advice and those that do may have been told that there is no help available. However, the nurse plays an important part in offering practical advice such as taking regular analgesia prior to the onset of periods, use of a hot water bottle or by being a friend – a familiar face who will listen, reassure and advise.

MENORRHAGIA

Normal menstruation is defined as menstruation occurring every 21–35 days and lasting 2–7 days with a loss of between 35 and 40 ml of blood. Menorrhagia is defined as menstrual loss of 80 ml or more. It is a common complaint experienced by up to 30% of women. One in 20 women between the ages of 30 and 49 consults their GP each year, resulting in more than 700 000 prescriptions (Coulter 1994), costing several million pounds. These figures have increased in recent years and it could be said that women in today's society are, understandably, less willing to suffer unacceptable bleeding. Changes in reproductive behaviour have led to an increase in menstrual cycles per woman per lifetime, giving rise to an increased incidence of menstrual problems (Rees & Turnbull 1989). In addition to fewer pregnancies and less breastfeeding, women are also remaining on the oral contraceptive pill for several years. Whilst on the pill the periods are light and regular, and natural, i.e. physiological, periods appear unacceptably heavy when the pill is stopped.

Menorrhagia is a very subjective complaint, which might not be confirmed if all menstrual loss was measured. Several studies have shown that the correlation between measured menstrual loss and the patient's perceived loss was not accurate. Cameron found that 50% of women who complained of menorrhagia actually had measured loss within the normal range (Cameron 1989). Accurate history into the amount of sanitary protection used, whether or not clots and flooding occurs and the frequency and regularity of menses may help diagnose menorrhagia. However, there is no simple means to quantify the patient's assessment of her loss. So how is a diagnosis made? Often it is made retrospectively after an evaluation of the prescribed treatment. Perhaps this is why the treatment of menorrhagia is frequently so unsatisfactory and why approximately 25 000 apparently normal uteri are removed each year (Coulter 1994).

Causes

The common causes of menorrhagia are listed in Box 6.3. However, in 60% of cases there is no organic cause for the excessive menstrual loss. This is referred to as dysfunctional uterine bleeding (DUB). In most cases of menorrhagia regular ovulatory cycles occur. Anovulatory cycles usually occur at either end of the menstrual life, i.e. soon after the menarche and prior to the menopause. However, when anovulation does occur the proliferative effect of progesterone on the endometrium is lost, thus putting women at risk of hyperplasia and endometrial carcinoma. Bleeding occurring in these types of anovulatory cycles usually occurs after a period of amenorrhoea followed by heavy persistent bleeding. When DUB occurs in ovulatory cycles the bleeding tends to be regular, heavy and associated with dysmenorrhoea. There is usually no abnormality of the hypothalamic–pituitary axis but menorrhagia is related to disorders of prostaglandins and their receptors within the endometrium. To understand this further we must look at the normal mechanisms that occur during menstruation.

Mechanism of normal menstruation

In normal menstruation (Box 6.4) approximately half of the loss is blood. The rest is made up of fragments of endometrial tissue, epithelial tissue and mucus. This menstrual blood is unusual – it does not clot readily due to a lytic substance produced by the endometrium. When the menstrual loss is excessive the amount of this lysin substance may be inadequate and the passage of large clots may occur. These clots are also unusual, they contain minimal fibrin and therefore tend to form in the vagina and not in the uterus.

It should be noted that anything that disturbs the equilibrium between the formation of the platelet plugs in the spiral arterioles and the lysin may result in excessive menstrual loss.

Box 6.3 Causes of menorrhagia

Gynaecological causes
- endometriosis/adenomyosis
- pelvic inflammatory disease
- uterine tumours – polyps, fibroids, endometrial hyperplasia, endometrial and cervical carcinoma
- intrauterine contraceptive device.

Endocrine and haematological causes
- thyroid disorders
- von Willebrand's disease
- idiopathic thrombocytopenia
- long-term anticoagulants.

Others
- poststerilization
- psychological.

Box 6.4 Physiology of menstruation

- Spiral arterioles are present in the uterus.
- These arterioles grow upwards and become more superficial with the endometrium during the proliferative phase.
- Following ovulation and formation of the corpus luteum, these spiral arterioles become dilated.
- If pregnancy does not occur, the corpus luteum starts to atrophy and spasm of the arterioles occurs.
- The bloodflow through the arterioles decreases and results in ischaemia.
- The resulting ischaemia causes the endometrium to shed down to the basal layer.

Gynaecological causes of menorrhagia

Gynaecological causes account for 35% of menorrhagia and include endometrial polyps, fibroids and endometrial hyperplasia.

Endometrial polyps (adenoma)

These are benign growths that protrude into the uterine cavity or endocervix (endocervical polyps). Endometrial polyps are a common disorder that can cause intermenstrual, postcoital and postmenopausal bleeding. They are frequently asymptomatic but may be associated with a vaginal discharge, especially in the case of endocervical polyps. Polyps are frequently multiple, especially before the menopause, and may be a component of endometrial hyperplasia.

Treatment. They are easily removed by dilatation and curettage (D&C). Direct vision with hysteroscopy is of value. A polyp may elude curettage particularly in the postmenopausal woman where there may only be a single polyp present. All polyps should be sent for histological examination to exclude malignant change.

Fibroids (leiomyoma)

These are the most common tumours of the female genital tract (see Plates 8 and 9). They occur in 20% of women over the age of 35 with a peak incidence between 35 and 45 years. Fibroids are benign tumours derived from fibrous and muscular tissue. They can vary in size and are usually multiple in number. They are generally firm but can be soft if they begin to degenerate. Malignant change within a fibroid is rare (less than 0.5% of cases) and growth is oestrogen dependent.

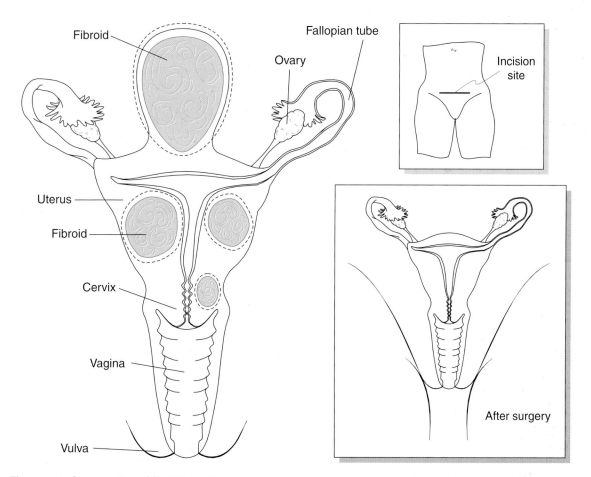

Figure 6.1 Common sites of fibroids and illustration of before and after myomectomy. From Stafford M 1996, Patient Pictures, Gynaecology Health Press, Oxford, with permission.

Sites of origin. Fibroids can occur throughout the female genital tract (Fig. 6.1):

- intramural – occurring within the muscle layer of the uterine wall
- subserous – projecting from the peritoneal surface of the uterus, they may become pedunculated
- Intraligamental – occurring between layers of ligaments, e.g. the broad ligament
- Submucous – occurring with the submucous layer indenting the uterine cavity and distorting the endometrium, these can become polypoidal.

Signs and symptoms. Most of the time, fibroids will go unnoticed and remain symptomless. Frequently they are discovered during a routine check-up or during investigations for other problems – most do not cause any problems. However, there may be increased menstrual loss caused by submucous fibroids distorting the endometrium. If multiple submucous fibroids occur then menstruation can be excessive. Intermenstrual bleeding, dysmenorrhoea and vaginal discharge can occur with polypoid fibroids, especially if these enter the cervical canal. Abdominal swelling or pressure effects may occur as the enlarging fibroids cause bladder and bowel symptoms. Large fibroids may also interfere with venous return and cause peripheral swelling. Fibroids do not usually cause pain unless they have become complicated (see Boxes 6.5 and 6.6). Degeneration occurs in most moderate to large-sized fibroids to some extent. Hyaline degeneration of the connective tissue and blood vessels can occur, in which the tumour becomes painful, enlarged and soft. Necro or red degeneration typically occurs during pregnancy. It is caused by localized death or infarct of the tissue in the centre of the fibroid. The fibroid suddenly enlarges and is very painful. This is particularly alarming for the pregnant woman and is frequently mistaken for an obstetric emergency such as placenta abruption. Pain from fibroids can also occur with malignant change. As previously mentioned, this is rare but in these cases the fibroids will be found to have enlarged and will be tender.

Treatment. The treatment of fibroids is largely influenced by the extent of the problem they are causing and the size of the fibroids. Other factors to be considered are the woman's age, i.e. is she near the menopause, and future fertility issues. Conservative measures are appropriate if the fibroids are small, asymptomatic, are found during pregnancy, if pregnancy likely and either near or postmenopause. Surgical options are usually indicated if the fibroids are very large, growing rapidly, causing problems such as anaemia and pain or if they are likely to complicate future fertility or future pregnancies (see, p. 101) (Box 6.7).

Myomectomy or 'shelling out' of the fibroids is usually performed in women who have not completed their families or in whom hysterectomy is not acceptable. Myomectomy, particularly if multiple fibroids are present, carries a significant risk of haemorrhage during surgery. It should be considered a major operation with pre- and postoperative care as for hysterectomy (see Chapter 20). Unfortunately, fibroids can recur after myomectomy but the procedure may allow time for conception to take place.

Resection of fibroids such as submucous or intramural may be via an operating hysteroscope with direct vision or via a laparoscopy. This reduces morbidity, i.e. there is no vertical or Pfannenstiel incision, a minimal stay in hospital and a return to normal lifestyle within 7–10 days.

GnRH analogues serve a valuable role in reducing fibroid size and vascularity. Either prior to a surgical

---

Box 6.5 Points to note regarding fibroids

- Fibroids are more common in nulliparous women or those with small families.
- They are common in black women.
- They become more frequent as women get older but do not start after the menopause.
- They are not related to any forms of contraception.
- There is no known means of prevention.

Box 6.6 Complications of fibroids

- Torsion of pedunculated fibroid.
- Haemorrhage.
- Infection.
- Degeneration.
- Calcification.
- Malignant change.

Box 6.7 Effects of fibroids on pregnancy

- Subfertility.
- Abortion and preterm labour.
- Malpresentation.
- Obstructed labour – rare.
- Delayed involution postpartum and risk of postpartum haemorrhage.

procedure to make surgery easier or to shrink fibroids to give a window of opportunity for conception to occur. Unfortunately, the shrinkage is only sustained during therapy and for a limited time thereafter. GnRH analogues act by suppressing LH and FSH, thereby making the ovaries 'dormant'. Oestrogen levels become very low and menopausal symptoms of hot flushes and night sweats are common; osteopenia also occurs. These effects can be minimized by HRT 'add-back'.

Fibroid embolization or uterine artery embolization is a technique in which both uterine arteries are catheterized and injected with microparticles, thus impairing the blood supply to the fibroid and causing it to shrink and the symptoms to resolve. Arterial embolization was first reported in the late 1970s when postpartum and postoperative haemorrhages were arrested using this technique (Oliver et al 1979, Pai et al 1980). Since then trials have been instituted in Paris, the United Kingdom and the United States into the treatment of fibroids by this method. It remains a treatment under development and evaluation and cannot be recommended as standard.

Preoperative evaluation for embolization is necessary and includes a thorough history and examination. An endometrial biopsy to exclude endometrial carcinoma and an ultrasound scan to exclude any pre-existing pathology, and in particular to rule out ovarian enlargement and for postoperative comparison, are required. Patients on GnRH analogues are required to stop therapy for a minimum of 6 weeks prior to the procedure (although the reason is unclear, the procedure appears to be less effective in those on GnRH analogues). Patients are counselled regarding the risks, benefits and alternative treatment, including the advantages and disadvantages of myomectomy, hysterectomy and hormonal therapies. Fertility issues should also be discussed. Although pregnancies have been reported following embolization, women should be informed that embolization may have a negative impact on their fertility (Goodwin & Walker 1998).

The procedure is performed under a local anaesthetic, administered into the right groin for the femoral puncture. In addition, intravenous sedation, intravenous antibiotics and an added analgesia for postoperative pain relief are administered. Postoperative pain can be fairly intense, probably due to ischaemia, and careful pain management is necessary. Non-steroidal anti-inflammatories and an antiemetic are also prescribed. Patients are usually discharged home with an oral, broad-spectrum antibiotic to reduce the risk of infection and consequent readmission.

Box 6.8 Possible complications following artery embolization

- Groin haematoma.
- Crampy pelvic/abdominal pain.
- Nausea and vomiting.
- Uterine/pelvic infection.
- Ischaemia/tissue infarction.
- Postembolization syndrome characterized by malaise, anorexia, nausea and vomiting, fever and raised white blood cell count.

Recovery is fairly quick and usually requires only a day or two in hospital. Normal physical activity is usually achieved within a fortnight and postoperative follow-up is at 6 weeks and 6 months to include a repeat ultrasound scan.

Uterine embolization appears to be a promising method for treating symptoms relating to fibroids. Clinical success is considered when the symptoms, i.e. pain, bleeding and pressure symptoms, improve so as to require no further operative therapy. However, it is not without its complications or risks (Box 6.8) but has the advantages of potential fertility preservation, avoidance of surgical risks and shorter hospitalization.

Endometrial hyperplasia

This occurs when the proliferative phase of the menstrual cycle, under the influence of oestrogen, does not transform to the secretory phase under the influence of progesterone. There is an overgrowth of the endometrium due to excessive cell formation and hyperplastic changes can occur. A woman is at risk of developing endometrial hyperplasia when either endogenous or exogenous oestrogens are stimulating the proliferative effects without being opposed by the protective effects of progesterone. This can occur when there are anovulatory cycles in cases such as PCOS or during the perimenopause, or in cases of unopposed oestrogen replacement therapy. It is now well known that women receiving HRT who have an intact uterus must receive a continuous or cyclical progestogen to prevent hyperplasia. Endometrial hyperplasia, if left untreated, is liable to progress to malignancy.

Intrauterine contraceptive device (IUCD)

The menstrual loss can increase significantly after insertion of an intrauterine contraceptive device (IUCD) by as much as 50%. This is often the main reason for requests for removal, although bleeding may be less of a problem with the use of smaller-sized devices. Historically, IUCDs have not been recommended for women suffering with heavy periods. However, with the introduction of the progesterone releasing device, these women are now being offered this as a form of treatment for heavy periods, in addition to a reliable form of contraception (see p. 103).

Investigations into menorrhagia

A comprehensive history and examination is essential and a menstrual diary may be useful. Further investigations are often required to confirm diagnosis and exclude serious pathology.

History

Type of loss: is it regular, cyclical, irregular, intermenstrual or postcoital? Type of contraception: possibly the IUCD, depot progesterone, oral contraceptive. Systemic disorders such as thyroid, diabetes, anticoagulant therapy.

Examination

Observe general health. Check for the possibility of anaemia. Give a bimanual examination for uterine enlargement, fibroids and ovarian cysts and use a speculum for cervical disease, protruding polyps or erosions.

Cervical smear

Particularly important with intermenstrual or postcoital bleeding, which raises the possibility of endometrial or cervical carcinoma.

Blood tests

Haemoglobin for anaemia, thyroid function and possible glucose. Endocrine check to determine hormonal status.

Ultrasound scan

Ultrasound examination can be particularly helpful, especially if there is evidence of uterine enlargement on pelvic examination or if, due to obesity, pelvic examination is difficult. The size and position of the ovaries may be observed and, in specific cases, the blood flow and vascularity can be measured when early ovarian disease is suspected or as a screening process. The endometrial thickness can be measured – the unstimulated postmenopausal endometrium is thin and atrophic. A thick endometrium measured in this case requires further investigation.

Endometrial biopsy

An endometrial biopsy (EB) is a diagnostic procedure to exclude endometrial hyperplasia and malignancy. It can replace the need to perform a dilatation and curettage (D&C) in most cases and has the advantages of a lower complication rate and being more cost effective. There is no therapeutic value in an EB unless, for example, an endometrial polyp is removed during the procedure. Indications for an EB are abnormal bleeding, including increased menstrual loss that is unresponsive to prescribed medical therapy, intermenstrual, postcoital or post menopausal bleeding. There is no requirement for routine EBs for women taking HRT but it is indicated in cases such as those who develop irregular bleeding patterns, a change in withdrawal bleeds or breakthrough bleeding. It is also indicated in a woman who is amenorrhoeic on 'no bleed' HRT and starts to bleed or does not stop bleeding after 4–6 months of taking continuous combined HRT. Bleeding should stop after a few weeks on this type of therapy. It is also indicated in women on unopposed oestrogens who have an intact uterus and who required annual biopsies irrespective of bleeding. Although this is not regular practice in the UK due to the significant increased risk of endometrial malignancy (Paganini-Hill et al 1989), it is occasionally reserved for women who cannot tolerate progestogens. It could be said that there is no place for this method of treatment with the introduction of new progestogen delivery systems such as the new progestogen-releasing IUCD (see p. 103).

How are endometrial biopsies performed? First, a pelvic examination is performed to determine the size, shape and position of the uterus. The cervix is visualized by means of a cuscos speculum. The uterus may need to be stabilized by a single toothed tenaculum or cervical hook, attached to the anterior lip of the cervix. The endometrial sampler is then inserted into the external cervical os. Occasionally the cervix may require dilatation and this can cause increased discomfort to the patient. An anaesthetic spray can be used to numb the cervix. There are different types and varieties of endometrial samplers from the Vabre vacuum aspiration curette (Rocket of London Ltd., Watford, UK) to the disposable plastic devices such as the Z-sampler

(Zinnanti Surgical Instruments, Chatsworth, CA, USA). The sample obtained is added to a histological fixative and sent for histological examination.

Complications. These are rare. However, the following have been reported: uterine perforation, cervical and uterine spasm, pain and occasional fainting and shock. In general, however, the procedure is well tolerated and minimal discomfort experienced. Stovall reported that endometrial sampling is accepted by 80% of patients, with only 5% experiencing severe pain and 15% experiencing moderate but tolerable pain (Stovall et al 1991). Analgesia may be administered prior to the procedure, particularly to those who are postmenopausal, nulliparous or very nervous and those in whom the procedure may be more difficult or not so well tolerated, for example in cases of vaginismus or a stenosed cervical canal. Although the EB is not without its limitations, it is reliable in terms of histopathological reproducibility, patient acceptability and it is cost effective (Cornier 1994, Henig et al 1989). Thus the combination of ultrasound examination and endometrial sampling will identify the majority of gynaecological pathology associated with menstrual disturbances (Reid & Gangar 1994). It should not, however, be performed in the presence of pregnancy, intrauterine infection or heavy vaginal bleeding where the result may be unreliable.

Dilatation and curettage

This is one of the most common procedures performed. It is a time-honoured operation – it is possible that even Hippocrates described the use of a set of dilators corresponding to the Hegar or Hanks of today (Ricci 1949)! Although it is gradually being replaced by outpatient procedures, there are still indications for its preference to the endometrial biopsy. These include: cervical stenosis; previous surgery, for example cervical diathermy, loop cone and Manchester repair; postmenopausal vaginal **atrophy**; severe vaginal irritation; obstruction due to vaginal/cervical lesions. It may also be preferable in a case where endometrial carcinoma is strongly suspected and an examination under anaesthetic is also required. The patient's preference should also be considered, especially in the older woman or the very nervous. However, some women who request a D&C because they have heard that a D&C will 'cure them' should have the myth dispelled. There is no evidence to suggest that a D&C has any long-term therapeutic benefit. The menstrual periods following the procedure might be lighter and the woman may report a significant improvement. This is generally short-lived and subsequent cycles revert to the previous pattern of menstrual loss (Gimes 1982).

Hysteroscopy

This is being increasingly used for the diagnosis and therapy of intrauterine disease. Whereas the previous procedures are performed 'blind', and can therefore miss lesions, hysteroscopy can inspect the uterine cavity under direct vision. A fine hysteroscope is passed through the dilated cervix, either under a general anaesthetic or as an outpatient procedure. Gas or fluid is pumped into the uterine cavity to separate the walls of the uterus. This enables submucous fibroids, endometrial polyps or structural abnormalities to be detected and biopsies from suspicious lesions may be obtained (see Plates 10–12). Bleeding hinders visibility and therefore the procedure should not be performed if the woman is menstruating. Hysteroscopy may be the investigation of choice in the case of persistent abnormal bleeding when endometrial biopsy is negative or abnormal endometrial thickness is detected on ultrasound.

The advantages of the diagnostic hysteroscopy are that it:

- is a simple and cost-effective method
- allows direct visualization of the uterine cavity
- enables the exact localization of pathological intrauterine findings
- has a high correlation with histological findings
- fills the diagnostic gap between vaginal sonography and curettage in abnormal uterine bleeding
- provides early information for the patient.

Aftercare

Following an endometrial biopsy, D&C and hysteroscopy, recovery is quick. The patient may experience some cramping pain, particularly if the cervix has been dilated. She may also notice some vaginal bleeding for a couple of days. The nurse should forewarn the patient and advise her to have sanitary protection and analgesia available. She should also be advised that if she experiences any severe cramping abdominal pain, heavy vaginal bleeding, offensive vaginal discharge or develops a temperature and feels generally unwell, she should seek medical attention. In rare cases intrauterine infection and endometritis may develop.

Treatment of menorrhagia

The treatment of choice very much depends on the individual woman and her particular circumstance. Her age, the severity of the problem, her beliefs and culture and whether she has completed her family – all

> **Box 6.9** Treatment options for the different age groups of women. They are listed in order of choice (from Reid & Gangar 1994, with permission.)
>
> **The younger woman (15–30 years)**
> • combined oval contraceptive pill (especially desogestrel and gestodene preparations)
> • mefenamic acid
> • danazol
> • levonorgestrel-releasing intrauterine device.
> **Middle reproductive years (30–40 years)**
> • mefenamic acid
> • danazol
> • levonorgestrel-releasing intrauterine device
> • combined oral contraceptive pill
> • hormone replacement therapy.
> **The older women (>40 years)**
> • norethisterone/medroxyprogesterone acetate
> • hormone replacement therapy
> • combined oral contraceptive pill.

of these things may influence her choice of preference in addition to the clinical indication (Box 6.9).

Non-hormonal therapies

These are useful in regular cyclical but heavy bleeding and include the following:

Mefenamic acid. Prostaglandins and the fibrinolytic system play an important role in uterine haemostasis, with studies observing an association between the quantity of prostaglandin production and the degree of menstrual loss, i.e. those women with an excessive blood loss having greater levels of prostaglandins. This led to the use of prostaglandin sythetase inhibitors such as mefenamic acid. It has been shown that mefenamic acid can reduce menstrual loss by up to 50% (Anderson et al 1976). It need only be taken during menses and, with its minimal side-effects, can result in a sustained beneficial effect. Side-effects can consist of nausea, indigestion, light-headiness, headaches and skin irritation.

Dose: 500 mg three times daily during menses is commonly used.

Tranexamic acid. The human endometrium possesses an active fibrinolytic system and women with menorrhagia tend to have greater levels of fibrinolysis in the endometrium. This abnormal fibrinolytic activity has led to the use of medical agents such as tranexamic acid, which impairs fibrinolysis. This antifibrinolytic medication has been highly effective in reducing menstrual blood loss. However, high doses are required and troublesome side-effects such as nausea, vomiting, diar-

rhoea, headaches, dizziness, weight gain and leg cramps can be experienced. There has been some concern over the risk of thrombosis with its use. However, studies in Scandinavia showed that the incidence of thrombosis in women treated by tranexamic acid was no different from spontaneous incident in untreated women (Rybo 1991). Thus it remains a suitable medication in fit healthy women in whom there is no known thromboembolic risk factors.

Dose: 1–1.5 g three to four times a day during menstruation.

Ethamsylate. This claims to reduce blood flow by acting via an antiprostaglandin mechanism and increasing capillary wall strength. It is promoted as a useful short-term treatment for menorrhagia associated with IUD use. However, there are few studies to confirm is efficacy.

Dose: 500 mg every 4–6 hours during menstruation.

Non-steroidal anti-inflammatory drugs. NSAIDs such as ibruprofen and naproxen appear to reduce menstrual loss.

Hormonal therapies

These are of particular value in irregular non-cyclical menorrhagia.

Oral progestogens. These are used frequently but are often ineffective in reducing menstrual flow; their principal value is as a menstrual regulator. The progestogen of choice is generally norethisterone. This is a potent progestogen, derived from testosterone. It may be prescribed cyclically as a regulator or in high doses to arrest horrendously heavy bleeding. Unfortunately, its unpleasant androgenic side-effects, such as breast tenderness, bloating, irritability and emotional lability, makes longer term use unpopular. A less potent progestogen, such as medroxyprogesterone acetate, may be helpful, with fewer side-effects. However, the menstrual control may be less effective.

Dose: norethisterone 5 mg two to three times a day for 7–10 days cyclically or up to 30 mg daily to control torrential bleeding.

Medroxyprogesterone acetate 2–20 mg daily for 7–10 days each menstrual cycle.

Danazol. This gonadotrophin inhibitor acts on the hypothalamic–pituitary–ovarian axis. It also acts directly on the endometrium, resulting in atrophy. The endometrial atrophy and the inhibition of ovulation should not, however, be relied upon for contraception and a barrier method of contraception should be used to avoid an unwanted pregnancy. Danazol is also a testosterone derivative. It can cause unpleasant side-effects such as weight gain, acne, muscular pain and headaches. These, with its metabolic effects of adversely influencing serum lipid levels, can limit long-term therapy.

Dose: 200–400 mg daily for 3–4 months.

Combined oral contraceptive pill. This can be particularly useful in women who also require contraception. It will, in the majority of cases, control menstrual flow (although the mode of action is unclear) and act as a menstrual regulator. Since the FDA's 1989 decision that fit, healthy, normotensive, non-smoking women may safely remain on the combined oral contraceptive pill until menopause, it is entirely appropriate and may be particularly helpful for women in the peri-menopausal years, in whom menstrual control, contraception and relief of early menopausal symptoms are necessary. The pill continues to be an appropriate therapy for the younger woman with the withdrawal bleed likely to be considerably lighter than a 'normal period'. It also gives the flexibility of continuous administration, i.e. taking three packets consecutively followed by a 7-day break and then a repeat of the regimen. This gives only four withdrawal bleeds per year, which may be more acceptable to some women, particularly those who have the additional problem of endometriosis.

Dose: ethinyloestradiol 20–30 mg and progestogen daily for 21 days followed by a 7-day break and repeat, or as discussed above.

Hormone replacement therapy. This can be particularly helpful in women who require menstrual control and menopause symptom relief. In the form of sequential combined preparations of oestradiol and progestogen, it is an effective, safe and largely underused therapy in the control of menstrual disorders. However, this is an area that requires further research and evaluation.

Gonadotrophin releasing hormone (GnRH) analogues. These include goserelin (Zoladex i.m. injection), nafarelin and buserelin (nasal spray) and are effective in controlling menorrhagia by inducing a 'medical menopause'. They work by producing pituitary desensitization and inhibition of gonadotrophin release. This results in suppressed ovarian activity and hence suppression of endometrial growth. This hypo-oestrogen state also triggers typical menopausal symptoms and can cause significant reduction in bone mass. However, this has not been correlated with an increased risk of bone fracture. Nevertheless, caution should be exercised and its use limited to 4–6 months. Thus, those at risk of osteoporosis should be identified, bone densitometry performed and HRT add-back (see Chapter 12) should be prescribed. Although GnRH analogues have a promising future in the management of menorrhagia, their relatively high cost prohibits more widespread use.

Progesterone-releasing intrauterine device. There is only one progesterone releasing intrauterine device available in the United Kingdom at present. This is the levonorgestrel intrauterine system (LNG–IUD) or Mirena (Schering Healthcare). It was introduced in Scandinavia as a contraceptive but its effects on the menstrual cycle soon become apparent. It is now licensed for both contraception and menorrhagia in European countries. However, in the United Kingdom it is currently licensed only for use in cases of menorrhagia in women who also require contraception. This is likely to change, as a licence for use in the treatment of menorrhagia is currently being applied for. The LNG-IUD consists of a plastic, T-shaped device. The stem carries a steroid reservoir, which controls the rate of release of LNG to 20 µg per 24 h, sustained over 5 years. The endometrium is markedly suppressed in response to its local effects on the endometrium, i.e. the high local tissue concentration, thus preventing endometrial proliferation. This strong suppression of endometrial growth causes a considerable reduction in blood loss. Menstruation becomes shorter, lighter and, in some cases, there is relief of dysmenorrhoea. This occurs because the inactive endometrium produces less prostaglandins and hence less dysmenorrhoea. As with all long-acting progestogen-only contraceptives, abnormal bleeding problems are the most common side-effect. Menstrual spotting and irregular bleeding are particularly common in the first 2–3 months following insertion. This tends to be light and within 3 months there is a uniform atrophic change. As the endometrium undergoes these changes under the influence of LNG the frequency and duration of bleeding lessens. Therefore, by 1 year, many users will have experienced amenorrhoea. However, preinsertion counselling regarding this unpredictable, inconvenient spotting is imperative. Although this irregular bleeding can be a nuisance, with good counselling and the minimal side-effects, the LNG-IUD can offer an acceptable alternative to both medical and surgical treatments of menorrhagia. It is low-cost (at £33 per year; it is used for 3 years), avoids surgery and conserves fertility. Some side-effects, consisting of headaches, nausea, breast tenderness, depression and weight gain, have been reported in a small number of users, but generally these are largely avoided due to its local action. Some levonorgestrel is absorbed into the systemic circulation but levels tend to be on par with, or less than, the progesterone-only pill. The levels tend to peak after insertion when side-effects tend to be experienced, then gradually decrease over its life span.

Case study Jackie

Jackie, a 25-year-old dental nurse, was referred to the gynaecology clinic by her GP with a long-standing history of dysmenorrhoea. During the history taking, it was ascertained that dysmenorrhoea had been a problem since the menarche and the periods had been getting progressively heavier over the past few years. Her periods were regular every 28 days and lasted 5–6 days. The symptoms she experienced were severe abdominal pain, backache, headaches and generally feeling unwell. These commenced about a week prior to the onset of the period and lasted for the duration of the period.

Jackie herself was a fit, healthy, married woman with no relevant past medical history. Her regular cervical smear tests were negative. She smoked two to five cigarettes a day and drank a couple of glasses of wine at the weekends.

In the past, Jackie had tried many types of medications, including Ponstan, Brufen and paracetamol. All had had limited benefit. She had also tried the oral contraceptive pill. This also had limited benefit such that Jackie had been prescribed the combined oral contraceptive pill to be taken continuously for 63 days followed by a 7-day break and repeat. This provided a solution but, during the seven pill-free days and for several days after, all the symptoms had returned with increased intensity.

Following a thorough history, a physical examination was performed. Pelvic examination revealed a normal anteverted mobile uterus with no abnormal masses palpable. After discussion is was decided a laparoscopy was required to exclude any uterine pathology such as endometriosis. If no abnormalities were found then a progesterone-releasing intrauterine device would be inserted. This would provide Jackie with good contraception and lighten the periods, therefore reducing the dysmenorrhoea. At laparoscopy the pelvis was found to be completely healthy and normal and a Mirena coil was inserted. Jackie made an uneventful recovery and was followed up in the gynaecology clinic 6 weeks later. She was advised to use another type of contraception, such as the sheath, until her coil was checked at her postoperative check up. At that visit Jackie reported that she had experienced some lower abdominal discomfort and some intermittent bleeding. The coil was checked and found to be correctly situated and Jacky was told that she could now rely on it for contraception. At her 3- and 6-month appointments following her operation, Jackie reported that she had had very light regular periods with no dysmenorrhoea and was absolutely delighted.

Surgical therapy

This may be indicated when medical therapies have failed or in women who have completed their families and do not relish taking medical therapy for many years. Surgical therapies range from minor procedures, such as hysteroscopy to remove polyps, to hysterectomy (see Plate 13) (for preoperative assessment and postoperative care see Chapter 20). Although hysterectomy is effective and the final cure for menorrhagia, many women choose to avoid it. Not only is there significant morbidity associated with hysterectomy, such as infection and haemorrhage, but many women have extreme anxieties regarding their sexuality and body image. A solution to this is to remove the endometrium by means of endometrial ablation.

Endometrial ablation. With the advent of the hysteroscope and direct vision of the uterine cavity, endometrial surgery via hysteroscopy has increased. A range of techniques were introduced in the mid-1980s and, by 1990, 83% of NHS hospitals were providing these techniques (Overton et al 1997) (Fig. 6.2):

- Laser ablation – laser energy is delivered along a flexible fibre, which is passed down the hysteroscope. Normal saline or glycine is used to distend the cavity and improve visibility during surgery. Tissue vaporization is achieved either by a non-touch technique or by dragging the laser across the endometrium.
- Electrodiathermy – coagulation of the endometrium is achieved using a rollerball electrode. This is commonly used in conjunction with a resection technique using a cutting loop. This procedure has been adapted from the technique used in the transurethral resection of the prostate for benign prostatic **hypertrophy**.
- Radiofrequency – irreversible thermal tissue damage to the endometrium occurs when the endometrium temperature is raised via a uterine sound placed in the uterine cavity. The radiofrequency waves generate an electric field around the probe via an external electrode placed around the woman's abdomen.

The minimally invasive nature of such techniques has clear advantages and requires only a day or so in hospital. The postoperative morbidity is less and consequently there is a more rapid convalescence.

The main limitation is that amenorrhoea cannot be guaranteed, many women need repeat procedures and may eventually require a hysterectomy. Although the aim is to destroy the endometrium, any residual endometrium can regenerate and cause bleeding. In

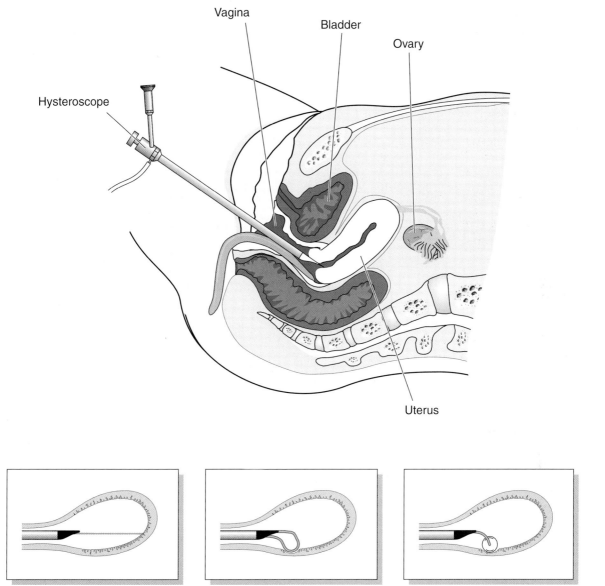

Vagina

Bladder

Ovary

Hysteroscope

Uterus

Laser

Wire loop

Revolving ball

Figure 6.2 Types and technique of endometrial ablation. From Stafford M 1996, Patient Pictures, Gynaecology Health Press, Oxford, with permission.

addition, any residual endometrium stimulated by oestrogen that is not opposed by progesterone can give rise to hyperplasia, which cannot always be accessed to rule out premalignancy and malignancy. Preoperative endometrial preparation may also be requested. Drug therapy such as progestogens, danazol or GnRH analogues are used to 'thin' the endometrium, potentially reducing the risk of intraoperative haemorrhage. It is also important to exclude endometrial hyperplasia and carcinoma by means of endometrial sampling. Prior to surgery the woman needs to be aware of the need for contraception. Although it is unlikely, following a successful ablation, pregnancy can occur and contraception needs to be discussed. Clip sterilization may be considered and performed in conjunction with the endometrial resection to avoid a further operation.

Although postoperative morbidity is less with endometrial ablation than with surgery such as hysterectomy, and although common complications (such as those discussed in Chapter 20) are avoided, the procedure is not without complications, which include uterine perforation, diathermy of intra-abdominal structures, haemorrhage, fluid overload and emergency hysterectomy. There is a risk that the flushing medium is absorbed, causing fluid overload. Careful observation should be made during the operation of the amount of fluid introduced and returned. The procedure may have to be halted if a large amount of fluid appears to have been absorbed. The place of endometrial ablation in gynaecological surgery is to provide an alternative to those women who are unable or unwilling to accept long-term medical therapy and as an alternative to hysterectomy. Its true efficacy and morbidity is yet to be defined, with ongoing audit and continuing research. However, results of the minimally invasive surgical techniques – laser, endothermal or endoresection survey, which ran from April 1993 to October 1994, showed that:

- the procedures generally have a low mortality and morbidity rate
- laser and rollerball techniques alone are the safest procedures.
- preoperative medical treatments are of little value in reducing complication rates.

Hysterectomy. The first hysterectomy was performed in 1812 in Milan by Dr G. Paletta; the woman died 3 days later from peritonitis. The first successful hysterectomy was carried out on 1 September 1853 in Boston, USA, by Gilman Kimball. This surgical procedure has come a long way since the nineteenth century, with many thousands of hysterectomies being performed annually in the UK. However, the 'hysterectomy' is surrounded by the most fundamental social and individual myths. It is an area where gynaecology nurses can shine, using their expert knowledge to expel fears and dismiss old wives' tales, and giving factual advice regarding morbidity and mortality and sensible advice regarding postoperative activity and care (for a further discussion, see Chapter 20).

POSTMENOPAUSAL BLEEDING

The perimenopause or climacteric is when a woman progresses from the reproductive to the non-reproductive phase in her life. When ovarian follicular activity declines and finally ceases, she will experience the menopause or the last menstrual bleed. The postmenopause is the phase in a woman's life when she is 12 months from that final menstrual period. Any bleeding that occurs after a woman has had 12 months of spontaneous amenorrhoea must be investigated. Investigations must include a thorough pelvic examination, a cervical smear, an endometrial biopsy and possible hysteroscopy.

However, the journey from the perimenopause to the postmenopause can take several years, with a very gradual decline in ovarian function. Women in the early postmenopause can experience surges of ovarian activity. This can give rise to an episode of bleeding, which may be preceded by typical prodromal symptoms of menstruation. Investigations in this situation will be normal. However, when a patient is undergoing investigations for postmenopausal bleeding, the nurse should be ever-mindful of the possible sinister diagnosis of endometrial carcinoma.

Cancer of the endometrium

Cancer of the endometrium is primarily a disease of the postmenopausal woman. Approximately 4200 women are diagnosed with this condition each year and of these only 5% are under the age of 45 (Cancer Statistics for England, Wales and Scotland 1992, Cancer Statistics for Northern Ireland 1995) (Office for National Statistics 1998).

Risk factors include:

- late menopause
- nulliparity
- obesity
- unopposed oestrogen therapy
- hereditary factors
- hormonal factors.

Signs and symptoms

The most common symptom is abnormal bleeding, which might be irregular and intermenstrual; 75% of cases have postmenopausal bleeding. The abnormal bleeding may be associated with a vaginal discharge that is usually brown, watery and often offensive. On examination the uterus may be enlarged and blood visible in the vagina. The endometrium will be thickened on ultrasound scan.

Screening

Unfortunately, no effective screening test is available for uterine cancer in asymptomatic women. Therefore any symptoms must be reported and investigated as soon as possible to allow early diagnosis and treatment.

CONCLUSION

The gynaecology nurse plays a vital role whilst women are undergoing gynaecological investigations and treatment. Women are often frightened or embarrassed and need the reassuring face of the nurse to help allay their fears. It is crucial that nurses keep abreast and up-to-date with the changes and developments within the field of gynaecology, then they can give women current information and help them face their problems with knowledge and confidence.

GLOSSARY

Atrophy: wasting away, diminished in size and function
Dysmenorrhoea: painful periods
Hypertrophy: increase in size independent of natural growth
Idiopathic: of unknown origin

Menarch: onset of menstruation
Myometrium: thick muscular wall of the uterus
Oligomenorrhoea: scanty, infrequent periods
Synechiae: abnormal union of parts, i.e. adhesions

REFERENCES

Anderson ABM, Haynes PJ, Guillebaud J 1976 Reduction of menstrual blood loss by prostaglandin synthetase inhibitors. Lancet i:774–776

Cameron IT 1989 Dysfunctional uterine bleeding. In: Drife JO (ed) Baillière's clinical obstetrics and gynaecology. WB Saunders, London, pp. 315–328

Cornier EG 1994 The Pipelle. A disposable device for endometrial biopsy. American Journal of Obstetrics and Gynecology 148:109–110

Coulter A 1994 Seminar of dysfunctional uterine bleeding. Royal Society of Medicine, London

Coulter A, Noone A, Goldacre M 1989 General practitioners' referrals to specialist outpatient clinic. British Medical Journal 299:304–308

Frisch RE, Revelle R, Cook S 1973 Components of weight at menarche and the initiation of the adolescent growth spurt in girls: estimated total water, lean body weight and fat. Human Biology 45:469

Gimes DA (1982). Diagnostic dilatation and curettage. American Journal of Obstetrics and Gynecology 142:1–6

Goodwin SC, Walker WJ 1998 Uterine artery embolization for the treatment of uterine fibroids. Current Opinion in Obstetrics and Gynecology 10:315–320

Henig I, Chan P, Redway DR, Maw GM, Gullett AJ, Cheatwood M 1989 Evaluation of the pipelle curettage for endometrial biopsy. Journal of Reproductive Medicine 34:786–789

Office for National Statistics 1998 Cancer statistics registrations 1992, MBI No 25. London: Her Majesty's Stationery Office

Oliver JA, Lance JS 1979 Selective embolization to control massive haemorrhage following pelvic surgery. American Journal of Obstetrics and Gynecology 135:431–432

Overton C, Hargreaves J, Maresh M 1997 A national survey of the complications of endometrial destruction for menstrual disorders: the MISTLETOE study. British Journal of Obstetrics and Gynaecology 104:1351–1359

Paganini-Hill A, Ross RK, Henderson BE 1989 Endometrial cancer and patterns of use of oestrogen replacement therapy: a cohort study. British Journal of Cancer 59:445–447

Pai SO, Glickman M, Schwartz PE, Pingoud E, Berhowitz R 1980 Embolization of pelvic arteries for control of postpartum haemorrhage. Obstetrics and Gynaecology 55:754–758

Rees MCP, Turnbull AC 1989 Menstrual disorders: an overview. In: Drife JO (ed) Baillière's clinical obstetrics and gynaecology. WB Saunders, London, pp. 217–226

Reid B, Gangar K 1994 Medical management of menorrhagia. In: Studd J (ed) The diplomate. Parthenon Press, London, vol 1(2), pp. 92–98

Ricci JV 1949 The development of gynaecology surgery and instruments. Blakiston Co, Philadephia, pp. 13, 297, 299, 300, 301

Rybo G 1991 Tranexamic acid therapy is effective treatment in heavy menstrual bleeding. Clinical update on safety. Therapeutic Advances 4:1–8

Shearman RP 1986 Secondary amenorrhoea. In: Whitfield CR (ed) Dewhurst's textbook of obstetrics and gynaecology for postgraduates. Blackwell, Oxford, pp. 70–79

Stafford M Patient's pictures – gynaecology. Health Press, Oxford

Stovall TG, Photopulos GJ, Poston WN, Ling FW, Sandles LG 1991 Pipelle endometrial sampling in patients with known endometrial carcinoma. Obstetrics and Gynaecology 77: 954–956

FURTHER READING

McPherson A 1993 Women's problems in general practice, 3rd edn. Oxford University Press, Oxford

Scambler A, Scambler G 1993 Menstrual disorders. Routledge, London

Stirrat GM 1997 Aids to obstetrics and gynaecology for MRCOG, 4th edn. Churchill Livingstone, Edinburgh

The diplomate series. Available from the Royal College of Obstetricians and Gynaecologists, London. Tel: 020 7772 6200

USEFUL ADDRESSES

Women's Health Information Centre & Hysterectomy Support Network
52 Featherstone Street, London EC1Y 8RT
Helpline: 020 7251 6580

Hysterectomy Support Group:
The Venture,
Green Lane, Upton, Huntingdon, Cambridgeshire PE17 5YE
Send SAE for nearest contact details.

Hysterectomy Advice Pack:
from The National Osteoporosis Society
PO Box 10, Radstock, Bath BA3 3YB
Tel: 01761 471771

Women's Health Concern
83 Earl's Court Road, London W8 6EF

Hospitals performing arterial embolization:
Royal Surrey Hospital, Guildford. Tel: 01483 571122
Guy's & St Thomas' Hospital, London. Tel: 020 7928 9292

7

Premenstrual syndrome

Kathy Suffling

Premenstrual syndrome (PMS) is a subject that has always generated a great deal of interest and publicity in both the lay and medical press. Regardless of the numbers of women who claim to suffer from it, most women would admit that they can relate to it in some way or another. Women today play a far more active role in their lives in terms of health issues than they used to, and they demand knowledge about PMS not only to understand about this condition but also to find ways of coping with it. Despite extensive research there is still much we do not understand about PMS and many controversies surround its cause, diagnosis and management. Some doctors maintain that it does not exist at all, and is 'all in the mind'. This attitude makes women feel frustrated and let down by the medical profession, especially if their lives are dominated and disrupted by the symptoms of PMS.

DEFINITION AND PREVALENCE

PMS is often thought of as a twentieth century disorder but, in fact, historical references about the symptoms of PMS were documented by Hippocrates as early as 460 BC (Chadwick & Mann 1950).

PMS was first formally described in 1931 in a group of women who all suffered cyclical symptoms of mood changes, headaches and weight gain (Frank 1931). The symptoms occurred 7–10 days premenstrually and were relieved with the onset of menstruation, giving it the term 'premenstrual tension'. This was then changed to 'premenstrual syndrome' in 1953 following work done by Greene and Dalton, as it became apparent that there was a much wider variety of symptoms associated with the menstrual cycle; this term is still used today.

The World Health Organization does not recognize PMS as an illness and therefore there is no WHO definition. A number of definitions have since been developed, of which the following are probably the most well quoted:

Distressing physical, psychological and behavioural symptoms not caused by organic disease which regularly recur during the same phase of the ovarian (or menstrual) cycle, and which significantly regress or disappear during the remainder of the cycle.

Magos & Studd 1984

A disorder of non-specific somatic, psychological or behavioural symptoms recurring in the premenstrual phase of the menstrual cycle. Symptoms must resolve completely by the end of menstruation leaving a symptom-free week. The symptoms should be of sufficient severity to produce social, family or occupational disruption. Symptoms must have occurred in at least four of the six previous menstrual cycles.

O'Brien 1990

The American Psychiatric Association has felt that PMS has such significant diagnostic criteria in some women with severe symptoms that they can be described as having a possible psychiatric condition requiring further study. PMS is recorded in the *Diagnostic and Statistical Manual of Mental Disorders* (DSM-IV) as 'late luteal dysphoric disorder' (American Psychiatric Association 1994).

It is believed that as many as 75–95% of women report some premenstrual changes, 20–50% of these women experience more significant symptoms sufficient to describe it as 'premenstrual syndrome' and approximately 3–5% of women suffer from severe symptoms to meet the criteria for late luteal dysphoric disorder.

There are unfortunately no biological markers to enable the medical profession to make a diagnosis of PMS. As the symptoms are cyclical in nature, daily diaries can assist as the symptoms should appear predominantly in the luteal phase of the cycle, up to 7–14 days before menstruation, gradually cease with the onset of menstruation and be virtually absent in the follicular phase of the cycle. Symptoms can vary from month to month in one individual so several diaries must be completed before a diagnosis can be made.

It is very easy to use the label of PMS to describe any fluctuations of a woman's mood or to explain their behaviour and performance at certain times. Women today lead very demanding lives, very often having to juggle the demands of a career and bringing up children with being a wife, lover and carer. PMS can be a good excuse when women feel they cannot live up to their own or others' expectations. It may well be the case that, for many women, cyclical changes *do* mean that they function less well than usual with the demands upon them, but we must be careful to differentiate this from true PMS.

AETIOLOGY

As previously stated, despite extensive research no definitive cause of PMS has ever been demonstrated and many different theories have been put forward, including dietary, genetic, social and evolutionary ideas. The idea that PMS is purely psychological and 'all in the mind' still exists, but various other medical hypotheses have been described, the most common include:

- progesterone deficiency
- oestrogen/progesterone imbalance
- **hyperprolactinaemia**
- increased **aldosterone** or renin–angiotensin activity
- **hypoglycaemia**
- prostaglandin deficiency/excess
- vitamin B6 deficiency.

All these possibilities have been explored, with sometimes conflicting but no conclusive evidence to support any of them.

More recent research has suggested that the cause of PMS might be neuroendocrine. Many of the symptoms and behavioural patterns of PMS are also common features of depression and other behavioural disorders. Typical symptoms might include low mood, irritability, aggression and disturbances of appetite and **cognition**. **Serotonin** is a neurotransmitter that is known to play an important role in our mood, appetite and behaviour patterns. Patients suffering from certain types of depression show decreased serotonergic activity. Some studies have demonstrated blood serotonin levels to be significantly lower in the luteal phase of the menstrual cycle of women with PMS than in control subjects, in whom there were increased levels of serotonin. It would appear that women with PMS may have an abnormal neurotransmitter response to normal ovarian function. The serotonergic system therefore has become a logical focus of study in PMS (Rapkin 1992).

Rapkin speculates that alterations in hormone levels following ovulation may cause deregulation of this system. It might be that some women are able to regulate their own serotonergic system by seeking appropriate social activities or 'serotonin fixes' that are mood enhancing, and this might in turn make them more immune from the symptoms of PMS. Alternatively, women who have an inability to seek or receive mood-enhancing behaviour could experience deregulation and resulting decreased serotonergic activity, and it may be that these women are those most likely to suffer from PMS.

Rapkin suggests that both oestrogen and progesterone may play a part in the regulation of the serotonergic system. Studies in animals have demonstrated that administration of oestrogen and progesterone increased serotonin **synthesis** in the brain in females but not in males. It is also known that repeated stress can cause defective serotonin synthesis and, potentially, lead to depressive symptoms.

Another study published in 1997 by Rapkin et al looked further at the link between stress and PMS. Allopregnanolone, a metabolite of progesterone, has anxiolytic effects. Repeated environmental stress has been shown to increase allopregnanolone concentrations. Rapkin et al suggests that women who met their criteria of PMS had lower serum concentrations of allopregnanolone in the luteal phase of the cycle than women with no PMS symptoms. A deficiency in this neurosteroid could therefore contribute to various mood symptoms, such as anxiety, tension and depression.

This work is speculative, but opens interesting avenues for future research for these theories to be validated.

What we do know for certain is that PMS is linked to cyclical ovarian activity and that PMS is experienced only between puberty and the menopause. Symptoms disappear during pregnancy and following hysterectomy, although if the ovaries are conserved the symptoms persist. Attempts to suppress ovulation with **gonadotrophin**-releasing hormone (GnRH) analogues or following bilateral oopherectomy will resolve symptoms of PMS completely.

PMS is prevalent regardless of parity, race, culture or socioeconomic group. It is likely that there is no single cause for PMS and that a combination of physiological, psychological and social factors are involved.

SYMPTOMS

Over 150 different symptoms of PMS have been described. Some women will only suffer physical symptoms, others only psychological effects, but most will have a combination of different symptoms, therefore every women could potentially have her own individual experience of PMS. The severity of symptoms may vary from cycle to cycle but the type of symptoms experienced will usually remain constant. Many women will experience only mild symptoms, which are not severe enough to bring her to her doctor's surgery, and yet they will essentially be the same as those reported by other women whose lives are totally incapacitated by them. The symptomatol-

---

Box 7.1 Physical symptoms

- Breast tenderness and swelling.
- Abdominal bloatedness.
- Oedema.
- Weight gain.
- Headaches/migraines.
- Appetite changes.
- Carbohydrate cravings.
- Abdominal/pelvic discomfort.
- Altered bowel habits.
- Clumsiness/lack of coodination.
- Hot flushes.
- Dizziness.
- Palpitations.
- Acne/skin blemishes.
- Tiredness.
- Nausea.
- Muscular stiffness/discomfort.
- Backache.
- Exacerbation of other medical conditions.

Box 7.2 Psychological symptoms

- Tension.
- Irritability/outbursts.
- Depression/low mood.
- Mood swings.
- Anxiety.
- Aggression.
- Tiredness/lethargy.
- Sleep disturbance.
- Changes in libido.
- Restlessness.
- Poor concentration.
- Tearfulness.
- Poor cognition.

Box 7.3 Behavioural symptoms

- **Agoraphobia**
- Absenteeism from work
- Poor work performance
- Social withdrawal
- Difficulty with personal relationships
- In extreme cases, criminal behaviour, suicide attempts, hospital and psychiatric admissions (Dalton 1961)

---

ogy being so complex makes diagnosis difficult and it is important to be aware that some of them could be explained by a variety of other causes or other medical disorders and therefore might not be directly related.

Diagnosis is important if we are to provide appropriate and effective treatment.

Symptoms can be be categorized in three ways: physical (Box 7.1), psychological (Box 7.2) and behavioural (Box 7.3).

PRESENTATION AND EFFECTS

As previously discussed, a large proportion of women suffer some effects of PMS to one extent or another. Many will see their symptoms as just a part of life as a female and would take the view that they 'just have to put up with it'. PMS will affect different people in a variety of different ways. Individuals have varying expectations of themselves and a number of factors will govern this.

The way we are brought up will influence our ability to cope with life and many coping mechanisms will be 'learnt' from our parents subconsciously. Our beliefs and attitudes to menstruation often stem from our mothers and other carers and, if attitudes to PMS have been presented to us in a negative way, then our own views will obviously be influenced.

For some women, symptoms will be of a sufficient nature to seek some relief from them. The majority of these women would try some form of self-help remedies, such as dietary or lifestyle changes. Some symptoms can often be relieved by relatively simple treatments and these women might not necessarily seek help from any other source. However, some women suffer symptoms that may cause such severe disruption within their personal, family or occupational relationships, that they may seek professional help.

Although it has been suggested that certain types of personality are more susceptible to PMS, there does not seem to be any particular 'type' of woman who is more likely to experience it. It does appear to be more common in women in their early thirties, and also in perimenopausal women. Symptoms often get progressively worse and can overlap with the onset of the menopause. Perimenopausal women can experience a whole range of distressing physical and psychological symptoms and it can be difficult to differentiate between worsening PMS and the onset of the menopause. PMS often first presents in women who have young children, which of course is a particularly stressful time for women generally. Stopping the oral contraceptive pill or following a pregnancy is often a time when the onset of PMS is seen, and women who have suffered from postnatal depression are also more susceptible. PMS is more likely to be experienced during times of stress in a woman's life, when other problems are present, than when life is relatively stress free and going well for her.

Many women will cope with physical symptoms but it is the psychological ones that are the most difficult to manage, particularly if these symptoms are affecting her life adversely – causing problems within her relationships and coping abilities at home or at work.

Despite some views that PMS is a complaint of 'neurotic' women, there is no consistent relationship between women's personalities and PMS. There do, however, appear to be links between PMS and general psychological health. Women with psychiatric illness may experience PMS more often, and symptoms can be more severe in these women than in psychologically well women.

Sexuality

Our mood and general wellbeing are closely linked to our sexuality, so PMS is likely to affect our feelings about this. Due to the natural fluctuations in hormone levels in the menstrual cycle many women will be less interested in sexual activity premenstrually, and this might be influenced further if she suffers from symptoms such as tiredness, breast tenderness and mood changes. This could potentially lead to tension within relationships and women and their partners need reassurance and explanation that these changes are not only common but also normal. Women may worry about symptoms like breast tenderness and whether it might indicate some problem, but their fears must be dispelled.

It is not unusual for women to present with symptoms of PMS instead of the 'real' reason they have consulted a doctor or nurse for. Sometimes, underlying deep-rooted psychosexual problems manifest themselves as physical or emotional symptoms, but the woman herself may have no conscious awareness of this. It may be necessary for a skilled counsellor to carefully explore these problems, and appropriate referral should be made if this is the case.

DIAGNOSIS AND DIARIES

Diagnosis of PMS is difficult but, as the timing of the symptoms in the menstrual cycle is significant, daily symptom diaries are a logical way to evaluate them. A full medical and gynaecological history and examination should be carried out, if possible, to exclude any other medical problems. An assessment of the woman's psychological state would be helpful, and details of her current life situation, with any stresses highlighted. A subjective account of a woman's symptoms, their severity and the effects on her life are obviously important, but it is difficult to assess them effectively in this way.

Presentation with a picture of severe symptoms is common but on evaluation of diaries they may not be so marked. This could be because when asked to focus on her symptoms they may not appear so severe and there might be a 'placebo' effect due to the perception that someone is taking them seriously and doing something constructive to help.

In spite of this, prospective diary information is probably the most helpful tool we have in assisting diagnosis, and retrospective information should not be used as a basis for instigating any treatment.

A minimum of two monthly diaries (ideally more) should be kept in order to demonstrate the variations in severity from one month to another. A daily rating of individual symptoms and bleeding patterns is kept

Menstrual diary chart

Name: _____   Year: _____

	Jan	Feb	Mar	Apr	May	Jun	Jul	Aug	Sep	Oct	Nov	Dec
1												
2												
3												
4												
5												
6												
7												
8												
9												
10												
11												
12												
13												
14												
15												
16												
17												
18												
19												
20												
21												
22												
23												
24												
25												
26												
27												
28												
29												
30												
31												

M = Menstruation   B = Breast tenderness
H = Headache   I = Irritability

Figure 7.1   Menstrual diary chart. From The National Association for Premenstrual Syndrome, with permission.

and will show whether there is any relationship between the two premenstrually. Additional useful information might include any illnesses or stressful events and also any medication the woman may have taken. Excluding any other underlying psychological cause for symptoms, such as a depressive illness or other emotional disorder, is important as these problems will further complicate the diagnosis of PMS. This type of information would also be difficult to ascertain from a woman's subjective reports of her symptoms, but would be much easier to demonstrate after assessment of her diaries as they would not demonstrate a typical cyclical pattern of symptoms.

Sampson (1989) has described three patterns of symptoms common in women complaining of PMS.

- *'Pure PMS'* – the symptoms are confined to the luteal phase of the menstrual cycle and decrease with the onset of menstruation, with complete resolution of symptoms in between. What we generally think of as 'classic PMS'.
- *Premenstrual exacerbations* – also known as 'perimenstrual distress'. Symptoms fluctuate throughout the whole menstrual cycle but are exacerbated premenstrually and do not resolve after menstruation. These women often have underlying psychological problems as well as a cyclical disorder.
- *Non-cyclical symptoms* – this might represent a generalized anxiety state with mood fluctuations unrelated to menstruation or may perhaps be part of another disorder, e.g. depression.

A variety of diaries are available and, once completed, they allow doctor, nurse and woman to see at a glance whether the symptoms are cyclical in nature. This will give the woman the opportunity to assess her own patterns of symptoms and, hopefully, lead to a greater understanding of PMS and how it is affecting her life. It may become apparent that certain stresses or situations exacerbate her symptoms and she may need to find alternative ways of dealing with these stresses in order to accommodate for her PMS symptoms.

This approach is obviously not scientific in any way, so for research purposes other more accurate means of evaluating diary data is necessary. Magos and Studd (1986) have adapted a method of time series analysis (Trigg's trend analysis), which can define PMS by a mathematical analysis. Time series analysis is the specific statistical approach to chronological data. This allows significant symptoms to be defined in terms of PMS trends, non-PMS trends and no trends, depending on the symptoms reported. Completed diary information is entered into a computer, then assessed using the Trigg's trend analysis. This method has been used in various research studies over recent years.

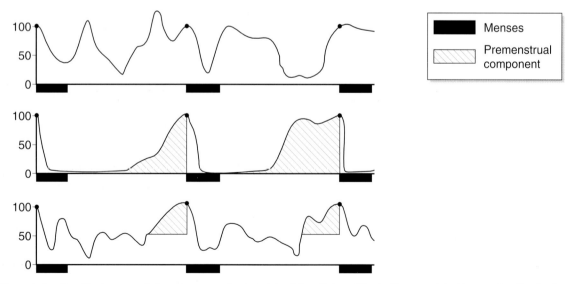

Figure 7.2 Graphical representation of a generalized anxiety state with mood fluctuations unrelated to menstruation (top), classical premenstrual syndrome (middle) and premenstrual distress (bottom). All cycles score 100 on day 1 of menstruation. The premenstrual component of symptoms is highlighted. From Sampson 1989, with permission.

Once diary information has been completed and assessed then a diagnosis can be made and the appropriate treatment options and management discussed.

TREATMENT OPTIONS AND MANAGEMENT

Treatment for PMS depends largely on the severity of the symptoms and also whether they are physical or psychological.

Women suffering mild to moderate symptoms will probably look at ways of relieving their symptoms without ever seeking any professional help. Many may view their experiences as a normal and acceptable part of life, but equally may find them a nuisance and therefore look at ways of minimizing them. Minor symptoms can be treated in a variety of simple ways and many lifestyle changes can be made, which will be a positive start. A number of over-the-counter pro-

ducts are are specifically designed for PMS sufferers and women might choose to pursue this type of option first.

Complementary therapies are a very popular choice, especially for those who do not wish to take any form of conventional medical treatment. Physical symptoms are generally much easier to treat and there are more options available for this. What is more difficult is trying to treat symptoms of a psychological nature, and the choices for this are more limited. Women are often not able to accept that there might be any psychological basis for their symptoms and may perceive this as a suggestion that their problems are 'all in their mind'. What may be more appropriate is a 'dual approach', with a combination of medical and psychological help. It should tactfully be suggested that the woman should try to recognize that some of her symptoms are of a 'psychological nature' and that they do exist, but that a different approach to treatment may be more helpful.

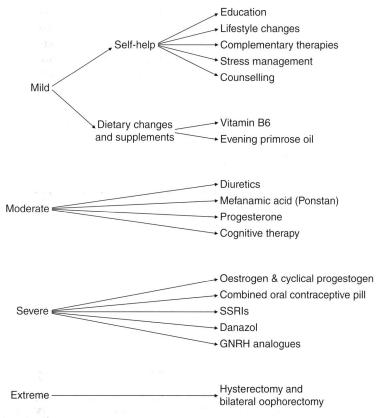

Figure 7.3   Guide to treatment options

Any symptoms appearing on a diary card that are not cyclical in nature will also need addressing in separate way.

If treatment options have been tried and have failed to control symptoms, or for any woman whom a GP feels it necessary, then referral to a specialist clinic must be made. In the case of severe forms of PMS or those with late luteal dysphoric disorder, then referral to a gynaecologist or psychiatrist would be more appropriate.

Self-help measures

There are numerous ways in which a woman can help herself, and this applies to all women regardless of the severity of their symptoms. Publicity in the lay press often presents PMS in an unhelpful way and women are led to believe that they are suffering from a 'syndrome', as if it is some kind of illness that needs radical treatment. The following section will describe some of the methods by which the problems and symptoms can be tackled sensibly and, by doing this herself, the woman will feel that she is more in control of her life in whatever approach she chooses.

Education

A sympathetic GP or nurse can be all that is needed to reassure a woman that what she is experiencing is normal. Knowledge of the menstrual cycle and the symptoms and effects of PMS is important. Time spent just 'talking' can be enormously beneficial and can provide the reassurance that she 'is not going mad'! Various support groups are available for women seeking more information and support, and helpful literature can be obtained through these sources. Some support groups may advocate specific treatments and some charge a fee for their literature and it might be useful to make women aware of this. Many books have been written on the subject but, with new research being published all the time, information can quickly become out of date. Many women prefer to talk to a female doctor, nurse, friend or colleague with the idea that they may have a greater understanding of these problems.

A consultation with a doctor or nurse can provide the woman with an opportunity to discuss any other issues that may be relevant, such as other stresses in her life that could be exacerbating her symptoms.

Diaries can be issued for completion if thought necessary to confirm a diagnosis and exclude other underlying problems. This is a very useful learning tool as the woman can observe on a daily basis how her symptoms throughout her cycle affect her life and those around her. It may highlight areas in which she can take positive steps to make changes that will help make her life easier, such as avoiding certain situations and decisions that cause her stress during the premenstrual phase of her cycle.

Discussing her expectations of treatment options should be included at a consultation as many women feel that their GP can provide a 'magic answer'. Women do have a responsibility to themselves in the management of their PMS but ideally both should work together to reach realistic goals that are achievable.

Lifestyle changes

A critical look at lifestyle will often highlight many factors that can be altered in some way. There are some very effective and simple changes that can be made that may go a long way to improving health and general wellbeing both physically and emotionally. Making allowances for PMS symptoms is helpful. Premenstrually it is common for a woman to find that the normal demands upon her become increasingly difficult and, if these demands are not met, her life can become a vicious circle as she gets more and more despondent about not being able to cope and tries even harder to achieve things that normally would be second nature to her. Recognizing this pattern of behaviour is vital if she is going to learn to live and cope with it. Time taken to reorganize her lifestyle to reduce the demands upon her will help and she should learn to set herself small but realistic goals that she will be able to achieve more easily. Measures such as putting off tasks that are not essential, whether it be housework, decisions or social events, can reduce the increased stress and demands that she might experience premenstrually and this in turn will make her feel more in control and therefore more able to cope at this particular time.

Taking some time out 'for herself', perhaps to indulge in an enjoyable hobby or pastime will be beneficial. Equally, some women wish to be 'left alone' and having understanding and supportive partners, family and friends can be very helpful at this time.

Advice on general health is obviously important, such as cutting down or giving up smoking. Reducing alcohol and caffeine intake may help to reduce anxiety, irritability and palpitations. Exercise is very therapeutic and increases the production of natural endorphins. It can, therefore, be useful in reducing stress whilst at the same time increasing general fitness levels. Adequate rest and a good night's sleep will not only help to reduce the symptoms of tiredness but may also result in improvement in symptoms such as irritability.

This may all seem common sense but minor changes combined with trying to maintain a positive attitude to life will go a long way to minimizing the impact of PMS on a woman's life.

Diet and supplements

Diet is another vital factor in maintaining optimum health. Many theories about the effects of diet and PMS exist and many nutritional supplements have been recommended for PMS over the years.

Frequent high carbohydrate meals. Advocated to reduce the symptoms of tiredness, irritability and headaches, frequent meals have been suggested based on the common belief that hypoglycaemia is a contributing factor in PMS.

In a study carried out by Wurtman et al (1989), consuming an evening high-carbohydrate, low-protein meal improved many mood symptoms in sufferers of PMS. The authors suggested that the positive mood that followed the intake of the carbohydrate was related to increases in the synthesis of serotonin levels. This has been shown by other studies also and is consistent with the theory of decreased blood serotonin levels during the luteal phase of the menstrual cycle in PMS patients.

Many women report cravings, particularly for sweet things such as chocolate and other carbohydrates premenstrually. This should be discouraged if possible as it could potentially contribute to weight gain unless the snacks can be substituted for healthier options such as fruit or vegetables.

Women must be encouraged to eat regularly and sensibly premenstrually. Skipping meals and eating 'junk food' is only likely to aggravate symptoms. Some studies have suggested that too much refined sugar increases fluid retention resulting in symptoms such as breast tenderness and abdominal bloating.

Vitamin A and zinc. Suggestions that vitamin A is helpful in treating PMS have not been substantiated by double-blind, placebo-controlled trials, although vitamin A and zinc have been demonstrated to be effective in controlling premenstrual oily skin and acne (Michaelson et al 1977).

Vitamin B6. Vitamin B6 has been widely advocated for the treatment of PMS based on the theory that it is involved in the synthesis of several neurotransmitters, including **dopamine** and serotonin. Several un-controlled studies have shown it to be helpful, but placebo-controlled studies have produced less conclusive results. Some studies have shown benefits on weight gain and fluid retention and others showed no effects at all in the symptoms of PMS. Vitamin B6 taken in large doses continuously carries a potential risk of **peripheral neuropathy**.

Evening primrose oil. Evening primrose oil has become a well-publicized and popular choice of treatment for PMS. It contains a high content of an essential fatty acid called gamma-linolenic acid. Fatty acid deficiencies are associated with some types of breast disease and double-blind studies have shown it to be more effective than placebo in the treatment of cyclical **mastalgia** (Khoo et al 1990). It is less effective, however, than danazol or **bromocriptine** but does have fewer side-effects. There is no real evidence that it is helpful for any other PMS symptoms and it is expensive, however it is available on prescription for mastalgia (Efamast).

All dietary supplements can be bought over-the-counter from most chemists, health food shops and some of the larger supermarkets, but cost is a consideration. Numerous vitamin and mineral deficiencies have been linked to PMS (calcium and magnesium are also involved in neurotransmitter synthesis) but many are difficult to study and evaluate. Many women do choose to supplement their diets in this way but it can prove costly and the general advice you would give anyone is that a healthy, well-balanced diet containing plenty of fresh food is the best way to get these important nutrients, although supplements will do no harm if taken in moderation. Benefits will not appear overnight and a sensible diet needs to be maintained long term.

Complementary therapies

Some women may consult practitioners who specialize in 'alternative' or 'complementary' therapies. These include: acupuncture, homeopathy, herbalism, aromatherapy, reflexology and hypnotherapy.

These approaches are often appealing but it must be remembered that, although helpful to many, there is little scientific evidence to say that they work, and the benefits could be placebo in nature. However, this does not matter if a woman is going to gain some symptom relief from them. Therapies can be very beneficial in treating specific symptoms rather than PMS as a whole and the therapies are often very relaxing in nature, which is always a good way of reducing stress and stress-related symptoms. Women often appreciate the 'time' that is given to them, and having the opportunity to talk and be listened to is always very therapeutic. Some of the therapies can be very costly but the benefits for some still make this a worthwhile choice.

Stress management

We all lead very busy and demanding lives and these days more and more women work, some through choice and others through necessity. Trying to cope with all the demands at home and at work can be very stressful and dealing with this stress in a constructive way is not always easy. A few enviable people always seem to be able to cope no matter what problems they have, but the majority have to try to find ways of 'coping' with life.

Acknowledging when we feel under pressure is the first step, as is accepting the fact that premenstrually we perhaps feel more pressured than usual.

Adapting our life to accommodate PMS will help to alleviate some of the symptoms experienced, rather than trying to struggle on and achieving what we might normally do easily. Lowering our expectations of ourselves will help make life easier. Some women, however, find this impossible and will aim to meet all the usual demands put upon them, and it may well be that these women suffer more because they are not prepared to make any allowance for their PMS in any way.

Finding ways of reducing stress is important to us all and there are many ways of doing this. Some of the self-help and lifestyle changes already discussed may help but any form of relaxation will be beneficial. Relaxation and stress management can be formally taught or experienced through any means we find helpful personally. Reading, watching television, relaxation techniques, gentle exercise like swimming, walking or yoga might be examples. Acupuncture, reflexology and aromatherapy or a combination of these complementary therapies (a massage or bath combined with aromatherapy oils) can have obvious positive benefits.

Some women feel very angry premenstrually and this can be a cause for concern, as it is a common perception that women should not display their anger. This in turn can create frustration and resentment, which can often be followed by outbursts of irrational and angry behaviour, which in turn can lead to feelings of guilt. It is helpful to find constructive ways of dealing with these feelings, rather than taking it out on the family or on colleagues at work. Sporting activities can be a useful outlet for these emotions, but it might also be helpful to warn those close to them that it is 'that time of the month'.

Women must try not to allow their whole lives to be governed by their PMS. It is easy to fall into this negative trap, but better to try to focus on those times of the month when they feel well and adopt a more positive approach to their lives at that time instead.

Psychological measures

Counselling

Counselling can be undertaken in many ways from simply talking to another individual, possibly a friend, work colleagues, family member or partner. It might take the form of more formalized counselling with a nurse, trained counsellor or doctor, and both can be very positive. Psychological symptoms of PMS are complex and a woman perhaps having pursued some of the self-help measures already outlined may find that this group of symptoms are not being helped sufficiently. At this point they may seek further professional help.

For those women who have many symptoms it can be difficult to distinguish which are due to PMS and which are caused by other precipitating factors. A careful and detailed history may help to determine what course of action needs to be taken. Diary cards can be helpful here and will highlight those symptoms that are genuinely due to PMS and those that may persist regardless of the cycle and need addressing separately. Both can be helped by counselling and the severity of the symptoms will determine whether counselling is enough or whether measures like **cognitive therapy** might be more appropriate.

GPs are usually very restricted in terms of time and may have to refer a patient on to a trained counsellor who will have not only the expertise but also the time to address their needs more effectively.

Cognitive therapy

Treatments for psychological disorders are difficult to evaluate and very few studies have been conducted but, recently, cognitive therapy has been studied as a form of treatment for PMS (Blake 1995).

Cognitive therapy is a particularly suitable form of treatment for PMS because it is largely common-sense. It has been shown to be an effective treatment for other psychological disorders such as anxiety and depression.

It is suggested that a woman with PMS experiences physiological changes that trigger negative thoughts based on her assumptions about how she should feel and behave at this time. She is influenced by previous experiences of PMS and she may predict that these changes are going to create difficulties for her, especially if she associates these symptoms with previous unpleasant exchanges with her partner or family. This in turn leads her to feel anxious and depressed about her responses, and causes further negative thoughts and behaviour.

There are beliefs and assumptions about the female role in society that are important in this. We are frequently brought up with the concept that women should be submissive, self-sacrificing and totally available. When our ability to cope premenstrually falls short of our expectations of ourselves and those of others around us we feel inadequate and try harder to keep up with the usual demands upon us, when we are unable to do this, we begin a vicious circle of negative patterns of thinking.

Cognitive therapy is based on the theory that if a woman focuses on her responses to any physical and emotional symptoms that she experiences, she can then challenge these unhelpful patterns of behaviour and look to find more constructive and positive ways of dealing with them.

Therapy usually consists of twelve sessions working with a trained therapist. A woman presenting for cognitive therapy has often exhausted many other avenues of treatment. She may have reservations about a non-pharmacological approach to treatment of her symptoms and may be uncomfortable about viewing her problems as 'psychological', especially if medical treatments have been tried unsuccessfully. The concept of cognitive therapy must be explained to her and her fears and thoughts acknowledged. The effectiveness of treatment will depend on establishing a trusting and understanding relationship with her therapist. Most women feel more comfortable and confident with a

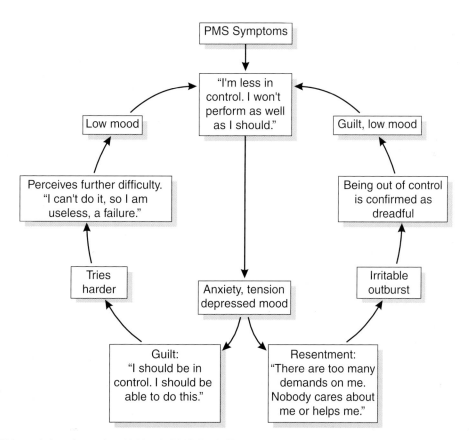

Figure 7.4 Vicious circles of negative thinking in PMS. From Blake 1995, with permission.

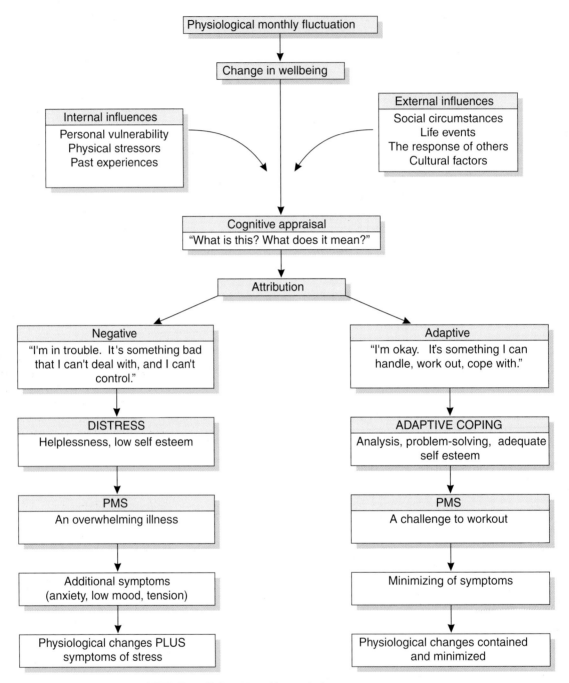

Figure 7.5 A cognitive model of PMS. From Blake 1995, with permission.

female therapist and, if a woman believes men cannot possible understand her PMS, a relationship with a male therapist is unlikely to be successful.

Initial assessment is made to highlight the main problem areas of difficulty. Symptoms and their impact on the woman's life must be discussed in detail. Social circumstances, the demands of her job and family and their response to her PMS are also important. Medical, gynaecological and psychological examinations should be carried out to exclude any other problems.

Diaries must be kept in order to confirm a diagnosis of PMS, ideally for at least two months, so that patterns of symptoms can emerge. Once this is done areas of concern can be identified and explored. Non-PMS patterns of symptoms can also be discussed. At this stage the woman and her therapist can draw up a vicious circle illustrating her problems and her responses to them, it may well be that her responses exacerbate the problems even more.

Once therapist and patient have identified usual responses, then alternative approaches can be suggested and practised. She may have to find ways of nurturing herself and looking after her own needs, and not feeling responsible for the needs of others. A pilot study (Blake et al 1995) demonstrated that cognitive therapy is an effective and acceptable way of helping women with PMS to help themselves.

Pharmacological treatments

Placebo effect

Comparing the effects of an active treatment to a non-active placebo is an important way of assessing the efficacy of a new therapy. Many treatments will have a large placebo response purely because a patient feels that something constructive is being done to help them. Many self-help principles will work in this way, from measures such as talking or counselling to the use of dietary supplements and alternative therapies. In order to provide evidence that any given treatment is effective, it must be tested using double-blind, placebo-controlled trials. A placebo might produce a response rate of improvement in symptoms of up to 40%, or possibly more. The placebo effects in treatments for PMS have been found to be very significant. This makes defining effective treatments more difficult and may also explain why so many different treatment options for PMS have been studied, but none of these being shown to be totally effective.

Taking part in a clinical trial, with the time and individual care that is given to women during this process, may be largely responsible for this high placebo effect, because of the psychological benefits that are gained from such support.

Women who have persistent symptoms of a more severe nature, which have persisted despite trying other treatment options, will need a more medical approach in the management of their PMS.

Diuretics

Women who experience symptoms attributed to fluid retention, such as abdominal bloating and breast tenderness, might be prescribed diuretics. There is no evidence that diuretics are helpful for any other symptoms of PMS and they should only be prescribed in extreme cases where there is significant weight gain during the luteal phase of the menstrual cycle. They must be used with caution under medical supervision as they can lead to problems of electrolyte imbalance. This can be minimized by the use of aldosterone **antagonists** such as spironolactone but, in general, their use is probably best avoided.

Prostaglandin inhibitors

Double-blind, placebo-controlled trials carried out using Ponstan (mefenamic acid) have shown that it is effective in relieving some PMS symptoms (Moline 1993), but results have been inconsistent and further work needs to be done. Mefenamic acid is a prostaglandin inhibitor with analgesic properties and can also reduce menorrhagia. Its use should be considered for any women suffering from symptoms of pain (including migraines) and other menstrual problems. It has not been shown to have any effect on breast symptoms.

Progesterone and progestogens

Progesterone has become the most widely used form of treatment for PMS. It is usually prescribed as vaginal suppositories or in the form of oral progestogen dydrogesterone (Duphaston).

Kathrina Dalton has enthusiastically recommended this form of treatment on the basis that women have a deficiency of progesterone premenstrually. She has written extensively on the subject and has done much to raise public awareness of PMS for women. However, claims of the efficacy of progesterone have not been substantiated. Clinical trials have not demonstrated progesterone to be any more effective than placebo and a well-controlled study carried out by Freeman et al (1990) showed that premenstrual symptoms were not significantly improved in any measure used in the study.

Some women do claim that progestogens are helpful but, in reality, there is limited evidence and indeed sense for the continued prescribing of progestogens.

Progestogen-releasing intrauterine system

An intrauterine coil containing the progestogen, levo-norgestrel, has been recently developed and although currently only licensed for contraceptive use, it can also be an effective treatment for other gynecological conditions such as menorrhagia. Progestogen given cyclically can cause side-effects but, with this treatment, progestogen contained in the stem of the coil is slowly and continuously released into the endometrium and, for many women, results in ammenorrhoea. There is minimal systemic absorption of progestogen and therefore side-effects, including PMS-type symptoms, can be reduced.

Ovulation is not prevented but the decrease or absence of cyclical bleeding can be an advantage, as the anticipation of PMS symptoms and a monthly bleed are removed. Oestrogen can be given in addition to the coil if needed and, if given in a sufficient dose, can suppress ovulatory function. It is therefore reasonable to suppose that a progestogen-releasing intrauterine system (IUS), given with continuous and sufficient oestrogen, might be beneficial for the treatment of PMS.

Oestrogen/progestogen therapy

More recently, another approach using oestrogen therapy has been of interest. Giving women sufficient doses of oestrogen will suppress ovulation and therefore help to resolve symptoms of PMS caused by the natural ovarian cycle. Oestrogen is given continuously and a progestogen added in cyclically to induce a bleed. Studies carried out using oestradiol implants and cyclical norethisterone showed encouraging results compared to placebo, but implants can have unpleasant side-effects as they wear off and blood levels of oestrogen need to be closely monitored as they can become abnormally high with repeated use (tachyphylaxis) and for these reasons long-term use is not advisable. The use of oestradiol patches may be a more acceptable way of achieving similar symptoms control and, unlike implants, the effects are easily reversible. Studies using patches have demonstrated the same improvement in symptoms compared to placebo (Watson et al 1989) and recent work has concentrated on finding a dose that suppresses ovulation without causing significant oestrogenic side-effects. Smith et al (1995) found that a dose of 100 μg oestradiol (twice weekly) is effective at suppressing ovulation and relieving PMS symptoms, but these results need confirming with a placebo-controlled trial in the

Case history

'I had always been aware of my PMS, but it wasn't until I started to record my moods and symptoms that I realised just how it affected my life. I knew that I would get snappy and grumpy in the week leading up to my period, but that was about it.

I would generally consider myself to be a happy, optimistic person. I will always try to find something to look forward to, but when the hormones kick in (about 4–5 days after ovulation) I tend to become miserable. I am not extreme in any sense of the word, but I tend to feel sorry for myself and become very pessimistic at this time. I also start to look a little rounder, or at least I *feel* fatter, and that makes me even more fed up. As a result, I tend to eat more and it becomes a bit of a vicious circle. Everything seems to be a real effort, I can almost hear myself whinging and whining when people ask me how I am, It must be really annoying for them.

I am not violent or dangerous in any way, but I do snap at people. I have very little patience at the best of times, but when I am premenstrual it is a nightmare.

It is difficult to explain how PMS affects me, it is not a big thing in my life, more of an irritation; I think it affects the people around me more.

My boyfriend would describe me as 'stroppy, withdrawn and uncommunicative', and he would say it affects me three weeks out of four!

In summary, when I am premenstrual I feel 'snappy, fat and miserable'.

same way as 200 μg has been studied. Trials are currently being carried out to look at this and there is also a possibility that even lower doses of oestrogen may be effective. The use of matrix patches is less likely to cause the unwanted side-effect of skin irritation.

Oestrogen can be given to women of any age but for perimenopausal women with PMS symptoms, this type of treatment could potentially be very helpful as they may also be lacking in oestrogen.

Oral contraceptive pill

The oral contraceptive pill is another treatment that is widely prescribed for PMS. Hormonal manipulation using contraceptives can be helpful in suppressing ovulation with the idea that PMS symptoms will therefore be reduced. However, placebo-controlled trials have failed to demonstrate any consistent effectiveness. Whilst some women find this treatment helpful, others have found that the progestogen phases of the pill can have the side-effect of reproducing some cyclical symptoms. Giving oral contraceptives continuously to prevent breakthrough bleeding would be a more logical

---

Case history

'My PMS began during the latter part of my teens, but because I was on the contraceptive pill I was informed that this was unlikely.

It seemed to subside during my 20s and returned after the birth of my second child, at the age of 34 years. It gradually worsened each month, the symptoms being mood swings, headaches, depression, irritability etc. It was like being a Jekyll and Hyde character, although you know you're being offensive, rude and irrational, your behaviour is impossible to control, especially if you're in a situation that if you were feeling 'normal' you would usually compromise. The slightest thing can trigger off this behaviour – inconsiderate motorists, children being nosier than usual, supermarket trolleys with minds of their own, computers going down, everyday situations that you would normally be quite capable of dealing with seem monstrous.

This character change happens approximately half-way through your cycle, so out of four weeks in the month you get one or two great weeks and then it's downhill all the way to your period.

I tried to 'get my act together' by various options such as 3-hourly carbohydrate meals, vitamin B6 and evening primrose oil, none of which helped and also cost a lot of money.

So I went to the GP (a woman of around the same age) and then was referred to a specialist clinic, a female team who took time to listen to me. After a careful history and filling out diary cards, treatment in the form of oestrogen patches and progestogen tablets (for 12 days out of 28) was recommended. Encouragement was given to persist with the treatment to allow it to work. I gained some weight but it could be that because I felt so well I was eating and drinking more!

The treatment really helped me and I'm a sceptic. I now feel I can take on whatever is thrown at me and be more or less in control of my actions. I am even writing this premenstrually!'

---

approach and can provide welcome relief for those women who suffer menstrual problems such as pain and heavy bleeding. At present no research supports this treatment and further work in this area is needed.

Selective serotonin re-uptake inhibitors

Modern antidepressants known as selective serotonin re-uptake inhibitors (SSRIs) have been studied with great interest as a form of treatment for PMS (Dimmock et al 2000). SSRIs have had a significant impact on the treatment of depression and other **affective disorders**. They work by increasing serotonin levels in the brain by inhibiting uptake of serotonin. If,

as already discussed, some of the new theories that women with PMS may be deficient in serotonin are further confirmed, then boosting serotonin levels with these drugs should improve symptoms (O'Brien & Chenoy 1995).

Fluoxetine (Prozac) has been shown to be effective for the treatment of premenstrual dysphoric disorder (PMDD) in several controlled studies compared to placebo (Ozeran et al 1997, Pearlstein et al 1997, Steiner et al 1995).

In 1999, Prozac became licensed as a treatment for PMDD or severe PMS. The effects of various doses have been studied, but 20 mg reduces the potential for side-effects whilst maintaining therapeutic efficacy (Steiner et al 1995). Side-effects can occur and include gastrointestinal irritability, insomnia and sexual dysfunction, but generally these seem to be well-tolerated (Ozeren et al 1997). Studies are underway to look at whether intermittent Prozac treatment could be given premenstrually. If this is possible, it might be useful for those women who do not like taking medication (particularly antidepressants) all the time (Steiner et al 1997). Several other SSRIs have been studied and Yonkers et al carried out a large trial in 1997 that showed that sertraline (Lustral) was significantly better than placebo for treatment of premenstrual dysphoria.

SSRIs show considerable promise in treating a range of PMS symptoms, but may be most beneficial for those women suffering from symptoms such as irritability and mood changes. They may also benefit those with any underlying depressive symptoms or illnesses.

GnRH analogues

Gonadotrophin-releasing hormone (GnRH) analogues, such as goserelin, buserelin, leuprorelin and naferelin, are given to create a 'medical oophorectomy'. They work by suppressing ovarian function and menstruation and therefore the cyclical PMS symptoms that would normally occur with the menstrual cycle. Oestrogen levels are reduced and cause a temporary menopausal state.

Several well-conducted studies have shown GnRH analogues to be effective compared to placebo. They are most effective if given by depot injection but their use is generally limited to 6 months because of the side-effects. Symptoms experienced by menopausal women such as hot flushes, night sweats, vaginal dryness and headaches are common but these are usually well tolerated if prior warning is given. Other more potentially serious side-effects, including the risks of osteoporosis and cardiovascular disease, are due to low oestrogen levels and can be prevented by the use of 'add-back therapy' (continuous combined therapy of oestrogen and progestogen as in HRT).

This type of treatment can have advantages in that if a women experiences complete resolution of her symptoms, as well as giving her 'a break' from PMS, it also provides her with the reassurance that her symptoms are due to her ovarian cycle.

Treatment with GnRH analogues is generally reserved for those women with severe symptoms for whom other treatment options have failed and if a definitive diagnosis is needed.

Danazol

Suppression of the ovarian cycle can be also achieved by the use of another GnRH analogue – danazol. This is a synthetic, oral steroid that works by inhibiting ovulation. It therefore often results in ammenorrhoea.

Placebo-controlled trials have shown danazol to be effective for women with PMS symptoms, although it can result in unpleasant **androgenic** side-effects such as weight gain, bloating, acne and hirsutism. These can be minimized by giving smaller doses, but trials suggest that lower doses are less effective on PMS symptoms other than mastalgia.

Prolonged use of danazol can adversely affect lipid profiles and, if its use is to be for more than 6 months, then these must be monitored. It is currently not licensed for the treatment of PMS.

Surgery

In very extreme cases of PMS, surgery is occasionally recommended. A hysterectomy and bilateral oophorectomy results in the relief of all genuine PMS cyclical symptoms. If symptoms are not shown to be cyclical then they are likely to persist and therefore this radical treatment should not be done. The ovaries will need to be removed otherwise PMS symptoms would persist despite the absence of bleeds.

HRT in the form of oestrogen must be given both to relieve short-term menopausal symptoms and to prevent the long-term consequences of the menopause such as coronary heart disease, osteoporosis and Alzheimer's disease. This is particularly important for these women as they are going to be undergoing a much earlier menopause than normal, so the long-term effects are going to be much more significant. A

progestogen need not be given as endometrial protection is not necessary in the absence of a uterus.

THE ROLE OF THE NURSE

PMS being an exclusively female disorder means that women can often relate to and would prefer to discuss this condition with other women. This means that female nurses (and female doctors) are potentially very central to the management of PMS. Nurses are often viewed as being more approachable than doctors, possibly because they are perceived to have more time, or perhaps women are more comfortable talking to them about issues that might be embarrassing. Many women do not understand much about PMS themselves, or even recognize that the problems that they have are related to their menstrual cycle. They may feel their symptoms are not severe enough to discuss with a doctor.

Routine check-ups such as cervical screening provide an opportunity for nurses to enquire about a woman's menstrual cycle and any problems she may be experiencing. Health visitors are also in a position to meet women postnatally and during the stressful years when children are small, when PMS often presents.

Nurses could potentially provide much of the initial support for these women, providing them with knowledge, information and if possible literature about PMS. The role of the nurse is continually being extended, and it is not unusual for nurses to have acquired many additional skills, such as counselling, which could be put into excellent use for these women. The therapeutic benefits of talking and 'being listened to' cannot be underestimated, and any stresses in a woman's life that might be exacerbating her symptoms can often be identified and then addressed during this time.

General advice on measures such as lifestyle changes, diet and supplements and complementary therapies can be given, as these do not require a medical practitioner to prescribe them. Most importantly, women should be given adequate information where possible, so that they have the choice about what type of treatment options they would like to pursue.

These approaches may be all that is needed, but if at any point it becomes apparent that medical intervention or advice is more appropriate then the nurse must refer a woman to her doctor for the necessary treatment.

There is scope for treating women in groups and setting up such a system might be possible. Alternatively, there are several support groups available already and information regarding these can be given if required.

The management of women with PMS can be a time-consuming commitment and, as most doctors are very restricted in this respect, nurses have the potential to be very central in the management of these women and, if time could be made available, this could be explored as a specific role.

CONCLUSION

Despite extensive research, PMS still has many unresolved questions surrounding its cause. Establishing an effective treatment is therefore going to remain difficult. There is limited scientific evidence to support many of the current medical treatment options advocated, and the non-medical treatment options are more difficult to assess accurately. PMS is known for having a significant placebo response, which should be taken into account.

There are self-help options for those women who wish to take this approach as well as a number of support groups available.

Education is a key factor and once a woman understands the implications of PMS on her life, she can then begin to accept that she has a role to play herself in the management of her symptoms. Learning to challenge negative patterns of behaviour and looking for more

positive ways of coping with her problems will enable her to feel more in control and responsible for the treatment of her PMS. Many psychological problems can manifest themselves as physical symptoms, and doctors and nurses who do not separate mind and body may be more appropriate for these women, who, at the end of the day, want help from a sympathetic and supportive source.

Cognitive therapy has been shown to be a helpful non-medical treatment for PMS and this could have potential for being used in general practice, if even in some modified form.

Recent advances in our understanding of the role of serotonin and other neurotransmitters has generated new interest and may lead to some new answers. Clinical trials of selective serotonin re-uptake inhibitors have shown promising results for women with psychological symptoms – the hardest group of symptoms to treat – and further work will be watched with interest.

Gynaecologists and psychiatrists continue to study this fascinating syndrome but neither speciality accepts total responsibility for it. Gynaecologists are not trained in psychiatry and vice versa, so perhaps we should be looking at ways of working together in a dual approach, so that the physical and psychological needs of these women can be met.

GLOSSARY

Affective disorder: pertaining to emotions or moods
Affective psychosis: major mental illness in which there is grave disturbance of emotions and moods
Agoraphobia: morbid fear of being alone or in large open places
Aldosterone: an adrenocortical steroid that, by its action on renal tubules, regulates electrolyte metabolism
Androgenic: masculinizing effect usually pertaining to androgens, the hormones secreted by the testes and adrenal cortex that control male secondary sex characteristics
Antagonist: a drug that exerts active opposition
Bromocriptine: a dopamine receptor agonist useful in hyperprolactinaemia
Cognition: the mental processes by which knowledge is acquired. These include perception, reasoning, acts of creativity, problem solving and possibly intuition.
Cognitive therapy: an approach to the psychological treatment of depression and anxiety-related disorders through correcting errors in thinking and poor problem solving

Dopamine: a catecholamine neurotransmitter closely related to adrenaline
Gonadotrophin: any gonad-stimulating hormone
Hyperprolactinaemia: excessive prolactin in the blood
Hypoglycaemia: decreased levels of glucose in the blood
Mastalgia: pain in the breast
Peripheral: pertaining to the outer part of an organ or of the body
Neuropathy: disease of the nervous system
Serotonin: a compound widely distributed in the tissues, particularly in the blood platelets, intestinal wall and central nervous system. Serotonin is thought to play a role in inflammation similar to that of histamine and it also acts as a neurotransmitter.
Synthesis: the process of building complex substances from simpler substances by chemical reaction

ACKNOWLEDGEMENT

The case histories used are descriptions from genuine patients and I would like to thank them for their time and contributes to this chapter.

REFERENCES

American Psychiatric Association 1994 Diagnostic and statistical manual of mental disorders (DSM-IV) 4th edn. American Psychiatric Association, Washington DC

Blake F 1995 Cognitive therapy for premenstrual syndrome. Cognitive and Behavioural Practice 2:167–185

Blake F, Gath D, Salkovskis P 1995 Psychological aspects of premenstrual syndrome: developing a cognitive approach. Treatment of Functional Somatic Symptoms 271–284 In: Mayou R, Bass C, Sharpe M. Oxford University Press, Oxford

Chadwick J, Mann WN 1950 The medical works of Hippocrates. Blackwell, Oxford, 267–268

Dalton K 1961 Menstruation and crime. British Medical Journal 2:1752

Dimmock PW, Wyatt KM, Jones PW et al 2000 Efficacy of selective serotonin-reoptane inhibitors in premenstrual syndrome: a systematic review. The Lancet vol 356: 1131–1136

Frank RT 1931 The hormonal basis of premenstrual tension. Archives of Neurological Psychiatry 26:1053–1057

Freeman E, Rickels K, Sondheimer SJ et al 1990 Ineffectiveness of progesterone suppository treatment for premenstrual syndrome. Journal of the American Medical Association 264(3):349–353

Greene R, Dalton K 1953 The premenstrual syndrome. British Medical Journal 1:1007–1014

Khoo SK, Munro C, Battistutta D 1990 Evening primrose oil and treatment of premenstrual syndrome. The Medical Journal of Australia 153:188–192

Magos AL, Studd JWW 1984 The premenstrual syndrome. In: Studd JWW (ed) Progress in obstetrics and gynaecology, vol 4. Churchill Livingstone, Edinburgh, pp. 334–350

Magos AL, Studd JWW 1986 Assessment of menstrual cycle symptoms by trend analysis. American Journal of Obstetrics and Gynecology 155:271–277

Michaelson G, Juhlin L, Vahlquist A 1977 Effects of oral zinc and vitamin A in acne. Archives of Dermatology 113:31

Moline ML 1993 Pharmacologic strategies for managing premenstrual syndrome. Clinical Pharmacy 12:181–196

O'Brien PMS 1990 The premenstrual syndrome. British Journal of Family Planning 15 (suppl.):13–18

O'Brien S, Chenoy R 1995 Premenstrual syndrome. The Diplomate (Review) 87–93

Ozeron S, Corakci A, Yucesoy I et al 1997 Fluoxetine in the treatment of premenstrual syndrome. European Journal of Obstetrics and Gynaecology Reproductive Biology 73(2):167–170

Pearlstein TB, Stone AB, Lund LA et al 1997 Comparison of fluoxetine, bupropion, and placebo in the treatment of premenstrual dysphoric disorder. Journal of Clinical Psychopharmacology 17(4):261–266

Rapkin AJ 1992 The role of serotonin in premenstrual syndrome. Clinical Obstetrics and Gynaecology 35(3):629–636

Rapkin AJ, Morgan M, Goldman L et al 1997 Progesterone metabolite allopregnanolone in women with premenstrual syndrome. Obstetrics and Gynaecology 90(5):709–714

Sampson GA 1989 Premenstrual syndrome. Baillière's Clinical Obstetrics and Gynaecology 3:687–704

Smith RNJ, Studd JWW, Zamblera D et al 1995 A randomised comparison over 8 months of 100 μg and 200 μg of transdermal oestradiol in the treatment of severe premenstrual tension. British Journal of Obstetrics and Gynaecology 102:475–484

Steiner M, Steinberg S, Stewart D et al 1995 Fluoxetine in the treatment of premenstrual dysphoria. Canadian Fluoxetine/Premenstrual Dysphoria Collaborative Study Group. New England Journal of Medicine 332(23):1529–1534

Steiner M, Korzekwa M, Lamout J et al 1997 Intermittent fluoxetine dosing in the treatment of women with premenstrual dysphoria. Psychopharmacology Bulletin 33(4):771–774

Watson NR, Studd JWW, Savvas M et al 1989 Treatment of severe premenstrual syndrome with oestradiol patches and cyclical oral norethisterone. Lancet ii:730–732

Wurtman J, Brzezinski A, Wurtman AJ et al 1989 Effect of nutrient intake on premenstrual tension. American Journal of Obstetrics and Gynecology 161:1128

Yonkers KA, Halbreich U, Freeman E et al 1997 Symptomatic improvement of premenstrual dysphoric disorder with sertraline treatment. Journal of the American Medical Association 278(12):983–988

FURTHER READING

Andrews G (ed) 1997 Premenstrual syndrome. In: Women's Sexual Health, Baillière Tindall, London, pp. 314–335

Blake F 1995 Cognitive therapy for premenstrual syndrome. Cognitive and Behavioural Practice 2(1):167–185

DeGraff Bender S, Kelleher K 1996 PMS: Women tell women how to control premenstrual syndrome. New Harbinger Publications, Oakland, CA

Gardner K, Sanders D 1997 Premenstrual syndrome. In: McPherson A, Waller D (eds) Women's health, 4th edn. Oxford Medical Publications, Oxford, pp. 280–302

Hayman S 1996 PMS the complete guide to treatment options. Judy Piatkus Publishers, London

USEFUL ADDRESSES

National Association for Premenstrual Syndrome
PO Box 72, Sevenoaks, Kent TN13 1XQ
Tel: 01732 741709

The Premenstrual Society (Premsoc)
PO Box 429, Addlestone, Surrey KT15 1DZ
Tel: 01932 872560

The Woman's Nutritional Advisory Service
PO Box 268, Lewes, East Sussex BN7 2QN
Tel: 01273 487366

8

Polycystic ovary syndrome

Hazel Watson

The original description of polycystic ovary syndrome (PCOS) was by Stein and Leventhal (1935). They defined a clinical syndrome of hirsutism, obesity and infertility associated with bilaterally enlarged polycystic ovaries. This original definition has been constantly modified as knowledge of the morphological and biochemical features of PCOS has increased with improvements in technology. In particular, the advancement in pelvic ultrasound scanning has enabled the identification of polycystic ovaries (PCO) in women who do not display the classic symptoms of the Stein–Leventhal syndrome. This has led to a recognition of the clinical and biochemical **heterogeneity** of the condition and the consequent diversity in clinical presentation. The heterogeneity has fuelled considerable controversy and debate regarding all aspects of this complex disorder. This chapter will address current concepts in its diagnosis, aetiology and management. However, the understanding of all aspects of PCO is continually improving, necessitating constant updating of knowledge.

DIAGNOSIS

Ovarian morphology

Histological examination of a portion of the ovary removed by wedge resection was previously the only means of identifying PCO. The advent of high resolution ultrasound scanning has provided a non-invasive, reliable method of diagnosis. Criteria may vary between centres but a widely accepted ultrasound definition of PCO (Adams et al 1986) requires that:

- Each ovary contains, in one plane, at least ten follicles of 2–8 mm in diameter distributed peripherally.
- There is an increase in the density of ovarian stroma, observed as an increase in echogenicity. The volume of stroma may also be increased.

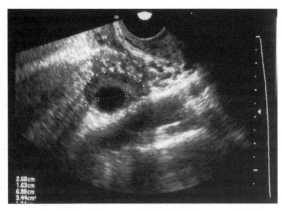
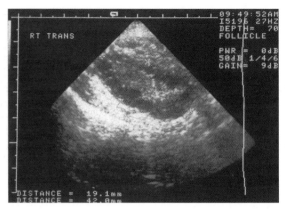

A   B

Figure 8.1   Transvaginal ultrasound scans showing (A) a normal ovary with a developing follicle and (B) a polycystic ovary. Photographs courtesy of Dr D M White.

- The mean ovarian volume may exceed the normal value of 8.7 ml.

These diagnostic criteria were based on transabdominal ultrasound scans. The advent of transvaginal ultrasound scanning has allowed closer inspection of the ovaries with improved resolution. Consequently, some groups now define the polycystic ovary as one that contains at least 15 cysts and usually more than 20 (Fox et al 1991).

Figure 8.1 shows transvaginal ultrasound scans of a normal (Fig. 8.1A) and a polycystic (Fig. 8.1B) ovary. Saxton et al (1990) demonstrated an excellent correlation between the histological analysis of ovarian morphology and that seen on transabdominal ultrasound scan.

The ultrasound diagnosis is considered by most centres to be the gold standard. However, where machines and expertise are not available, diagnosis by endocrine profiles combined with clinical presentation may be employed.

Uterine area and endometrial thickness

The uterine area is slightly increased and the endometrium thicker in women with PCO (Adams et al 1988). In anovulatory cycles, this is due to stimulation by oestrogen unopposed by progesterone. This can result in heavy bleeding and, in the long term, in an increased risk of endometrial carcinoma (Sherman & Brown 1979). However, the endometrium is also thicker in the follicular phase of ovulatory cycles, strongly suggesting that additional as yet unknown factors are involved (Adams et al 1988).

Endocrine indices

Androgens

Hyperandrogenaemia is the most consistent biochemical abnormality in women with PCO (Franks 1991). Studies of the incidence of raised androgen concentrations have given variable results. These can be accounted for by factors such as the selection criteria for study and the referral bias of the clinics from which they are obtained. Although individual random serum samples are often normal (< 2.6 nmol/L) mean serum testosterone concentrations are raised in all groups of women with ultrasound evidence of PCO compared to those of women with normal ovaries (Franks 1991) and increase with the severity of the clinical symptoms. Conway et al (1989) found a raised serum concentration of testosterone in 22% of women with PCO; Balen et al (1995) found that in 28.9% of 1741 women with PCO serum testosterone concentrations were above the normal range. As serum testosterone concentration increased, there was an increased risk of hirsutism, infertility and menstrual cycle disturbance.

Alterations in the rate of androgen production, clearance and bioavailability are additional important factors to be considered as they also affect clinical presentation. Both the rates of androgen production and clearance by peripheral tissues are raised in some women (Bardin & Lipsett 1967, Kirschner & Bardin 1972, Kirschner et al 1983). This results in overall normal testosterone concentrations even though symptoms of hyperandrogenism, such as hirsutism, may be present (Conway et al 1989, Franks 1989, Lobo 1991).

The serum concentration of sex-hormone binding globulin (SHBG) affects the bioavailability of testosterone (Anderson 1974, Rosner 1990). Low SHBG levels result in an increase in free testosterone and hence greater clinical effect. Insulin suppresses SHBG production, therefore hyperinsulinaemic women with PCOS have lower SHBG levels (Kiddy et al 1990). Hyperinsulinaemia and insulin resistance are exacerbated by obesity; SHBG concentrations are therefore lower in obese women, consequently the symptoms of hyperandrogenism are more severe.

Should serum testosterone concentrations exceed 5 nmol/L on two or more occasions, congenital adrenal hyperplasia, Cushing's syndrome and adrenal or ovarian tumours should be excluded.

Luteinizing hormone and follicle stimulating hormone

The second recognized biochemical abnormality in women with PCO is a raised serum luteinizing hormone (LH) concentration. As with testosterone, there is biochemical heterogeneity; thus levels are not always elevated in women who have PCO diagnosed by ultrasound scanning. Moreover, as LH is secreted in a pulsatile fashion, results depend on the frequency of sampling and can be affected by the assay systems employed (Fauser et al 1992). The prevalence of raised LH concentrations is also affected by the way in which the study population is selected, and on referral bias. The mean (SD) early–mid-follicular phase serum LH concentration in a group of 277 women with PCO was 13.6 (8.8) u/L compared to 6.3 (2.4) u/L in a group of women with normal ovaries (Franks 1989). A raised concentration of serum LH was found in 44% of women diagnosed as having PCO on ultrasound or clinical findings by Conway et al (1989). Balen et al (1995) found that 39.8% of 1741 women with PCO had elevated serum LH concentrations and concluded that the rates of infertility and cycle disturbance increased as serum LH concentrations rose.

Serum concentrations of follicle stimulating hormone (FSH) are typically normal, resulting in a raised LH:FSH ratio in some women with PCO (Adashi 1988).

Oestrogens

In anovulatory women with PCOS, the pattern of secretion of oestrogen differs from that of the normal menstrual cycle. Although serum concentrations of oestradiol lie within the normal range for the early and mid-follicular phases of the cycle (Polson et al 1987)

there is no preovulatory or mid-luteal rise. In obese women, serum levels of oestrone may be raised due to the increased aromatization of androgens to oestrone in adipose tissue (Polson et al 1987). Oestrogen concentrations in women with PCO who are ovulating are within the normal range.

Prolactin

Hyperprolactinaemia has been noted in 5–30% of women with polycystic ovaries (Franks 1989, Futterweit 1983, Murdoch et al 1986). The significance and cause are unknown, although it may be due to the unopposed action of oestrogen on the pituitary gland (McKenna 1988).

Growth hormone

Although an impairment of growth hormone secretion has been noted in women with PCOS, this seems to be as a result of coexistent obesity and not due to PCOS per se (Slowinska-Srzednicka et al 1992).

PREVALENCE OF PCO IN THE NORMAL POPULATION

In order to discover the background incidence of polycystic ovaries, Polson et al (1988a) carried out ultrasound scans on 257 women recruited from the general population. Although none of these women had complained of menstrual disturbance, infertility or acne, 22% had PCO. Regular cycles were defined as having an intermenstrual interval of not less than 21 and not more than 35 days, with not more than a 4-day variation from cycle to cycle. Although none of the women with PCO had found it necessary to seek medical advice, a detailed menstrual history questionnaire revealed that 75% of the women with PCO had irregular cycles and six of the eight women with regular cycles had unwanted facial hair. Clayton et al (1990) found a 21% prevalence of PCO in a normal population, again diagnosed by ultrasound, and an identical prevalence was found in a community in New Zealand by Farquar et al (1994).

THE CLINICAL SPECTRUM

It can be seen from the preceding sections that a women may have polycystic ovaries on ultrasound scan without having any biochemical abnormalities or clinical symptoms. It is important therefore to make a distinction between having polycystic ovaries (PCO)

Box 8.1 The difference between PCO and PCOS

Polycystic ovaries + Biochemical abnormality **and/or** Clinical symptoms:
on ultrasound   raised androgens and/or   hirsutism
(PCO)   raised LH and/or   menstrual
                           raised LH:FSH ratio   irregularity

↓

Polycystic ovary syndrome (PCOS)

Box 8.2 Definitions of PCO and PCOS

The biochemical and clinical heterogeneity of PCO make a universal definition difficult to establish. The following have been suggested:
• 'Polycystic ovaries' – the ovarian morphology that may occur regardless of symptoms (Franks 1998).
• 'Polycystic ovary syndrome' – the typical ovarian morphology plus at least one presenting symptom of hyperandrogenism (hirsutism, acne, alopecia) anovulation (oligomenorrhoea) or amenorrhoea (Conway et al 1989, Franks 1989).
• 'Polycystic ovary syndrome' – the association of hyperandrogenism with chronic anovulation in patients without specific diseases of the adrenal or pituitary gland (Zawadski & Dunaif 1992).

---

and polycystic ovary *syndrome* (PCOS) (Boxes 8.1 and 8.2). The classic definition of polycystic ovary syndrome is the association of hyperandrogenism with chronic anovulation in patients without specific diseases of the adrenal or pituitary glands (Zawadski & Dunaif 1992). In the light of ultrasonographic studies, a modification has been suggested such that the term 'polycystic ovaries' refers to the ovarian morphology that may occur regardless of symptoms and 'polycystic ovary syndrome' can be defined as the typical ovarian morphology plus at least one presenting symptom of hyperandrogenism (hirsutism, acne, alopecia) anovulation (oligomenorrhoea) or amenorrhoea (Conway et al 1989; Franks 1989).

It is perhaps easiest to regard PCO as a clinical spectrum with women having regular ovulatory cycles and no symptoms or problems at the lower extreme, and women with anovulation and/or hirsutism at the opposite extreme, with various grades of presentation in between.

CLINICAL PRESENTATION

The biochemical and clinical heterogeneity seen in women with PCO results in diverse clinical presentation. Women may attend gynaecology, infertility or endocrine clinics, depending on which symptoms they have found to be problematic. The clinical features of 300 women with an ultrasound diagnosis of PCO are shown in Table 8.1 (Gilling-Smith & Franks 1993).

Anovulation

Anovulation is diagnosed by subnormal mid-luteal phase progesterone concentrations (< 30 nmol/L) and/or the absence of follicular development during cycle monitoring by ultrasound.

PCOS is a major cause of anovulation and therefore infertility. As there is no regular cyclical stimulation and shedding of the endometrium without ovulation, women who are anovulatory are either amenorrhoeic

Table 8.1 Clinical features of 300 women with polycystic ovaries diagnosed by ultrasound scanning ('total' indicates the total number of women who were found to have the clinical abnormalities listed following history and/or examination). (From Gilling-Smith & Franks 1993, with permission.)

	Presenting features (%)	Total (%)
Hirsutism	34	64
Acne	9	27
Obesity (BMI > 25 kg/m^2)	10	35
Infertility	41	42
Amenorrhoea	23	28
Oligomenorrhoea/irregular cycle	38	52
Dysfunctional uterine bleeding	6	14

or, more commonly, oligomenorrhoeic. In a series of women presenting to a gynaecology clinic, 32% of those with secondary amenorrhoea and 87% of those with oligomenorrhea had PCO (Franks 1989).

Menstrual disturbances

A consequence of anovulation is irregular menstrual bleeding. This may therefore be the presenting feature in women who are not concerned with issues of fertility. As oestrogen is unopposed by progesterone during anovulatory cycles, the uterus is often enlarged and the endometrium thicker, resulting in heavy, often painful, bleeding. This constant exposure of the endometrium to unopposed oestrogen can result in endometrial hyperplasia and carcinoma. In a study of 1741 women with PCO diagnosed by ultrasound scan, 47% had oligomenorrhoea, 19.2% had amenorrhoea, 2.7% had polymenorrhoea, 1.4% had menorrhagia and 29.7% had a normal menstrual cycle (Balen et al 1995).

A more disturbing finding was reported by Coulam et al (1983): namely, a three-fold increased risk of endometrial cancer in anovulatory women. Furthermore, most women who develop endometrial cancer before the age of 40 have PCOS (Farhi et al 1986). The risk of endometrial hyperplasia can be eliminated by the use of cyclical progesterone to induce regular endometrial shedding.

Unexplained infertility

When the women of couples presenting to an infertility clinic underwent diagnostic ultrasound scans, 54% of those with unexplained infertility were found to have PCO (Kousta et al 1994).

Early pregnancy loss

Sagle et al (1988) determined the prevalence of PCO in women with recurrent early pregnancy loss who ovulate spontaneously. Using ultrasound scanning as their diagnostic tool, they identified PCO in 80% of women in this group. A larger study of 500 women with recurrent early pregnancy loss revealed a 54% incidence of PCO (Clifford et al 1994).

The aetiology of miscarriage in women with PCO remains unknown. However, early pregnancy loss has been recognized as a distressing complication of ovulation induction in women with PCOS (Garcia et al 1980, Gemzell & Wang 1980). A high rate of miscarriages (33%) was observed in women with PCOS

undergoing ovulation induction with pulsatile gonadotrophin releasing hormone (GnRH) compared to women with hypergonadotrophic hypogonadism (5%) (Homburg et al 1989). Women with PCOS receiving low-dose gonadotrophins suffered a 35% rate of early pregnancy loss (Hamilton Fairley et al 1991). However, in a large analysis of 109 pregnancies in 225 women having the same ovulation induction protocol the miscarriage rate was around 20% (White et al, 1996). This approaches the reported sporadic rate of 10–15%.

Hirsutism, acne and alopecia

The skin is a target organ for androgen action, excess exposure resulting in hirsutism, alopecia and acne. These clinical conditions are therefore associated with PCOS. Hirsutism is measured using the Ferriman–Galwey score. This is a semi-quantatitive measurement of hair growth, a score of less than eight being normal and the maximum value being 36. Of 175 anovulatory women presenting to a reproductive endocrinology clinic, more than 60% were hirsute (Adams et al 1986). More surprisingly, PCO were found in 87% of women presenting with hirsutism but with regular cycles who had previously been classified as having 'idiopathic hirsutism' (Adams et al 1986, Franks 1989). However, non-hirsute women with PCO may have hyperandrogenaemia and hirsute women may have normal testosterone levels (Conway et al 1989, Franks 1989, Givens 1976). This is because the bioavailability of androgens at peripheral tissues is the major determinant of hirsutism. The biologically active androgens in the skin are the 5α-reduced metabolites. The rates of conversion of testosterone and androstenedione to these metabolites therefore influences the degree of hirsutism in individual women. Moreover, the lower concentration of SHBG in some women with PCOS results in an increased concentration of free testosterone being available to exert its effects (Yen 1980).

Although obese women with PCOS may have similar testosterone concentrations to lean women, they are more likely to be hirsute. As body mass index (BMI) increases, **insulin resistance** and hyperinsulinaemia increase. Insulin reduces SHBG concentrations, resulting in an elevated free testosterone fraction and therefore increased hirsutism.

The sensitivity of the hair follicle to androgens is variable, meaning that different women will have different degrees of hirsutism despite similar serum testosterone concentrations (Barth 1988, Lobo 1991). The sensitivity of the pilosebaceous unit to androgen action varies partly on a genetic basis (Carmina et al 1992).

'Androgenetic alopecia' (male pattern baldness with frontal hair loss) also results from exposure of the hair follicle to excess androgens. This is thought to occur only in genetically predisposed women with PCOS (Rosenfield 1997).

Acne has been noted in 27% of women with PCO by Franks (1989) and in 24% by Conway et al (1989). The prevalence of PCO in women with acne vulgaris has been found to be 83% (Bunker et al 1989), 45% (Peserico et al 1989) and 52% (Betti et al 1990).

METABOLIC ABNORMALITIES AND THEIR LONG-TERM CONSEQUENCES

Insulin resistance, hyperinsulinaemia, type 2 diabetes mellitus and obesity

An extreme form of insulin resistance is associated with acanthosis nigricans, a pigmentation of the skin that affects the neck, axilla and groin (Khan et al 1976). Serum insulin concentrations are up to 100 times greater than normal. Moreover, polycystic ovaries are present in almost all of those women in whom ovarian morphology has been defined. This has led to the investigation of the connections between insulin and ovarian function, and the implications for women with PCO.

Burghen et al (1980) noted that women with PCOS were hyperinsulinaemic, even those without acanthosis nigricans, but many of the women in the group were obese. This was a confounding factor, because hyperinsulinaemia and insulin resistance are associated with obesity. When Chang et al (1983a) studied a group of lean women with PCOS, they discovered that they too were hyperinsulinaemic when compared to a group of women with normal ovaries. Insulin resistance was demonstrated in lean women with PCOS by Dunaif et al (1989) and Holte et al (1994). Conway (1990) found that fasting insulin concentrations were higher in women with PCOS than those with normal ovaries. Furthermore, insulin concentrations were significantly higher in women with irregular menstrual cycles than in women whose cycles were regular. A study by Robinson et al (1993) supported these findings by demonstrating that women with PCOS who are anovulatory are more insulin resistant and hyperinsulinaemic than women with normal ovaries when matched for weight. Between 35 and 40% of women with PCO are obese, that is their BMI exceeds $25\,kg/m^2$. The presence of obesity compounds insulin resistance and hyperinsulinaemia, so exacerbating clinical symptoms such as hirsutism and menstrual

disturbances (Conway et al 1989, Kiddy et al 1990). Weight reduction in obese oligomenorrhoeic women with PCO reduces insulin and raises SHBG concentrations. This can reduce hirsutism, restore menstrual regularity, induce ovulation and, in some cases, achieve pregnancy (Kiddy et al 1992). It is important to note that the insulin resistance in women with PCO is peripheral and not hepatic. Moreover, ovarian cells are able to respond to insulin in vitro. This has led to one proposed hypothesis for the mechanism of anovulation as described on page 137.

Insulin resistance is associated with type 2 diabetes mellitus. Accordingly, the risk of developing type 2 diabetes mellitus appears to be increased in women with PCOS. Both impaired glucose tolerance or frank diabetes were found in 20% of obese young women with PCOS by Dunaif et al (1987). In a cohort of women who had undergone ovarian wedge resection 20–30 years earlier, Dahlgren et al (1992a) found that 13% had previously diagnosed non-insulin-dependent diabetes mellitus (NIDDM) compared with an incidence of 2.3% in a large, matched, reference population. In other words, the incidence of NIDDM was almost seven times higher in the PCOS group.

In a group of 122 women with PCOS, the prevalence of type 2 diabetes mellitus was 12% and of its precursor, impaired glucose tolerance (IGT), was 35%; the progression of IGT to type 2 diabetes mellitus was accelerated in women with PCOS (Ehrmann et al 1999). Legro and co-workers also concluded that women with PCOS are at significantly increased risk for IGT and type 2 diabetes mellitus at all weights and at a young age (Legro et al 1999). A converse study of premenopausal women with type 2 diabetes mellitus found that 82% had polycystic ovaries identified by ultrasound scanning (Conn et al 2000).

The body fat distribution in women with PCOS is characteristically central (central adiposity) resulting in a high waist:hip ratio (Rebuffe-Scrive et al 1989, Talbott et al 1995). Central adiposity is associated with raised plasma insulin and triglyceride levels and lower high-density lipoprotein (HDL) cholesterol concentrations (Pasquali et al 1994). Therefore both the presence of obesity and its distribution increase the risks of type 2 diabetes mellitus and possibly vascular disease in women with PCOS.

Hyperlipidaemia, hypertension and coronary artery disease

The association of insulin resistance with NIDDM, hypertension and abnormal lipid profiles has prompted investigations into the lipid profiles of women with PCOS and their risk of developing early coronary artery disease. Although coronary artery disease is the most common cause of death in postmenopausal women (Bush et al 1988), screening for risk factors in premenopausal women is not considered to be useful. Conway et al (1992) have suggested that women with PCOS may constitute a group in which preventive measures may be effective. They found that lean women with PCOS were hyperinsulinaemic and had low serum HDL and HDL_2 concentrations when compared to women with normal ovaries. Low HDL-cholesterol, especially HDL_2 cholesterol, is a risk factor for vascular disease. Serum insulin levels correlated positively with blood pressure measurements. Obese women with PCOS had higher systolic blood pressure and serum triglyceride levels than lean women with PCOS or controls. Wild et al (1990) found that hirsute women were more likely to have significant atheroma detailed by coronary angiography than non-hirsute women. The long-term follow-up study by Dahlgren et al (1992a,b) of women who had previously undergone wedge resection found that their lipid concentrations were above the normal range and suggested that they may have an increased risk of developing cardiovascular disease. Robinson et al (1996) found increased serum triglyceride and decreased HDL cholesterol in obese PCOS women compared to weight-matched controls. Moreover, HDL_2 cholesterol concentrations were lower in lean women with PCOS and were associated with insulin insensitivity. They concluded that, as hyperinsulinaemia, insulin insensitivity, impaired glucose tolerance, a reduced HDL_2 cholesterol and an increased waist:hip ratio are associated with cardiovascular morbidity, prospective studies of women with PCO are needed in order to assess their long-term health.

Polycystic ovaries were present in 42% of 163 women aged 60 years and younger who were under-

going coronary catheterization and the women with PCO had more extensive coronary atherosclerosis (Birdsall et al 1997). However, in a study investigating cardiovascular mortality in women with PCOS over long-term follow-up, the ratio of observed to expected deaths as a result of all circulatory disease was lower than expected (Pierpoint et al 1998). Although current data is conflicting, and prospective data to confirm the incidence of circulatory disorders is lacking (for a review, see Solomon, 1999), Amowitz & Sobel (1999) have stressed that aggressive management of obesity and insulin resistance is imperative in decreasing the risk of cardiovascular disease in women with PCOS.

AETIOLOGY

Elucidation of the cause of PCO(S) has fuelled much debate. The hypothalamus, ovary and adrenal gland have been proposed as sites of the principal defect. More recently, genetic studies have shed new light on this complex and fascinating puzzle, which nevertheless is yet to be solved.

Ovarian morphology

The typical morphology of the PCO is of unknown aetiology. One of the defining features of the PCO is the clearly visible peripheral arrangement of 10 or more follicles of 2–10 mm in diameter. On microscopic examination, however, twice the number of primary and secondary follicles can be seen than in normal ovaries (Hughesdon 1982), suggesting that a defect occurs at an early stage of follicular development. This early stage does not appear to be under endocrine control but may be influenced by as yet unknown local factors, resulting in altered activity during the later developmental stages. The intriguing possibility of an intrinsic difference in the programming of **folliculogenesis** between the PCO and normal ovary is suggested by these findings (Franks et al 1998a).

The cause of the increased stroma in the PCO is at present unknown. Hughesdon (1982) attributed the thicker cortical and subcortical stroma to both increased regression of numerous old follicles and to stromal hyperplasia. Dewailly et al (1994) used computerized quantification of ovarian stroma to demonstrate that its increase is specific for the clinical phenotype and concluded that it is the most valuable diagnostic probe for PCO. However, because its assessment is subjective, they recommend that the total ovarian area be used, as this is proportional to stromal area. The area of stroma in their study

---

Box 8.3 Possible long-term consequences of PCOS

- The risk of developing NIDDM in later life is six to seven times that in the appropriate control population.
- Dyslipidaemia suggests a predisposion to cardiovascular disease, but more studies are needed.
- There is an increased risk of endometrial cancer if prolonged exposure to oestrogen during repeated anovulatory cycles is unchallenged by progesterone.

correlated well with serum androstenedione and 17-hydroxyprogesterone, but not with serum LH or fasting insulin. Pache et al (1993) found that stromal volume and echogenicity correlated positively with serum insulin and testosterone concentrations. However, a causal relationship between increased hormone concentrations and increased stroma has not yet been established.

Hyperandrogenism

PCO is associated with an overproduction of androgens both in women who are ovulating and anovulatory (Conway et al 1989, Franks 1989, Stein and Leventhal 1935). Although some controversy still exists as to the origin of these androgens, most available data indicates that the ovary, not the adrenal gland, is the primary site of excess androgen production.

Adrenal androgens

Dehydroepiandrosterone sulphate (DHAS) and excretion of the urinary metabolites of cortisol and adrenal androgens have been reported to be increased in some women with PCO (Hoffmann et al 1984, Rodin et al 1994). However, the adrenal-specific metabolite of androstenedione, 11β-hydroxyandrostenedione were found to be the same in women with PCO and normal ovaries (Polson et al 1988b). Similar controversy has arisen following studies in which adrenal androgen secretion was suppressed using dexamethasone and the effect on total androgen concentrations was determined. In two studies, dexamethasone normalized androgen concentrations in women with PCOS (Loughlin et al 1986, McKenna & Cunningham 1992) whilst in another, androgen concentrations remained elevated (Lachelin et al 1982).

Ovarian androgens

There is now much evidence to suggest that the ovary is the main source of the elevated androgens present in women with PCOS. The suppression of ovarian androgen production using a GnRH analogue resulted in a reduction of circulating androgen concentrations to those seen postoophorectomy (Change et al 1983b).

The reason why PCO secrete more androgen than normal ovaries is unclear. Increased accumulation of androstenedione, 17-hydroxyprogesterone and progesterone in the medium of ovarian **theca cells** from PCO was found in the in vitro studies of Gilling-Smith

et al (1994). Levels were raised in both ovulatory and anovulatory PCO, indicating that hyperandrogenaemia is neither a sole cause, nor the result of, anovulation. Androgen production is stimulated by LH, although the hyperandrogenaemia in PCO can occur in the absence of raised LH. Moreover, increased androgen production is not due to hyper-responsiveness to LH, either in vitro (Gilling-Smith et al 1993) or in vivo (White et al 1995).

Insulin stimulates theca cell androgen production but, as with LH, the degree of augmentation is the same in both PCO and normal ovaries (Gilling-Smith et al 1993). Moreover, as insulin is raised only in women who are anovulatory (see p. 134) it cannot be the sole cause of hyperandrogenaemia. Current data therefore supports the hypothesis that there is an intrinsic abnormality in ovarian androgen production due to dysregulation of key enzymes in the steroidogenic pathway.

Hypersecretion of LH

The secretion of LH and FSH from the anterior pituitary gland is regulated by the release of GnRH from the hypothalamus (see Chapter 1). Whether alterations in GnRH secretion, resulting in hypersecretion of LH, occur due to a primary defect in hypothalamic function or secondarily as a result of abnormal steroid feedback is controversial. In women with PCOS, higher concentrations of LH are produced in response to GnRH than in women with normal ovaries (Yen et al 1975). However, equivalent amounts of FSH are secreted.

Several studies have demonstrated that an increase in the amplitude of GnRH pulses results in an increased amplitude of LH pulses and therefore contributes to the increased mean serum LH concentrations seen in some patients with PCOS (for review, see Futterweit 1995). However, investigations of pulse frequency in women with PCOS have given conflicting results (for review, see Filicori & Flamagni 1992).

The weight of evidence suggests that the disturbances in GnRH pulsatility seen in women with PCOS occur as a result of disordered ovarian feedback. In a study by Christman et al (1991) LH pulse frequency and amplitude, mean serum LH and incremental LH response to GnRH all decreased following administration of mid-luteal phase concentrations of oestradiol and progesterone. The exaggerated response to GnRH secretion found in PCOS returns to normal following an ovulatory cycle (Blankstein et al 1987). Moreover, the falls in serum testosterone, androstenedione, oestrone and oestradiol concentrations that follow ovarian diathermy are accompanied by a lowering of LH pulse amplitude and a reduction in response to GnRH challenge (Rossmanith et al 1991). These data suggest that if feedback by the ovarian steroids is restored then LH concentrations are lowered.

Evidence for disordered central dopaminergic, opoidergic, noradrenergic or serotoninergic pathways has proved elusive, hindering the formulation of a unifying neuroendocrine disorder in PCOS (for review, see Soule 1996). Currently, the weight of evidence points to inappropriate gonadotrophin secretion being a consequence of altered feedback due to the abnormalities in ovarian steroid concentrations seen during ovulatory disturbances (Soule 1996). However, the causes of the more subtle alterations in LH concentrations in women who are ovulating remain to be determined.

An intriguing suggestion has been that the pituitary glands of women with PCO have been 'masculinized' by exposure to excessive androgens during development in utero (Rosenfield et al 1990). Hence they have an enhanced LH response to GnRH. Evidence to support this has been provided by patients who have a history of neonatal exposure to high androgen concentrations due to 21-hydroxylase deficiency. In a study by Barnes et al (1993) the LH response to GnRH was enhanced in women with 21-hydroxylase deficiency.

Insulin resistance, hyperinsulinaemia and type 2 diabetes mellitus

If peripheral insulin resistance is present, the β-cells of the pancreas increase their secretion of insulin in order to compensate. Type 2 diabetes mellitus will develop if this increase does not maintain euglycaemia. Studies in women with PCOS are focused on abnormalities of insulin action and/or insulin secretion.

The cause of insulin resistance in women with PCOS is at present unclear. Dunaif et al (1995) has found abnormal serine phosphorylation of the insulin receptor in 50% of PCOS skin fibroblasts. This could cause defects in the early steps of the insulin signalling pathway, which would result in insulin resistance. Interestingly, Zhang et al (1995) have found that serine phosphorylation of the enzyme P450c17, which regulates androgen biosynthesis, increases its activity. Therefore the same factor could cause both hyperandrogenism and insulin resistance (Dunaif 1997).

Abnormalities of first phase insulin secretion in women with PCOS during glucose tolerance tests were reported which persist after weight reduction even though there is an improvement in insulin sensitivity (Holte et al 1995). Ehrmann et al (1995) have also found insulin secretory defects. Thus a disorder of pancreatic β-cell function may coexist with insulin resistance in women with PCOS.

Anovulation

The mechanism of anovulation in PCOS is at present unknown. The biochemical markers of raised LH and raised testosterone occur in women with PCO who are ovulating, therefore they cannot be the cause of anovulation. Although follicles are characteristically arrested at the 5–10 mm stage, they are not atretic (Erickson et al 1992). In fact the **granulosa cells** from follicles of anovulatory ovaries hypersecrete oestradiol (Mason et al 1994). Increased concentrations of androstenedione, 17-hydroxyprogesterone and progesterone accumulate in the medium of thecal cells from PCO (Gilling-Smith et al 1994) in both ovulatory and anovulatory PCO. This would suggest that androgens cannot be the cause of anovulation, although they may be involved in the mechanism.

Current research is focused on discovering the agent or agents responsible for causing the arrest of follicle growth. Inhibitors of FSH action include epidermal growth factor (EGF) and transforming growth factor α (TGFα), which inhibit aromatase action in vitro (Hsueh et al 1981). However, no differences have been found in their concentrations in the follicular fluid of women with PCO compared to those with normal ovaries (Mason et al 1995). It is unlikely, therefore, that these growth factors have a role in the mechanism of anovulation in PCOS. The insulin-like growth factors (IGFs), IGF receptors, IGF binding proteins and their proteases are important regulators of follicular development. Although they change at the time of follicle selection, **atresia** and arrest of development, it is not clear whether these changes contribute to, or are a consequence of, follicle selection; their roles in the mechanism of anovulation in PCOS are yet to be elucidated (see Giudice 1999 and references therein).

The striking endocrine difference between women with PCO who are either ovulating or anovulatory is an elevated serum insulin concentration in the anovulatory women (Sharp et al 1991). The in vitro studies of Willis et al (1996) have shown that insulin sensitizes granulosa cells to the effects of LH. This has given rise to a proposed mechanism of anovulation in PCOS. In ovulatory cycles, the granulosa cells of the dominant follicle acquire LH receptors at a follicle diameter of approximately 10 mm. LH is then able to bind to its receptors and initiate terminal differentiation, allowing the follicle to grow to approximately 20 mm in diameter prior to growth arrest and ovulation. The involvement of insulin in the acquisition of LH receptors has been proposed (Hattori & Horiuchi 1992). Willis et al (1998) have therefore suggested that follicles from the ovaries of women with PCOS who are anovulatory acquire LH receptors at an earlier stage due to exposure to high concentrations of insulin. They demonstrated that granulosa cells of follicles from the ovaries of women with ovulatory cycles (either normal or PCO) reach 9.5–10 mm before a response can occur; however, small follicles (>4 mm diameter) with the ovaries of women with PCOS who were anovulatory can respond to LH in culture. This would allow terminal differentiation to proceed earlier, resulting in prematurely arrested growth of the follicle at <10 mm diameter and thus anovulation.

The preovulatory follicle is thought to switch from growth to terminal differentiation due to a rise in cyclic adenosine monophosphate (cyclic AMP) concentrations above a threshold level (Hillier 1994), normally initiated by the onset of the LH surge. Androgens augment LH-induced cyclic AMP production in granulosa cell cultures (Harlow et al 1988). Therefore it has been proposed that a combination of raised LH and/or insulin and/or testosterone may generate preovulatory levels of cyclic AMP in PCOS, causing early growth arrest and anovulation (Franks et al 1996).

Miscarriage and PCO

The link between PCO and miscarriage is currently unknown. It has been suggested that elevated LH levels in the follicular phase could prematurely mature the oocyte, which is then 'aged' at ovulation (Stanger & Yovich 1985). This may then give rise to problems in fertilization and implantation. In a study of spontaneously ovulating women conducted by Regan et al (1990), elevated LH in the follicular phase of conception cycles was more common in women who subsequently miscarried than in those whose pregnancies proceeded to term. However, Clifford et al (1996) used a GnRH analogue to suppress LH levels in women with PCO, elevated LH and a history of recurrent early pregnancy loss. Ovulation was then induced using the low-dose human menopausal gonadotrophin (hMG) protocol and the luteal phase was supported using progesterone pessaries. Miscarriage rates were compared to those in women with the same selection criteria but who were allowed to ovulate spontaneously with either luteal phase progesterone support

or placebo pessaries. No difference in miscarriage rates between the three groups was observed. The reasons why over 50% of women with recurrent early pregnancy loss have PCO are yet to be established.

Obesity is an independent risk factor for miscarriages. Hamilton-Fairley et al (1992) compared the miscarriage rate in lean (BMI 19–24 kg/m²) and obese (BMI 25–27.9 kg/m²) women with PCOS having ovulation induction with low-dose gonadotrophins. The miscarriage rate in the lean group was 27% but in the obese group was 60%. Data from the North West Thames Health Region obstetric database was analysed and, although the ovarian morphology of the women was not known, the risk of miscarriage was increased in moderately obese women. The link between obesity in PCO and increased risk of miscarriage is unknown.

GENETICS OF PCO

Several studies have indicated that PCO is a familial disorder (Cooper et al 1968, Givens 1988, Simpson 1992). However, its genetic basis remains to be determined. The difficulties of assigning affection status to postmenopausal women and of defining a male phenotype have hindered the elucidation of the mode of inheritance.

One suggested male phenotype has been premature male pattern baldness, a hyperandrogenic disorder (Ferriman & Purdie 1979). Several studies have suggested that there is an autosomal dominant mode of inheritance (Carey et al 1993, Cooper et al 1968, Ferriman & Purdie 1979, Lunde et al 1989). One has suggested an X-linked model (Givens 1988) and another found that the prevalence of PCO among siblings was too high to indicate a simple dominant model (Hague et al 1988). The heterogeneity of PCOS suggests that it is unlikely to be a single gene disorder. Simpson (1992) suggested that it should be treated as a **quantitative trait disorder** and Franks et al (1998b) have proposed that it has an **oligogenic** basis.

The candidate gene approach has been employed in attempts to discover the genes involved in its aetiology.

Genes coding for steroidogenic enzymes

As hyperandrogenaemia is a consistent biochemical abnormality and theca cell androgen production is increased in PCO, it has been proposed that PCOS is a genetically determined disorder of ovarian androgen secretion (Franks et al 1998b). An upregulation of the enzymes involved in steroidogenesis is likely, therefore the genes encoding these enzymes were considered to be appropriate candidates.

The first gene to be investigated was *CYP17*, encoding cytochrome P450c17α (17α-hydroxylase/17–20 lyase), the enzyme that catalyses the conversion of progesterone to androstenedione. This has been excluded as a major causative gene (Gharani et al 1996, Techatraisak et al 1997). Attention was therefore focused on *CYP11a*, which encodes P450 side-chain cleavage. This catalyses the removal of the side-chain from cholesterol to form pregnenolone. Gharani et al (1997) suggest that *CYP11a* may be a major genetic susceptibility locus for PCOS.

Genes involved in insulin secretion or action

Although impaired sensitivity to insulin action suggests a defect in the insulin receptor in women with PCOS, no abnormality in the insulin receptor gene has been detected (Conway et al 1994, Talbot et al 1996). Increased first phase insulin secretion in women with PCOS (Ehrmann et al 1995, Holte et al 1994, O'Meara et al 1993) that persists after weight reduction (Holte et al 1995) has suggested a primary abnormality in pancreatic β-cell function. This points to a defect in the insulin gene itself. A sequence of DNA near to the insulin gene variable number tandem repent (VNTR)

has been implicated in the regulation of insulin secretion and in the susceptibility to NIDDM (Bennett & Todd 1996). Waterworth et al (1997) found an association between specific alleles of this locus and PCOS, with the strongest association in anovulatory women with PCOS. This is in accordance with the finding of hyperinsulinaemia in anovulatory women with PCOS.

These data suggest that the steroid synthesis gene *CYP11a* and the insulin gene VNTR regulatory **polymorphism** are important factors in the genetic basis of PCOS. Variation in androgen production and its sequelae, such as hirsutism, could be explained by differences in expression of *CYP11a*, whilst class III alleles of the insulin gene VNTR may confer hyperinsulinaemia and therefore anovulation (Franks et al 1998b).

The clinical heterogeneity could therefore be explained by the variable expression of these and other as yet unidentified genes, together with environmental factors, such as nutrition, which modify the presentation and symptoms (Franks et al 1997) (Fig. 8.2).

MANAGEMENT

The management of patients with PCO depends on their presentation and individual areas of concern. However, as knowledge of the metabolic disorders increases, important long-term health issues may need to be addressed in all patients.

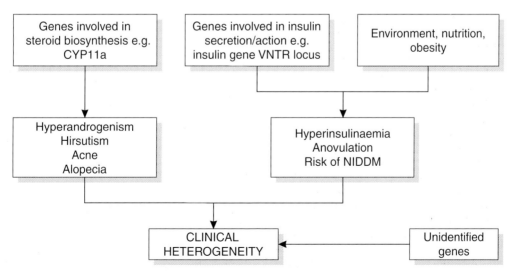

Figure 8.2 Possible interactions between genetic and environmental factors in the aetiology of PCO, adapted from Franks et al 1997, with permission.

> **Case study:** Anne
>
> Anne presented to the gynaecological endocrinology clinic with prolonged and irregular bleeding, which she found distressing and unmanageable. Her cycles were 14–30 days in length but the duration of bleeding was variable.
>
> Anne was obese, with a BMI of 31 kg/m^2 (normal range 20–25 kg/m^2). A pelvic ultrasound scan revealed polycystic ovaries. Her LH was 7.2 iu/L, FSH was 5.6 iu/L and testosterone was 4 nmol/L (normal range 0.5–3.0 nmol/L). Her Ferriman–Galway score was 16, indicating moderate hirsutism.
>
> She was advised to begin a calorie-restricted diet and was referred to a dietitian for a dietary regime and continued follow-up. Medroxyprogesterone acetate (Provera, Upjohn) was prescribed (10 mg/day for 10 days in every calendar month) to induce a regular withdrawal bleed. She also decided to undergo electrolysis to reduce her facial hirsutism.
>
> After 6 months, Anne's BMI was reduced to 27 kg/m^2. She ceased taking Provera and commenced taking Dianette (Schering). This contains 30 µg of ethinyl oestradiol and 2 µg of cyproterone acetate. The latter is an antiandrogen, which acts at the hair follicle to reduce hirsutism. After 3 months her serum testosterone was < 1 nmol/L and her Ferriman–Galway score was 12.

Menstrual disturbances

Periodic progestin therapy is essential in anovulatory women to prevent endometrial hyperplasia or carcinoma. A three-fold increase in endometrial cancer has been reported in anovulatory women (Coulam et al 1983). Bayer and DeCherney (1993) recommend that an endometrial biopsy be carried out in women who have been anovulatory for more than a year before beginning therapy. The treatment of choice is the oral contraceptive pill, as this both inhibits endometrial proliferation and suppresses androgen production, so reducing androgenic symptoms. Alternatively, a non-androgenic progestagen such as medroxyprogesterone acetate may be given for 12 days per month. The treatment of menstrual disturbance is dealt with in detail in Chapter 6.

Anovulation

In a large population study of 708 couples who needed specialist help for infertility, Hull et al (1985) reported that 21% suffered from ovulation failure. Kousta et al (1997) found that over 30% of patients presenting to their infertility clinic had an ovulatory disorder as a major cause of their infertility.

The aims of all methods of ovulation induction are to develop one follicle, which will release one oocyte and produce one healthy baby. Careful ultrasound monitoring of follicular development is essential, as women with PCOS are especially liable to over-respond, resulting in multiple follicular development and possible ovarian hyperstimulation syndrome (OHSS) and/or multiple pregnancy (see Chapter 3). Levine et al (1992) have indicated that there were more triplet pregnancies following ovulation induction than in vitro fertilization (IVF). Clomiphene citrate therapy was responsible for 58% of these compared to 42% following human menopausal gonadotrophin. Careful monitoring of stimulated cycles by ultrasound scanning detailing the number and size of follicles is essential for appropriate patient management. In addition to alerting the practitioner to the dangers of OHSS and multiple pregnancy, ultrasound monitoring has the added benefits of enabling assessment of endometrial thickness, length of luteal phase and accurate timing of mid-luteal progesterone measurement. A single, mid-luteal phase progesterone concentration of more than 30 nmol/L has shown to be an adequate confirmation of ovulation (Hull et al 1982, Talbert 1983).

Ovulation induction should be commenced only if the semen analysis of the woman's partner has excluded severe male factor infertility (see Chapter 3). It should be the first line of treatment in women with PCOS who are anovulatory. However, more invasive infertility investigations, such as hysterosalpingogram, laparoscopy and dye test, should be considered if pregnancy has not occurred after a reasonable number of ovulatory cycles.

Weight reduction

The beneficial effects of weight reduction were demonstrated in a study by Kiddy et al (1992) in which obese women with PCOS undertook a weight-reducing diet. Thirteen women with oligomenorrhoea lost > 5% of their original weight. Their reproductive function improved such that six experienced more regular cycles and five became pregnant. Fasting serum insulin concentrations fell, therefore SHBG concentrations rose (Plymate et al 1988). This resulted in lower circulating free testosterone and thus reduced hirsutism in 40% of these women. Only one of the eight women who lost < 5% of their initial weight noted an improvement in menstrual function and none experienced a reduction in hirsutism. A 6-month programme promoting healthy lifestyle factors but without rapid weight loss led to a reduction of central fat, improved insulin sensitivity and a restoration of ovulation in overweight infertile women with PCOS (Huber-Buchholz et al 1999). Obesity significantly reduces the success of ovulation induction therapy (Hamilton-Fairley et al 1992, Kousta et al 1997, White et al 1996) (see p. 143).

Weight reduction should therefore be strongly encouraged in obese, anovulatory women with PCOS. This may be sufficient to achieve pregnancy; if not, the subsequent likelihood of successful ovulation induction therapy will be increased. Dietary advice and support from a dietitian, if available, is extremely beneficial both in designing specific eating plans for individual women, and in motivating the women to achieve their target weights. The inability to conceive may already have lowered the self-esteem of the women, therefore sensitive handling of weight-related issues by all practitioners is essential.

Medical ovulation induction

Antioestrogens. Antioestrogens such as clomiphene citrate and tamoxifen are the first choice of treatment in women with PCOS who are infertile due to anovulation. The most commonly prescribed is clomiphene citrate. Antioestrogens are thought to act by displacing endogenous oestrogen from hypothalamic and pituitary oestrogen receptors. Thus negative feedback is alleviated, pulsatile GnRH secretion is altered favourably and a 50% increase in endogenous FSH secretion occurs. This then stimulates the development of a dominant follicle and ovulation proceeds.

The recommended dose of clomiphene citrate is 50 mg per day, orally, on days 2 to 6 of the menstrual cycle. Before commencing treatment, menses should be induced in oligomenorrhoeic or amenorrhoeic patients whose endometrium is more than 8 mm thick. Should the endometrium be thin, clomiphene citrate can be taken at any time to initiate the first menstrual cycle. Careful monitoring of the first induced cycle by ultrasound scanning is essential to ensure that the ovaries are responding but not developing multiple follicles. The frequency of scans will depend on the rate of follicular growth. Patients who develop two dominant follicles should be advised of the possibility of a twin pregnancy. If three follicles develop, the decision to have intercourse should be carefully considered in view of the poor outcome of triplet pregnancies and the potential health risks for the mother. When more than three dominant follicles develop, pregnancy should be avoided due to the serious risks of OHSS and multiple pregnancy. Following multiple follicular development, the patient should be monitored care-

fully for signs of OHSS, namely, abdominal pain, thirst, nausea and dehydration. Ultrasound scanning of the ovaries should be carried out frequently until they return to their normal size. Ovulation induction can be recommenced only when the ovaries return to their normal size with only follicles of < 10 mm being present. In patients who over-respond, the dose of clomiphene citrate in the subsequent cycle should be reduced to 25 mg on days 2 to 6. The cycle should be again monitored by ultrasound scanning to ensure unifollicular development.

Of the women who ultimately respond to clomiphene therapy, 30% fail to respond to a dose of 50 mg. For these women the dose may be increased to 100 mg per day, again on days 2 to 6 of the cycle. The first cycle on this higher dose should again be monitored. If the ovaries do not respond to 100 mg of clomiphene, increasing the amount further confers no advantage (Kousta et al 1997), therefore alternative methods of ovulation induction should be commenced.

Ovulation occurs in 75–80% of women with PCOS taking clomiphene citrate and cumulative conception rates approach normal (Franks et al 1985, Hull 1992). A study of 128 women by Kousta et al (1997) reported cumulative conception rates of 51.4% at six cycles and 56.6% beyond six cycles of treatment. The overall pregnancy rate was 11% per cycle, with 71% of pregnancies occurring within the first three cycles of treatment. The miscarriage rate was 23.6%.

Miscarriage rates of 13–25% have been reported following clomiphene citrate therapy. These are similar to the sporadic rate, which is estimated to be up to 15%. A large series reported by Dickey et al (1996) indicated that biochemical and clinical abortion rates were similar in women who had become pregnant spontaneously and those who had conceived following clomiphene citrate therapy.

The multiple pregnancy rate in the study by Kousta et al (1997) was 11%. Multiple pregnancy rates of between 18 and 13% have been reported (Scialli 1986) emphasizing the need for careful monitoring of at least the first treatment cycle.

The duration of treatment requires careful consideration. A retrospective report by Rossing et al (1994) suggested that more than 12 cycles of clomiphene citrate treatment may be associated with an increased risk of borderline or invasive ovarian tumour. Whilst there is no prospective data to confirm this initial report, long-term use of clomiphene is not recommended.

It has been reported in various studies that between 15 and 40% of women do not respond to clomiphene citrate therapy. Should antioestrogen therapy be unsuccessful, the clinician and patient have a choice between proceeding to gonadotrophin therapy or surgical ovulation induction.

Exogenous gonadotrophin therapy. If women do not ovulate when on antioestrogen therapy, or ovulate but do not conceive, exogenous gonadotrophins may be employed to induce ovulation. These have a direct stimulatory effect on the ovary in the same way as endogenous gonadotrophins. They induce ovulation by providing the early to mid-follicular phase rise in FSH, which is absent in anovulatory women with PCOS, thus allowing follicle recruitment to proceed.

Human menopausal gonadotrophin (hMG) preparations such as Pergonal (Serono) and Menagon (Ferring), derived from the urine of postmenopausal women, have been used for more than 30 years. They contain 75 international units (iu) of both LH and FSH per vial in powdered form and are dissolved in water or saline prior to intra-muscular (i.m.) injection. Success rates are variable but a pregnancy rate of 30% has been reported in the largest study using the so-called 'conventional' dose regime (Lunenfeld & Insler 1978, Wang & Gemzell 1980). However, problems with multiple follicular development, multiple pregnancy and OHSS have led to the development of 'low-dose regimens' (Kamrava et al 1982, Seibel et al 1985). A chronic low dose of gonadotrophins is used to find a threshold level of FSH that will stimulate the development of a single follicle but avoid the recruitment of a large cohort. Thus the serious complications of conventional therapy are circumvented. In the protocol employed by White et al (1996), doses of between 37.5 and 52.5 iu (0.5–0.7 ampoule) were used daily for up to 2 weeks during the first cycle of treatment. Follicular development was monitored by ultrasound scanning; treatment with hMG was stopped when a leading follicle of 18 mm in diameter had developed. If no response had occurred after 2 weeks, that is, no follicle of more than 10 mm in diameter was present, the dose was increased to 75 iu (one ampoule) per day for up to 1 week, then the dose increased weekly by half an ampoule until a dominant follicle emerged. Ultrasound scans were carried out at least twice per week throughout treatment. When a dominant follicle had developed and the endometrium was more than 8 mm in diameter, hMG was stopped and 5000 iu of human chorionic gonadotrophin (hCG) was given by intramuscular injection to cause follicle rupture. If either two or three dominant follicles developed, the decision to give hCG was made jointly with the clinicians and patient, due to the possibility of a twin or triplet pregnancy. If more than three follicles developed, the

cycle was abandoned in order to avoid multiple pregnancy and/or OHSS and the couple advised to use contraception. In subsequent cycles, the starting dose was maintained for 1 week, and doses increased by half an ampoule weekly thereafter. If follicle development occurred at a dose of 112.5 iu (1.5 ampoles) or greater, the starting dose was 75 iu (one ampoule). Blood was taken for progesterone measurement 1 week after hCG administration and an utrasound scan performed to measure endometrial thickness and monitor corpus luteum development.

In most women, doses of 52.5–75 iu per day were sufficient to induce ovulation. The average length of the follicular phase was 15 days and clinic visits averaged only six per cycle. In 225 patients, 72% of cycles were ovulatory and, of these, 77% were unifollicular. The overall pregnancy rate was 45%; only 6% were twins, with no higher order pregnancies. The miscarriage rate was 20%. This is lower than the 32% incidence reported in previous studies (Hamilton-Fairley et al 1991). Eighteen per cent of cycles were abandoned, mostly due to multiple follicular development; mild or moderate OHSS developed in 8% of completed cycles and 26% of abandoned cycles. Only one of these patients required hospital admission for observation. This large study illustrates the safety and efficacy of the low-dose protocol, with high rates of pregnancy accompanied by low incidences of OHSS, multiple pregnancy and miscarriage.

The presence of LH in hMG does not appear to adversely affect the outcome of treatment. Sagle et al (1991) demonstrated that a urinary preparation containing FSH and an extremely small amount of LH (Metrodin, Serono) conferred no advantage over hMG in terms of ovulation, pregnancy or miscarriage rates. Recently developed recombinant human FSH (Gonadal F, Serono; Puregon, Organon) contains no LH and is free of urinary proteins. It is well tolerated, consistent from batch to batch and may be injected subcutaneously (s.c.) A large multicentre trial comparing recombinant FSH with urinary-derived FSH demonstrated no difference in follicular development, ovarian steroid production, ovulation or pregnancy rates (Homburg et al 1994).

Pulsatile GnRH therapy. The physiological secretion of GnRH occurs in a pulsatile fashion. This can be mimicked by delivering 15 µg pulses every 90 min using a pump attached to an s.c. needle or intravenous (i.v.) canula. Whilst this therapy is usually reserved for women with hypogonadotrophic hypogonadism, it can be used to induce ovulation in women with PCOS. It has the advantages of producing unifollicular devel-

Anita and Bob presented to the infertility clinic with 2 years of primary infertility. Bob's semen analysis was normal; Anita's menstrual cycles were irregular, being from 2 months to 6 months in length. A pelvic ultrasound scan revealed that Anita had polycystic ovaries. Her serum LH and FSH concentrations were 11.1 iu/L and 5.4 iu/L respectively and her serum testosterone was 3.0 nmol/L. Cycle monitoring detected no follicular development with serum progesterone concentrations of 3 nmol/L. The couple agreed that Anita should commence ovulation induction.

Anita's endometrium was 10 mm thick, therefore she was given 5 mg medroxyprogesterone acetate (Provera, Upjohn) per day for 5 days to induce bleeding. She then commenced taking 50 mg of clomiphene citrate per day from day 2 of bleeding until day 6. Her response was monitored by twice weekly ultrasound scanning. There was no follicle growth until day 12, when one follicle of 11 mm diameter was noted in the left ovary; her endometrium was 8 mm thick. The follicle was 17 mm in diameter on day 15 and her endometrium 10 mm. By day 17 the follicle was 21 mm and the endometrium 11 mm, the couple were therefore made aware of their fertile time. On day 24, Anita's endometrium was 12 mm thick and echogenic, a corpus luteum of 21 mm diameter was seen in her left ovary and her serum progesterone concentration was 54 nmol/L. She menstruated on day 31.

Anita took clomiphene citrate for two further cycles; cycle monitoring was not necessary as she had responded satisfactorily. Her mid-luteal progesterone concentrations were 45 nmol/L and 49 nmol/L. As no pregnancy occurred, the couple were reviewed in the infertility clinic. Athough they were rather disappointed, no problems were highlighted and clomiphene citrate therapy was continued for three further cycles.

Despite having a further three ovulatory cycles, Anita did not become pregnant. The couple were again reviewed in the infertility clinic and agreed that a hysterosalpingogram (HSG) should be carried out to ensure tubal patency. The results of the HSG were completely normal, therefore a further six cycles of clomiphene citrate were prescribed. Anita still did not conceive and, following a long discussion in the infertility clinic and having identified no other factors that could contribute to their conception delay, the couple decided to commence hMG therapy.

An ultrasound scan on day 3 of bleeding showed that Anita's endometrium was 5 mm thick and her ovaries did not contain any follicles of more than 10 mm in diameter. A dose of 52.5 iu hMG (0.7 ampoule Pergonal, Serono) per day was commenced and twice weekly scans for the following 2 weeks showed no follicular development. The dose of hMG was increased to 75 iu per day until day 17 of treatment, when an 11 mm follicle was noted in the left ovary and the endometrium was 8 mm thick; on day 20 of treatment they had increased to 15 mm and 9 mm, respectively. On day 24, the endometrium was 11 mm and the follicle 21 mm, therefore hMG was stopped and 5000 iu hCG (Profasi, Serono) were given to cause follicle rupture. One week later, an ultrasound scan revealed a corpus luteum of 22 mm in diameter in the left ovary, and an echogenic endometrium of 12 mm in diameter. Anita's serum progesterone concentration was 52 nmol/L. Her period commenced 1 week later.

The following cycle was again monitored by twice weekly ultrasound scanning. The starting dose of hMG was 52.5 iu and in the absence of follicular development this was increased to 75 iu after 1 week. A dominant follicle of 20 mm had developed by day 16 of treatment and the endometrium was 10 mm thick; hCG was given. One week later, an ultrasound scan revealed a corpus luteum of 20 mm in diameter and an echogenic endometrium of 12 mm in diameter. Anita's serum progesterone concentration was 50 nmol/L but her period commenced 1 week later. She was becoming very anxious about the amount of time she had to take from work so decided to take a break in treatment of 2 months.

On her return she underwent a further cycle of hMG therapy. Fifteen days after ovulation, a pregnancy test was positive; the pregnancy proceeded to term and Anita gave birth to a healthy 3.5 kg boy.

opment, thus avoiding multiple pregnancy and OHSS. However, the observed ovulation rates of 50% per cycle are relatively low (Shoham et al 1990a).

Factors affecting the outcome of medical ovulation induction

Body mass index. In a prospective study of 158 anovulatory women, Lobo et al (1982) noted that body weight was positively correlated with the dose of clomiphene citrate required to induce ovulation. Polson et al (1989) found that overweight women responded less well to clomiphene citrate than lean women. In a study of 128 patients receiving clomiphene citrate therapy, Kousta et al (1997) found that women who did not respond had a significantly higher BMI than those who ovulated. However, BMI did not influence miscarriage rates in this series.

An increased BMI has been reported to have an adverse effect on several outcomes of ovulation induction with hMG. In a study of 100 women with PCOS who were anovulatory and resistant to clomiphene therapy, larger doses of hMG were required by the obese group to achieve ovulation (Hamilton-Fairley et al 1992). Moreover, the proportion of ovulatory cycles was lower in the obese group than the lean group (57%

versus 77%). Forty-seven per cent of women who were obese suffered a miscarriage compared to 27% of lean women. The study by White et al (1996) also demonstrated that an increased BMI had an adverse effect on outcome of hMG therapy in women with PCOS. The number of abandoned cycles in women whose BMI was greater than 25 kg/m^2 was 31% compared to a rate of 15% in women of normal weight. The overall cumulative conception rate was 57%, but reduced to 46.8% in the overweight group. The miscarriage rate was higher in the overweight group, being 31.3% compared to the overall rate of 20%. Moreover, the ongoing pregnancy rate in the overall group was 40% but only 10% in the few women whose BMI was > 27 kg/m^2. These studies confirm the desirability of weight reduction prior to the commencement of ovulation induction therapy.

LH concentrations. A reduced conception rate following clomiphene citrate therapy has been reported in women whose serum LH concentrations were high in the follicular phase (Shoham et al 1990b). Basal LH concentrations prior to commencing therapy in the study by Kousta et al (1997) influenced neither the response to therapy nor the risk of miscarriage. However, LH concentrations immediately following clomiphene citrate, that is in the mid-follicular phase of the cycle of treatment, were higher in those women who miscarried than in those whose pregnancies proceeded to term. As there was a wide overlap in LH concentrations between these two groups, however, the LH concentration did not predict miscarriage in an individual woman.

Following treatment with pulsatile GnRH, both failure to ovulate and occurrence of miscarriage were increased in women whose follicular phase LH levels were elevated (Homburg et al 1988). In a series of 100 clomiphene-resistant women with PCOS undergoing low-dose hMG therapy, Hamilton-Fairley et al (1991) found that the presence of a raised baseline or mid-follicular phase LH concentration was associated with anovulation, failure to conceive and early pregnancy loss. However, in the larger series of 109 pregnancies in 225 women reported by White et al (1996) there was no difference in the serum LH concentrations of those women whose pregnancy proceeded to term compared to women who did not conceive or those who miscarried. Moreover, as the overall miscarriage rate of 20% was close to the expected spontaneous abortion rate of 12–15% and obesity appeared to be the only observed adverse factor, the authors concluded that the concurrent use of GnRH analogues to suppress endogenous LH levels was not necessary when the 'low dose' protocol is employed.

The use of GnRH analogues to suppress endogenous gonadotrophins prior to superovulation is widely used in IVF–embryo transfer (ET) programmes (see Chapter 3). It was thought that the use of this regimen to reduce LH concentrations would be advantageous in women with PCOS undergoing ovulation induction. Retrospective analyses by Homburg et al (1993) of women undergoing ovulation induction or superovulation for IVF–ET indicated that the miscarriage rate in women who received GnRH analogue was 17.6% compared to a rate of 39.1% in those who received hMG alone. However, prospective randomized studies have demonstrated neither improved responses to gonadotrophins nor increased pregnancy rates as a result of pituitary downregulation with GnRH agonists (Buckler et al 1989, Kupferminc et al 1991).

Surgical ovulation induction

Historically, the first treatment for anovulation in women with PCOS was ovarian wedge resection (Stein & Leventhal 1935). This involved the removal of a wedge-shaped piece of each ovary at laparotomy. Although the mechanism by which this induces ovulation is not understood, several studies have reported successful outcomes of between 25 and 86.7% (Donesky & Adashi 1995). However, this invasive surgical procedure can result in adhesion formation and consequent impairment of fertility (Adashi et al 1981, Kistner 1969).

More recently, interest in surgical procedures has been revived by the discovery that laparoscopic diathermy or laser 'drilling' of the ovaries can induce ovulatory cycles (Armar et al 1990, Gjonnaess 1984). These procedures damage the ovary in several sites, inducing ovulation by as yet unknown mechanisms. Following laparoscopic procedures, oestradiol and LH levels fell in most studies and testosterone levels fell in almost all studies (for review, see Donesky & Adashi 1996). It has therefore been proposed that, by destroying portions of the ovarian stroma and releasing androgens from punctured follicles, androgen levels are reduced. This decreases the amount of substrate for aromatization, so causing a decrease in oestradiol concentrations. This in turn prevents negative feedback on FSH release and positive feedback on LH release at the pituitary, so normalizing the LH:FSH ratio and restoring ovulation. Pituitary secretion of LH in response to GnRH infusions are reduced postoperatively (Sumioki et al 1988) and greatest ovulation rates are achieved when preoperative LH levels were high (Abdel Gadir et al 1990) or follicular fluid is high in androgens (Keckstein et al 1990). An alternative proposal is that damaging the ovary releases paracrine factors, which are then able to gain access to areas where they exert local control over ovulation (for review, see Donesky & Adashi, 1996). Although these suggested mechanisms are speculative, it would seem that the effects on ovulation are mediated systemically. This was illustrated in a study by Balen and Jacobs (1994), which showed that when only one ovary was treated, ovulation could occur postoperatively from either ovary.

Donesky and Adashi (1996) have reviewed 35 reports of ovulation and pregnancy rates following laparoscopic ovulation induction. Analysing the 947 patients revealed an overall 82.1% ovulation rate, either spontaneously or with additional medication to which they had been resistant preoperatively. The overall pregnancy rate was 59.2%; when those patients who did not ovulate were excluded, the pregnancy rate was 72.1%. However, these are not randomized controlled studies. One controlled trial of ovarian electrocautery versus exogenous gonadotrophin therapy showed that there was no difference in outcome between the two treatment options (Abdel Gadir et al 1990). Comparisons between miscarriage rates following electrocautery or gonadotrophin therapy have not as yet been made in prospective controlled trials.

Although these laparoscopic procedures are less invasive than ovarian wedge resection, they nevertheless carry the risks of adhesion formation and anaesthetic complications. Studies by Gurgan et al (1991) revealed that adhesion formation occurs in the majority of patients. However, in a follow-up study, patients who underwent lysis of adhesions had the same pregnancy rate as those without lysis (Gurgan et al 1992). Although these small studies may suggest that the adhesions are not severe enough to cause problems in conception, further, larger, studies are needed in order to establish their safety and complications.

Assisted conception – in vitro fertilization and embryo transfer

If conception does not occur in women with PCOS following an appropriate trial of all methods of ovulation induction, the couple may choose to proceed to IVF and ET (see Chapter 3). Again, the problem of OHSS is heightened in this group of women, therefore superovulation should be carefully managed. A study by MacDougall et al (1993) compared outcomes in 76 patients with and 76 without PCOS undergoing IVF–ET. Patients with PCO received less hMG but

developed more follicles and produced more oocytes. However, fertilization rates were lower in the PCOS patients but there were no differences in embryo cleavage rates or pregnancy rates per embryo transfer. Three of the PCOS patients had higher order multiple pregnancies compared to none of those with normal ovaries. Moderate to severe OHSS occurred in 10.5% of the patients with PCOS compared with none of those with normal ovaries. This study indicates that patients with PCO have similar pregnancy and live birth rates to those of patients with normal ovaries, but underlines the problems of OHSS and multiple pregnancy in this group. It is therefore important that PCO are diagnosed prior to IVF–ET in order to alert practitioners to their potential problems.

Hyperandrogenism: hirsutism, acne, alopecia

Although adrenal and ovarian tumours are rare causes of hyperandrogenism, in women with high androgen levels (testosterone > 5 nmol/L) their presence should be excluded before commencing therapy.

Hirsutism

The management of hirsutism depends on the degree of the problem as perceived by the patient. Some women will be unable to tolerate mild hair growth, whereas others may not be distressed by even excessive hirsutism. It is important that the patient decides the type of treatment, if any, which they feel will adequately fulfil their individual needs and improve their own body image. Beneficial effects of drug therapy for hirsutism usually take at least 5 months to appear, and may not be maximal until 18 months. Such treatment therefore requires patience on the part of both the patient and practitioner.

Weight reduction Weight reduction can significantly reduce hirsutism in obese women with PCOS (Kiddy et al 1992). In women who lost > 5% of their original weight, fasting serum insulin concentrations fell, therefore SHBG concentrations rose (Plymate et al 1988). This resulted in lower circulating free testosterone and thus reduced hirsutism in 40% of these women. None of the eight women who lost < 5% of their initial weight experienced a reduction in hirsutism.

Cosmetic therapy In mild cases, depilatory treatment, shaving or electrolysis may be effective. More severe hirsutism may require medical treatment, either alone or in combination with cosmetic therapy.

Androgen receptor antagonists The most commonly used antiandrogen in Europe is cyproterone acetate. As it is also progestogenic, when taken in combination with ethinyl oestradiol it acts as a contraceptive and regulates menses. Whilst this is an added benefit in some women, it also means that this therapy is inappropriate for women with PCOS who are also receiving infertility treatment. Cyproterone acetate was found to reduce hirsutism in about 70% of women (Hammerstein et al 1975, van Weyjen & van den Ende 1995). An alternative antiandrogen is spironolactone, also used in conjunction with the oral contraceptive pill. About 70–90% of patients showed a reduction in hirsutism following treatment with spironolactone (McMullen & van Herle 1993). Flutamide has been shown to have beneficial effects in 19 of 20 women when used in combination with the oral contraceptive pill (Cusan et al 1990).

The side-effects of antiandrogens may be distressing and include mood swings, lethargy and loss of libido. Some patients may find that the severity of their side-effects outweighs the benefits of these drugs and may therefore elect to discontinue or take a break from treatment. The serious problem of liver dysfunction as a result of antiandrogen therapy is rare (Wyowski et al 1993) but necessitates regular monitoring of liver function in all patients.

Inhibitors of androgen production Any form of low-dose oral contraceptive pill induces ovarian suppression and decreases androgen production. Whilst being less effective than other methods of androgen suppression, this treatment is recommended for mild cases (Azziz et al 1995). Androgen production by the ovaries may be suppressed using the GnRH analogues. These can be given as a daily subcutaneous injection, intranasally or as a monthly depot injection. It requires the replacement of oestrogen and progesterone to prevent menopausal symptoms and to maintain bone density, making it rather cumbersome and relatively expensive. Several studies have suggested that approximately 75% of hirsute women will respond to GnRH therapy (Barnes 1997).

Acne

The management of acne again requires a sensible assessment of the benefits of therapy versus the severity of side-effects. Initially, broad-spectrum antibiotics may be the treatment of choice, followed by hormone therapy or retinoic acid derivatives if the acne persists. The oral contraceptive pill is very effective in the treatment of acne. Lemay et al (1990) reported that 70% of patients with moderate acne experienced at least a 50% decrease in the number of lesions. The oral contraceptive pill alone or in combination with dexamethazone resulted in a complete resolution of cystic acne in 75% of patients and an improvement in the remaining 25% (Marynick et al 1983). Cyproterone acetate has been shown to reduce the severity of acne in about 90–95% of patients (Hammerstein et al 1975, van Weyjen & van den Ende 1995).

Alopecia

Androgen-dependent alopecia may be treated with antiandrogen therapy. However, symptoms are rarely reversed and improvement is limited. Studies by Hammerstein et al (1975) and van Weyjen & van den Ende (1995) indicated that alopecia was reduced in 45% of patients following cyproterone acetate treatment for 9 months.

Obesity and metabolic sequelae

As has already been stated, the presence of obesity exacerbates pathology and adversely affects the outcome of fertility treatments in women with PCO. Therefore even modest weight loss can reduce symptoms such as menorrhagia, irregular cycles, anovulation and infertility. Hirsutism is also reduced if obese women with PCOS lose weight. Weight reduction should therefore be encouraged. Support and advice regarding calorie-restricting diets may need to be sought from dietitians.

As weight is reduced there is typically a reduction in hyperinsulinaemia and hyperandrogenaemia. This has stimulated interest in the therapeutic application of insulin-sensitizing drugs in the treatment of symptoms in both lean and obese hyperinsulinaemic women with PCOS. Metformin is a biguanide that reduces hepatic glucose production. Improvement in insulin sensitivity is also seen during metformin therapy mainly, however, due to the weight loss that often occurs (DeFronzo et al 1991). In two studies, treatment with metformin caused a reduction in insulin and androgen levels (Nestler & Jakubowicz 1996, Velazquez et al 1994). However, in the study by Velazquez et al (1994) the patients also lost weight, so confounding the results. When metformin was given to obese women with PCOS in whom weight was maintained for the duration of a 3 month study, Ehrmann et al (1997a) found no improvement in glucose or insulin responses to an oral glucose tolerance test or in insulin resistance. Other studies have found that metformin has no effect on hyperinsulin-aemia or hyperandrogenaemia in obese normal (Fendri et al 1993) or obese hirsute (Crave et al 1995) women. Metformin decreased insulin secretion in obese women with PCOS and increased the ovulatory response to clamiphene (Nestler et al 1998). No effect of metformin on insulin-stimulated thecal cell androgen production was demonstrated in vitro (Duleba et al 1993). The conflicting results from these studies indicate that the therapeutic value, if any, of metformin is yet to be determined. Further randomized controlled trials in selected subgroups are required.

Troglitazone is a thiazolidinedione insulin-sensitizing agent currently not available in the UK. It improves oral glucose tolerance, insulin resistance and β-cell function in individuals with impaired glucose tolerance (Cavaghan et al 1997). When anovulatory obese women with PCOS were treated with troglitazone, their insulin sensitivity improved and testosterone concentrations decreased, even though their weight did not change (Dunaif et al 1996, Ehrmann et al 1997b). In the study of Dunaif et al (1996) two of the 25 women had ovulatory menses. The authors conclude that insulin sensitizing agents may provide a novel therapy for women with PCOS.

Hyperprolactinaemia

The reported incidence of hyperprolactinaemia in women with PCO varies between 5 and 30% (Franks 1989, Futterweit 1983, Murdoch et al 1986). If prolactin is > 1000 mu/L on two occasions, a pituitary tumour should be excluded. In the absence of a tumour, dopamine agonists such as bromocriptine may be used to return prolactin levels to normal. This may result in a return to ovulatory cycles (Franks 1989).

NURSING CARE

Most of the clinical problems associated with PCO can be dealt with on an outpatient basis. Patients may present to endocrine clinics but have associated gynaecological problems, or vice versa. The diagnosis of PCO can be alarming and distressing. Nulliparous women who seek treatment for hirsutism or menstrual disturbance may well be concerned about their future fertility following a diagnosis of PCO. Women attending an infertility clinic may be relieved at the identification of a potential problem that may be resolved with treatment. However, they will certainly have anxieties concerning its implications and their likelihood of becoming pregnant. It is very important,

therefore, that all nursing staff have a full understanding of the characteristics of PCO and can discuss patients' fears and worries with tact and sensitivity. Both the physical and psychological wellbeing of these women must be monitored and addressed.

Hirsutism, acne, alopecia

Symptoms of hyperandrogenism such as hirsutism, alopecia and acne may be very distressing and embarrassing. Nurses should ensure that women are fully informed about the treatment options and their side-effects. Women will differ in the amount and type of treatment they prefer or are willing to tolerate, so individual needs should be perceived and fulfilled. The length of time taken for signs of improvement to appear can lead to frustration. Altered body image may lead to loss of confidence, social withdrawal and depression. It is very important, therefore, that nurses listen to the problems and anxieties of individual women and refer those requiring more specialist help, for example from counsellors, when requested.

Obesity

Improvements in the symptoms of PCOS following weight loss have been emphasized throughout this chapter. However, weight reduction is often difficult to achieve, especially in women whose self-esteem may already be low. The advice and support of dietitians is extremely beneficial in designing individual eating plans, setting realistic targets and increasing motivation. Nursing staff should be encouraging and supportive, but also sensitive to the associated difficulties and frustrations.

Subfertility and miscarriage

The care of subfertile women with PCOS undergoing infertility investigations and ovulation induction provides exciting opportunities for nurses to extend their roles.

Phlebotomy and the administration of injections are nursing tasks. Treatment regimens are often time-consuming, requiring patients to take time off work. This can lead to much anxiety, especially if patients are unwilling to disclose their situation to colleagues. However, if patients or their partners are taught to give injections, their clinic visists are minimized and the treatment becomes more manageable.

Following appropriate training, in some units nurses carry out pelvic ultrasound. This is used to measure follicle size, uterine area and endometrial thickness during spontaneous cycles to pinpoint ovulation and to monitor response to treatment in induced cycles.

Nurses may be closely involved in patient management, making decisions regarding treatment regimens according to predesigned protocols.

Supporting the patient and her partner during this stressful and emotional experience is of paramount importance. The uncertainty of the outcome leads to great anxiety; containing this anxiety whilst maintaining realistic expectations requires great skill on the part of the nursing staff. Some couples may wish to be referred to a counsellor.

Procedures

Nurses have an important role to play whilst the woman undergoes the various investigations and procedures. Women with PCOS may be admitted to gynaecology wards for surgery. This may be investigative, for example laparoscopy and dye, or therapeutic, for example ovarian diathermy. The nursing care involved in gynaecological surgery is discussed in detail in Chapter 20. It is important that nurses are aware of the specific anxieties of the subfertile patient. Full explanations of the investigations and procedures should be given. The results of investigations may be

distressing and their implications profound, therefore time should be spent in their discussion. When subfertile women are admitted following miscarriage or for evacuation of retained products of conception, nurses should be sensitive to the extreme grief caused by the loss of a much wanted pregnancy.

CONCLUSION

In summary, PCO are a common finding in the general population. The definitive diagnosis is by ultrasound scanning, though this will be an incidental finding in those women who are experiencing no problems. The presentation and symptoms are heterogeneous, creating a clinical spectrum including symptoms of hyperandrogenism (hirsutism, acne, alopecia) and/or menstrual disturbances and anovulation. Those women with a biochemical abnormality and/or menstrual irregularity can be said to have PCOS. The hyperinsulinaemia associated with PCOS has important implications for long-term health. In the absence of data to allow informed management, it is important to ensure that obese women with PCOS are encouraged to lose weight. Further insights into the genetic basis of this disorder may assist in the elucidation of its aetiology. The management and care of women with this complex disorder presents nurses and clinicians with fascinating challenges, which are changing and developing as new information is gained.

GLOSSARY

Atresia: the degenerative process by which oocytes and follicles are eliminated from the ovary if they are not involved in ovulation
Folliculogenesis: the growth and development of a follicle
Granulosa cells: the inner layer of cells within the follicle; they synthesize oestrogen
Heterogeneity: made up of dissimilar elements; mixed, varied
Insulin resistance: a diminished effect of a given dose of insulin on glucose homeostasis

Oligogenic: meaning that a small number of genes are responsible for a disorder
Polymorphism: having several different forms, controlled by a series of alternative alleles
Quantitative trait disorder: a trait that is brought about by the action of many genes each having a small effect and causing a gradual change in a characteristic
Theca cells: the androgen-producing layer of cells within the follicle

REFERENCES

Abdel Gadir A, Mowafi RS, Alnaser HM, et al 1990 Ovarian electrocautery versus human menopausal gonadotrophins and pure follicle stimulating hormone therapy in the treatment of patients with polycystic ovarian disease. Clinical Endocrinology (Oxford) 33:585–592

Adams J, Polson DW, Franks S 1986 Prevalence of polycystic ovaries in women with anovulation and idiopathic hirsutism. British Medical Journal 293:355–359
Adams JM, Tan SL, Wheeler MJ, et al 1988 Uterine growth in the follicular phase of spontaneous ovulatory cycles and

during luteinising hormone-releasing hormone-induced cycles in women with normal or polycystic ovaries. Fertility and Sterility 49:52–55

Adashi EY 1988 Hypothalamic–pituitary dysfunction in polycystic ovary disease. Endocrinology and Metabolism Clinics of North America 17:549–666

Adashi EY, Rock JA, Guzick D, et al 1981 Fertility following bilateral ovarian wedge resection: a critical analysis of 90 consecutive cases of the polycystic ovary syndrome. Fertility and Sterility 35:320–325

Amowitz LL, Sobel BE 1999 Cardiovascular consequences of polycystic ovary syndrome. In: Dunaif A (ed) Polycystic ovary syndrome. Endocrinology and Metabolism Clinics of North America 28(2):439–458

Anderson DC 1974 Sex-hormone binding globulin. Clinical Endocrinology (Oxford) 3:69–96

Armar NA, McGarrigle HH, Honour J, et al 1990 Laparoscopic ovarian diathermy in the management of anovulatory infertility in women with polycystic ovaries: endocrine changes and clinical outcome. Fertility and Sterility 53:45–49

Azziz R, Ochoa TM, Bradley Jr, EL et al 1995 Leuprolide and oestrogen versus oral contraception pills for the treatment of hirsutism: a prospective randomised study. Journal of Clinical Endocrinology and Metabolism 80:3406–3411

Balen AH, Jacobs HS 1994 A prospective study comparing unilateral and bilateral laparoscopic ovarian diathermy in women with the polycystic ovary syndrome. Fertility and Sterility 62:921–925

Balen AH, Conway GS, Kaltsas G, et al 1995 Polycystic ovary syndrome: the spectrum of the disorder in 1741 patients. Human Reproduction 10:2107–2111

Bardin CW, Lipsett MB 1967 Testosterone and androstenedione blood production rates in normal women and women with idiopathic hirsutism or polycystic ovaries. Journal of Clinical Investigation 46:891–902

Barnes RB, Ehrmann DA, Rosenfield RL 1993 Ovarian hyperandrogenism in 'late-onset' congenital adrenal hyperplasia. Proceedings of the Endocrine Society 75th Annual Meeting 1993, Abstract 128

Barnes RB 1997 Diagnosis and therapy of hyperandrogenism. In: Rosenfield RL (ed) Hyperandrogenic states and hirsutism: Baillière's Clinical Obstetrics and Gynaecology 11(2):369–396

Barth JH 1988 Alopecia and hirsutes: current concepts in pathogenesis and management. Drugs 35:83–91

Bayer SR, DeCherney AH 1993 Clinical manifestations and treatment of dysfunctional uterine bleeding. Journal of the American Medical Association 269:1823–1828

Bennett ST, Todd JA 1996 Human type 1 diabetes and the insulin gene: principles of mapping polygenes. Annual Review of Genetics 30:343–370

Betti R, Bencini PL, Lodi A, et al 1990 Incidence of polycystic ovaries in patients with late-onset or persistent acne: hormonal reports. Dermatologica 181:109–111

Birdsall MA, Farquar CM, White HD 1997 Association between polycystic ovaries and extent of coronary artery disease in women having cardiac catheterisation. Annals of Internal Medicine 126(1):32–35

Blankstein J, Rabinovici J, Goldenberg M, et al 1987 Changing pituitary reactivity to follicle-stimulating hormone and luteinising hormone-releasing hormone after induced ovulatory cycles and after anovulation in

patients with polycystic ovarian disease. Journal of Clinical Endocrinology and Metabolism 65:1164–1167

Buckler HM, Phillips SE, Kovacs GT, et al 1989 GnRH agonist administration in polycystic ovary syndrome. Clinical Endocrinology 31:151–165

Bunker CB, Newton JA, Kilborn J, et al 1989 Most women with acne have polycystic ovaries. British Journal of Dermatology 121:675–680

Burghen GA, Givens JR, Kitabchi AE 1980 Correlation of hyperandrogenism with hyperinsulinism in polycystic ovarian disease. Journal of Clinical Endocrinology and Metabolism 50:113–116

Bush TL, Fried LP, Barrett-Bonnor E 1988 Cholesterol, lipoproteins and coronary heart disease in women. Clinical Chemistry 34:B60–B70

Carey AH, Chan KL, Short F, et al 1993 Evidence for a single gene effect in polycystic ovaries and male pattern baldness. Clinical Endocrinology 38:653–658

Carmina E, Koyama T, Chang L, et al 1992 Does ethnicity influence the prevalence of adrenal hyperandrogenism and insulin resistance in polycystic ovary syndrome? American Journal of Obstetrics and Gynaecology 167:1807–1812

Cavaghan M, Ehrmann D, Burne M, Polonsky K 1997 Treatment with the oral antidiabetic agent troglitazone improves beta cell responses to glucose in subjects with impaired glucose tolerance. Journal of Clinical Investigation 100(3):530–537

Chang RJ, Nakamura RM, Judd HL, Kaplan SA 1983a Insulin resistance in nonobese patients with polycystic ovarian disease. Journal of Clinical Endocrinology and Metabolism 57:356–359

Chang RJ, Laufer LR, Meldrum DR, et al 1983b Steroid secretion in polycystic ovarian disease after ovarian suppression by a long-acting gonadotrophin-releasing hormone agonist. Journal of Clinical Endocrinology and Metabolism 56:897–903

Christman GM, Randolph JF, Kelch RP, Marshall JC 1991 Reduction of GnRH pulse frequency is associated with subsequent selective follicle stimulating hormone secretion in women with polycystic ovarian disease. Journal of Clinical Endocrinology and Metabolism 72:1278–1285

Clayton RN, Rodin DA, Robinson S, et al 1990 Epidemiology, clinical and hormonal diagnosis of polycystic ovaries and polycystic ovarian syndrome. In: Shaw RW (ed) Polycystic ovaries – a disorder or symptom? Advances in Reproductive Endocrinology, vol 3. Parthenon Publishing, Lancaster, pp. 1–16

Clifford K, Rai R, Watson H, Regan L 1994 An informative protocol for the investigation of recurrent miscarriage: preliminary experience of 500 cases. Human Reproduction 9:1328–1332

Clifford K, Rai R, Watson H, et al 1996 Suppressing luteinising hormone secretion does not reduce the miscarriage rate. British Medical Journal 312:1508–1511

Conn JJ, Jacobs HS, Conway GS 2000 The prevalence of polycystic ovaries in women with type 2 diabetes mellitus. Clinical Endocrinology (Oxf) 52(1):81–86

Conway GS 1990 Insulin resistance and the polycystic ovary syndrome. Contemporary Reviews in Obstetrics and Gynaecology 2:34–39

Conway GS, Honour JW, Jacobs HS 1989 Heterogeneity of the polycystic ovary syndrome: clinical, endocrine and ultrasound features in 556 patients. Clinical Endocrinology (Oxford) 30:459–470

Conway GS, Agrawal R, Betteridge DJ, Jacobs HS 1992 Risk factors for coronary artery disease in lean and obese women with the polycystic ovary syndrome. Clinical Endocrinology 37:119–125

Conway GS, Avey C, Rumsby G 1994 The tyrosine kinase domain of the insulin receptor gene is normal in women with hyperinsulinaemia and polycystic ovary syndrome. Human Reproduction 9:1681–1683

Cooper HE, Spellacy WN, Prem KA, Cohen WD 1968 Heredity factors in the Stein–Leventhal syndrome. American Journal of Obstetrics and Gynaecology 100:371–387

Coulam CB, Annegers JF, Kranz JS 1983 Chronic anovulation syndrome and associated neoplasia. Obstetrics and Gynaecology 61:403–407

Crave J-C, Fimbel S, Lejeune H, et al 1995 Effects of diet and metformin administration on sex hormone binding globulin, androgens and insulin in hirsute and obese women. Journal of Clinical Endocrinology and Metabolism 80:2057–2062

Cusan L, Duport A, Belanger A, et al 1990 Treatment of hirsutism with the pure antiandrogen flutamide. Journal of the American Academy of Dermatology 23:462–469

Dahlgren E, Johansson S, Leadstedt G, et al 1992a Women with polycystic ovary syndrome wedge resected in 1956 to 1965: a long term follow up focusing on natural history and circulating hormones. Fertility and Sterility 57:505–513

Dahlgren E, Janson PO, Johansson S, et al 1992b Polycystic ovary syndrome and risk for myocardial infarction. Acta Obstetrica et Gynecologica Scandinavica 71:599–604

DeFronzo RA, Barzilai N, Simonson DC 1991 Mechanism of metformin action in obese and lean noninsulin-dependent diabetic subjects. Journal of Clinical Endocrinology and Metabolism 73:124–130

Dewailly D, Robert Y, Helin I, et al 1994 Ovarian stromal hypertrophy in hyperandrogenic women. Clinical Endocrinology 41:557–562

Dickey RP, Taylor SN, Curole D, et al 1996 Incidence of spontaneous abortion in clomiphene pregnancies. Human Reproduction 11:2623–2628

Donesky BW, Adashi EY 1995 Surgically induced ovulation in the polycystic ovary syndrome: wedge resection revisited in the age of laparoscopy. Fertility and Sterility 63:439–463

Donesky BW, Adashi EY 1996 Surgical ovulation induction: the role of ovarian diathermy in polycystic ovary syndrome. In: Jacobs HS (cd) Polycystic ovary syndrome. Baillière's Clinical Endocrinology and Metabolism 10(2): pp. 293–309

Duleba AJ, Pawelczyk LA, Ho Yuen B, Moon YS 1993 Insulin actions on idogenesis are not modulated by metformin. Human Reproduction 8:1194–1198

Dunaif A 1997 Insulin resistance and the polycystic ovary syndrome: mechanism and implications for pathogenesis. Endocrine Reviews 18:774–800

Dunaif A, Graf M, Mandeli J, et al 1987 Characterisation of groups of hyperandrogenic women with acanthosis nigricans, impaired glucose tolerance and/or hyperinsulinaemia. Journal of Clinical Endocrinology and Metabolism 65:499–507

Dunaif A, Segal KR, Futterweit W, Dobrianski A 1989 Profound peripheral insulin resistance, independent of obesity, in polycystic ovary syndrome. Diabetes 38:1165–1174

Dunaif A, Xia J, Book C, et al 1995 Excessive insulin receptor serine phosphorylation in cultured fibroblasts and in skeletal muscle: a potential mechanism for insulin resistance in the polycystic ovary syndrome. Journal of Clinical Investigation 96:801–810

Dunaif A, Scott D, Finegood D, et al 1996 The insulin sensitising agent troglitazone: improves metabolic and reproductive abnormalities in the polycystic ovary syndrome. Journal of Clinical Endocrinology and Metabolism 81:3299–3306

Ehrmann D, Sturis J, Byrne M, et al 1995 Insulin secretory defects in polycystic ovary syndrome: relationship to insulin sensitivity and family history of non-insulin-dependent diabetes mellitus. Journal of Clinical Investigation 96:520–527

Ehrmann DA, Cavaghan MK, Imperial J, et al 1997a Effects of metformin on insulin secretion, insulin action and ovarian steroidogenesis in women with polycystic ovary syndrome. Journal of Clinical Endocrinology and Metabolism 82:524–530

Ehrmann DA, Schneider DJ, Sobel BE, et al 1997b Troglitazone improves defects in insulin action, insulin secretion, ovarian steroidogenesis, and fibrinolysis in women with polycystic ovary syndrome. Journal of Clinical Endocrinology and Metabolism 82:2108–2216

Ehrmann DA, Barnes RB, Rosenfield RL, et al 1999 Prevalence of impaired glucose tolerance and diabetes in women with polycystic ovary syndrome. Diabetes Care 22(1):141–146

Erickson GF, Magoffin DA, Garzo GV, et al 1992 Granulosa cells of polycystic ovaries: are they normal or abnormal? Human Reproduction 7:293–299

Farhi DC, Nosanchuk J, Silverberg SG 1986 Endometrial adenocarcinoma in women under 25 years of age. Obstetrics and Gynaecology 68:741–745

Farquar CM, Birdsall M, Manning P, et al 1994 The prevalence of polycystic ovaries on ultrasound scanning in a population of randomly selected women. Australian and New Zealand Journal of Obstetrics and Gynaecology 34:67–72

Fauser BC, Pache TD, Hop WC, et al 1992 The significance of a single serum LH measurement in women with cycle disturbances: discrepancies between immunoreactive and bioactive hormone estimates. Clinical Endocrinology (Oxford) 37:445–452

Fendri S, Debussche X, Puy H, et al 1993 Metformin effects on peripheral sensitivity to insulin in non diabetic obese subjects. Diabetes and Metabolism 19:245–249

Ferriman D, Purdie AW 1979 The inheritance of polycystic ovarian disease and a possible relationship to premature balding. Clinical Endocrinology (Oxford) 11:291–300

Filicori M, Flamagni C 1992 Hypothalamic–pituitary abnormalities in polycystic ovary syndrome. In: Hershmann JM (ed) Current issues in endocrinology and metabolism. Blackwell Scientific Publications, Boston, pp. 31–38

Fox R, Corrigan E, Thomas PA, Hull MGR 1991 The diagnosis of polycystic ovaries in women with oligo-amenorrhoea: predictive power of endocrine tests. Clinical Endocrinology 34:127–131

Franks S 1989 Polycystic ovary syndrome: a changing perspective. Clinical Endocrinology 31:87–120

Franks S 1991 The ubiquitous polycystic ovary. Journal of Endocrinology 129:317–319

Franks S 1998 Oligomenorrhoea and polycystic ovary syndrome. In: Cameron IT, Fraser IS, Smith SK (eds) Clinical disorders of the endometrium and menstrual cycle. Oxford University Press, Oxford.

Franks S, Adams J, Mason H, Polson D 1985 Ovulatory disorders in women with polycystic ovary syndrome. Clinics in Obstetrics and Gynaecology 12:605–632

Franks S, Mason H, White D, Willis DS 1996 Mechanisms of anovulation in polycystic ovary syndrome. In: Filicori M, Flamagni C (eds) The ovary: regulation, dysfunction and treatment. Elsevier, Amsterdam, pp. 183–186

Franks S, Gharani N, Waterworth D, et al 1997 The genetic basis of polycystic ovary syndrome. Human Reproduction 12:2641–2648

Franks S, Mason H, White D, Willis D 1998a Etiology of anovulation in polycystic ovary syndrome. Steroids 63:1–2

Franks S, Gharani N, Waterworth D, et al 1998b Current developments in the molecular genetics of the polycystic ovary syndrome. Trends in Endocrinology and Metabolism 9:51–54

Futterweit W 1983 Piuitary tumours and polycystic ovarian disease. Obstetrics and Gynaecology 62 (suppl.):745–795

Futterweit W 1995 Pathophysiology of polycystic ovary syndrome. In Redmond GP (ed) Androgenic disorders. Raven Press, New York, pp. 77–166

Garcia JE, Jones GS, Wentze AC 1980 The use of clomiphene citrate. Fertility and Sterility 33:479–486

Gemzell C, Wang CF 1980 The use of human gonadotrophins for the induction of ovulation in women with polycystic ovarian disease. Fertility and Sterility 33:479–486

Gharani N, Waterworth DM, Williamson R, Franks S 1996 5′ polymorphism of the CYP17 gene is not associated with serum testosterone levels in women with polycystic ovaries [Letter]. Journal of Clinical Endocrinology and Metabolism 81:4174

Gharani N, Waterworth D, Batty S, et al 1997 Association of the steroid synthesis gene CYP11a with polycystic ovary syndrome and hyperandrogenism. Human Molecular Genetics 6:397–402

Gilling-Smith C, Franks S 1993 Polycystic ovary syndrome. Reproductive Medicine Review 2:15–32, Cambridge University Press

Gilling-Smith C, Willis DS, Mason HD, Franks S 1993 Effects of insulin and insulin-like growth factors on androstenedione production by human theca cells. Journal of Endocrinology 139 (suppl.):OC35

Gilling-Smith C, Willis DS, Beard RW, Franks S 1994 Hypersecretion of androstenedione by isolated theca cells from polycystic ovaries. Journal of Clinical Endocrinology and Metabolism 79:1158–1165

Giudice LC 1999 Growth factor action on ovarian function in polycystic ovary syndrome. In: Dunaif A (ed) Polycystic ovary syndrome. Endocrinology and Metabolism Clinics of North America 28(2):325–341

Givens JR 1976 Hirsutism and hyperandrogenism. Advances in Internal Medicine 21:221–247

Givens JR 1988 Familial polycystic ovarian disease. Endocrinology and Metabolism Clinics of North America 17:771–783

Gjonnaess H 1984 Polycystic ovarian syndrome treated by ovarian electrocautery through the laparoscope. Fertility and Sterility 41:20–25

Gurgan T, Kisnisci H, Yarali H, et al 1991 Evaluation of adhesion formation after laparoscopic treatment of polycystic ovarian disease. Fertility and Sterility 56:1176–1178

Gurgan T, Urman B, Aksu T, et al 1992 The effect of short-interval laparoscopic lysis of adhesions on pregnancy rates following Nd:YAG laser photocoagulation of polycystic ovaries. Obstetrics and Gynaecology 80:45–47

Hague WM, Adams J, Reeders ST, et al 1988 Familial polycystic ovaries: a genetic disease? Clinical Endocrinology 29:593–605

Hamilton-Fairley D, Kiddy DS, Watson H, et al 1991 Low dose gonadotrophin therapy for induction of ovulation in 100 women with polycystic ovary syndrome. Human Reproduction 6:1095–1099

Hamilton-Fairley D, Kiddy DS, Watson H, et al 1992 Association of moderate obesity with a poor pregnancy outcome in women with polycystic ovary syndrome treated with low dose gonadotrophin. British Journal of Obstetrics and Gynaecology 99:128–131

Hammerstein J, Meckies J, Leo-Rossberg I, et al 1975 Use of cyproterone acetate (CPA) in the treatment of acne, hirsutism and virilism. Journal of Steroid Biochemistry 6:827–836

Harlow CR, Shaw HJ, Hillier SG, Hodges JK 1988 Factors influencing FSH-stimulated steroidogenesis in marmoset granulosa cells: effects of androgens and stages of follicular development. Endocrinology 122:2780–2787

Hattori M, Horiuchi R 1992 Biphasic effects of exogenous ganglioside GM3 on follicle-stimulating hormone-dependent expression of luteinising hormone receptor in cultured granulosa cells. Molecular and Cellular Endocrinology 88:47–54

Hillier SG 1994 Current concepts of the roles of follicle stimulating hormone and luteinising hormone in folliculogenesis. Human Reproduction 9:188–191

Hoffmann DL, Klove K, Lobo RA 1984 The prevalence and significance of elevated dehydroepiandrosterone sulfate levels in anovulatory women. Fertility and Sterility 42:76–81

Holte J, Bergh T, Berne C, et al 1994 Enhanced early insulin response to glucose in relation to insulin resistance in women with polycystic ovary syndrome and normal glucose tolerance. Journal of Clinical Endocrinology and Metabolism 78:1052–1058

Holte J, Bergh T, Berne C, et al 1995 Restored insulin sensitivity but persistently increased early insulin secretion after weight loss in obese women with polycystic ovary syndrome. Journal of Clinical Endocrinology and Metabolism 80:2586–2593

Homburg R, Armar NA, Eshel A, et al 1988 Influence of serum luteinising hormone concentrations on ovulation, conception and early pregnancy loss in polycystic ovary syndrome. British Medical Journal 297:1024–1026

Homburg R, Eshel A, Armar NA, et al 1989 One hundred pregnancies after treatment with pulsatile luteinising hormone to induce ovulation. British Medical Journal 298:809–812

Homburg R, Levy T, Berkovitz D, et al 1993 Gonadotrophin-releasing hormone agonist reduces the miscarriage rate for pregnancies achieved in women with polycystic ovary syndrome. Fertility and Sterility 59:527–531

Homburg R, Giroud D, Howles C, Loumaye E 1994 Efficacy of recombinant human follicle stimulating hormone, Gonal-F, for inducing ovulation in WHO group II anovulatory patients. Preliminary results of a comparative multicentre study. In Mori T, Tominanga T, Hiroi M (eds) Perspectives on assisted reproduction. Raven Press, New York, pp. 463–467

Hsueh AJW, Welsh TH, Jones PBC 1981 Inhibition of ovarian and testicular steroidogenesis by epidermal growth factor. Endocrinology 108:2002–2004

Huber-Buchholz MM, Carey DGP, Norman RJ 1999 Restoration of reproductive potential by lifestyle modification in obese polycystic ovary syndrome: role of insulin sensitivity and luteinising hormone. Journal of Clinical Endocrinology and Metabolism 84(4):1470–1471

Hughesdon PE 1982 Morphology and morphogenesis of the Stein–Leventhal ovary and the so-called 'hyperthecosis'. Obstetric and Gynaecological Survey 37:59–77

Hull MGR 1992 The causes of infertility and relative effectiveness of treatment. In: Templeton AA, Drife JO (eds) Infertility. Springer-Verlag, London, pp. 33–62

Hull MG, Savage PE, Bromham DR, et al 1982 The value of a single serum progesterone measurement in the midluteal phase as a criterion of a potentially fertile cycle ('ovulation') derived from treated and untreated conception cycles. Fertility and Sterility 37:355–360

Hull MRG, Glazener CMA, Kelly NJ, et al 1985 Population study of cases, treatment and outcome of infertility. British Medical Journal 291:1693–1697

Kamrava MM, Seibel MM, Berger MJ, et al 1982 Reversal of persistent anovulation in polycystic ovarian disease by administration of chronic low-dose follicle-stimulating hormone. Fertility and Sterility 37:520–523

Keckstein G, Wolf AS, Borchers K, et al 1990 [Pelviscopic use of the CO$_2$ laser in the treatment of polycystic ovary syndrome.] Zentralblatt fuer Gynaekologie 112:361–368

Khan CR, Flier JS, Bar RS, et al 1976 The syndromes of insulin resistance and acanthosis nigricans. New England Journal of Medicine 294:739–745

Kiddy DS, Sharpe PS, White DM, et al 1990 Differences in clinical and endocrine features between obese and non-obese subjects with polycystic ovary syndrome; an analysis of 263 consecutive cases. Clinical Endocrinology 32:213–220

Kiddy DS, Hamilton-Fairley D, Bush A, et al 1992 Improvement in endocrine and ovarian function during dietary treatment of obese women with polycystic ovarian syndrome. Clinical Endocrinology 36:105–111

Kirschner MA, Bardin CW 1972 Androgen production and metabolism in normal and virilised women. Metabolism 21:667–688

Kirschner MA, Samojlik E, Silber D 1983 A comparison of androgen production and clearance in hirsute and obese women. Journal of Steroid Biochemistry 19:607–614

Kistner RW 1969 Peri-tubal and peri-ovarian adhesions subsequent to wedge resection of the ovaries. Fertility and Sterility 20:35–42

Kousta E, White D, Franks S 1994 Significance of polycystic ovaries in women with unexplained infertility. Journal of Endocrinology 140 (suppl.): p. 219

Kousta E, White DM, Franks S 1997 Modern use of clomiphene citrate in induction of ovulation. Human Reproduction 3:359–365

Kupferminc MJ, Lessing JB, Peyser MR 1991 Ovulation induction with gonadotrophins in women with polycystic ovary disease. Journal of Reproductive Medicine 36:61–64

Lachelin GCL, Judd HL, Swanson SC, et al 1982 Long term effects of nightly dexamethasone administration in patients with polycystic ovarian disease. Journal of Clinical Endocrinology and Metabolism 55:768–773

Legro GS, Kunselman AR, Dodson WC, Dunaif A 1999 Prevalence and predictors of risk for type 2 diabetes mellitus and impaired glucose tolerance in polycystic ovary syndrome: a prospective, controlled study in 254 affected women. Journal of Clinical Endocrinology and Metabolism 84(1):165–169

Lemay A, Dewailly SD, Grenier R, Huard J 1990 Attenuation of mild hyperandrogenic activity in postpubertal acne by a triphasic oral contraceptive containing low doses of ethinyloestradiol and d, 1-norgestrel. Journal of Clinical Endocrinology and Metabolism 71:8–14

Levine M, Wild J, Steer P 1992 Higher multiple births and the modern management of infertility in Britain. British Journal of Obsterics and Gynaecology 99:607–613

Lobo RA 1991 Hirsutism in polycystic ovary syndrome: current concepts. Clinical Obstetrics and Gynaecology 34:817–826

Lobo RA, Gysler M, March CM, et al 1982 Clinical and laboratory predictors of clomiphene response. Fertility and Sterility 37:168–174

Loughlin T, Cunningham S, Moore A, et al 1986 Adrenal abnormalities in polycystic ovary syndrome. Journal of Clinical Endocrinology and Metabolism 62:142–147

Lunde O, Magnus P, Sandvik L, Hoglo S 1989 Familial clustering in the polycystic ovary syndrome. Gynaecological and Obstetric Investigation 28:23–30

Lunenfeld B, Insler V 1978 Diagnosis and treatment of functional infertility. Gross Verlag, Berlin

MacDougall MJ, Tan SL, Balen A, Jacobs HS 1993 A controlled study comparing patients with and without polycystic ovaries undergoing in-vitro fertilisation. Human Reproduction 8:233–237

Marynick SP, Chakmakjian ZH, McCaffree DL, Herndon JH Jr 1983 Androgen excess in cystic acne. New England Journal of Medicine 380:981–986

Mason HD, Willis DS, Beard RW, et al 1994 Estradiol production by granulosa cells of normal and polycystic ovaries: relationship to menstrual cycle history and concentrations of gonadotrophins and sex steroids in follicular fluid. Journal of Clinical Endocrinology and Metabolism 79:1355–1360

Mason HD, Carr L, Leake R, Franks S 1995 Production of transforming growth factor-α by normal and polycystic ovaries. Journal of Clinical Endocrinology and Metabolism 80:2053–2056

McKenna TJ 1988 Pathogenesis and treatment of polycystic ovary syndrome. New England Journal of Medicine 318:558–562

McKenna TJ, Cunningham SK 1992 Adrenal abnormalities in polycystic ovary syndrome and the impact of their correction. In: Dunaif A, Givens JR, Haseltine FP, Merriam GR (eds) Polycystic ovary syndrome. Blackwell Scientific Publications, Oxford, pp. 183–193

McMullen GR, van Herle AJ 1993 Hirsutism and the effectiveness of spironolactone in its management. Journal of Endocrinological Investigation 16:925–932

Murdoch AP, Dunlop W, Kendall-Taylor P 1986 Studies of prolactin secretion in polycystic ovary syndrome. Clinical Endocrinology (Oxford) 24:165–175

Nestler JE, Jacubowicz DJ 1996 Decreases in ovarian cytochrome P450c17α activity and serum free testosterone after reduction in insulin secretion in polycystic ovary syndrome. New England Journal of Medicine 355:617–623

Nestler JE, Jakubowicz DJ, Evans WS, Pasquali R 1998 Effects of metformin on spontaneous and clomiphene-induced ovulation in the polycystic ovary syndrome. New England Journal of Medicine 338(26):1876–1880

O'Meara N, Blackmann JD, Ehrmann DA, et al 1993 Defects in β-cell function in functional ovarian hyperandrogenism. Journal of Clinical Endocrinology and Metabolism 76:1241–1247

Pache TD, de Jong FH, Hop WC, Fauser BCJM 1993 Association between ovarian changes assessed by transvaginal sonography and clinical and endocrine signs of the polycystic ovary syndrome. Fertility and Sterility 59:544–549

Pasquali R, Casimirri F, Venturoli S, et al 1994 Body fat distribution has weight independent effects on clinical, hormonal and metabolic features of women with polycystic ovary syndrome. Metabolism 43:706–713

Peserico A, Angeloni G, Bertoli P, et al 1989 Prevalence of polycystic ovaries in women with acne. Archives of Gynaecological Research 281:502–503

Pierpoint T, Mckeigue PM, Issacs AJ et al 1998 Mortality of women with polycystic ovary syndrome at long-term follow-up. Journal of Clinical Endocrinology and Metabolism 51:581–586

Plymate SR, Matej LA, Jones RE, Friedl KE 1988 Inhibition of sex-hormone binding globulin production in human hepatoma (Hep G2) cell line by insulin and prolactin. Journal of Clinical Endocrinology and Metabolism 67:460–464

Polson DW, Franks S, Reed MJ et al 1987 The distribution of oestradiol in plasma in relation to uterine cross-sectional area in women with polycystic or multifollicular ovaries. Clinical Endocrinology (Oxford) 26:581–588

Polson DW, Adams J, Wadsworth J, Franks S 1988a Polycystic ovaries – a common finding in normal women. Lancet ii:870–872

Polson DW, Reed MJ, Franks S, et al 1988b Serum 11-β hydroxyandrostenedione as an indicator of the source of excess androgen production in women with polycystic ovaries. Journal of Clinical Endocrinology and Metabolism 66:946–950

Polson DW, Kiddy DS, Mason HD, Franks S 1989 Induction of ovulation with clomiphene citrate in women with polycystic ovary syndrome: the difference between responders and non-responders. Fertility and Sterility 51:30–34

Prelevic GM, Wurzburger MI, Balint PL, Puzigaca Z 1989 Effects of a low-dose estrogen–antiandrogen combination (Diane-35) on clinical signs of androgenisation, hormone profile and ovarian size in patients with polycystic ovary syndrome. Gynaecological Endocrinology 3:269–280

Rebuffe-Scrive M, Cullberg G, Lundberg PA, et al 1989 Anthropometric variables and metabolism in polycystic ovarian disease. Hormone Metabolic Research 21:391–397

Regan L, Owen E, Jacobs HS 1990 Hypersecretion of luteinising hormone, infertility and miscarriage. Lancet 336:1141–1144

Robinson S, Kiddy D, Gelding SV, et al 1993 The relationship of insulin insensitivity to menstrual pattern in women with hyperandrogenism and polycystic ovaries. Clinical Endocrinology 39:351–355

Robinson S, Henderson AD, Gelding SV, et al 1996 Dyslipidaemia is associated with insulin resistance in women with polycystic ovaries. Clinical Endocrinology 44:277–284

Rodin A, Thakkar H, Taylor N, Clayton R 1994 Hyperandrogenism in polycystic ovary syndrome: evidence of dysregulation of 11β hydroxysteroid dehydrogenase. New England Journal of Medicine 330:460–465

Rosenfield RL 1997 Current concepts of polycystic ovary syndrome. In: Hyperandrogenic states and hirsutism. Rosenfield RL (ed) Baillière's clinical obstetrics and gynaecology, vol 11(2). Baillière Tindall, London, pp. 307–335

Rosenfield RL, Barnes RB, Cara JF, Lucky AW 1990 Dysregulation of cytochrome P450c17 alpha as the cause of polycystic ovarian syndrome. Fertility and Sterility 53:785–791

Rosner W 1990 The functions of corticosteroid binding globulin and sex-hormone binding globulin; recent advances. Endocrine Reviews 11:80–91

Rossing MA, Daling JR, Weiss NS, et al 1994 Ovarian tumours in a cohort of infertile women. New England Journal of Medicine 331:771–776

Rossmanith WG, Keckstein J, Spatzier K, Lauritzen C 1991 The impact of ovarian laser surgery on the gonadotrophin secretion in women with polycystic ovarian disease. Clinical Endocrinology 34:223–230

Sagle M, Bishop K, Ridley N, et al 1988 Recurrent early miscarriage and polycystic ovaries. British Medical Journal 297:1027–1028

Sagle MA, Hamilton-Fairley D, Kiddy DS, Franks S 1991 A comparative, randomised study of low-dose human menopausal gonadotrophin and follicle-stimulating hormone in women with polycystic ovarian syndrome. Fertility and Sterility 55:56–60

Saxton DW, Farquar CM, Rae T, et al 1990 Accuracy of ultrasound measurements of female pelvic organs. British Journal of Obstetrics and Gynaecology 97:695–699

Scialli AR 1986 The reproductive toxicity of ovulation induction. Fertility and Sterility 45:315–323

Seibel MM, McCardle C, Smith D, Taylor ML 1985 Ovulation induction in polycystic ovary syndrome with urinary follicle-stimulating hormone or human menopausal gonadotrophin. Fertility and Sterility 37:520–523

Sharp PS, Kiddy DS, Reed M, et al 1991 Correlation of plasma insulin and insulin-like growth factor-I indices of androgen transport and metabolism in women with poycystic ovary syndrome. Clinical Endocrinology 35:253–257

Sherman AI, Brown S 1979 The precursors of endometrial carcinoma. American Journal of Obstetrics and Gynaecology 135:947–956

Shoham Z, Homburg R, Jacobs HS 1990a Induction of ovulation with pulsatile LHRH. Baillière's Clinical Obstetrics and Gynaecology 4:589–608

Shoham Z, Borenstein R, Lunenfield B, Pariente C 1990b Hormone profiles following clomiphene citrate therapy in conception and non-conception cycles. Clinical Endocrinology 33:271–278

Simpson JL 1992 Elucidating the genetics of polycystic ovary syndrome. In: Dunaif A, Givens JR, Haseltine FP, Merriman GR (eds) Polycystic ovary syndrome. Blackwell Scientific, Oxford, pp. 265–278

Slowinska-Srzednicka J, Zgliczynski W, Makowska A, et al 1992 An abnormality of the growth hormone/insulin-like growth factor-I axis in women with polycystic ovary syndrome due to coexistent obesity. Journal of Clinical Endocrinology and Metabolism 74:1432–1435

Solomon CG 1999 The epidemiology of polycystic ovary syndrome: prevalence and associated disease risk. In: Dunaif A (ed) Polycystic ovary syndrome. Endocrinology and Metabolism Clinics of North America 28(2):247–264

Soule SG 1996 Neuroendocrinology of the polycystic ovary syndrome. In: Jacobs HS (ed) Polycystic ovary syndrome, Baillière's Clinical Endocrinology and Metabolism 10(2):205–219. Balliere Tindall, London

Stanger JD, Yovich JL 1985 Reduced in-vitro fertilisation of human oocytes from patients with raised basal LH levels during the follicular phase. British Journal of Obstetrics and Gynaecology 92:385–393

Stein IF, Leventhal ML 1935 Amenorrhea associated with bilateral polycystic ovaries. American Journal of Obstetrics and Gynecology 29:181–191

Sumioki H, Utsunomyiyo T, Matsuoka K, et al 1988 The effects of laparoscopic multiple punch resection of the ovary on hypothalamo–pituitary axis in polycystic ovary syndrome 50:567–572

Talbert LM 1983 Clomiphene citrate induction of ovulation. Fertility and Sterility 39:742–743

Talbot JA, Bicknell EJ, Rajkhowa M, et al 1996 Molecular scanning of the insulin receptor gene in women with polycystic ovary syndrome. Journal of Clinical Endocrinology and Metabolism 81:1979–1983

Talbott E, Guzick D, Clerici A, et al 1995 Coronary heart disease risk factors in women with polycystic ovary syndrome. Arteriosclerosis and Thrombosis 15:821–826

Tetchatraisak K, Conway GS, and Rumsby G 1997 Frequency of a polymorphism in the regulatory region of the 17α-hydroxlase-17,20 lyase (CYP17) in hyperandrogenic states. Clinical Endocrinology 46:131–134

van Weyjen RGA, van den Ende A 1995 Experience in the long-term treatment of patients with hirsutism and/or acne with cyproterone acetate-containing preparations: efficacy, metabolic and endocrine effects. Experimental and Clinical Endocrinology 103:241–251

Velazquez EM, Mendoza S, Hamer T, et al 1994 Metformin therapy in polycystic ovary syndrome reduces hyperinsulinaemia, insulin resistance,

hyperandrogenaemia and systolic blood pressure while facilitating normal menses and pregnancy. Metabolism 43:647–654

Wang CF, Gemzell C 1980 The use of human gonadotrophins for induction of ovulation in women with polycystic ovarian disease. Fertility and Sterility 33:479–486

Waterworth DM, Bennett ST, Gharani N, et al 1997 Linkage and association of insulin gene VNTR regulatory polymorphism with polycystic ovary syndrome. Lancet 349:986–989

White DM, Leigh A, Wilson C, et al 1995 Gonadotrophin and gonadal steroid response to a single dose of a long-acting agonist of gonadotrophin-releasing hormone in ovulatory and anovulatory women with polycystic ovary syndrome. Clinical Endocrinology 42:475–481

White DM, Polson DW, Kiddy DS, et al 1996 Extensive personal experience. Induction of ovulation with low-dose gonadotrophins in polycystic ovary syndrome: an analysis of 109 pregnancies in 225 women. Journal of Clinical Endocrinology and Metabolism 81:3821–3824

Wild RA, Van Nort JJ, Grubb B, et al 1990 Clinical signs of androgen excess as risk factors for coronary artery disease. Fertility and Sterility 54:255–259

Willis DS, Mason HD, Gilling-Smith C, Franks S 1996 Modulation by insulin of follicle stimulating hormone and luteinising hormone actions in human granulosa cells of normal and polycystic ovaries. Journal of Endocrinology and Metabolism 81:302–309

Willis DS, Watson H, Mason HD, et al 1998 Premature response to luteinising hormone of granulosa cells from anovulatory women with polycystic ovary syndrome: relevance to mechanism of anovulation. Journal of Clinical Endocrinology and Metabolism 83:3984–3991

Wyowski DK, Freiman JP, Tourtelot JB, Horton ML 1993 Fatal and non fatal hepatotoxicity associated with flutamide. Annals of Internal Medicine 118:860–864

Yen SSC 1980 The polycystic ovary syndrome. Clinical Endocrinology 12:177–207

Yen SSC, Lasley BL, Wang CF, et al 1975 The operating characteristics of the hypothalamic-pituitary system during the menstrual cycle and observation of biological action of somatostatin. Recent Progress in Hormone Research 31:321–363

Zawadski JK, Dunaif A 1992 Diagnostic criteria for polycystic ovary syndrome; towards a rational approach. In: Dunaif A, Givens JR, Haseltine FP, Merriman GR (eds) Polycystic ovary syndrome, Blackwell Scientific, Oxford, pp. 337–340

Zhang L, Rodriquez H, Ohno S, Miller W 1995 Serine phosphorylation of human P450c17 increases 17,20 lyase activity: implications for adrenarche and the polycystic ovary syndrome. Proceedings of the National Academy of Sciences USA 92:10619–10623

USEFUL ADDRESSES

CHILD, The National Infertility Support Network
Charter House, 43 St Leonards Road, Bexhill-on-Sea, East
Sussex TN40 1JA
Fertility Nurses Interest Group
c/o Womens' Issues, Royal College of Nursing,
Cavendish Square, London W1M 0AB
Issue
509 Aldridge Road, Great Bar, Birmingham
B44 8NA

Miscarriage Association
c/o Clayton Hospital, Northgate, Wakefield, West
Yorkshire WF1 3JS
Society for Endocrinology
17–18 The Courtyard, Woodlands, Bradley Stoke, Bristol
Society for the Study of Fertility
82A High Street, Sawston, Cambridgeshire CB2 4HJ
Verity
Tindle Manor, 52–54 Featherstone Street, London EC1 8RT

9

Benign ovarian cysts

Barbara Walters

This chapter will concentrate on ovarian cysts other than ovarian cancer, chocolate cysts as found in endometriosis and polycystic ovarian syndrome, as these are covered in other chapters.

Benign ovarian cysts are often asymtomatic with the woman being unaware of their presence as they resolve spontaneously. In those women where symptoms do prevail, this tends to be when the cyst has grown so as to cause pressure symptoms. Pelvic and abdominal discomfort may eventually lead the woman to consult her general practitioner, or some women suffer pain as a result of rupture or torsion of an ovarian cyst. Benign ovarian cysts are the fourth most common gynaecological cause of hospital admissions (Girling & Soutter 1997).

PATHOLOGY

Box 9.1

- Non-neoplastic distension cysts
    - Follicular cysts
    - Theca-lutein cysts
    - Corpus luteum cysts.
- Cystic neoplasms
    - Serous cystadenoma
    - Mucinous cystadenoma
    - Brenner tumour
    - Fibroma.
- Germ cell tumours
    - Dermoid cyst.
- Gonadal stromal tumours
    - Theca cell tumour
    - Sertoli–Leydig cell tumour
    - Mixed.

Non-neoplastic distension cysts

Follicular cysts

These are the most frequently diagnosed ovarian cysts and are often found incidentally (see Plate 14). Large follicular cysts are uncommon before puberty (Creatsas et al 1992). A follicular cyst will develop if the normal atresia fails in a non-dominant follicle or if there is non-rupture of a dominant follicle (Girling & Soutter 1997). A thin layer of granulosa cells line the wall of a follicular cyst. Most follicular cysts do not require treatment because they regress spontaneously (Andrews 1997).

Theca-lutein cysts

These present as a type of follicular cyst. There is luteinization of the theca interna and they are often associated with hydatidiform mole (Crosignani et al 1992).

Corpus luteum cysts

These can cause pain as they occasionally rupture, resulting in intraperitoneal bleeding; most, however, regress. They are less common than follicular cysts. Corpora lutea are only considered to be luteal cysts when greater than 3 cm in diameter (see Plate 15).

Cystic neoplasms

Serous cystadenoma

In women over 40, this is the most common ovarian cyst arising from the ovarian surface epithelium. Often bilateral, they are usually unilocular with a smooth outer surface (Girling & Soutter 1997).

Mucinous cystadenoma

These constitute 16–30% of all ovarian cysts and manifest themselves as large, multilocular cysts with a smooth inner surface. Columnar mucus-secreting cells are present in the lining epithelium and produce a glutinous fluid. *Pseudomyxoma peritonei* is a rare complication, which can be present before the cyst is removed.

Brenner tumours

The majority of these are benign. It is thought that they arise from the surface epithelium – Wolffian metaplasia. They have a solid appearance consisting of islands of transitional epithelium in a dense fibrotic stroma. They can cause abnormal vaginal bleeding. They are bilateral in 10–15% of cases.

Fibroma

These are unusual, being derived from stromal cells. Approximately 10% of cases are bilateral and they present as glistening large tumours. In 1% of cases women develop Meig's syndrome, whereby the fibroma is associated with ascites and a pleural effusion.

Germ cell tumours

Dermoid cyst

Thirty per cent of benign tumours are ovarian teratomas (see Plate 16) (Dubuisson & Chapron 1992). Women are often asymptomatic but torsion or rupture can occur. Dermoid cysts are lined by stratified squamous epithelium and may contain cartilage, alimentary and respiratory epithelium, teeth, neural tissue, hair, sebaceous and sweat glands and active thyroid tissue (see Plate 17) (Andrews 1997). Occasionally only a single tissue may be present and the term monodermal teratoma is then used. Rupture can occur acutely, causing a chemical peritonitis, or slowly, causing chronic granulomatous peritonitis.

Gonadal stromal tumours

Theca cell tumour

Granulosa, theca, Leydig and Sertoli cells can differentiate into any cells or tissues arising from the mesenchyme of the gonad. Theca cells may produce oestrogen-causing systemic effects. They are usually solid and unilateral.

Sertoli–Leydig cell tumour

These are usually small, rare and may produce androgens.

Mixed cell tumour

These contain a mixture of granulosa and Sertoli–Leydig cells.

EPIDEMIOLOGY

As previously stated, benign ovarian cysts are often asymptomatic and are found incidentally as a result of ultrasound scanning or pelvic examination (Girling & Soutter 1997). They are most common in young women, although they may occur in any premenopausal woman and, at ultrasound scanning, 7% of 5678 asymptomatic English volunteers aged 45 or over had enlarged ovaries (Crosignani et al 1992).

The link between the oral contraceptive pill and functional ovarian cysts has been investigated, although none of the research has distinguished between follicle and corpus luteum cysts (Vessey et al 1987). The Boston Collaborative Drug Surveillance Programme (Ory 1974) and The Royal College of General Practitioners (1974) demonstrated that oral contraceptives afforded protection against functional ovarian cysts.

However, further studies undertaken on women to consider the risk factors for serous, mucinous and endometrioid ovarian cysts found no relationship between incidence and body mass, smoking habit, life-long menstrual pattern, use of the oral contraceptive pill or number of miscarriages. The risk of ovarian cysts did increase, however, with a longer interval between first intercourse and age at first live birth (Parazzini et al 1992). It had been thought that the use of the oral contraceptive pill offered some degree of protection from functional cysts but variations in the composition and frequency of use of oral contraceptives suggest that the risk of developing a cyst is not appreciably reduced. It is suggested, however, that the pill may be responsible for up to half of the observed reduction in hospital discharge rates for women aged 15–44 with a main diagnosis of ovarian cyst (Crosignani et al 1992).

In those women with dermoid cysts, there was found to be no significant association with oral contraceptive use, but protection was afforded by pregnancies, the pregnancy-induced hormonal changes directly deterring the growth of benign teratomas (Westhoff et al 1988).

Treatment

The major concern on finding a cyst is to exclude malignancy and to avoid any possible complications arising from the presence of the cyst. Morbidity and impaired future fertility are the two main concerns (Girling & Soutter 1997).

Most simple cysts will resolve spontaneously. They should be observed over a 2–3 month period. Gonadotrophin suppression by an oral contraceptive pill will further encourage the resolution of physiological cysts.

OVARIAN CYSTS IN PREGNANCY

Ovarian cysts associated with pregnancy are usually functional. During pregnancy, asymptomatic patients have ultrasonography performed and the detection of ovarian cysts is increased by transvaginal ultrasonography, with its direct visualization of the ovaries (Struyka & Treffers 1984).

In early pregnancy, ovarian activity promotes ovarian cyst development, and the ultrasound and gynaecological examinations that would not have been performed if the woman had not been pregnant, result in the frequent diagnosis of ovarian cysts (Hedon et al 1992). Management of the patient in all cases is not to endanger the pregnancy in any way.

Most ovarian cysts resolve spontaneously during the first trimester. Complications can occur later on in the pregnancy if the cyst has persisted causing torsion, rupture or infection. Occasionally, cysts can cause a mechanical obstruction of labour, necessitating caesarean section (Hess et al 1988).

Surgical intervention should be avoided during the first trimester. If an organic ovarian cyst is suspected, laparoscopy should be performed after this period but before the enlarging uterus makes the intervention too difficult. Where it is not possible to perform a laparoscopy a microlaparotomy should be done. During the third trimester, if an ovarian cyst is detected and does not require emergency intervention, surgery should be deferred until the fetus has developed sufficiently.

PREPUBERTAL OVARIAN CYSTS

Prepubertal ovarian cysts are uncommon, although ovarian cysts can be identified in the fetus thanks to the improvement in ultrasonographic techniques. Follow-up during childhood shows that most of these cysts regress automatically when the maternal endocrinological influence stops (Creatsas et al 1992). Thus there is no need for immediate surgery unless there are prominent signs of precocious puberty or a palpable large mass.

In infants and neonates, ovarian cysts can be diagnosed easily in cases of precocious puberty. Pain is the most common sign. Diagnosis is facilitated by the history and by clinical examination and laparoscopy in childhood; these are difficult to undertake during infancy. Exclusion of ovarian malignancy is the most important aspect of diagnosis. It accounts for 1% of all cancers in the age group (Muram et al 1992). For this reason tumour markers such as alpha-feto protein and **CA 125** must be tested. Laparoscopy or **fine needle aspiration** under ultrasound guidance is recommended. The aim is to avoid reproductive disability. It is essential to preserve ovarian tissue and it is recommended that the management of these children should be undertaken in specialist centres.

Juvenile primary hypothyroidism is another cause of ovarian cysts but these usually regress following treatment of the condition (Pringle et al 1988).

It is unlikely that nurses working in the field of gynaecology will care for these children as they will be nursed in paediatric units that specialize in meeting the needs of such children. Occasionally an adolescent may be treated on the gynaecological ward and therefore nurses must be aware of the special needs of this client group. Adolescents and their parents should be nursed with supportive reassurance and observation as ovarian cysts in the teenage years can cause considerable concern for the young adolescent and her parents (Lumsden et al 1997).

DIAGNOSIS

Signs and symptoms

Ovarian cysts may cause gastointestional or urinary symptoms. These result from the effects of pressure. Oedema of the legs, haemorrhoids and varicose veins may result in extreme cases. However, the most common presenting symptoms, as already mentioned, are pain and abdominal swelling.

Pain may result from torsion, rupture, haemorrhage or infection. Torsion can cause ischaemia of the cyst and areas may become infarcted. The pain is sharp and constant (Girling & Soutter 1997). A detailed history should be taken from the woman, including whether she is undergoing infertility treatment. Any woman undergoing infertility treatment is at risk of ovarian hyperstimulation syndrome. This is an iatrogenic condition and is a side-effect of infertility treatment, usually with **gonadotrophins** alone, with human chorionic gonadotrophin administration, or in combination, in super-ovulation regimes for assisted conception treatments (Luesley & Watts 1997). Ovarian hyperstimulation syndrome may be mild, moderate or severe. If severe, it can be fatal and hospital admission is essential for rest and observation. Torsion, haemorrhage and rupture of the ovaries can arise, resulting in a laparotomy. Conservative management should be adopted, unless life threatening.

Investigations

Investigation is aimed at excluding conditions with similar presentations, e.g. pelvic inflammatory disease, ectopic pregnancy, appendicitis and torsion of an ovarian cyst.

First, an abdominal and pelvic examination is undertaken. It may be possible to palpate an ovarian mass but, if the pain is severe, pelvic examination may well be unrewarding.

Pelvic pain produces anxiety and fear. Women should be made fully aware of the therapeutic steps that may be required. Tact and sympathetic handling is essential. Any potential gynaecological condition may threaten a woman's femininity and any hopes of future childbearing (Pickrell 1997).

To exclude pregnancy, and particularly an ectopic pregnancy, a beta human chorionic gonadotrophin (hCG) should be performed. A positive blood hCG assay indicates an ongoing pregnancy or recent miscarriage. A high (greater than 6000 iu/L) or rising hCG level without ultrasound evidence of an intrauterine pregnancy means that an ectopic pregnancy is a real possibility.

Next, transvaginal ultrasonography is performed (Fig. 9.1). This procedure uses high resolution images that can detect abnormalities within the pelvis (Gould 1998). Better definition is achieved with transvaginal scanning, although if the woman is in a lot of pain this approach can be difficult. The bladder should be empty for a transvaginal scan. The ultrasound can demonstrate the presence of an ovarian cyst with reasonable sensitivity and fair specificity. Colour-flow Doppler usage may increase the reliability of ultrasound in this area (Bourne et al 1993). Computerized tomography (CT) scanning and magnetic resonance imaging (MRI) are both more expensive and neither has significant advantages over ultrasound in this situation (Girling & Soutter 1997).

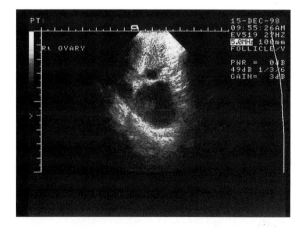

Figure 9.1   Ultrasound scan showing a right-sided 6 cm cyst ovarian swelling. Laparoscopy revealed a chocolate cyst with endometriotic deposits.

Ultrasound-guided diagnostic ovarian cyst aspiration has gradually been introduced into gynaecological practice. The role is to distinguish between functional and benign cysts and to determine the type of benign cyst. However, this is not always reliably achieved and is not to be recommended as a first-line diagnostic tool (Diernaes et al 1987).

The gynaecological examination

Bimanual examination is an essential component of the assessment. During the examination the patient can be depersonalized by a series of rituals. Pelvic examination has particularly distinctive features because there are more pronounced questions of modesty and privacy than in other medical examinations (Meerabeau 1999). A woman's body integrity and sense of herself should be maintained by the presence of a female nurse as a chaperone if being examined by a male doctor (RCN 1991).

Blood test and serum markers

Serum markers have yet to establish a role in the routine management of most ovarian cysts, although a raised serum CA 125 is suggestive of ovarian carcinoma and, in all cases, malignancy should be excluded.

TREATMENT

When an ovarian cyst is larger than 6 cm there is greater risk of torsion occurring due to the increased pedicle length. The common ovarian cyst associated with torsion arises from the germ cell and is a cystic teratoma. Torsion result initially in obstruction of venous return and stretching of the ovarian capsule. In some instances, the torsion can be corrected and the ovarian cyst removed, thus conserving ovarian function. This is important if the contralateral ovary is damaged or missing. However, it is often necessary to remove the affected ovary. Laparoscopic treatment of ovarian torsion has been reported but recurrence rates are high (Pickrell 1997).

Nursing management

The United Kingdom Central Council for Nursing, Midwifery and Health Visiting (UKCC 1992) states that, in exercising professional accountability, the registered nurse/midwife must:

...recognize and respect the uniqueness and dignity of each patient and client, and respond to their need for care irrespective of ethnic origin, religious beliefs, personal attributes, the nature of their health problems or any other factor...
    UKCC (1992: Clause 7) Code of Professional Conduct

In gynaecology, where care is of an intimate nature, it is important to ensure that this is provided in a manner that is sensitive to the needs of the individual patient. The UKCC (1996) also advises that nurses must obtain consent prior to the delivery of any treatment or care and that the person who is to carry out the procedure obtains consent from the patient (UKCC 1996). In this particular case, a woman needs to know that everything possible will be done to conserve her ovary, but she must consent to surgery and its removal should it become infarcted or life threatening.

Intravenous analgesia can be given if the pain is severe. An appropriate antiemetic should also be administered, either intramuscularly or rectally via suppositories.

The advantages of laparoscopic surgery are that in general there is less postoperative pain. The patient's hospital stay is shorter and they are able to resume normal activities quicker (Girling & Soutter 1997). However, the disadvantages are that the cyst contents can spill, the cyst wall can be incompletely excised and unexpected malignancy can be found. Laparoscopic surgery also requires appropriate training.

Nursing issues

The specific pre- and postoperative care for patients undergoing gynaecological surgery has been covered elsewhere in this book.

For women with torsion of an ovarian cyst there are specific nursing care issues to consider. First, the emergency nature of the surgery. Gynaecological nurses should allow the woman to explore and express any feelings of relief, happiness, guilt or anger. If she has undergone an oophorectomy she may be angry at the loss of part of her reproductive system and concerned as to her future fertility. Equally, she may be relieved that the pain and vomiting have now subsided. Gynaecological nurses need to adopt an uncritical and non-threatening approach and attitude, which will promote an open interaction with their patients.

Second, the woman may have concerns that the cyst is cancerous. Again, she should feel supported in exploring her feelings and she should be told the histological findings as soon as possible.

Advice and counselling should be available if required.

Melanie, aged 24, is admitted to the Accident and Emergency department with a history of intermittent colicky iliac fossa pain and vomiting. The pain is severe and her partner had telephoned for an ambulance because he was unsure what else to do.

Melanie is triaged in the Accident and Emergency department. Her observations are:

- temperature: 37°C
- pulse: 90 beats per min
- blood pressure: 110/60 mmHg
- respirations: 20 per min.

The investigations that Melanie undergoes are aimed at excluding conditions with similar presentations, e.g. pelvic inflammatory disease, ectopic pregnancy, appendicitis and torsion of an ovarian cyst. Melanie is given an abdominal and pelvic examination, which reveals a tender adnexal mass. Her lower abdomen is tender, with guarding and rigidity. To make sure that she isn't pregnant, Melanie's levels of beta human chorionic gonadotrophin (hCG) are checked; Melanie's hCG assay is negative. She is then given transvaginal ultrasonography, which discovers an ovarian swelling 12 cm in diameter.

Melanie's presenting signs and symptoms are indicative of torsion of an ovarian cyst. She needs to be prepared for theatre for a laparoscopy, with consent to proceed to laparotomy if necessary. She must be prepared speedily as the whole appendage may infarct. Her haemoglobin and white blood cell count are ascertained and blood is taken for cross-matching. The doctor explains that everything possible will be done to conserve Melanie's ovary but that she must consent to surgery and its removal should it become infarcted or life threatening.

Because Melanie's pain is severe she has been given intravenous analgesia. An appropriate antiemetic is also administered and Melanie goes into theatre for a laparotomy.

OVARIAN HYPERSTIMULATION SYNDROME

As mentioned, ovarian hyperstimulation syndrome (OHSS) can occur as a result of the increasing use of ovulation induction, particularly for assisted fertilization. An extremely serious complication is clinical hyperstimulation, the risks being increased if there is a history of hypothyroidism, hyperprolactinaemia and polycystic ovarian disease.

The World Health Organization (WHO) recognizes that the severe form of hyperstimulation of the ovaries represents the greatest worry. Enlarged ovaries with multiple follicular cysts, stromal oedema and large cystic corpora lutea are the key characteristics of the condition (Pickrell 1997). Ascites, oliguria, electrolyte disturbances, hypovolaemia and a pleural effusion could develop if it is left untreated.

Nursing management

Women with OHSS will have an intravenous infusion *in situ* and their circulatory volume should be assessed via a central venous pressure line.

Vital signs of temperature, pulse, respiration and blood pressure should be taken hourly in the first instance until the condition stabilizes. The woman may be hypertensive and tachycardic as a result of fluid loss from the vascular into the extravascular space and dyspnoea may arise as a result of pleural effusions. As the abdomen is distended, daily girth measurements should be taken and daily weight measurements will show evidence of fluid retention.

These women also require careful monitoring of their fluid intake and output, together with a daily electrolyte imbalance. Diuretics should be avoided as the fluid is in the extravascular space. Albumin infusions may improve the urinary output.

Bed-rest and analgesia should be prescribed and administered for the abdominal pain and an anti-emetic should be given for the nausea. Twice weekly ultrasound scans will determine and monitor ovarian size and the extent of the ascites; a beta hCG should also be done.

Thromboembolic deterrent stockings should be prescribed because of the risk of thrombus formation due to haemoconcentration, which occurs as a result of hypovolaemia as a result of the ascites. The stockings should be worn at all times. It may also be necessary to administer prophylactic subcutaneous heparin.

Ovarian torsion, rupture and haemorrhage are all complications that could arise. Any change in the nature of the pain could be indicative of any of these. The medical staff should be informed immediately as a laparotomy may be necessary. Should the ascites increase, abdominal paracentesis is advised. This should be performed under ultrasound control so as to avoid damage to the ovaries. The drainage tube can be left in for several days. Drainage of ascites can simultaneously improve renal function (Luesley & Watts 1997). However, if there is evidence of oliguria a catheter should be inserted and hourly urine measurements taken.

Another complication is adult respiratory distress syndrome (ARDS), which will necessitate transfer to the intensive care unit.

Throughout this period the woman may be anxious and indeed frightened about what is happening to her.

<table>
<tr><td>

Case study: Julie

Julie is a 35-year-old woman who has been given follicle stimulating hormone and luteinizing hormone as part of a superovulation regime for assisted conception treatment. She is admitted to the ward for observation as she has developed a degree of associated ascites. She has some abdominal pain and distension and is feeling nauseous.

Julie is given an intravenous infusion *in situ* and a central venous pressure line is inserted to assess her circulatory volume. Her temperature, pulse, respiration and blood pressure are taken hourly and she is prescribed bed-rest, analgesia for her abdominal pain and an antiemetic for her nausea.

Julie will remain on the ward for observations. She will require careful monitoring of fluid intake and output and her electrolyte imbalance will be checked daily. Twice-weekly ultrasound scans will determine the size of her ovaries and the extent of her ascites. Julie will need to wear thromboembolic deterrent stockings because she is susceptible to thrombus formation. She is asked to tell the ward staff immediately if there is any change in the nature of her pain because this could indicate ovarian torsion, rupture and haemorrhage, which are all complications of ovarian hyperstimulation syndrome.

</td></tr>
</table>

She may have thoughts that she will never be able to become pregnant or indeed she may think that she is going to die. Psychological nursing care should be aimed at providing the emotional support that these women need at this time.

CONCLUSION

Most benign ovarian cysts are asymptomatic and resolve spontaneously. Surgery is necessitated in those women who present with pain as a result of torsion, rupture, haemorrhage or infection. There is debate over whether the oral contraceptive pill offers women some degree of protection from ovarian cysts. Ovarian cysts in pregnancy are usually functional. If surgery is necessary the aim is always not to endanger the pregnancy. Ovarian cysts before puberty are uncommon. However, if diagnosed and surgery is required the child should be nursed in a specialist unit. Ovarian hyperstimulation syndrome can occur as a result of women undergoing superovulation regimes for assisted conception treatments. Investigations performed for women thought to have an ovarian cyst include a bimanual pelvic examination, transvaginal ultrasonography, a serum beta hCG and a serum CA 125. In all women where ovarian cysts are found, malignancy needs to be excluded and cyst accidents avoided. The woman's future fertility should also not be impaired. Nursing care should be holistic and the woman's needs met physically, psychologically, socially, culturally and spiritually.

GLOSSARY

CA 125: the associated antigen for ovarian cancer
Fine needle aspiration: via ultrasound, especially transvaginal ultrasonography, a fine needle is inserted into the pelvic organs. Individual cells and small pieces of tissue can be obtained.

Gonadotrophins: the hormones, follicle stimulating hormone and luteinizing hormone

REFERENCES

Andrews G 1997 Women's sexual health. Baillière Tindall, London

Bourne TH, Campbell S, Reynolds KM 1993 Screening for early familial ovarian cancer with transvaginal ultrasonography and colour flow imaging. British Medical Journal 303:1025–1029

Creatsas G, Hassan E, Aravantinos D 1992 Prepubertal ovarian cysts. In: Bruhat MA (ed) The management of adnexal cysts. Blackwell Scientific Publications, Oxford

Crosignani PG, Vercellini P, Ragni G, Trespidi L, Colombo A, Parazzini F 1992 Epidemiology of ovarian tumours. In:

Bruhat MA (ed) The management of adnexal cysts. Blackwell Scientific Publications, Oxford

Diernaes E, Rasmussen K, Soersen T, Hasche E 1987 Ovarian cysts: management by puncture? Lancet:1084

Dubuisson JB, Chapron C 1992 Complications of dermoid cysts: spillage and dissemination. In: Bruhat MA (ed) The management of adnexal cysts. Blackwell Scientific Publications, Oxford

Girling JC, Soutter WP 1997 Benign tumours of the ovary. In Shaw RW, Soutter WP, Stanton SL (eds) Gynaecology, 2nd edn. Churchill Livingstone, London

Gould D 1998 Uterine problems: the menstrual cycle. Nursing Standard 50(12):38–43

Hedon P, Nagy P, Dechaud H, Laffargue F, Viala JL 1992 Ovarian cysts in pregnancy. In: Bruhat MA (ed) The management of adnexal cysts. Blackwell Scientific Publications, Oxford

Hess LW, Peaceman A, O'Brien WF, Winkel CA, Cruikshank DP, Morrison JC 1988 Adnexal mass occurring with intrauterine pregnancy: report of fifty four patients requiring laparotomy for definitive management. American Journal of Obstetrics and Gynecology 158:1029–1034

Luesley D, Watts J 1997 Basic gynaecology: a trainee's companion. RCOG Press, London

Lumsden MA, Norman J, Critchley H 1997 Menstrual problems. RCOG Press, London

Meerabeau E 1999 The management of embarrassment and sexuality in healthcare. Journal of Advanced Nursing 29(6):1507–1513

Muram D, Gale GL, Thompson E, Marina N 1992 Ovarian cancer in children and adolescents. Adolescent Paediatrics & Gynaecology 5:21–26

Ory H 1974 Functional ovarian cyst and oral contraceptives. Journal of the American Medical Association 228:68–69

Parazzini F, La Vecchia C, Franceschi S, Negri E, Cecchetti G 1992 Risk factors for endometrioid, mucinous and serous benign ovarian cysts. International Journal of Epidemiology 18:108–112

Pickrell D 1997 Gynaecological emergencies. In: Luesley DM (ed) Common conditions in gynaecology: a problem-solving approach. Chapman & Hall, London

Pringle PJ, Stanhope R, Hindmarsh P, Brook CGD 1988 Abnormal pubertal development in primary hypothyrodism. Clinical Endocrinology 28:479–486

Royal College of General Practitioners 1974 Oral contraceptives and health. Pittman Medical Publishing, Tunbridge Wells

Royal College of Nursing 1991 Standards of care for gynaecological nursing. RCN, London

Struyka A, Treffers PE 1984 Ovarian tumours in pregnancy. Acta Obstetrica Gynaecologica Scandinavica 63:421–424

United Kingdom Central Council for Nursing, Midwifery and Health Visiting (UKCC) 1992 Code of professional conduct. London

United Kingdom Central Council for Nursing, Midwifery and Health Visiting (UKCC) 1996 Guidelines for professional practice. London

Vessey M, Metcalfe A, Wells C, McPherson K, Westhoff CL, Yeates D 1987 Ovarian neoplasm, functional ovarian cyst and oral contraceptives. British Medical Journal 294:1518–1520

Westhoff CL, Pike M, Vessey M 1988 Benign ovarian teratomas: a population-based case-control study. British Journal of Cancer 58:93–98

USEFUL ADDRESSES

British Association for Counselling
1 Regent Place, Rugby CV21 2PJ
Tel: 01788 578328
Women's Health
52 Featherstone Street, London EC1Y 8RT
Tel: 020 7251 6580

Women's Health Concern (WHC)
83 Earl's Court Road, London W8 6EF
Send on SAE with your enquiry.

10

Chlamydia and pelvic inflammatory disease

Alison Sutton

In the last 20 years the significance of genital chlamydial infection has been recognized worldwide. However, control of infection with *Chlamydia trachomatis* is much more difficult to achieve, given the high rate of asymptomatic infection in both women and men. In the developed world, *C. trachomatis* is now the most common bacterial sexually transmitted infection (STI) and, in 1994, genital chlamydia, associated infections and the sequelae were estimated to cost the UK at least £50 million a year for diagnosis and management (Taylor-Robinson 1994). However, there is no national screening programme for chlamydia in place in the UK and many healthcare professionals are unaware of the care and implications of chlamydia and of the severe personal and economic cost of sequelae such as pelvic inflammatory disease (PID) to many women and their partners. These factors led to various major governmental and clinical reports and guidelines in the 1990s.

CHLAMYDIA

Incidence, prevalence and risk factors

In 1997, 22 527 women and 16 105 men were diagnosed with chlamydia in genitourinary medicine (GUM) clinics in England (Hughes et al 1998). The breakdown in age groups is shown in Table 10.1, from which it can be seen that young women aged 16–24 have the highest number of infections. From 1992 to 1996 uncomplicated chlamydial infections diagnosed in GUM in women aged 16–24 increased by approximately 43% (Simms et al 1998). Overall, for women aged 15–59 the incidence of genital chlamydia diagnosed in GUM increased by 16% between 1993 and 1995, with an incidence of 104 cases per 100 000 population in 1995 in this group of women, according to the Chief Medical Officer's (CMO's) Expert Advisory Group (1998).

Table 10.1 1997 Data for England for uncomplicated chlamydia diagnosed in GUM clinics (PHLS, unpublished)

Age	Male	Female
<15	16	135
15	33	366
16–19	1772	7221
20–24	5273	7989
25–34	6986	5541
35–44	1631	971
45–64	357	203
65+	26	19
Not known	11	83
Total	16 105	22 527

Unfortunately, data from other settings such as gynaecology clinics, general practice and family planning clinics are not readily available, although a large number of chlamydial infections are diagnosed and managed outside GUM clinics.

The prevalence of chlamydia in the UK is difficult to calculate as available data are not complete and the infection is so frequently asymptomatic, but median prevalence from various surveys was summarized by the CMO's Expert Advisory Group (1998) as shown in Table 10.2 below.

Stokes (1997) reviewed reports of chlamydia diagnosed in general practice and concluded that the estimated prevalence was 3–4% (with a range of 2–12%). The Central Audit Group in Genitourinary Medicine (1997) – referred to hereafter as the CAG – suggests that chlamydia is found in 4% of the sexually active women attending general practitioners (GPs) and 25% of teenagers attending for termination of pregnancy.

Table 10.2 Median prevalences reported from various clinical settings (CMO's Expert Advisory Group 1998)

Survey population	Median prevalence (%)	Range
General practice attenders	4.5	1–12
Antenatal clinic or obstetric unit attenders	4.6	2–7
Gynaecology clinic attenders	4.8	3–6
Family planning clinic attenders	5.1	3–7
Women seeking terminations	8.0	7–12
GUM clinic attenders	16.4	7–29

Box 10.1 Factors associated with genital chlamydial infection (CMO's Expert Advisory Group 1998)

- Younger age, particularly 25 years old or less
- Being single
- Using oral contraceptives or no contraception
- A recent new sexual partner, particularly within the last 3 months
- Ethnic group
- Young age on leaving school
- No previous births

Although anyone who is sexually active is at risk of chlamydia, certain factors appear to carry more risk.

Hammerschlag et al (1987) believe that the strongest predictor of *C. trachomatis* infection is the presence of another STI, particularly gonorrhoea. In addition, they note that the risk of chlamydia is inversely correlated to age, with 30% of adolescent patients attending urban family planning clinics or STI clinics in America and 15% of sexually active middle-class adolescents infected. Harrison et al (1985) argue that chlamydial infection is more prevalent in women with **ectopy**. Certainly, more susceptible columnar epithelial cells are exposed in ectopy, which makes infection more likely and may increase the shedding of chlamydia from the cervix. Ectopy is seen in 30–50% of women up to 28 years of age and then abruptly decreases in prevalence (Harrison et al 1985). This age-related link may be one factor in chlamydia being so prevalent in younger women (Stamm & Holmes 1990). The CAG (1997) suggests that other risk factors for chlamydia are a recent change of sexual partners or more than two partners in a year and not using barrier contraception. The CMO's Expert Advisory Group (1998) summarizes the risk factors for chlamydia as shown in Box 10.1, with recent sexual partner change, two or more partners in the last year and age as the risk factors that are most frequently reported.

Biology of chlamydia

Chlamydiae are microorganisms that have characteristics of both viruses and bacteria. They are classified as bacteria and *Chlamydia trachomatis* is one of the two species in the genus. Schachter (1990) describes how *C. trachomatis* is specific only to humans and that it has 15 serotypes in total: types A, B, Ba and C cause eye infections (trachoma), types D to K are responsible for genital infections and also for eye infections in adults and babies when transmitted from the genital tract, and types L1, L2 and L3 cause lymphogranuloma venereum. *Chlamydia psittaci,* the other species in the chlamydiae genus, is a common pathogen in birds and can cause a pneumonitis referred to as psittacosis in humans, leading to moderate to severe systemic symptoms (Saunders 1988). Church & Sutton (1996) note that psittacosis can be found in elderly people who keep birds in their living rooms.

Schachter (1990) describes chlamydia as an 'obligate intracellular parasite' because it is restricted to an intracellular lifestyle for replication. Chlamydiae rely on the host cell to supply them with energy and nutrients as they are unable to synthesize high-energy compounds themselves and they lack a system for transport of electrons. This intracellular lifestyle led to chlamydiae originally being thought of as viruses (Saunders 1988). Chlamydiae have a unique growth cycle involving two highly specific morphological life forms summarized by Schachter (1990) as follows. Initially there is attachment and penetration of a susceptible host cell by the infectious particle or elementary body (EB), which can live extracellularly but is metabolically inactive. Once inside the host cell the EB undergoes a morphological change to a reticulate body (RB). It grows and multiplies, using energy from the cell, for 18–24 h after entering the host cell. From this time on there is another morphological change to infectious EBs and, 48–72 h after the process first starts, the cell ruptures, releasing new EBs into the host.

Chlamydia is composed of approximately 40–50% lipid and 35% protein and both RNA and DNA are found, with RBs having more RNA because they are metabolically active. Finally, it is worth noting that, uniquely among bacteria, chlamydia has a cell wall lacking in muramic acid, however, it seems to represent a specialized structure and morphological lifestyle compatible with the special requirements of the growth cycle of chlamydia (Schachter 1990).

The CAG (1997) notes that there is an incubation period of 1–3 weeks for chlamydial infection before symptoms appear, if any do. However, many patients may remain asymptomatic for many years before an associated syndrome appears (Church & Sutton 1996).

Clinical features and complications

One of the most striking features about chlamydia in women is that up to 70% of infected women are asymptomatic (CMO's Expert Advisory Group 1998). However, about 30% of women have local signs of infection on examination (Harrison et al 1985). The most commonly observed sign is mucopurulent cervical discharge, found in 37% of women; and hypertrophic ectopy where the ectopy is congested, oedematous and bleeds easily, found in 19% of women (Stamm & Holmes 1990). It is important to distinguish this **cervicitis** from normal ectopy, which, as previously discussed, is found in many sexually active adolescents – up to 60–80% and particularly in those on oral contraception. Stamm & Holmes (1990) state that a careful cervical examination and a high index of suspicion are needed for clinical recognition of chlamydial cervicitis. Harrison et al (1985) examined a number of variables relating to cervicitis and discharge and found a heavy discharge in 33% of women, green discharge in 50% and purulent discharge in 23%. Friability of the cervix with bleeding on touch was seen in 25% of women with chlamydia. When a Gram-stain of the cervical mucus or discharge is undertaken, a finding of 30 or more polymorphonuclear leucocytes or pus cells per 1000 field is usually indicative of chlamydia (Stamm & Holmes 1990). However, it should be noted that without infection being present, women have a wide range of pus cell values, which may relate to the menstrual cycle, sexual activity and contraceptive practices, as oral contraceptives alter the consistency of cervical mucus. Crowley et al (1997) analysed the menstrual cycle of women tested for chlamydia and found significant variations in detection of chlamydia related to the cycle. There was increased detection from the cervix after the second week in women on combined oral contraceptives but only after the third week in women who did not have ectopy.

Urethritis can be a further clinical feature of chlamydial infection in women with dysuria, pyuria and frequency, although many women with chlamydial urethritis will be asymptomatic (Stamm & Holmes 1990). Paavonen (1979) studied 99 female partners of men with non-gonococcal urethritis and found that only 54% of women with urethral chlamydia actually reported any urethral symptoms, although a higher proportion of women who had urethral chlamydia complained of urethral symptoms than those women who only had cervical chlamydia. Twenty-five per cent of women were chlamydia-positive only from the urethra and not the cervix. Hay et al (1994) also examined urethral samples in women with cervical chlamydia and found that the urinary tract was positive for chlamydia almost as often as the cervix. They concluded that both sites need to be tested to confirm whether a woman is infected with chlamydia.

Hammerschlag et al (1987) note that chlamydia can be found rectally in 35% of women with cervical chlamydial infection. They believe that such infections are almost always asymptomatic and a result of contamination from the vagina rather than from anal intercourse. Pharyngeal chlamydial infection is also seen in women who practice oral sex – fellatio – on an infected partner without using a condom, though Østergaard et al (1997) suggest that the incubation time can be over 3 months for pharyngeal infection. Other clinical features in women include dyspareunia, abdominal pain, vaginal discomfort, purulent infection of the Bartholin glands with discharge from the ducts, alterations to the menstrual cycle, such as postcoital or intermenstrual bleeding, and rebound tenderness and cervical excitation on pelvic examination, with the latter often related to PID, which is discussed later in this chapter (CAG 1997, Cameron & Blakely 1993, Hammerschlag et al 1987, Horner & Caul 1999, Stamm & Holmes 1990).

In some patients, genital chlamydial infection is diagnosed only because the patient is found to have chlamydial conjunctivitis. Postema et al (1996) found that 74% of women and 54% of men with chlamydial conjunctivitis had positive cervical and urethral chlamydial tests, respectively, and concluded that the eye infection was a result of autoinoculation from the genital region. Genital chlamydial infection in pregnant women may lead to premature birth, postpartum endometritis, neonatal conjunctivitis and neonatal pneumonia (Jensen et al 1997). Brunham et al (1990) suggest that 2–30% of pregnant women may have chlamydia infection, although it is not known whether pregnancy influences shedding of *C. trachomatis* from the cervix. Sixty per cent of babies exposed to their mother's chlamydial infection will be infected, even though maternal antibodies to chlamydia have been transferred through the placenta. Whelan (1988) states that 18–50% of babies born to infected women will develop unilateral or bilateral conjunctivitis with mucopurulent discharge and inflammation 1–3 weeks after delivery, although the symptoms may be missed if they are mild and even the more severe forms of the infection appear to be self-limiting. Also, 3–18% of infants will develop chlamydial pneumonia, usually between 1 and 3 months of age (Whelan 1988). Obviously, if chlamydial infection is found in neonates, it is extremely important that the mother and father are tested for chlamydial infection. Equally, pregnant women found to have chlamydia should be treated to prevent neonatal infection (Church & Sutton 1996).

Given the very high asymptomatic rate of chlamydial infection in women, it is important that gynaecology nurses are aware of the clinical features of infection in men, as many women are only diagnosed as having chlamydia because they are the sexual contacts of infected men. Hammerschlag et al (1987) note that 10–20% of men with chlamydia are asymptomatic, although the CAG (1997) puts this figure at 50%. In men, the principal signs and symptoms are mild dysuria and urethral discharge, which tends to be less purulent than a gonococcal urethral discharge. **Epididymitis** with unilateral scrotal pain, tenderness, swelling and fever may be present in young men with chlamydia, previously described as ideopathic epididymitis (Berger et al 1978), although the link between prostatitis and chlamydial infection is more controversial (Stamm & Holmes 1990). More important and serious complications of chlamydia in men are Reiter's syndrome and reactive arthritis, which manifests as genital tract inflammation, ocular inflammation and peripheral arthritis (Keat & Rowe 1990). Dysuria and discharge are accompanied or followed by joint symptoms and synovitis within 30 days of infection in 90% of patients, with uveitis and lesions on the mucous membranes and skin. Symptoms may last up to 1 year and may recur for several years. Women with sexually acquired reactive arthritis are frequently not diagnosed quickly because of the asymptomatic nature of their genital chlamydia (Church & Sutton 1996). It should also be noted that male infertility can be linked to asymptomatic, untreated genital chlamydia (Greendale et al 1993).

It can be seen that the very unspecific nature of the clinical features of chlamydia make diagnosis clinically difficult, exacerbated by the frequency of asymptomatic infection in both women and men. Therefore, a high index of suspicion is required by all healthcare workers looking after young, sexually active women regardless of the setting.

Testing for chlamydia

Methods of testing for chlamydia and the collection of different specimens has come a long way since chlamydiae were first grown in culture cells in the 1960s (Taylor-Robinson 1992). As chlamydia is an intracellular organism it has to be grown by cell culture, which is expensive, time-consuming and only available in some laboratories (Ridgway & Taylor-Robinson 1992) and, although cell culture used to be the gold standard for chlamydia testing, it is only 75–85% sensitive at best and may be as low as 55%

sensitive (CAG 1997). It is only now used in the UK for medicolegal cases such as assault and rape, as noted by Horner & Caul (1999), who have written national guidelines on chlamydia for clinicians on behalf of the Clinical Effectiveness Group for the Medical Society for the Study of Venereal Diseases (MSSVD) and the Association for Genitourinary Medicine (AGUM).

Another older test for chlamydia used direct staining of specimens with vital dyes but, as it is an insensitive method, and open to operator error, it is no longer used (Taylor-Robinson 1992). The next testing process to be used was direct fluorescent antibody (DFA) testing, which uses fluorescin-conjugated monoclonal antibodies to stain extracellular EBs and is generally 68–100% sensitive in women, although it is dependent on the skill and experience of laboratory staff in interpreting results (Ridgway & Taylor-Robinson 1992). This method is very fast, which makes it useful in cases of chlamydial ophthalmia neonatorum (CAG 1997).

All the above test processes use specimens taken by swab from the cervix or the urethra. The next development was that of enzyme immunoassay (EIA) tests, which are automated, convenient and useful for large numbers of samples but only 64–98% sensitive when compared with culture, which is only 60% sensitive to start with (Taylor-Robinson 1992). As there are a significant number of false-positive results with EIA testing, all positive results should be confirmed by another method, such as DFA (CAG 1997). However, EIA has the significant advantage that it can be undertaken on a first void urine (FVU) sample in men, which is a much more acceptable specimen to patients than a urethral swab (Crowley et al 1992, Hay et al 1993), although EIA is not generally considered sensitive enough to be done on urine samples from women (Ridgway & Taylor-Robinson 1992).

The latest methods developed for testing for chlamydia are based in molecular biology – polymerase chain reaction (PCR) and ligase chain reaction (LCR) are methods of amplifying DNA so that even very small amounts of chlamydia will be detected, giving very specific and sensitive tests (Davies & Ridgway 1997). Although both PCR and LCR are relatively expensive they may well prove cost-effective, as they can be carried out on non-invasive specimens such as urine and vulval swabs (CAG 1997). There are now a number of studies showing that LCR carried out on vaginal swabs or urine samples are very sensitive and specific at detecting chlamydia in women (Chernesky et al 1994, Lee et al 1995, Ridgway et al 1996, Thomas et al 1998), although Jensen et al (1997)

sound a note of caution that urine samples from pregnant women contain inhibitors to LCR assays and should therefore not be used. Horner & Caul (1999) reviewed new testing methods and concluded that PCR and LCR systems give high specificity, and that urine should not be used with EIA systems when testing women. The CMO's Expert Advisory Group (1998) point out that equivocal results from urine samples should be confirmed by taking an endocervical specimen for testing. Finally, Welsh et al (1997) note that variations in quality of specimens has a significant impact on results and prevalence figures for chlamydia within a population.

Screening and epidemiological control

At present there is no programme of screening for chlamydia in the UK, although there is much discussion on the value and feasibility of screening. However, in Sweden a programme screening all women under 30 years old for chlamydia when they attend for family planning, termination of pregnancy or antenatal care has been running since 1982 with considerable effect (Ripa 1990). Since 1984 the prevalence of the infection in 15–29-year-old Swedish women has been reduced by 50% and a 44% reduction in calculated expenditure has been achieved. There has also been a significant reduction in cases of PID in Sweden (Kamwendo et al 1998). It is interesting to note that chlamydia has been a reportable disease in Sweden since 1988 (Ripa 1990). As a result, much more accurate data are available than in the UK. Although GUM clinics in the UK use KC60 forms to report all incidences of chlamydia that they diagnose, there is no obligation for other areas to report cases of chlamydia. Therefore accurate UK national figures are not available. Overall, Sweden's epidemiological programme has resulted in a 30–50% decrease in genital chlamydial infection (Ripa 1990).

Mårdh (1997) considered whether Europe is ready for an STI screening programme and concluded that a major obstacle to the introduction of screening is the lack of knowledge about chlamydia and its sequelae by the medical profession and other healthcare workers, and that not only the medical community but also the general population need to accept the necessity of such a screening programme. He suggests that combining STI screening with cervical screening and counselling on general health risks such as smoking, exercise and weight may help reduce the costs of a screening programme, along with the actual cost reduction achieved by screening. In the UK, Caul et al (1997) suggest that LCR offers the chance of a non-invasive test that allows a screening programme to be advocated. Dean et al (1998) believe that EIA testing with DFA, PCR or LCR for verification offers an acceptable sensitivity and specificity at a reasonable cost for low-to-moderate-risk populations and could therefore be extended to wider at-risk populations. Recently, the CMO's Expert Advisory Group (1998) has addressed three options for screening:

- testing as part of the diagnostic process for those with symptoms
- a register based screening with call and recall
- opportunistic screening of target populations.

Box 10.2 Recommendations for chlamydia screening (CMO's Expert Advisory Group 1998)

Testing offered as part of the diagnostic process for those with symptoms, regardless of age or any other factors
- women with mucopurulent cervicitis
- women with acute PID
- women with vaginal discharge
- women with lower abdominal pain
- women with postcoital or intermenstrual bleeding
- men with non-specific urethritis (NSU) and epididymitis
- men with urethral discharge
- men with reactive arthritis
- the sexual partners of the above patients because of the risk of asymptomatic infection
- infants with neonatal pneumonitis or ophthalmia neonatorum and their parents
- couples having infertility investigation or treatment
- women having procedures requiring instrumentation of the uterus, such as IUD fitting, colposcopy
- semen donors

Specific target populations for screening
- all GUM clinic attenders and their partners
- women seeking termination of pregnancy and their partners
- asymptomatic women aged 25–35-years-old who have a new sexual partner or who have had two or more partners in a year
- asymptomatic sexually active women under 25 years old, especially teenagers

Settings for opportunistic screening of asymptomatic populations of appropriate age and sexually active
- general practice
- family planning clinics
- antenatal clinics for women under 25

They felt that a register with call and recall was not suitable and favoured screening in settings where a person's risk could be assessed before screening was offered, or selective screening based on risk factors such as age and frequent partner change. Their recommendations are set out in Box 10.2.

Treatment of chlamydia

Since chlamydia was first recognized, the treatment of choice has been erythromycin and tetracyclines, although chlamydia is also susceptible to sulphonamides and trimethoprim but not penicillin (Schachter 1990). However, newer antibiotics are now recommended for use. Certain issues are of importance to encourage compliance when choosing a regime for patients. The CAG (1997) highlights that treatments should be easy to take and, ideally, should be taken not more than twice daily. They should have a low side-effect profile, cause minimal interference with the patient's lifestyle and achieve a microbiological cure rate in excess of 95% for effective treatment. There have been a number of studies into the efficacy of treatment for chlamydia, but most of these have been small scale and have used culture methods to detect the organism (Horner & Caul 1999), which is not the situation in clinical practice.

Table 10.3 summarizes the recommendations for treatment given by the CAG (1997), by Horner & Caul (1999) in their guidelines for clinicians and by the Centers for Disease Control in America, described by Zenilman (1998). It should be noted that certain drugs have different dosages in America. Various points should be remembered in relation to patient compliance versus cost and efficacy, as outlined by the CAG (1997) as follows:

- doxycycline: cannot be used in pregnancy; causes about 20% gastrointestinal (GI) side-effects and occasional photosensitization
- Deteclo (triple tetracycline): cannot be used in pregnancy; causes photosensitization; cannot be taken with milk
- erythromycin: less than 95% efficacy; 20–25% GI upset; lengthy or frequent dosing
- azithromycin: only a one-off dose but expensive; may be justified in patients where compliance is an issue (Handsfield & Stamm 1998); safety in pregnancy not known; possible cure rate of less than 95% although Ridgway (1996) suggests a virtual 100% cure rate
- tetracyclines: cannot be used in pregnancy; not with milk; frequent dosing
- ofloxacin: cannot be used in pregnancy; expensive.

Table 10.3 Treatment recommendations for chlamydia

CAG (1997)	Horner & Caul (1999)	Centers for Disease Control (Zenilman 1998)
First line		
doxycycline 100 mg b.d. for 7 days **or** deteclo 300 mg b.d. for 7 days	doxycycline 100 mg b.d. for 7 days **or** azithromycin 1 g single dose	azithromycin 1 g single dose **or** doxycycline 100 mg b.d. for 7 days
Second line or alternative regime		
erythromycin 500 mg q.d.s. for 7 days **or** erythromycin 500 mg b.d. for 14 days **or** azithromycin 1 g single dose **or** tetracycline 500 mg q.d.s. for 7 days **or** ofloxacin 400 mg o.d. for 7 days	erythromycin 500 mg q.d.s. for 7 days **or** erythromycin 500 mg b.d. for 14 days **or** deteclo 300 mg b.d. for 7 days **or** ofloxacin 200 mg b.d./400 mg o.d. for 7 days **or** tetracycline 500 mg q.d.s. for 7 days	erythromycin 500 mg q.d.s. for 7 days **or** erythromycin ethyl succinate 800 mg t.d.s. for 7 days **or** ofloxacin 300 mg b.d. for 7 days
Pregnancy		
erythromycin 500 mg q.d.s. for 7 days **or** erythromycin 500 mg b.d. for 14 days **or** amoxycillin 500 mg t.d.s. for 7 days	erythromycin 500 mg q.d.s. for 7 days **or** erythromycin 500 mg b.d. for 14 days **or** amoxycillin 500 mg t.d.s. for 7 days	

Management and nursing intervention

Perhaps the most important aspect of the management of chlamydial infection is the **contact tracing** or partner notification of sexual contacts. Church & Sutton (1996) believe that the importance of contact tracing is difficult to overemphasize. Both the patient and any contacts should be advised not to have sexual intercourse until all parties have been tested for chlamydia and treated as necessary. Horner & Caul (1999) point out that even if the tests from a contact are negative, epidemiological treatment may be given as it is known that no test is 100% accurate in diagnosing chlamydia and also that a large proportion of patients are asymptomatic. The CAG (1997) advise that:

- contact tracing of all partners of women and asymptomatic men over the last 6 months or until the last previous sexual partner, whichever is the longer time, should be undertaken
- contact tracing of all partners of symptomatic men in the 4 weeks before symptoms started should be carried out
- contacts should be treated regardless of the results because difficulty in testing means that infection is not excluded by a negative result.

Follow-up of all patients with chlamydia, regardless of where the patient is treated, is vitally important to: (i) assess the compliance with treatment and abstention from intercourse and therefore the risk of reinfection; (ii) reinforce health education; (iii) provide reassurance; and (iv) continue the contact tracing process (Horner & Caul, 1999). The CAG (1997) recommends that **test-of-cure** (TOC) does not need to be undertaken when treatment with a cure rate of at least 95% has been given for uncomplicated infection, although TOC should be performed if the woman is pregnant. TOC should be taken 3 weeks after treatment with erythromycin, as earlier testing may detect non-viable organisms and give a false result. It is not needed after treatment with azithromycin or doxycycline unless reinfection is suspected or symptoms persist (Horner & Caul 1999).

Contact tracing and treatment of contacts are frequently not carried out when patients attend areas other than GUM clinics (Church & Sutton 1996). It is therefore a vital part of the nursing intervention to educate and encourage patients to make sure that their sexual contacts attend for testing, ideally to a GUM clinic. Unless contact tracing is carried out, transmission of chlamydia will not be controlled, particularly given the asymptomatic nature of the infection, and

---

Case study: Caitlin

Caitlin attended the GUM clinic as a sexual contact of her regular boyfriend, who had been diagnosed with genital warts. She gave no history of infection of any kind.

On examination, Caitlin was found to have vaginal candida, which was treated that day and although genital warts were not seen, a cervicitis and cervical discharge were noted. The endocervical swab was positive and she was diagnosed as having asymptomatic chlamydia.

Caitlin was treated with deteclo 300 mg b.d. for 14 days and a TOC taken 2 weeks after the end of treatment proved negative.

Contact tracing was undertaken and, as she had had no other partners within the last 6 months, only her regular boyfriend was treated, even though his test was negative for chlamydia on his initial visit to the clinic.

---

therefore the physical and emotional effects and sequelae will not be reduced (Church & Sutton 1996). Nurses should also encourage patients with chlamydia to be tested for other STIs, as co-infection with other pathogens is a problem. The CAG (1997) recommends that all patients with chlamydia should be given written information about the infection, its diagnosis, treatment and importance.

It is important that nurses in healthcare settings such as obstetrics and gynaecology clinics, family planning units, termination of pregnancy services and general practice are well educated about all aspects of chlamydia and its sequelae. They should be able not only to assess the risk of chlamydia for a particular patient and to educate and care for patients but also to educate the general public and other health professionals. In conclusion, knowledge of genital chlamydial infection needs to be part of the practice of every nurse who cares for sexually active patients, and particularly of those who care for women, and accurate information needs to be given to patients and the general public alike by intelligent use of the media (Church & Sutton 1996).

PELVIC INFLAMMATORY DISEASE (PID)

Prevalence and risk factors

Pelvic inflammatory disease (PID) is generally caused by infection ascending from the lower genital tract to the upper genital tract; this is often a bacterial infection. Hare (1990a) defines PID as inflammation of the upper genital tract, with MacLean (1995) describing pelvic infection of the uterus, fallopian tubes, overlying pelvic peritoneum and adjacent parametria. Pelvic abscesses, either tubal or tubo-ovarian, are also included in the definition of PID (Weström & Mårdh 1990). Therefore the organs involved are the uterus, ovaries, fallopian tubes and the surrounding tissue. The terms **salpingitis** and PID are often used interchangeably when referring to pelvic infection but PID will generally be used in this chapter.

The KC60 reports from GUM clinics in England show that, in 1997, 10 420 women were diagnosed with PID, of which 86% were related to non-specific non-gonococcal infection, 12% from complicated chlamydial infection and only 1.8% were complications of gonococcal infection (Hughes et al 1998). However, as women with PID are seen across a wide range of fragmented services, the condition is difficult to diagnose with accuracy and other data are generally derived from inpatient hospital figures although many patients are managed only as outpatients (Mann et al 1996), accurate national figures for PID are not available. However, Catchpole (1992) notes a 50% increase in women aged 20–24 diagnosed with PID between 1975 and 1985, based on hospital discharge data, with no decrease seen since then.

A number of risk factors may contribute to the development of PID. Certainly sexual activity is linked to the risk of PID and MacLean (1995) notes that PID is much more likely in women who have had a number of sexual partners and is very rare in virgins. Weström & Mårdh (1990) state that even if the cause of PID is neither gonorrhoea or chlamydia, the relationship between PID and sexual activity is valid. Another major risk for PID is that of age, as it is rarely seen in postmenopausal women and never in prepubertal girls (MacLean 1995). Rome (1994) states that the risk of developing an STI and of PID is highest in adolescents. Although Weström & Mårdh (1990) believe that no one explanation is proved to relate to the age-dependent risk of PID, there are certain factors that appear relevant. These include less regular use of barrier contraception, quicker rate of partner change, higher rates of infection within partners, low levels of antibodies from lack of previous exposure to STIs, high rates of ectopy and early age of first intercourse (Mann et al 1996, Rome 1994).

The role of intrauterine devices (IUDs) as a risk factor for PID is unclear. They were originally thought to lead to an increased risk of PID but it now appears that any risk is usually only within a few months of insertion. However Wølner-Hanssen et al (1990) suggest that chronic endometritis and endosalpingitis are often seen in IUD users but that these changes may not be caused solely by infection. As a general rule, Rome (1994) believes that IUDs are not a good form of contraception for adolescents who often have a sexual activity pattern of serial monogamy, multiple partners and frequent exposure to STIs. PID following procedures such as termination of pregnancy, dilatation and curettage, tubal insufflation and IUD insertion has been noted, although the risk appears to be small when procedures are correctly performed (Weström & Mårdh 1990).

Causative agents

Pelvic infection has been known of for hundreds of years and the large number of organisms implicated in PID has also been noted, with gonorrhoea discovered in the late nineteenth century. PID was originally classified as being either tuberculous or non-tuberculous, but nowadays it is often described as being a gonococcal or a non-gonococcal infection (MacLean 1995). However, Weström & Mårdh (1990) classify causes of PID as either sexually transmitted, exogenous agents or organisms that live naturally in the lower genital tract, endogenous agents.

PID is very often found to be of non-specific origin and Weström & Mårdh (1990) note that the lack of access for sampling from the tubes and the multitude of species found naturally in the lower genital tract of women make diagnosing a causative agent for PID very difficult at times. Difficulties of diagnosis will be discussed later. Since its discovery, *Neisseria gonorrhoea* has been recognized as producing a classical PID, which, without antibiotics, is self-limiting, lasting 10–14 days, unless there is secondary infection or an acute crisis from rupture of an abscess (Hare 1990a). Gonococci disappear from the fallopian tubes as the length of infection increases (Weström & Mårdh 1990). There is a 2–14-day incubation time for gonococcal infection and 60% of women will be asymptomatic, although men will generally have symptoms. Toxin released by gonococci reduces the activity of the cilia lining the tubes and probably causes some of the tubal damage seen in PID (MacLean 1995). He goes on to state that, after the initial infection and damage with gonorrhoea, there is often secondary infection with other organisms. It appears that the damaged tubes are less resistant to further damage by the types of anaerobic and aerobic organisms found in the lower genital tract (Hare 1990b). However, in Europe, the prevalence of gonococcal PID is falling, although this is not the case elsewhere in the world (Hare 1990a), where an important cause of morbidity continues to be gonococcal sepsis (Mann et al 1996). This correlates with the reduction in cases of gonorrhoea diagnosed in the UK since the early 1990s (Simms et al 1998). However Kamwendo et al (1993) found gonorrhoea in 43% of men whose partners had acute PID with gonorrhoea and it is important to consider this aspect when diagnosing PID.

Chlamydia is now well established as the most important cause of acute and chronic PID in the developed world (Mann et al 1996), with at least 30% of women having laparoscopies found to have chlamydia in the fallopian tubes (Hare 1990a). When antibody studies and cervical chlamydial infection are also considered, then up to 60% of PID cases in developed countries may be due to chlamydia. Certainly, the ratio of chlamydia–PID is increasing in Europe in relation to gonococcal–PID (Weström & Mårdh 1990). Tait et al (1997) describe a small study where 40% of the women having laparoscopies were found to have 'silent' chlamydial upper genital tract infection with no symptoms or signs of either gonorrhoea or chlamydia and, in some cases, no tubal pathology observed. It appears that chlamydial PID tends to be milder but longer lasting than gonococcal PID and may even persist if antibiotic treatment does not include a specific antichlamydial agent (Hare 1990a). Although there may be an absence of signs and symptoms in chronic chlamydial PID, severe tubal damage may occur (Hare 1990b). Bevan et al (1995) found that women with chlamydial PID were younger than those with non-chlamydial PID and that a number of women were infected with both gonorrhoea and chlamydia in their tubes. As with gonorrhoea, tubes damaged by chlamydia can be overgrown with endogenous organisms, which may lead the patient to seek help due to a rapid exacerbation of symptoms (Hare 1990a). Hare (1990a) notes that ureaplasmas and mycoplasmas are also thought to be involved in pelvic abscess formation and PID, although their role as pathogens in the upper genital tract is unclear. Antibody to *Mycoplasma hominis* has been noted in up to 30% of women with PID and, although it is rarely isolated from the fallopian tubes, it is often found on the cervix (Weström & Mårdh 1990). Bevan et al (1995) also noted *M. hominis* in 38% of the women with acute salpingitis in their study group. However, as ureaplasmas and mycoplasmas are frequently isolated from healthy women, Hare (1990b) suggests that it is difficult to decide whether the organisms act as incidental colonizers, pathogens or opportunistic pathogens. Weström & Mårdh (1990) believe that cultures from the upper genital tract are needed to help study the role of various STI agents in PID, particularly as a number of women have mixed infection PID with more than one STI identified.

Various endogenous anaerobic and aerobic bacteria have been found in women with **bacterial vaginosis** and many authors report isolating such organisms from women with severe PID, particularly where there is abscess formation (Hare 1990b). Weström & Mårdh (1990) suggest that the following species have been isolated from the upper genital tract: *Escherichia coli*; *Bacteroides* species, particularly *B. melaninogenicus* and *B. bivius*; facultative and anaerobic streptococci including peptostreptococci and group B streptococci; and actinomyces and clostridial species. However, Hare (1990a) believes that *Actinomyces israeli* is only relevant in women with IUDs who have PID. Infection with a number of different organisms has often been seen at laparoscopy and Hare (1990b) believes that anaerobic infections may develop in fallopian tubes damaged by previous gonococcal or chlamydial infection.

It appears that viruses may have a role in PID, although this is difficult to define as few researchers try and isolate viruses from the upper genital tract of women with PID (Weström & Mårdh 1990) and further studies are needed. Hare (1990a) believes that herpetic PID may be a possibility, as *Herpes simplex* lesions on the genital tract are seen in women with PID. Respiratory tract and mouth organisms, among other miscellaneous agents, have been isolated in women with PID and some techniques used in oral sex, such as blowing air into the vagina, might lead to organisms already present or those from the sexual partner's mouth being spread upwards (Hare 1990a). Weström & Mårdh (1990) also note that tropical diseases such as schistosomiasis and filariasis may be associated with upper genital tract infection. It is important to remember that in any given case of PID it can be difficult to pinpoint the organism involved (Stacey et al 1992) and in many cases no organism is isolated.

Disease spread

The mechanism of disease spread is thought to be due to various factors but the basis is that of canalicular spread, that is from the cervix via the endometrial cavity to the fallopian tubes by ascending infection, with spread via the lymphatic system as a rare alternative pathway (Hare 1990a). However, the cervical canal is generally narrow and mucus is moved by the action of cilia downwards through the cervix to form the mucus plug, both of which are believed to act as a natural barrier. It has been noted previously that cervi-

cal ectopy seems to increase the risk of chlamydial infection and may be involved in disease spread (Weström & Mårdh 1990). Hare (1990a) notes that sperm may act as a vector for other organisms as they progress to the tubes, as research has shown that the sexual partners of men with low sperm counts or who are azoospermic have much lower rates of PID. The insuck phenomenon has also been well researched in recent years and it appears that uterine contractions causing pressure changes during intercourse lead to sperm and other material being sucked up into the uterus from the vagina (Hare 1990a, Weström & Mårdh 1990).

It is known that menstrual blood can flow from the uterus to the tubes in a retrograde manner and that microorganisms may be spread with the blood, leading to PID (Weström & Mårdh 1990). Hare (1990a) notes that the only barrier to infection spreading from the uterus to the tubes, once the endometrium is infected, is the small size of the tubal opening and the downward flow of mucus facilitated by cilial movement. Primary, secondary and recurrent PID have been described by Hare (1990a) and are shown in Table 10.4.

Other authors describe PID as either acute or chronic. MacLean (1995) suggests that acute PID is normally bilateral, although the tubes can look different to each other. Weström (1988) describes how tubal infection begins in the mucosa and the inflammatory reaction leads to oedema and an increase in volume of the mucosa and submucosal layers of the wall of the

Table 10.4 Types of PID (Hare 1990a)

Type of PID	Description
Primary	An infection that usually occurs in a young woman with no previous damage to the upper genital tract. A mechanism of transport is required for the organism to penetrate the cervical barrier. Often started by STI agents, although vaginal and bowel organisms may later colonize inflamed tissues
Secondary	Normally occurring when the cervical barrier has been breached or damaged, by childbirth, surgery, termination of pregnancy, miscarriage, etc. More often caused by anaerobic and aerobic organisms than with primary PID
Recurrent	Recurrent infection with non-STI organisms, as the woman is at high risk from a previous episode of PID. No definite link between the type of organism found and the clinical presentation

tube. Pressure increases with volume, resulting in damage to the serosa and swelling of the entire tube and causing the tubal fimbriae to be drawn together. Exudate containing microorganisms leaks into the pelvic cavity from the tube at the fimbrial end and can lead to infection and inflammation of the ovaries and adjacent organs and peritoneum (Weström 1988). Macroscopically, the tubal mucosa appears red and congested at the fimbrial ends and the serosa is reddened with swelling of the tubes (Weström & Mårdh 1990). As the infection progresses, the exudate covering the serosal surfaces acts like glue and tubes can become stuck to nearby structures and involve the pelvic peritoneum (Weström 1988, Weström & Mårdh 1990). At this stage, laparoscopy may show an inflammatory mass involving the entire pelvic cavity with actual structures difficult to see individually (Weström & Mårdh 1990).

In chronic PID MacLean (1995) notes that the tubes become very distorted, with extensive dilatation, and a **hydrosalpinx** or **pyosalpinx** may form. Often, the fimbrial end of the tube is obstructed or the tube may be fibrosed and blocked at a point along its length. Pelvic adhesions from the tube can involve the bowel, peritoneum, uterus, tubes and ovaries, reducing pelvic organ mobility and even leading to pelvic abscesses (MacLean 1995, Weström & Mårdh 1990).

Diagnosis and clinical features

PID is frequently difficult to diagnose and the accuracy of diagnosis of lower abdominal pain is low in women of childbearing age (Hare 1990b). Stacey & Munday (1994) believe that pain may resolve and recur without a definite diagnosis being made or specific treatment being given because the signs and symptoms are often vague in women of this age. It appears that acute PID can range from a life-threatening condition to an asymptomatic problem and the patient is not usually seriously ill with gonococcal or chlamydial PID (Weström & Mårdh 1990). As previously noted, it is difficult to sample from the upper genital tract without an operative procedure and, in addition, many microbial species are normally found in the lower genital tract which affects the diagnosis of PID. There are often differences between the organisms isolated from the lower and upper genital tracts in PID, which is partly explained by the fact that it appears that endogenous infections colonize the tubes following initial infection by gonorrhoea or chlamydia (Hare 1990a, b, Weström & Mårdh 1990). Lower genital tract infections are often asymptomatic or cause mild and

Table 10.5 Clinical critera for diagnosis of salpingitis (Hager et al 1983)

Clinical importance	Criteria for diagnosis
All of these are necessary for a diagnosis of salpingitis	Abdominal tenderness on palpation, rebound tenderness may or may not be present Moving the cervix and uterus causes excitation tenderness Adnexal tenderness on bimanual palpation
One or more of these are also required	Gram-negative intracellular diplococci (gonococci) seen on Gram stain from endocervix Pyrexia of more than 38°C White cell count more than 10 000 WBC/mm Fluid containing pus cells and white cells obtained from the peritoneal cavity at laparoscopy (or culdocentesis) Pelvic abscess or inflammation detected by bimanual examination or ultrasound

short-lived symptoms, as previously noted, and Weström & Mårdh (1990) suggest that lower genital tract infection can be present for months before PID becomes a problem.

Once a diagnosis of PID is made it tends to stick and further episodes of pain are often diagnosed as recurrent PID without alternatives being considered or investigated, even when the original diagnosis was unsubstantiated (Hare 1990a). The difficulty of diagnosing PID led Hager et al (1983) to suggest rigid criteria for diagnosis, as shown in Table 10.5.

As chlamydia was not widely recognized when these criteria were written, Hare (1990b) suggests that an acceptable alternative to the presumptive finding of gonococci is the finding of chlamydia. Recently Ross wrote (1999) draft guidelines for the Clinical Effectiveness Group of MSSVD/AGUM, in the series for chlamydia, and summarizes the diagnostic features of PID as shown in Box 10.3 (Ross 1999).

Abdominal pain is the most important presenting symptom. When describing patients' histories, Westcott (1992) suggests that many women have severe acute pain when they see a doctor. However, Weström & Mårdh (1990) note that pain may be dull, bilateral, pelvic or low abdominal and subacute in onset. Also,

---

Box 10.3 Diagnosis of PID (Ross 1999)

Features that are highly suggestive of PID as a diagnosis
- *Symptoms*
- lower abdominal pain
- abnormal bleeding
- dyspareunia
- abnormal cervical or vaginal discharge
- *Signs*
- adnexal tenderness on bimanual examination
- lower abdominal tenderness
- tenderness when the cervix is moved during bimanual examination
- pyrexia of more than 38°C
Features that are supportive of a diagnosis of PID
- elevated ESR or C reactive protein
- laboratory confirmed endocervical infection with chlamydia or gonorrhoea

---

not all patients with pain have PID, although women with PID usually have pain (MacLean 1995). It is important to establish the site, nature and pattern of pain and any associations with intercourse, micturition and menstruation. Although some studies describe women with PID as having deep dyspareunia, Stacey & Munday (1994) found that women with PID in their study were more likely to describe the pain as stabbing, and that deep dyspareunia was more common in women without PID.

Irregular bleeding may be seen in 35% of women with PID (MacLean 1995) and Weström & Mårdh (1990) note that it is more often associated with chlamydial PID than with PID from other causes. They also note that irregular bleeding of recent onset should always suggest genital endometrial infection in young women, particularly those not taking an oral contraceptive. Increased or altered vaginal discharge is reported in 50% of women with PID (Weström & Mårdh 1990) and Bevan et al (1995) believe that a mucopurulent vaginal discharge is the only useful sign for diagnosing PID, although many patients do not report a discharge and genital infection may go unnoticed.

Dysuria and proctitis have been noted in women with PID (Bevan et al 1995, Weström & Mårdh 1990) and MacLean (1995) suggests that patients with a severe infection and pyrexia may be acutely ill with nausea and vomiting. Weström & Mårdh (1990) summarize by noting that women with gonococcal PID generally have abdominal pain of short duration, palpable adnexal swelling, are young and are from a low social class, whereas women with chlamydial PID are

also young but may appear clinically well. A woman with a mixed infection often has an IUD, is older and may have recurrent PID and patients with endogenous PID have more obvious signs and symptoms than those with chlamydial or gonococcal infection.

Although the diagnosis of PID is more accurate with severe disease (Stacey & Munday 1994), clinical criteria appear to vary greatly and the use of laparoscopy for diagnosis has been investigated widely. Stacey & Munday's (1994) study found PID on laparoscopy in 14% of women with clinical PID, endometriosis in 16% and adhesions in 11% and they suggest that women with other diagnoses or no obvious cause were clinically indistinguishable from women with PID. Weström & Mårdh (1990) suggest a finding of PID on laparoscopy in 65% of women with PID on clinical diagnosis, while Bevan et al (1995) confirmed PID laparoscopically in 71% of women and Morcos et al (1993) achieved a figure of 76% in their study. Finally, Weström & Mårdh (1990) note that women with clinical PID and with evidence of endosalpingitis or endometritis may occasionally have normal laparoscopic findings.

In the UK, laparoscopy is not routinely undertaken on women given a presumptive diagnosis of PID in GUM or gynaecology. Ross (1999) suggests in his guidelines that, given the potential difficulty in identifying endometritis or mild tubal inflammation, and given the cost of the procedure, laparoscopy is not routinely justified, although it may strongly support a diagnosis of PID. However, differential diagnoses of appendicitis, ectopic pregnancy, bleeding from the corpus luteum and other pelvic conditions may be made by laparoscopy (Church & Sutton 1996). Patients in whom it is desirable to do a laparoscopy are summarized by Hare (1990a) and shown in Box 10.4.

Box 10.4 Cases when it is desirable to undertake a laparoscopy (Hare 1990a)

- In a woman who is severely ill, particularly if there is concern about cardiovascular shock
- In an older woman, as the incidence of malignant disease or endometriosis is greater
- If an ectopic pregnancy is suspected because of a history of menstrual irregularity
- If a women claims never to have had sexual intercourse
- If there is little or no response 72 h after starting antibiotic treatment

---

CHLAMYDIA AND PELVIC INFLAMMATORY DISEASE **177**

Complications

The short-term complication of PID – abscess formation – has already been mentioned. Fitz-Hugh–Curtis syndrome or gonococcal perihepatitis causes patients to have tenderness in the right upper abdominal quadrant, radiating to the right shoulder and giving a pleuritic pain. On laparoscopy adhesions like piano-wire or violin-strings are seen between the peritoneum and liver capsule and oedema of the liver capsule is noted (Hare 1990a). Chlamydia has also been known to cause this syndrome following PID (MacLean 1995). Van Dongen (1993) described how two patients had been diagnosed by ultrasound as having the piano-wire adhesions, and also that ascites were noted.

The long-term sequelae of PID generally relate to the damage done by infection to various structures in the pelvis. Weström (1988) notes that long-term pain is often cycle-related, getting worse at ovulation and afterwards. It is described as continuing and dull pain, often one-sided, that causes patients to have severe dyspareunia, which can lead to problems with sexual relationships. Weström & Mårdh (1990) report that chronic pain of more than 6 months duration was seen in 5% of controls and 18% of patients who had had PID in their study. Stacey et al (1992), in their longitudinal study of women with PID, found that 56% of them complained of pain 1–3 years later. Painkillers and long-term antibiotics offer little help. MacLean (1995) suggests that the formation of scar tissue means that movements of the reproductive organs caused by such things as the bladder or rectum filling, the menstrual cycle and deep coital penetration cause pain. He suggests that treatment that reduces cyclical variation, such as danazol or progesterone, may help. However, many women eventually ask for a hysterectomy and

---

removal of tubes and ovaries if they are involved, even though this means they will be sterile (Weström 1988).

Infertility is a well-reported consequence of PID. Stacey et al (1992) found that 33% of women in their study were having difficulty becoming pregnant 1–3 years after PID. Moore & Cates (1990) suggest that one episode of PID leads to an 11% risk of infertility, two episodes to 23% risk and three episodes to more than 50% risk. Various points noted by Weström (1988) are shown in Box 10.5.

Ectopic pregnancy is the last well-documented sequelae of PID noted over many years. Although the diagnosis of tubal pregnancy has also increased since the 1960s, Weström & Mårdh (1990) extrapolate from various studies that there is a 7–10-fold increased risk of ectopic pregnancy after PID. Weström (1988) suggested that 25–33% of the increased numbers of ectopic pregnancies between 1960 and 1988 might relate to PID, and this proportion might be doubled given the size of the large silent PID epidemic.

Treatment

Admission to hospital or outpatient treatment will affect the treatment regimen and patients in whom the diagnosis is unsure or who have severe infection are generally admitted. Hare (1990a) notes that antibiotics will be started before the full microbiological picture is known in most cases of PID. Multiple drug regimens with a wide spectrum of action are therefore required to cover chlamydia, gonorrhoea, aerobic and anaerobic infections (MacLean 1995). A large number of studies have looked at different regimens for hospitalized patients treated satisfactorily with clindamycin–gentamicin or cefoxitin–doxycycline (e.g. The European Study 1992). Wendel et al (1991) found treatment with ofloxacin or cefoxitin with probenecid–doxycycline effective in treating outpatients with PID, as did Martens et al (1993). Walker et al's (1993) meta-analysis concluded that ciprofloxacin was the cheapest effective treatment. The recommendations for treatment made by Ross (1999) in his guidelines and those made by the Centers for Disease Control in America described by Zenilman (1998) are shown in Table 10.6.

Management of outpatients must include the woman resting at home, monitoring her temperature and avoiding intercourse (Weström & Mårdh 1990). An IUD should be removed from a woman with PID, unless there is a risk of pregnancy following sexual intercourse when the patient is at or just after

---

Box 10.5 Factors relating to infertility following PID (Weström 1988)

- The prognosis for fertility is better the younger a woman is when she first has PID
- The chance of an individual woman becoming infertile doubles with each new episode of PID
- The prognosis is significantly better with a mild infection than with a severe or moderately severe episode of PID
- PID associated with gonorrhoea has a better prognosis for fertility than PID associated with chlamydia or other causes

Table 10.6 Treatment recommendations for PID

Ross (1999)	Zenilman (1998)
Inpatient regimens	
Option A	*Option A*
i.v. cefoxitin 2 g t.d.s. **plus** i.v. doxycycline 100 mg b.d. (oral doxycycline if it is tolerated)	i.v. cefotetan 2 g b.d. **or** i.v. cefoxitin 2 g q.d.s. **plus** i.v. doxycycline 100 mg b.d. (oral doxycycline if it is tolerated)
followed by	
oral doxycycline 100 mg b.d. **plus** oral metronidazole 400 mg b.d. for a total of 14 days	*Option B*
	i.v. clindamycin 900 mg t.d.s. **plus** i.v. gentamycin 1.5 mg/kg t.d.s.
Option B	
i.v. clindamycin 900 mg t.d.s. **plus** i.v. gentamycin 2 mg/kg loading dose followed by 1.5 mg/kg t.d.s. (or single daily dose)	*Other options*
	i.v. ofloxacin 400 mg b.d. **plus** i.v. metronidazole 500 mg b.d.
followed by either	**or**
oral clindamycin 450 mg q.d.s. to complete 14 days **or** oral doxycycline 100 mg b.d. **plus** oral metronidazole 400 mg b.d. to complete 14 days	i.v. ampicillin/sulbactam 3 g q.d.s. **plus** i.v./oral doxycycline 100 mg b.d.
	or
	i.v. ciprofloxacin 200 mg b.d. **plus** i.v./oral doxycycline 100 mg b.d. **plus** i.v. metronidazole 500 mg t.d.s.
Other options	
i.v. ofloxacin 400 mg b.d. **plus** i.v. metronidazole 500 mg t.d.s.	
or	
i.v. ciprofloxacin 200 mg b.d. **plus** i.v./oral doxycycline 100 mg b.d. **plus** i.v. metronidazole 500 mg t.d.s.	
Outpatient regimens	
Option A	*Option A*
oral ofloxacin 400 mg b.d. **plus** oral metronidazole 400 mg b.d. for 14 days	oral ofloxacin 400 mg b.d. **plus** oral metronidazole 500 mg b.d. for 14 days
Option B	*Option B*
i.m. ceftriaxone 250 mg stat **or** i.m. cefoxitin 2 g stat with oral probenicid 1 g **followed by** oral doxycycline 100 mg b.d. **plus** oral metronidazole 400 mg b.d. for 14 days	i.m. ceftriaxone 250 mg stat **or** i.m. cefoxitin 2 g stat with oral probenicid 1 g **plus** oral doxycycline 100 mg b.d. for 14 days

ovulation (Hare 1990a). Surgery to treat life-threatening infection if there is an abscess or if conservative treatment has failed, or surgery to remove retained products of conception, may be needed in some cases. Such surgery should be as conservative as possible and should include peritoneal toilet and division of adhesions (MacLean 1995, Weström & Mårdh 1990). Analgesia should be given as required to all patients (Ross 1999).

Follow-up and nursing intervention

As with chlamydial infection, contact tracing of the sexual partners of women with PID is very important and a sexual history must be taken. Weström & Mårdh (1990) note that testing, particularly for chlamydia and gonorrhoea, and suitable treatment as required should be undertaken on the sexual partners of all women with PID. Tait et al (1997) investigated silent upper genital tract chlamydial infection and state that contact tracing, investigation and treatment are mandatory when asymptomatic cervical chlamydia is diagnosed to prevent the sequelae of PID. Reid et al (1997) and Wales et al (1997) audited treatment and advice given to women diagnosed with PID in Accident and Emergency (A&E) and gynaecology clinics and noted the nearly universal lack of advice to women to abstain from intercourse and the lack of sexual history-taking and contact-tracing.

It can be seen, therefore, that the most important nursing intervention in PID is to encourage clinicians to refer the patient to a GUM clinic for contact tracing and management of the woman's sexual partners, or to undertake this process themselves when they see the patient. The nurse must support and encourage the

---

Case study: Gillian

Gillian, 36 years old, had two sexual partners in the 8 weeks before she attended the GUM clinic. She had been treated with Diflucan and Canestan for vaginal candida over the 4 months before her attendance.

On history, Gillian said she had had lower abdominal pain and dyspareunia for the last 2 weeks. On examination, she was tender abdominally, had a left adnexal mass and a mucopurulent cervical discharge. Specimens were negative for gonorrhoea but positive for candida and chlamydia and she was diagnosed as having PID and candidiasis.

Treatment with metronidazole 400 mg b.d. for 14 days, doxycycline 100 mg b.d. for 14 days and Sporanox 200 mg b.d. for 1 day was started.

Gillian was admitted to hospital via the gynaecology clinic 4 days later when she was still tender abdominally and not responding well. Laparoscopy showed signs of tubal infection but chlamydia was not isolated from the tubal specimens.

Her sexual partners were contact traced and both were treated for chlamydia, although only her previous partner was found to be positive for chlamydia. Her present partner was treated in case he had undiagnosed chlamydia and to prevent him reinfecting Gillian.

Gillian was seen on completion of treatment when her pain was resolving. At a later follow-up, her test for chlamydia was negative.

---

woman to understand the importance of treating partners in preventing reinfection and further episodes of PID (Weström & Mårdh 1990). Health education in the use of condoms, particularly by young women, is another part of the nurses' role, as is education of the general public about the serious consequences of PID and of asymptomatic chlamydial infection. Nurses need to help develop guidelines for management of patients with PID in settings such as A&E and gynaecology, to ensure that contact tracing and sexual health advice is given to patients along with suitable management of the condition (Wales et al 1997). Finally, nurses need to ensure their own knowledge base and skills relating to sexual history taking are up-to-date to enable women with PID to obtain good quality follow-up in all settings.

Conclusion

It can be seen that control of gonorrhoea and chlamydia transmission are vital to control PID infection in women. Even clinically mild disease must be treated early and effectively to prevent the sequelae of PID (Wales et al 1997). Kamwendo et al (1998) believe that primary, secondary and tertiary prevention is needed to reduce PID and its consequences. Targeted screening of women having operative procedures breaching the cervical barrier and populations at risk of chlamydia are part of the strategy needed (Weström & Mårdh 1990). Public awareness and the regular use of condoms are vital and Weström (1988) sums up by noting that only by education, day-to-day efforts to fight STIs and continuing research will the serious long-term effects of PID be decreased for the benefit of many young women and their partners.

GLOSSARY

Bacterial vaginosis: an overgrowth of naturally occurring vaginal bacteria causing a fishy smelling discharge
Cervicitis: inflammation of the cells of the cervix
Contact tracing: the process of identifying and contacting the sexual contacts of a patient with a sexually transmitted infection, in order to test and treat the contacts to break the chain of transmission of the infection. Contact tracing can be carried out by the patient or by the provider (usually genitourinary medicine clinic staff)

Ectopy: when the squamocolumnar junction (SCJ) of the different types of cells lining the cervix moves down and out onto the vaginal surface of the cervix
Epididymitis: inflammation of the epididymis in men
Hydrosalpinx: fluid in the fallopian tubes
Pyosalpinx: pus in the fallopian tubes
Salpingitis: inflammation of the fallopian tubes
Test-of-cure (TOC): test taken for a specific sexually transmitted infection following treatment for the infection, to confirm that the infection has been eradicated

REFERENCES

Berger RE, Alexander ER, Monda GD, Ansell J, McCormick G & Holmes KK 1978 *Chlamydia trachomatis* as a cause of acute 'idiopathic' epididymitis. The New England Journal of Medicine 298(6):301–304

Bevan CD, Johal BJ, Mumtaz G, Ridgway GL & Siddle NC 1995 Clinical, laparoscopic and microbiological findings in acute salpingitis: report on a United Kingdom cohort. British Journal of Obstetrics and Gynaecology 102:407–414

Brunham RC, Holmes KK & Embree JE 1990 Sexually transmitted diseases in pregnancy. In: Holmes KK, Mårdh P-A, Sparling PF & Wiesner PJ (eds) Sexually transmitted diseases, 2nd edn. McGraw-Hill, New York, ch 64

Cameron S & Blakely A 1993 A protocol for the detection of chlamydia. Nursing Standard 8(5):25–27

Catchpole M 1992 Sexually transmitted diseases in England and Wales 1981–1990. Communicable Disease Report Review 2(1):1–7

Caul EO, Horner PJ, Leece J, Crowley T, Paul I & Davey-Smith G 1997 Population-based screening programmes for *Chlamydia trachomatis*. The Lancet 349:1070–1071

Central Audit Group in Genitourinary Medicine 1997 Clinical guidelines and standards for the management of uncomplicated genital chlamydia infection. Health Education Authority, London

Chernesky MA, Jang D, Lee H et al 1994 Diagnosis of *Chlamydia trachomatis* infections in men and women by testing first-void urine by ligase chain reaction. Journal of Clinical Microbiology 32(11):2682–2685

Chief Medical Officer's Expert Advisory Group 1998 *Chlamydia trachomatis* summary and conclusions of CMO's Expert Advisory Group. Department of Health, London

Church N & Sutton A 1996 Chlamydia and pelvic inflammatory disease. In: Sutton A & Payne S (eds) Genito-urinary medicine for nurses. Whurr Publishers, London, ch 6

Crowley T, Milne D, Arumainayagam JT, Paul ID & Caul EO 1992 The laboratory diagnosis of male *Chlamydia trachomatis* infections – a time for change? Journal of Infection 25(suppl 1):69–75

Crowley T, Horner P, Hughes A, Berry J, Paul I & Caul O 1997 Hormonal factors and the laboratory detection of *Chlamydia trachomatis* in women: implications for screening? International Journal of STD & AIDS 8(1):25–31

Davies PO & Ridgway GL 1997 The role of polymerase chain reaction and ligase chain reaction for the detection of *Chlamydia trachomatis*. International Journal of STD & AIDS 8(12):731–738

Dean D, Ferrero D & McCarthy M 1998 Comparison of performance and cost-effectiveness of direct fluorescent-antibody, ligase chain reaction, and PCR assays for verification of chlamydial enzyme immunoassay results for populations with a low to moderate prevalence of *Chlamydia trachomatis* infection. Journal of Clinical Microbiology 36(1):94–99

European Study Group 1992 Comparative evaluation of clindamycin/gentamycin and cefoxitin/doxycycline for treatment of pelvic inflammatory disease: a multi-center trial. Acta Obstetrica Gynecologica Scandinavica 71:129–134

Greendale GA, Haas ST, Holbrook K, Walsh B, Schachter J & Phillips RS 1993 The relationship of *Chlamydia trachomatis* infection and male infertility. American Journal of Public Health 83(7):996–1001

Hager WD, Eschenbach DA, Spence MR & Sweet RL 1983 Criteria for diagnosis and grading of salpingitis. Obstetrics and Gynecology 61(1):113–114

Hammerschlag MR, Handsfield HH & Judson FN 1987 When to suspect chlamydia. Patient Care (Nov. 15):64–78

Handsfield HH & Stamm WE 1998 Treating chlamydial infection: compliance versus cost. Journal of Sexually Transmitted Diseases 25(1):12–13

Hare J 1990a Pelvic inflammatory disease. In: Csonka GW & Oates JK (eds) Sexually transmitted diseases – textbook of genitourinary medicine. Baillière Tindall, London, ch 17

Hare J 1990b Pelvic inflammatory disease: current approaches and ideas. International Journal of STD & AIDS 1:393–400

Harrison HR, Costin M, Meder JB et al 1985 Cervical *Chlamydia trachomatis* infection in university women: relationship to history, contraception, ectopy, and cervicitis. American Journal of Obstetrics and Gynecology 153(3):244–251

Hay PE, Thomas BJ, McKenzie P & Taylor-Robinson D 1993 Detection of *Chlamydia trachomatis* in men: sensitive tests for sensitive urethras. Sexually Transmitted Diseases 20(1):1–4

Hay PE, Thomas BJ, Horner PJ, MacLeod E, Renton AM & Taylor-Robinson D 1994 *Chlamydia trachomatis* in women: the more you look, the more you find. Genitourinary Medicine 70:97–100

Horner PJ, Caul EO 1999 National guideline for the management of *Chlamydia trachomatis* genital tract infection. Sexually Transmitted Infections 75(suppl 1):54–58

Hughes G, Simms I, Rogers PA, Swan AV, Catchpole M 1998 New cases seen at genitourinary medicine clinics: England 1997. Communicable Disease Report 8(suppl 7)

Jensen IP, Thorsen P & Møller BR 1997 Sensitivity of ligase chain reaction assay of urine from pregnant women for *Chlamydia trachomatis*. The Lancet 349(Feb 1):329–330

Kamwendo F, Johansson E, Moi H, Forslin L & Danielsson D 1993 Gonorrhoea, genital chlamydial infection, and nonspecific urethritis in male partners of women hospitalized and treated for acute pelvic inflammatory disease. Sexually Transmitted Diseases 20(3):143–146

Kamwendo F, Forslin L, Bodin L & Danielsson D 1998 Programmes to reduce pelvic inflammatory disease – the Swedish experience. The Lancet 351(suppl 111):25–28

Keat A & Rowe I 1990 Reiter's syndrome and reactive arthritis. In: Csonka GW & Oates JK (eds) Sexually transmitted diseases – textbook of genitourinary medicine. Baillière Tindall, London, ch 6

Lee HH, Chernesky MA, Schachter J et al 1995 Diagnosis of *Chlamydia trachomatis* genitourinary infection in women by ligase chain reaction assay of urine. The Lancet 345(8944):213–216

MacLean A 1995 Pelvic infection. In: Whitfield C (ed) Dewhurst's textbook of obstetrics and gynaecology for postgraduates, 5th edn. Blackwell Science, Oxford, ch 38

Mann SN, Smith JR & Barton SE 1996 Pelvic inflammatory disease. International Journal of STD & AIDS 7(5):315–321

Mårdh P-A 1997 Is Europe ready for STD screening? Genitourinary Medicine 73(2):96–98

Martens MG, Gordon S, Yarborough DR et al 1993 Multicenter randomized trial of ofloxacin versus cefoxitin and doxycycline in outpatient treatment of pelvic inflammatory disease. Southern Medical Journal 86(6):604–610

Morcos R, Frost N, Hnat M, Petrunak A & Caldito G 1993 Laparoscopic versus clinical diagnosis of acute pelvic inflammatory disease. Journal of Reproductive Medicine 38(1):53–56

Moore DE & Cates W Jr 1990 Sexually transmitted diseases and infertility. In: Holmes KK, Mårdh P-A, Sparling PF & Wiesner PJ (eds) Sexually transmitted diseases, 2nd edn. McGraw-Hill, New York, ch 63

Østergaard L, Agner T, Krarup E, Johansen UB, Weismann K & Gutschik E 1997 PCR for detection of *Chlamydia trachomatis* in endocervical, urethral, rectal, and pharyngeal swab samples obtained from patients attending an STD clinic. Genitourinary Medicine 73(6):493–497

Paavonen J 1979 *Chlamydia trachomatis*-indued urethritis in female partners of men with nongonococcal urethritis. Sexually Transmitted Diseases 6(2):69–71

Postema EJ, Remeijer L & van der Meijden WI 1996 Epidemiology of genital chlamydial infections in patients with chlamydial conjunctivitis; a retrospective study. Genitourinary Medicine 72:203–205

Reid S, Glucksman E, Blott M & Welch J 1997 Do women with pelvic inflammatory disease receive adequate treatment? International Journal of STD & AIDS 8(7):466–467

Ridgway GL 1996 Azithromycin in the management of *Chlamydia trachomatis* infections. International Journal of STD & AIDS 7(suppl 1):5–8

Ridgway GL, Mumtaz G, Robinson AJ et al 1996 Comparison of the ligase chain reaction with cell culture for the diagnosis of *Chlamydia trachomatis* infection in women. Journal of Clinical Pathology 49:116–119

Ridgway GL & Taylor-Robinson D 1992 Current problems in microbiology: 1 Chlamydial infections: which laboratory test? Journal of Clinical Pathology 44:1–5

Ripa T 1990 Epidemiologic control of genital *Chlamydia trachomatis* infections. Scandinavian Journal of Infectious Disease (suppl 69):157–167

Rome ES 1994 Pelvic inflammatory disease in the adolescent. Current Opinion in Pediatrics 6:383–387

Ross JDC 1999 National guideline for the management of pelvic infection and perihepatitis. Sexually Transmitted Infections 75(suppl 1):S54–S56

Saunders J 1988 Chlamydia infection. Nursing Times 84(49):35

Simms I, Hughes G, Swan AV, Rogers PA & Catchpole M 1998 New cases seen at genitourinary medicine clinics: England 1996. Communicable Disease Report 8(suppl 1)

Schachter J 1990 Biology of *Chlamydia trachomatis*. In: Holmes KK, Mårdh P-A, Sparling PF & Wiesner PJ (eds)

Sexually transmitted diseases, 2nd edn. McGraw-Hill, New York, ch 15

Stacey CM, Munday PE, Taylor-Robinson D et al 1992 A longitudinal study of pelvic inflammatory disease. British Journal of Obstetrics and Gynaecology 99:994–999

Stacey CM & Munday PE 1994 Abdominal pain in women attending a genitourinary medicine clinic: who has PID? International Journal of STD & AIDS 5:338–342

Stamm WE & Holmes KK 1990 *Chlamydia trachomatis* infections of the adult. In: Holmes KK, Mårdh P-A, Sparling PF & Wiesner PJ (eds) Sexually transmitted diseases, 2nd edn. McGraw-Hill, New York, ch 16

Stokes T 1997 Screening for chlamydia in general practice: a literature review and summary of the evidence. Journal of Public Health Medicine 19(2):222–232

Tait IA, Duthie SJ & Taylor-Robinson D 1997 Silent upper genital tract chlamydial infection and disease in women. International Journal of STD & AIDS 8(5):329–331

Taylor-Robinson D 1992 The value of non-culture techniques for diagnosis of *Chlamydia trachomatis* infections: making the best of a bad job. European Journal of Microbiological Infectious Diseases 11(6):499–503

Taylor-Robinson D 1994 *Chlamydia trachomatis* and sexually transmitted disease. British Medical Journal 308:150–151

Thomas BJ, Pierpoint T, Taylor-Robinson D & Renton AM 1998 Sensitivity of the ligase chain reaction assay for detecting *Chlamydia trachomatis* in vaginal swabs from women who are infected at other sites. Sexually Transmitted Diseases 74(2):140–141

van Dongen PWJ 1993 Diagnosis of Fitz-Hugh–Curtis syndrome by ultrasound. European Journal of Obstetrics & Gynecology and Reproductive Biology 50:159–162

Wales NM, Barton SE, Boag FC, Booth SJ & Smith JR 1997 An audit of the management of pelvic inflammatory disease. International Journal of STD & AIDS 8(6):409–411

Walker CK, Kahn JG, Washington AE, Peterson HB & Sweet RL 1993 Pelvic inflammatory disease: metaanalysis of antimicrobial regimen efficacy. Journal of Infectious Diseases 168:969–978

Welsh LE, Quinn TC & Gaydos CA 1997 Influence of endocervical specimen adequacy on PCR and direct fluorescent-antibody staining for detection of *Chlamydia trachomatis* infections. Journal of Clinical Microbiology 35(12):3078–3081

Wendel GD Jr, Cox SM, Bawdon RE, Theriot SK, Heard MC & Nobles BJ 1991 A randomized trial of ofloxacin versus cefoxitin and doxycycline in the outpatient treatment of acute salpingitis. American Journal of Obstetrics and Gynecology 164(5):1390–1396

Westcott P 1992 Pelvic inflammatory disease and chlamydia. Thorsons, London

Weström L 1988 Long-term consequences of pelvic inflammatory disease. In: Hare MJ (ed) Genital tract infection in women. Churchill Livingstone, Edinburgh, ch 21

Weström L & Mårdh P-A 1990 Acute pelvic inflammatory disease (PID). In: Holmes KK, Mårdh P-A, Sparling PF & Wiesner PJ (eds) Sexually transmitted diseases, 2nd edn. McGraw-Hill, New York, ch 49

Whelan M 1988 Nursing management of the patient with *Chlamydia trachomatis* infection. Nursing Clinics of North America 23(40):877–883

Wølner-Hanssen P, Kiviat NB & Holmes KK 1990 Atypical pelvic inflammatory disease: subacute, chronic, or subclinical upper genital tract infection in women. In: Holmes KK, Mårdh P-A, Sparling PF & Wiesner PJ (eds) Sexually transmitted diseases, 2nd edn. McGraw-Hill, New York, ch 50

Zenilman JM 1998 Update of the CDC STD treatment guidelines: changes and policy. Sexually Transmitted Infections 74(2):89–92

USEFUL ADDRESSES

PID Support Network
c/o Women's Health Research and Information Centre, 52 Featherstone Street, London, EC1Y 8RT
Tel: 020 7251 6580.

Open Monday, Wednesday, Thursday and Friday, 10–4. Support group for women with PID. Information leaflet, PID newsletter and telephone support network.

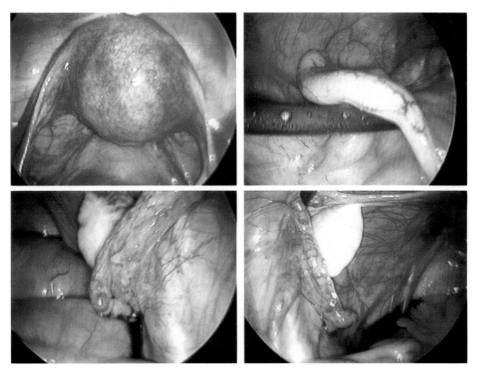

Plate 1   Normal healthy pelvis showing healthy uterus, fallopian tubes and ovaries.

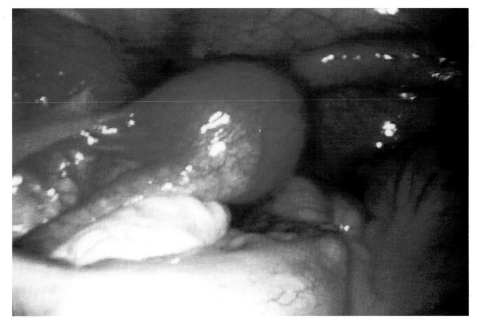

Plate 2   View at laparoscopy of rudimentary left uterine horn. The rest of the uterus, cervix and upper vagina are absent. Both ovaries are present and function normally.

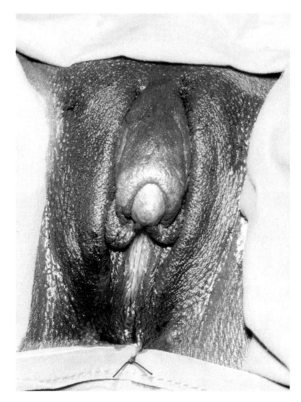

Plate 3 Genitalia of a 14-year-old girl presenting with virilization. She had normal female genitalia as a child and presented at puberty with clitoromegaly, hirsutism and voice breaking. She underwent gonadectomy and clitoral reduction. A vaginoplasty is planned at a second procedure.

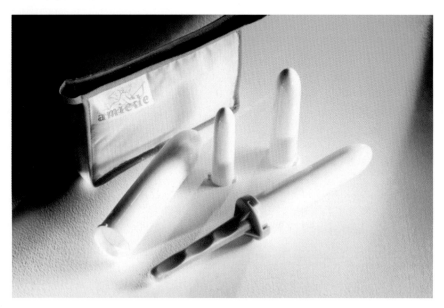

Plate 4 Set of Amielle dilators.

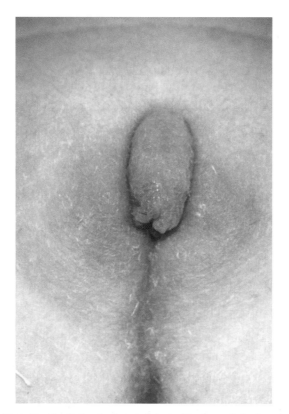

Plate 5 Genitalia of a female infant with congenital adrenal hyperplasia.

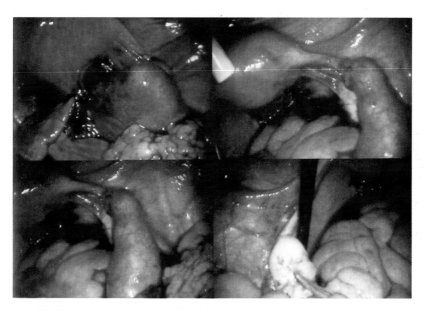

Plate 6 Tubal pregnancy visualized on laparoscopy.

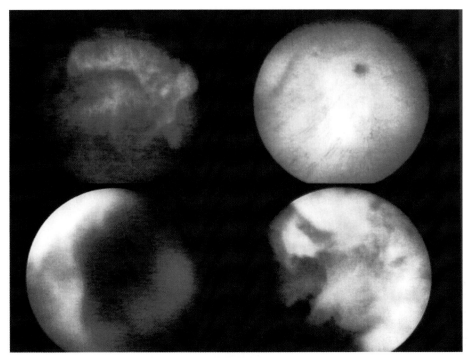

Plate 7   Hysteroscopic illustration of uterine adhesions present in Asherman's syndrome.

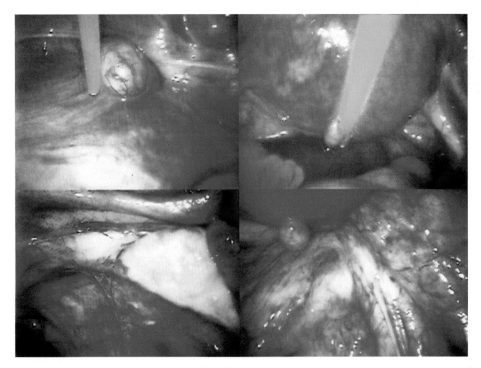

Plate 8   Laparoscopic illustration of multiple fibroid uterus.

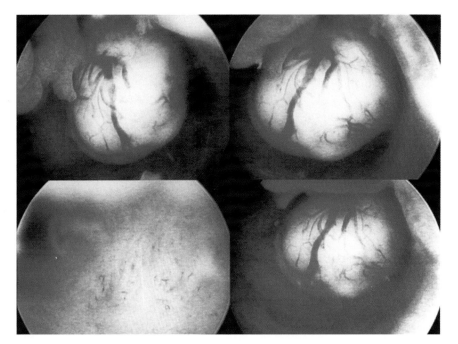

Plate 9 Hysteroscopic illustration of large submucous fibroid.

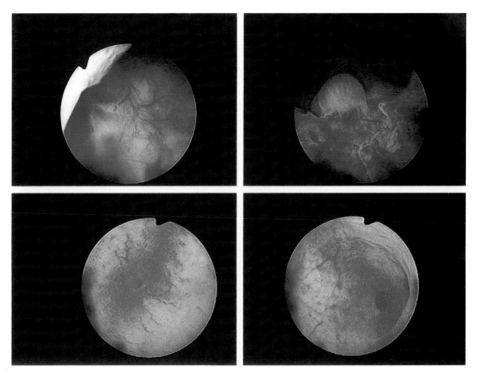

Plate 10 Hysteroscopic illustration of a very vascular, easily bleeding endometrium.

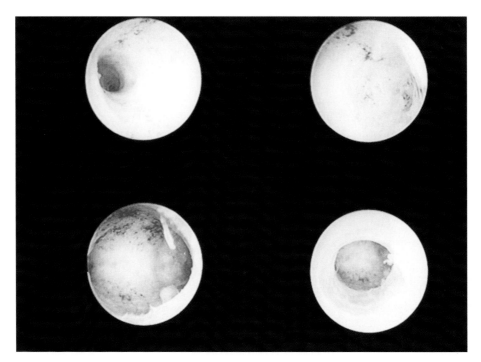

Plate 11 Hysteroscopic illustration of an atrophic endometrium.

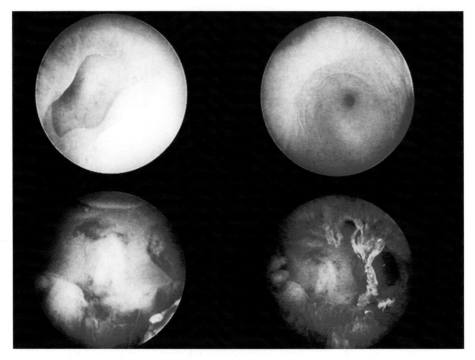

Plate 12 Hysteroscopic illustration of a normal endometrial cavity.

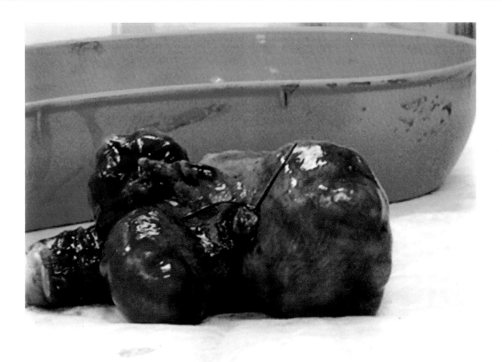

Plate 13 Uterus enlarged with multiple fibroids. Cervix visible to the extreme left and distorted fundus to the right of the picture.

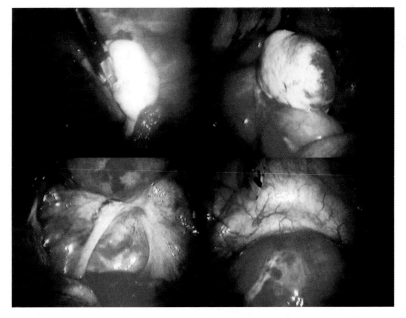

Plate 14 Normal ovary, top left, compared with ovaries with follicular cysts as seen in the other three photos.

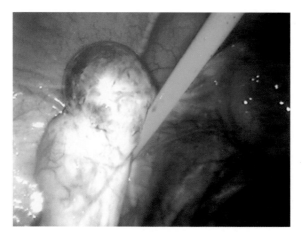

Plate 15   Corpus luteum cyst.

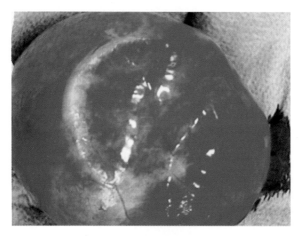

Plate 16   10-cm benign cystic teratoma (dermoid cyst).

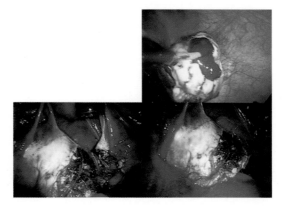

Plate 17   Dermoid cyst showing hair and other solid matter.

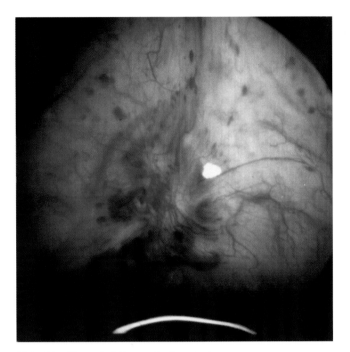

Plate 18 Characteristic powder-burn lesions

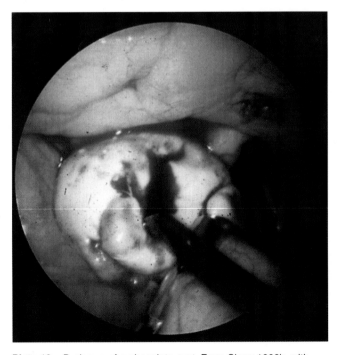

Plate 19 Drainage of a chocolate cyst. From Shaw 1992b, with permission.

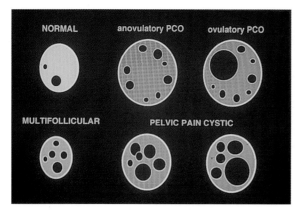

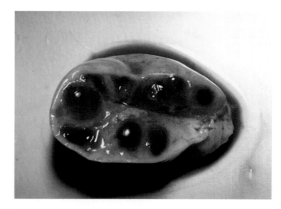

Plate 20 Comparison of cystic ovaries during the menstrual cycle.

Plate 21 Dissected section of a pelvic congestion cystic ovary.

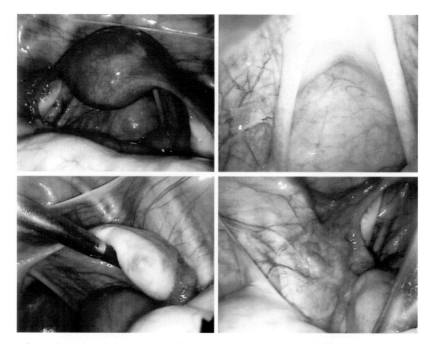

Plate 22 Pictures taken at laparoscopy in a patient with early pelvic venous congestion showing:
(a) congested uterus,
(b) normal utero-sacral ligaments,
(c) right ovary – early polycystic damage,
(d) varicocele of the left ovarian vein.

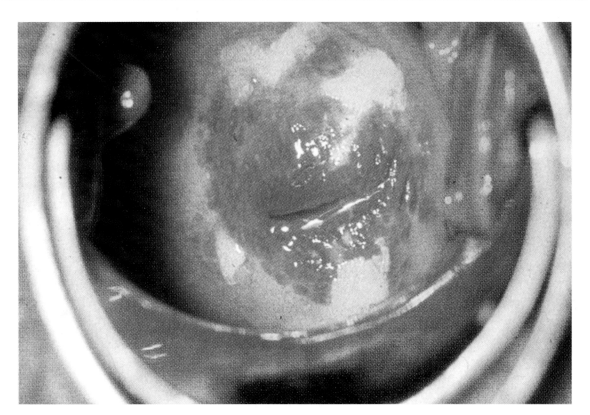

Plate 23 Colposcopic appearance of a normal cervix with candida infection

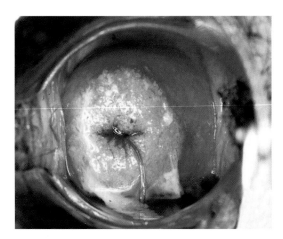

Plate 24 Photograph of the cervix taken using cervicography. Shows a large ectropian

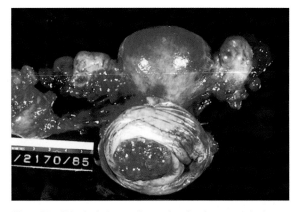

Plate 25 Wertheim's specimen showing large cervical tumour.

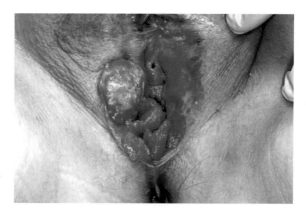

Plate 26 Squamous cell carcinoma of the vulva.

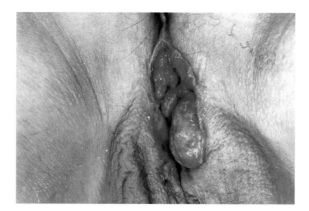

Plate 27 Squamous cell carcinoma of the vulva.

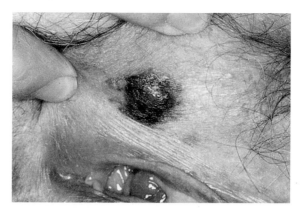

Plate 28 Melanoma of the vulva.

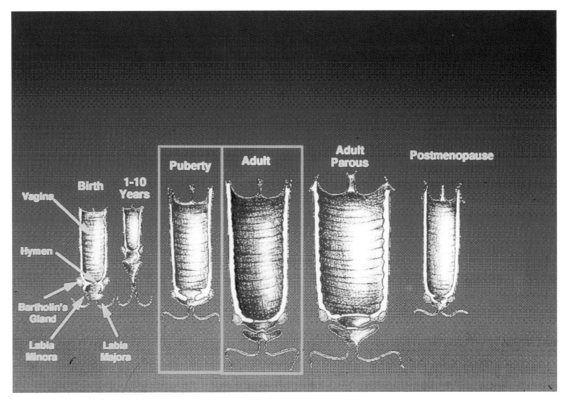

Plate 29 Anatomy of the vulva and the vagina illustrating the relative dimensions before, during and after the reproductive years.

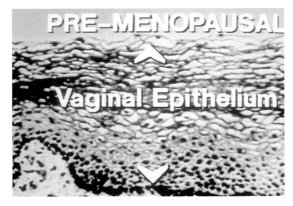

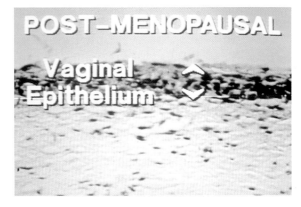

Plate 30 Microscopic appearances of cross section taken through the vaginal epithelium in pre-menopausal and post-menopausal (Plate 31) women showing the markedly reduced superficial cell thickness of the vaginal epithelium.

Plate 31

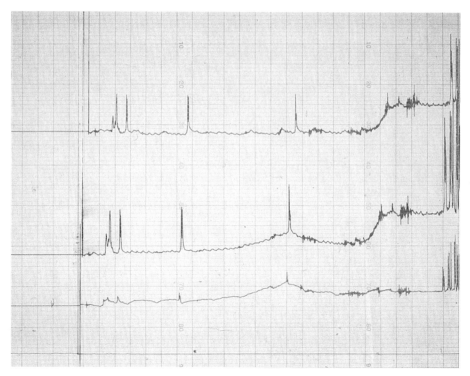

Plate 32 A urodynamic trace demonstrating a non-compliant bladder.

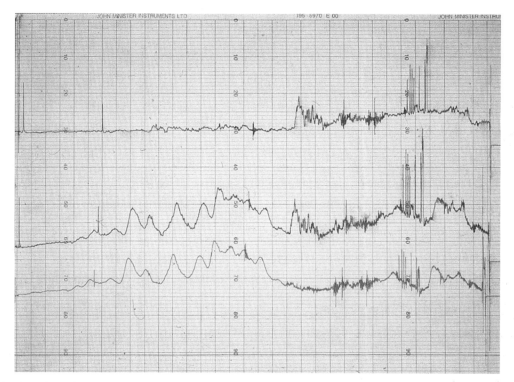

Plate 33 A urodynamic trace demonstrating systolic detrusor instability.

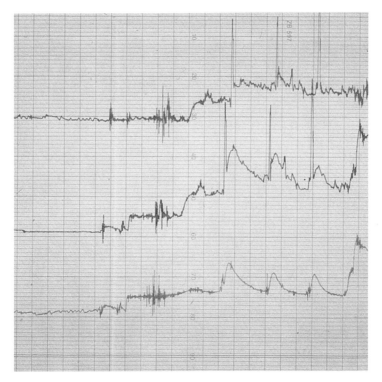

Plate 34 A urodynamic trace demonstrating provoked detrusor instability.

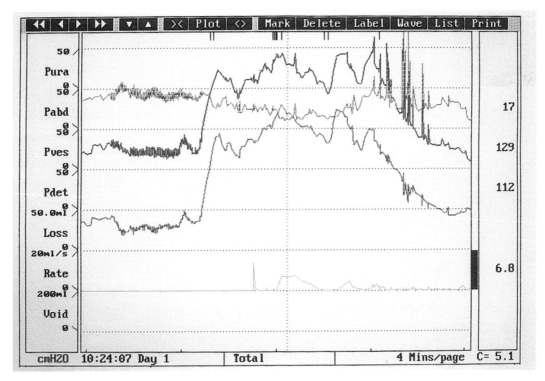

Plate 35 Demonstration of a high voiding pressure with a low flow rate indicating obstruction.

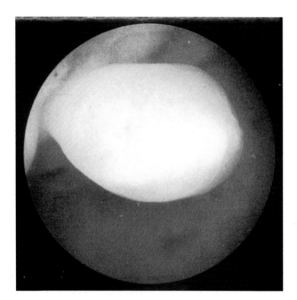

Plate 36   Hysteroscopic view of the endometrial cavity showing an endometrial polyp.

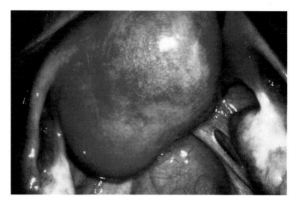

Plate 37   Laparoscopic view of the pelvis showing the uterus enlarged by fibroids.

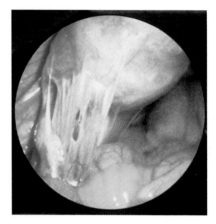

Plate 38   Laparoscopic view of the pelvis showing adhesions between the uterus, ovary and other pelvic organs.

11

Endometriosis

Maggie Barron

The condition of endometriosis – ectopic endometrial transplantation – has been documented since the nineteenth century. It is the second most common gynaecological, surgical abnormality after fibroids (Henderson & Studd 1991) and yet there is still much to understand of its aetiology and long-term history. Endometriosis is rarely life threatening (Mangtani & Booth 1993) but it is the diverse and unpredictable nature of this benign condition that raises the question of the need for specialist attention.

Endometriosis is characterized predominantly by pain and, for the majority of women, is mild and controllable. It is not known why it progresses in severity in a small subgroup of women, causing structural damage with far-reaching consequences for wellbeing and fertility. In the short term, it would appear to be fluctuating and self-limiting in that distribution of disease in pelvic areas is equal in the older and younger woman and does not progress inevitably with age (Redwine 1987a). It is thought to occur in most women at some time in their reproductive life (Thomas 1995), has not been documented prior to menarche (Lim 1996) and is uncommon after the menopause unless re-activated by hormone replacement therapy (HRT) or endogenous oestrogen due to obesity. There is little data to show economic or ethnic differences but it is thought to occur more frequently in the higher socio-economic groups, either because of delayed childbearing or perhaps because, as a group, they are more health conscious. There is a suggestion of a higher incidence of endometriosis in oriental women and particularly in Japanese women (Miyazawa 1976).

One hypothesis is that the condition is a normal physiological process in menstruating women and should be called a disease only when chronic bleeding becomes deeply and structurally invasive (Brosens 1997). Ironically, a major disadvantage against early referral to a specialist can be the cyclical nature of the symptoms. Dysmenorrhoea, even when acutely disabling, can still be considered a normal facet of menstruation and, when coupled with the diversity of symptoms, the problem of when to refer can apply to both patient and medical practitioner.

DEFINITION

Endometriosis is a common, benign, symptom-led, oestrogen-dependent condition of women, mainly in their reproductive years, which can be recurrent and for which there is no cure. It is defined as tissue histologically proven to be like the endometrium (endometrial glands and stroma) growing ectopically – that is, outside the uterine cavity where it sets up an independent existence.

Adenomyosis – endometrial glands and stroma within the myometrium – was originally called 'endometriosis interna' with the term 'endometriosis externa' referring to the pelvic condition we now know as endometriosis. Adenomyosis is thought to have a different pathology, it does not bleed cyclically and affects a different age group, thereby constituting a different disease. It can be superficial, lying close to the endometrium, and symptomless. Adenomyosis deep within the myometrium causes symptoms of menorrhagia, dysmenorrhoea and uterine enlargement and can be found in approximately 26% of uterine specimens (Outwater et al 1998).

AETIOLOGY

There are two main theories for the presence of endometrial cells in the pelvic cavity: either they are carried there by menstrual effluent and implant – metastasia – or they are there because the peritoneal mesothelium undergoes tissue transformation – metaplasia. There are reports in the literature of endometriosis of the bladder in men following prolonged oestrogen therapy (Oliker & Harris 1971, Pinkert et al 1979), which suggests that tissue similar to peritoneal epithelium can change under certain (hormonal) stimulation, which would support the metaplasia theory. However, viable endometrial cells have been found in bloody peritoneal fluid and in vitro work has strongly supported endometrium as the epithelia of origin (Mellor & Thomas 1994, Prentice et al 1992). For women with more than mild disease, it is possible that the endometrium either has a greater capacity to grow or the pelvic environment in some way favours the nurture of endometriosis (Smith 1991). The response to foreign bodies, in this case endometrial cells in the peritoneal fluid, is to use the defence mechanism –

macrophages, the body's scavengers – to remove cells and, whether it is the amount of menstrual debris or the failure of the defence system to cope (Evers 1996) and so enable the endometriosis to progress in severity, is unknown.

Endometriosis is found most commonly in the pelvic cavity and would appear to need both menstruation and oestrogen to develop. Extrapelvic endometriosis, sometimes far removed from the site of origin, is a phenomenon difficult to explain. As a disease outside the pelvic cavity, endometrial cells would need a different form of transportation and it is thought this may be either by vascular or lymphatic spread. Endometriosis has been noted microscopically both in lymph nodes and in well vascularized organs. There is also a suggestion of an autoimmune disease but, as yet, there is no strict consensus of opinion. For pelvic endometriosis, tubal retrograde menstruation is the accepted means by which endometrial cells are found in the abdomen. Pathogenesis of extrapelvic disease has yet to be proved and may be a combination of the above theories.

Retrograde menstruation

Endometrial implantation and haemorrhage of the ovaries has been documented since the early 1920s, when the condition was given the name 'endometriosis' (Sampson 1921). In 1927, Sampson proposed his theory of tubal retrograde flow as a means of menstrual effluent entering the pelvic cavity when he observed blood escaping from the fimbrial end of the fallopian tube during surgery. During the perimenstrual time of the cycle, over 90% of normal and infertile women with patent tubes have blood in their peritoneal fluid (Halme et al 1984). This is regularly reported at surgery and viable endometrial cells have been found in bloody peritoneal fluid (Haney 1991) taken at menses. Endometrial cells implant and proliferate, setting up their own existence. They produce pain chemicals, become inflamed, bleed, heal and eventually scar whilst remaining under the influence of cyclical hormones. These implants can be seen as small coloured spots (or lesions), which are thought to represent different stages of the disease (Redwine 1987b) – from active to non-active – reinforcing the belief that endometriosis is a fluctuating condition and does not necessarily progress with age. Self-limitation does not occur in a small subgroup of women and there is progression to severe disease, with possible bowel involvement and the formation of adhesions and ovarian cysts, which can mechanically impact on fertility. Several different lesions can be recognized and classified as endometriotic, however, the main lesions are:

- white, non-pigmented, early papules invading into tissue
- red, well-vascularized, active lesions
- blue–black 'powder-burn' lesions (see Plate 18) representing old inactive disease.

Sites

Common sites for endometriosis are the ovaries (bilateral or unilateral), the pelvic peritoneum, the uterosacral ligaments, the posterior of the uterus and the rectovaginal septum (Fig. 11.1). Ovaries lie directly under the fimbrial ostia and gravity dictates that peritoneal fluid settles at the bottom of the pelvis, hence the anatomical preference for the uterosacral ligaments. Endometriosis has been found in many different areas of the body, as can be seen in Table 11.1. Extrapelvic endometriosis, although relatively uncommon, has been found in virtually every organ and tissue of the female body (Markham 1991). It is of note that fixed structures are more likely to be affected than mobile ones.

Endometriomas

An endometrioma is an invaginated cyst of the ovary, thought to be formed when adhesions enclose and seal off an active endometriotic implant. The cyst remains largely on the outside of the ovary and contains an unmistakable fluid similar to that of thick chocolate sauce – a 'chocolate cyst' (Sampson 1921). Gradual

Table 11.1 List of sites

Common	Other	Rare
Ovary	Bowel	Lung
Uterosacral ligaments	Appendix	Bone
Peritoneum	Vagina	Muscle
Rectovaginal septum	Bladder	Eye
Posterior of uterus	Surgical scars (e.g. episiotomy)	Skin
	Umbilicus	Brain
	Cervix	

enlargement of the cyst pushes the ovary inwards but generally does not invade the ovarian cortex. The chocolate fluid may be the result of debris left from cyclical bleeding. Another school of thought is that the contents may not originate only from bleeding but are a combination of cyst wall exudation, congested cyst wall blood vessels and from inflammation around persistent foci of endometriosis (Donnez et al 1994). Not all haemorrhagic cysts are necessarily endometriotic but may be purely a sign that chronic bleeding has taken place. Positive histology should be obtained before any treatment commences. Plate 19 shows the drainage of a chocolate cyst.

DIAGNOSIS

More women are diagnosed with mild to moderate than severe disease (Redwine 1987a). The true incidence is impossible to ascertain but the number of women scheduled for laparoscopy can give an indication: endometriosis has been found in 4–24% of women undergoing laparoscopic sterilization and in

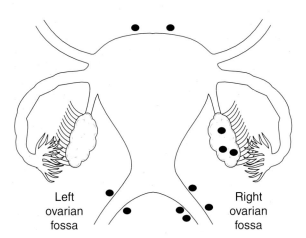

Figure 11.1 Common sites where endometriosis may be found.

Left ovarian fossa

Right ovarian fossa

Case Study: Samara

Samara, a fit 32-year-old, was admitted for routine laparoscopic sterilization at day surgery, having completed her family. At operation, scattered spots of endometriosis were seen in the anterior Pouch of Douglas: the rest of the pelvis was free of disease. This represented minimal disease on the rASRM scoring system – Stage I.

The findings at operation were subsequently conveyed to Samara and she was encouraged to talk through endometriosis, discuss the implications and read an information leaflet before leaving the department. In the absence of symptoms, and with the knowledge that the amount of endometriosis found was a common finding, Samara endorsed the decision to take no further action and was discharged to the care of her GP.

AMERICAN SOCIETY FOR REPRODUCTIVE MEDICINE
REVISED CLASSIFICATION OF ENDOMETRIOSIS

Patient's Name _____ Date _____

Stage I   (Minimal)   - 1–5
Stage II   (Mild)   - 6–15   Laparoscopy_____ Laparotomy_____ Photography_____
Stage III (Moderate)   - 16–40   Recommended treatment _____
Stage IV (Severe)   - >40   _____
Total _____   Prognosis _____

	ENDOMETRIOSIS	<1 cm	1–3 cm	>3 cm
PERITONEUM	Superficial	1	2	4
	Deep	2	4	6
OVARY	R Superficial	1	2	4
	Deep	4	16	20
	L Superficial	1	2	4
	Deep	4	16	20
	POSTERIOR CULDESAC OBLITERATION	Partial		Complete
		4		40
	ADHESIONS	<1/3 Enclosure	1/3–2/3 Enclosure	>2/3 Enclosure
OVARY	R Filmy	1	2	4
	Dense	4	8	16
	L Filmy	1	2	4
	Dense	4	8	16
TUBE	R Filmy	1	2	4
	Dense	4*	8*	16
	L Filmy	1	2	4
	Dense	4*	8*	16

*If the fimbriated end of the fallopian tube is completely enclosed, change the point assignment to 16
Denote appearance of superficial implant types as red [(R), red, red-pink, flamelike, vesicular blobs, clear vesicles], white [(W), opacifications, peritoneal defects, yellow-brown], or black [(B) black, hemosiderin deposits, blue]. Denote percent of total described as R___%, W___% and B___%. Total should equal 100%

Additional Endometriosis: _____   Associated Pathology: _____
_____   _____
_____   _____

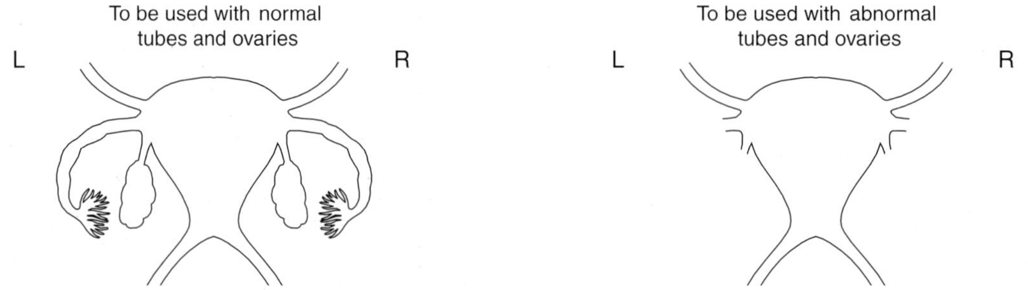

To be used with normal
tubes and ovaries

L   R

To be used with abnormal
tubes and ovaries

L   R

Figure 11.2 American Society for Reproductive Medicine revised classification. From American Society for Reproductive Medicine 1997, with permission

EXAMPLES AND GUIDELINES

STAGE I (MINIMAL)

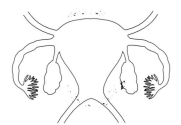

PERITONIUM
Superficial Endo - 1.3 cm - 2
R. OVARY
Superficial Endo - <1 cm - 1
Filmy Adhesions - <1/3 - 1
TOTAL POINTS 4

STAGE II (MILD)

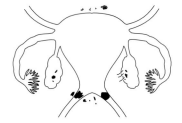

PERITONEUM
Deep Endo - >3 cm - 6
R. OVARY
Superficial Endo - <1 cm - 1
Filmy Adhesions - <1/3 - 1
L. OVARY
Superficial Endo - <1 cm - 1
TOTAL POINTS 9

STAGE III (MODERATE)

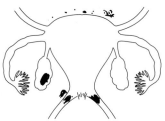

PERITONEUM
Deep Endo - >3 cm - 6
CULDESAC
Partial Obliteration - 4
L. OVARY
Deep Endo - 1.3 cm - 16
TOTAL POINTS 26

STAGE III (MODERATE)

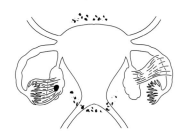

PERITONIUM
Superficial Endo - >3 cm - 4
R. TUBE
Filmy Adhesions - 1/3 - 1
R. OVARY
Filmy Adhesions - <1/3 - 1
L. TUBE
Dense Adhesions - 1/3 - 16*
L OVARY
Deep Endo - <1 cm - 4
Dense Adhesions - <1/3 - 4
TOTAL POINTS 30

STAGE IV (SEVERE)

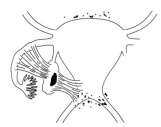

PERITONEUM
Superficial Endo - >3 cm - 4
L. OVARY
Deep Endo - 1.3 cm - 32**
Dense Adhesions - <1/3 - 8**
L. TUBE
Dense Adhesions - <1/3 - 8**
TOTAL POINTS 52

*Point assignment changed to 16
**Point assignment doubled

STAGE IV (SEVERE)

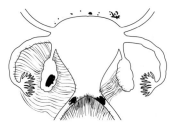

PERITONEUM
Deep Endo - >3 cm - 6
CULDESAC
Complete Obliteration - 40
R. OVARY
Deep Endo - 1.3 cm - 16
Dense Adhesions - 1/3 - 4
L. TUBE
Dense Adhesions - 2/3 - 16
L. OVARY
Deep Endo - 1/3 cm - 16
Dense Adhesions - >2/3 - 16
TOTAL POINTS 114

Determination of the stage or degree of endometrial involvement is based on a weighted point system. Distribution of points has been arbitrarily determined and may require further revision or refinement as knowledge of the disease increases.

To ensure complete evaluation inspection of the pelvis in a clockwise or counter clockwise fashion is encouraged. Number, size and location of endometrial implants, plaques, endometriomas and/or adhesions are noted. For example, five separate 0.5 cm superficial implants on the peritoneum (2.5 cm total) would be assigned 2 points. (The surface of the uterus should be considered peritoneum). The severity of the endometriosis or adhesions should be assigned the highest score only for peritoneum, ovary, tube or culdesac. For example, a 4 cm superficial and a 2 cm deep implant of the peritoneum should be given a score of 6

(not 8). A 4 cm deep endometrion of the ovary associated with more than 3 cm of superficial disease should be scored 20 (not 24).

In those patients with only one adenexa, points applied to disease of the remaining tube and ovary should be multiplied by two.' 'Points assigned may be circled and totaled. Aggregation of points indicates stage of disease (minimal, mild, moderate, or severe).

The presence of endometriosis of the bowel, urinary tract, fallopian tube, vagina, cervix, skin etc should be documented under 'additional endometriosis'. Other pathology such as tubal occlusion, leiomyomata, uterine anomaly, etc, should be documented under 'associated pathology'. All pathology should be depicted as specifically as possible on the sketch of pelvic organs and means of observation (laparoscopy or laparotomy) should be noted.

24–85% of laparoscopies for infertility (Evers 1996). The high rate in infertile women may merely be a reflection that more periods have been experienced, hence more occasions for cells to implant and proliferate. As a potential long-term condition, the need to have a positive diagnosis and an accurate extent of any endometriosis is necessary before therapy is commenced as treatment is generally hormonal, contraceptive and can have marked, unpleasant side-effects. Currently, absolute diagnosis can only be done on visual sighting, that is at laparoscopy or laparotomy, although suspected diagnosis can be strongly supported by a good and thorough history-taking and an abdominal and vaginal examination, the latter providing valuable information on the state of the pelvis. Dyspareunia can be mimicked by pressing on lesions that are knocked at intercourse – collision pain; a fixed retroverted uterus and nodules felt in the rectovaginal pouch can indicate adhesions and advanced disease. The use of routine ultrasound has a place in identifying endometrioma but not any underlying pathology (Stones & Thomas 1995) and should be used in conjunction with laparoscopy. Magnetic resonance imaging may prove to be a more effective diagnostic tool and could have a place in establishing and monitoring adolescent disease, where invasive surgery needs to be limited (Lim 1996). CA 125 (normal values 0–30 Ku/L), the serum tumour marker high in malignant disease (Muyldermans et al 1995), is also raised in severe endometriosis as in other disorders, for example pelvic inflammatory disease. It is known to fluctuate in mild disease and is slightly raised in pregnancy and during menstruation. There is therefore a potential for results to be misconstrued and, as severe disease is generally symptomatic anyway, the diagnostic benefit of this blood test has yet to be proved. A prospective study evaluating colour Doppler energy imaging (Guerriero 1998) plus serum Ca125 against the use of transvaginal ultrasonography alone suggested that by detecting the amount of arterial blood flow, difference between endometriomas and other adnexal masses could be detected. This could be a useful test. If cyclical rectal bleeding is a symptom and bowel involvement is thought likely, colonoscopy may be requested and should, ideally, be done at menses to visualize any bleeding areas. Laparoscopy currently remains the 'gold standard' for diagnosing disease.

Endometriosis is classified as minimal, mild, moderate or severe disease and is currently staged using the revised American Society for Reproductive Medicine (ASRM) (1997) classification system for pain and infertility, from Stage I (minimal) to Stage IV (severe) disease.

(Fig. 11.2). As an indicator of pain this system can be misleading, as there would appear to be no correlation between severity of pain and amount of disease seen (Fedele et al 1990, Vercellini et al 1996): the smallest lesion can give the most exquisite pain, yet a patient with a pelvis full of disease may be asymptomatic and endometriosis discovered only at surgery for other reasons. Red active lesions have been found to produce more prostaglandins which may explain the significant symptoms which undoubtedly do occur with a minimal or mild diagnostic score. It is a useful practice to keep a baseline record in the notes of initial staging of disease in order to monitor its progression or regression. Examples of staging are:

- Minimal (1–5): few superficial lesions on one ovary, uterosacral ligaments or peritoneum
- Mild (6–15): superficial lesions on two or more of the above structures or extensive on one ovary
- Moderate (16–40): ovarian cysts, adhesions and scarring
- Severe (> 40): deeply invasive endometriosis and/or severe adhesions.

If menstrual flow is a risk factor in endometriosis, the diameter of the cervical os and length of menses may play a part in the severity of the disease (Barbieri et al 1992). In a mechanical test it was shown that if the diameter of the os was under 0.2 mm it forced a

Mild endometriosis

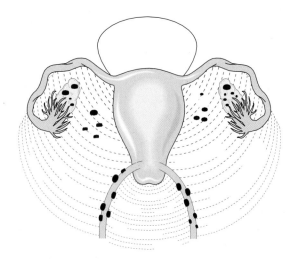

Figure 11.3 Mild endometriosis. Reproduced with kind permission of the Royal College of Obstetricians and Gynaecologists.

Severe endometriosis

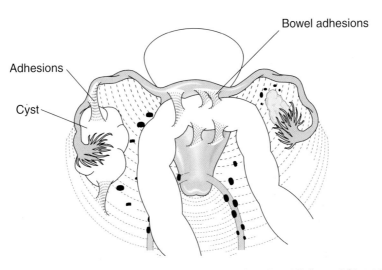

Figure 11.4 Severe endometriosis. Reproduced with kind permission of the Royal College of Obstetricians and Gynaecologists.

greater volume of refluxed menstrual debris back down the fallopian tubes, the only other exit being the vagina. It has also been suggested that a marked change in intra-abdominal pressure is produced by the sudden removal of tight clothing during menses (Dickinson 1999) contributing to retrograde menstrual flow and by implication endometriosis. It is known that childbearing has a protective role to play in endometriosis, as has the use of the oral contraceptive pill (OCP) (Vessey et al 1993), and that, conversely, delayed childbearing is implicated as a risk factor in the development of endometriosis. It can certainly be seen more frequently in the mid-20- to mid-30-year age group as more women, previously nulliparous, stop taking the OCP to conceive, have more periods and thus more occasions for cells to implant. Figures 11.3 and 11.4 are illustrative of mild and severe disease.

SIGNS AND SYMPTOMS

Physical signs of endometriosis are pelvic tenderness, induration, nodules in the rectovaginal pouch and a fixed uterus, all of which can be detected at abdominal and vaginal examination. Symptoms are less rigid, being subjective and individual but, in the main, are dysmenorrhoea, dyspareunia and pelvic pain just before and just after a period. All three cardinal symptoms do not have to be present for diagnosis as much will

depend on the site of the disease. As can be seen from Table 11.2, other symptoms are back pain, pain on micturition and pain on defecation, with intermittent constipation and diarrhoea. A ruptured ovarian cyst can give severe, acute abdominal pain and can frequently be mistaken for appendicitis or irritable bowel syndrome.

Dyspareunia

Dyspareunia can be either superficial or deep and one can lead to the other to the point of apareunia. As a symptom of endometriosis it should not be underestimated, but accepted as a distressing and life-altering condition. Superficial dyspareunia attributed to vaginismus, painful muscle spasms of the vaginal wall, can exclude coitus as much as pain on deep penetration. The use of a vaginal lubricant, positional changes and,

Table 11.2 Symptoms of endometriosis (in no preferential order)

Main	Other
Dysmenorrhoea	Pain on defecation
Dyspareunia – deep	Pain on micturition
and superficial	Constipation/diarrhoea
Pelvic pain	Back pain
Infertility	Pain at ovulation
	Depression
	Tiredness

Case study: Anne

Anne, a 36-year-old, requested referral to a specialist gynaecological clinic because of severe pelvic pain, always present but significantly worse prior to and immediately after a period, severe dysmenorrhoea and dyspareunia. She had never been pregnant.

Anne had had rheumatoid arthritis from her teenage years, necessitating daily medication. A diagnosis of minimal endometriosis had been made when she was aged 33, for which she was given a 6-month course of danazol. Noted side-effects were of significant hair growth and voice changes. Contraception following treatment was initially the OCP and the sheath. Laparoscopy for fertility investigations some time after revealed a normal pelvis.

In conjunction with the symptoms of pelvic pain, dysmenorrhoea and dyspareunia, Anne was also complaining of pain on defecation and pain at micturition, with possible haematuria at menses, all of which were impacting on work commitments. Her previous diagnosis of endometriosis had prompted referral to outpatient clinic and, on vaginal examination, she was markedly tender in both iliac fossae. Diagnostic laparoscopy, which had been performed prior to clinic visit, was normal apart from numerous peritoneal endometriotic deposits around the Pouch of Douglas and both uterosacral ligaments – a plausible explanation for deep dyspareunia – score 4, Stage I on the rASRM classification system. Treatment initiated was Provera 10 mg t.d.s. for 4 months, which produced amenorrhoea but little change in symptomatology and Anne returned to outpatient clinic.

In view of the lack of efficacy of previous treatments and the adverse effect on Anne's working life, a 6-month course of a GnRH analogue was prescribed and started at the beginning of a period. Despite her lack of conception in the past, Anne was advised to use an alternative means of contraception for the first 6 weeks of treatment.

Side-effects after 3 months' therapy were hot flushes, night sweats increasing in severity, headaches and some vaginal dryness. Anne was amenorrhoeic and her symptoms had improved.

After 6 months treatment Anne felt very well both physically and mentally. Vaginal examination was normal. Return of menses came 79 days from the last hormonal injection and she reported it as very painful.

Anne was followed up after 12 months. Her periods were regular and were less painful, with some dysmenorrhoea on the first day of the cycle and mild pelvic pain for 2 days after her period. Dyspareunia was not a problem. Abdominal examination showed slight discomfort in the left iliac fossa; vaginal examination was normal.

Two years from the end of her GnRHa therapy, all symptoms had returned to an unacceptable level and Anne requested a hysterectomy.

as importantly, an ability to discuss the problem with the patient can all be of help.

Deep dyspareunia can be attributed to:

- collision pain
- tethering of the ovaries by adhesions
- scarring on the uterosacral ligaments
- a fixed and retroverted uterus by adhesions
- bowel adhesions and scarring.

TREATMENT

Treatment is aimed primarily at alleviation of symptoms and, secondarily, at aiding fertility, depending on the wishes of the patient and the severity of disease. It is either medical or surgical. Endometriosis does not have to be treated just because it is there (Thomas 1993), as the finding of mild disease may be coincidental to pain and medical treatment is hormonal with possible unpleasant side-effects. Minimal or mild disease with little symptomatology may be best dealt with by analgesia of choice or the OCP, either monthly or tricyclically, to maintain control of symptoms. Medical therapy is effective for relieving pain but is unlikely to eradicate lesions completely, merely suppress them, and there will always be a risk that the disease will return. It does not appear to be an effective therapy for endometriomas larger than 3 cm, as drugs are unable to penetrate the fibrous cyst wall. If the maintenance of endometriosis depends on menstruation and oestrogen, suppression of ovarian function and endometrial atrophy are requisites of medical treatment.

Medical

Medical therapies are designed to reduce or abolish bleeding by direct action on the endometrium or by preventing the ovaries from producing oestrogen. Both should result in amenorrhoea. All have side-effects, some of which can be more problematic than the pain, and costs vary considerably, which can be a limiting factor for some general practices. The non-steroidal anti-inflammatory drugs (NSAIDs) can be taken for relief of pain in conjunction with a recognized drug regime. Overdosage can occur and care should be taken not to exceed the stated dose. A contraceptive intrauterine device (IUD), also used for menorrhagia, has potential for long-term use in endometriosis by its reduction of menstrual loss. A pilot study of patients with endometriosis-induced dysmenorrhoea, reported that the use of a levonorgestrel-releasing IUD (Mirena IUS), produced a marked reduction in menstrual pain plus a high degree of patient satisfaction (Vercillini 1999). Current drugs on the market are:

- progestogens: daily tablets
- antiprogesterone: tablets twice a week
- a synthetic androgen: daily tablets
- gonadotrophin releasing hormone analogues (GnRHa): daily intranasally or monthly subcutaneous/intramuscular injection, or an implant.

Daily medication has the advantage of ease of administration and discontinuation if side-effects become intolerable; monthly administration, though well tolerated, can be a disadvantage for some women as the above points cannot apply.

Progestogens

For example, medoxyprogesterone acetate 30 mg daily, norethisterone 10–25 mg daily, dydrogesterone 20–30 mg daily. Progestogens cause decidualization of the endometrium, bleeding stops and endometrial lesions atrophy. Side-effects are breakthrough bleeding, nausea, breast tenderness, fluid retention and depression.

Antiprogesterone

For example gestrinone 2.5 mg twice a week. Gestrinone has androgenic activity and is an antiprogesterone and antioestrogen. By interacting with hypothalamic and pituitary receptors it decreases the secretion of luteinizing hormone (LH) and follicle stimulating hormone (FSH), which, in turn, reduces the levels of oestrogen and progesterone with its effect on endometriotic tissue and the endometrium. Its action and side-effects are similar to danazol.

Danazol

Danazol (at an initial dose of 200 mg b.d.) is a synthetic derivative of the male hormone testosterone, an androgen, and has androgenic side-effects. Danazol abolishes release of LH and FSH and binds to active androgen receptors, leading to endometrial atrophy. It has proved effective for reducing implants but is not well tolerated as male-like side-effects are unacceptable to many women. It should not be given to pregnant women.

Danazol is absorbed directly from the gut and can be taken long term, although liver function tests are advised as it has adverse changes on serum lipids (Lindsay 1995). It has proved effective for reducing the majority of implants and has a recurrence rate of 29–30%.

The side-effects of danazol include weight gain, bloating, hirsutism, headache, breast reduction, acne, mood swings, fluid retention and deepening of the voice. More than 75% of women taking danazol will complain of side-effects at some time during therapy.

GnRH analogue

For example twice daily nasal spray or monthly subcutaneous/intramuscular injection or implant, into the anterior abdominal wall. GnRH analogues are usually given as a 6 month course and cannot be given orally as they are destroyed by enzymes (denatured) in the stomach. Their mode of action is to alter the hypothalamic receptors and pituitary response and, ultimately, to stop the production of oestrogen (down-regulation). An initial response is to produce a surge of FSH, which makes the ovaries produce more oestrogen and bleeding occurs – a breakthrough bleed. A few women will need 2 months' treatment before periods cease and the production of oestrogen falls to menopausal levels. Injections of GnRHa are designed to be given every 28 days, which should be adhered to at the beginning of a course or ovarian hormones will start to be secreted and bleeding may occur. Return to menses is individual – the age of the patient does not appear to be a factor – and is between 6 weeks and 3 months from the last injection.

GnRHa are effective drugs but generally restricted in use to a 6 month course as a certain amount of bone loss does occur (Fogelman 1992); long-term use could be detrimental for both osteoporosis and cardiovascular disease. Bone loss is approximately 3–5%, similar to pregnant or breastfeeding women, and is reversible. Values should return to normal 6–9 months after the end of therapy. As side-effects are the result of low oestrogen levels, a very low dose of HRT can be prescribed – addback therapy – which helps alleviate symptoms but should not induce bleeding.

This is best given in tablet form or as a patch, as both will provide a steady dose of oestrogen. Implants, which give an initial burst of hormone, are not ideal as there is potential for endometriosis to flare up. The addition of HRT to GnRHa therapy could therefore

Table 11.3 Examples of the cost of 4 weeks of therapy. UK National Health service 1999 net price of drugs used in endometriosis.

Generic name		Proprietary name	Dose	Cost (£)
Progestogens	Medoxyprogesterone acetate	Provera	30 mg daily	23.20 (90 day pack)
	Dydrogesterone	Duphaston (21-day cycle)	30 mg daily	11.87 (60 day pack)
Androgen	Danazol	Danol (start dose)	400 mg daily	35.34 (30 day)
Antiprogesterone	Gestrinone	Dimetriose	2.5 mg twice weekly	116.99 (8 caps)
GnRHa	Goserelin (implant)	Zoladex	3.6 mg	122.27
	Triptorelin	Decaptyl (injection)	3 mg	110.00
	Buserelin (nasal spray)	Suprecur	300 µg t.d.s. approx.	65.80

Source: *British National Formulary* No. 38

mean long-term use is a possibility (Gangar et al 1993), especially where conservation of the uterus is required for fertility. Bisphosphonates, which inhibit mobilization of calcium from the skeleton, can also be used where it is imperative not to add oestrogen. Although effective and well tolerated drugs, the cost of GnRHa can determine usage; the differences in a month's course of medication can be seen in Table 11.3. Results in clinical trials have not shown any difference in efficacy between danazol or GnRHa therapy (Rock et al 1993, Shaw 1992a).

Side-effects are menopausal in nature, perceived to be female, generally well tolerated and include: hot flushes/night sweats, mood swings/depression, loss of libido/vaginal dryness, headaches, breast reduction, joint pains and hair loss. Side-effects of the nasal spray include: headaches and mucosal irritation.

Surgical

Surgical treatment is by diathermy laser, laparoscopy, or formal laparotomy.

Laser laparoscopy

Laser treatment, by a trained specialist in the technique, is used to eradicate lesions with pin-point accuracy, leaving the surrounding tissue unharmed, and for cutting through adhesions. It is effective for implants causing deep dyspareunia and for separating adhesions that are likely to be mechanically impeding

fertility. Improvement in pain can take up to 3 months to be apparent. One follow-up report showed that laser treatment can be beneficial for up to 12 months in 90% of women with mild or moderate disease (Sutton et al 1997).

Advantages It is a one-stop therapy (Stones & Thomas 1995) and can be repeated in conjunction with medical therapy if and when necessary. Infection is less likely than at an open procedure.

Laparotomy

A formal laparotomy may be needed for:

- hysterectomy with or without bilateral salpingo-oophorectomy
- reconstructive surgery
- removal of large endometriomas
- bowel surgery if disease has involved colon/rectum.

Total abdominal hysterectomy (TAH) is usually performed for intractable pain, where other treatments have failed and/or where fertility is no longer an issue. Removal of both ovaries may be an intraoperative decision and will depend on the wishes of the patient, her age and severity of disease.

Increasingly, women appear to be questioning the merits of 'blanket' hysterectomy and there is an opinion that, as medical therapy does not eradicate disease, laparoscopic excision, for all but the most severe endometriosis, is the way forward (Garry 1997).

Case study: Clara

Clara, a nulliparous women in her late 30s, presented in clinic with a 2-year history of severe dysmenorrhoea and deep dyspareunia, bowel disturbances and ovulation pain.

Past medical history
Diagnostic laparoscopy in her early 20s for dyspareunia was normal apart from a retroverted uterus for which a ring pessary was fitted. Clara had a regular cycle and was not taking any drugs, including the OCP. In her early 30s, Clara had been investigated for primary infertility; at the time she had also complained of dysmenorrhoea. Diagnostic laparoscopy with dye insufflation revealed spots of endometriosis on the uterosacral ligaments, left ovary and peritoneum and a patent tube on the right but not on the left. This represented mild disease on the revised ASRM classification system – Stage II. A 6-month course of danazol was commenced, initially 200 mg t.d.s. Side-effects were weight gain, abdominal bloating and headaches. No significant disease was seen at repeat laparoscopy 1 year later. Despite treatment, Clara was now complaining of pelvic pain, dysmenorrhoea and occasional dyspareunia. Her infertility was addressed by prescribing clomiphene to boost ovulation but was not tolerated well. This was discontinued and Clara adopted two children.

Clara presented in clinic with symptoms of severe dysmenorrhoea and dyspareunia affecting her relationship, pelvic pain and pain on defecation during menses. Further investigations were requested. Diagnostic laparoscopy revealed a very injected uterus with a marked neovascular pattern, old scarring on both uterosacral ligaments, a left tube and ovary stuck firmly to the pelvic sidewall and small patches of disease on her right ovary. This represented Stage III on the revised ASRM classification system – score 37 – moderate disease. A written comment from the surgeon was that she would probably be best treated by a pelvic clearance. Lack of conception had been accepted but Clara was not emotionally ready for hysterectomy and a 6-month course of a subcutaneous GnRHa was commenced. Side-effects were hot flushes, night sweats, tiredness, loss of libido and headaches. Return to menses came nearly 3 months from her last injection. To her delight, Clara became pregnant and successfully delivered at term, approximately 2 years after completing her hormonal therapy.

Currently pelvic clearance is generally considered to be the definitive answer for endometriosis, removing precipitating factors – oestrogen and bleeding – with complete removal of all ovarian tissue the goal. Any small remnant of ovary remaining can be the cause of continuing disease, bleeding after hysterectomy being not only difficult to understand but manage effectively. Oestrogen-only HRT will need to be prescribed according to the age of the patient for both osteoporotic and cardiovascular cover.

ENDOMETRIOSIS AND INFERTILITY

The connection between endometriosis and infertility remains unclear, with the exception of adhesions and endometriotic cysts causing mechanical problems. It is hard to understand how a few spots of disease on, for example, the uterosacral ligaments – unless causing apareunia – can be responsible for lack of fertility. A study to assess the impact of treatment in women with mild disease was unable to show that either treatment or elimination affected future fertility (Thomas & Cooke 1987) and the finding of endometriosis may be coincidental.

It is possible that immune abnormalities may create an environment that is hostile to the fertilization (Thomas 1991) and development of the oocyte. Another factor could be that endometrial cysts disturb the follicular maturation and rupture of the follicle. This may provoke adhesions and be the cause of mechanical failure to conceive by not allowing normal movement of tubes and ovaries to pick up the egg.

RESEARCH
Genetics

The aetiology of endometriosis is reminiscent of malignant disease. The risk of malignant transformation of endometriosis is rare (possibly 1%) but there is an association with endometrial carcinoma from the observation of cancer arising from within endometrial cysts (McMeekin et al 1995). Recent research has shown molecular genetic alterations and inactivation of a tumour suppressor gene on certain ovarian chromosomes, suggesting the notion of an underlying genetic component in the development of endometriosis (Jiang et al 1996) and that genetic abnormalities are the precursor to certain ovarian carcinomas (Jiang et al 1998). It is known that endometriosis may be familial; genetic studies have shown disease in approximately 7% of first degree relatives with a 2% risk for second degree female relatives (Haney 1991).

Growth factors

There is growing evidence to suggest that growth factors may be associated with the disease process of endometriosis (Choi 1996). Active implants of endometriosis and their surrounding tissue are highly vascularized and research has shown that higher levels of vascular endothelial growth factor (VEGF) in the peritoneal fluid of women with endometriosis may have a part to play in the pathogenesis of the disease (McLaren et al 1996a). Further studies (McLaren et al 1996b, 1997) have demonstrated activated macrophages to be a major source of VEGF in endometriosis and that lack of their suppression may therefore contribute to the disease process. There is considerable ongoing research into the roles VEGF's (Donnez et al 1998) and angiogenesis (Healy et al 1999) play in the pathogenesis of endometriosis.

Aromatase inhibitors

Aromatase is an enzyme that changes androgen into oestrogen and a new medical treatment using non-steroidal aromatase inhibitors is the subject of clinical trials. It is hoped this treatment will lower oestrogen levels sufficiently to reduce or stop bleeding but not enough to produce menopausal side-effects. This could be a very useful addition to medical therapy already on the market.

ALTERNATIVE THERAPY

There are many products on the market for relief of symptoms. Medical practitioners may argue that, as a hormone-dependent condition, manipulation of hormones has somehow to be part of the treatment process. How they work is less important than the fact some women report a significant reduction of symptoms and generally feel much better.

Oil of Evening Primrose can be taken for pain; vitamins B6, E and C can counter depression, help prevent scar formation and the control of heavy bleeding, respectively. Selenium can be taken as an anti-inflammatory.

Traditional Chinese Medicine (TCM)

TCM with its holistic approach, which includes acupuncture and hoemeopathy, is being found helpful for the relief of symptoms and promotion of health issues.

NURSING MANAGEMENT

In general, patients with endometriosis are not ill in the accepted sense but can feel unhappy and alone with their symptoms. Management is therefore largely one of good communication, emotional support and continuity of care. The latter requirement is particu-

larly important as, for a few women, endometriosis is an uphill battle against acute and chronic pain and involves long-term management.

Fertility is a difficult area for newly diagnosed women to cope with and needs sensitive and careful handling. Patients need to be told the truth and be given accurate information and, above all, hope. For women in their late 20s and early 30s with obvious ovarian disease, advice, if applicable, would be to put conception to the test sooner rather than later, as progression of endometriosis is unpredictable. A take-home information leaflet, with contact numbers if possible, is a useful addition to patient care.

It is important to remember that chronic pain can be physically and emotionally draining, with detrimental effects on personal relationships at home and in the workplace. One study comparing psychological differences found that women with symptomatic, albeit mild, disease exhibited depressive symptoms and mild disorders of sexual functioning as compared with asymptomatic women, who showed no psychological abnormalities (Waller & Shaw 1995). A further study (Peveler et al 1996) showed that after a negative laparoscopy, with no outpatient follow-up given, women can be left feeling dismissed. For some, this may be as difficult to cope with as with their pain. The majority of women, however, will learn to cope with their symptoms and need only the reassurance of knowing that a clinic visit is their decision if symptoms reach an unacceptable level.

Points to remember

GnRHa therapy

- It is not a fertility treatment
- A bleed is likely 10–14 days after the first injection
- Main side-effects are hot flushes, night sweats, headaches and vaginal dryness
- A local anaesthetic may be used prior to Zoladex implant
- Use of alternative contraception for the first 6 weeks of therapy should be encouraged
- Return to menses can take anything from 6 weeks to 3 months from the last injection
- The first period may be very painful.

Danazol therapy

- Either tolerated well or not at all
- Main side-effects are weight gain, abdominal bloating and acne.

Laser treatment

- Noticeable improvement may take up to 3 months
- Short stay in hospital
- Less risk of infection.

CONCLUSION

Endometriosis is a benign, difficult-to-understand condition, the aetiology of which is not fully known. For the majority of women it will go unrecognized or be a minor disease. In a small subgroup of women, endometriosis will progress to severe disease, causing major problems in their lives. The complex nature of management in this minority of women calls for expert knowledge and attention. They would be best served in centres where specialist treatment is available and, as importantly, where nursing staff are able to provide up-to-date information and continuity of care. Recognition and acknowledgement of symptoms can be the first helpful step towards patient – and their partner's – understanding of endometriosis. Wingfield et al (1997) reported the formation of an endometriosis clinic running in conjunction with a self-help group, a combination that produced high rates of patient satisfaction. Ideally, this should be available for all women with endometriosis.

GLOSSARY

Analogue: similar to, like
Angiogenesis: a fundamental process by which blood vessels are formed.
Denature: change the property of
Exudation: fluid from capillary walls
Induration: hardening of tissue

Invagination: a pushing inward forming a pouch; not an active invasion of the ovary
Metaplasia: neogenesis of tissue
Metastasia: implantation of cells from one part of the body to another
Pathogenesis: origin and development of disease

REFERENCES

American Society for Reproductive Medicine 1997 Revised American Society for Reproductive Medicine classification of endometriosis: 1996. Fertility and Sterility 67:817–821

Barbieri L, Callery M, Perez S 1992 Directionality of menstrual flow: cervical os diameter as a determinant of retrograde menstruation. Fertility and Sterility 57(4):727–730

Brosens I 1997 Endometriosis: a disease because it is characterised by bleeding. American Journal of Obstetrics and Gynecology 176(2):263–267

Choi YM 1996 Growth factor gene expression in endometriotic tissue. In: Minaguchi H, Sugimoto O (eds) Endometriosis today – advances in research and practice. Parthenon, Carnforth, Lancashire, vol 13, ch 26, pp 174–180

Dickinson CJ 1999 Could tight garments cause endometriosis? British Journal of Obstetrics and Gynaecology 106, 1003–1005

Donnez J, Nissole M, Clerkx F, Casanas-Roux F, Saussoy P, Gillerot S 1994 Advanced endoscopic technique used in dysfunctional uterine bleeding, fibroids and endometriosis and the role of gonadotrophin releasing hormone agonist therapy. British Journal of Obstetrics and Gynaecology 101(suppl 10):2–9

Donnez J, Smoes P, Gillerot S, Casanas-Roux F, Nisolle M 1998 Vascular endothelial growth factor (VEGF) in endometriosis. Human Reproduction 13(6): 1686–1690

Evers JLH 1996 Do all women have endometriosis? Reflections on pathogenesis. In: Minaguchi H, Sugimoto O (eds) Endometriosis today – advances in research and practice. Parthenon, Carnforth, Lancashire, vol 13, ch 2, pp 14–20

Fedele L, Parazzini F, Bianchi S 1990 Stage and location of pelvic endometriosis and pain. Fertility and Sterility 53:155–158

Fogelman I 1992 Gonadotrophin hormone releasing hormone agonist and the skeleton. Fertility and Sterility 57(4):715–724

Gangar KF, Stones RW, Saunders D, Rogers V, Rae T, Cooper S, Beard RW 1993 An alternative to hysterectomy – GnRH analogue combined with hormone replacement therapy. British Journal of Obstetrics and Gynaecology 100(4):360–364

Garry R 1997 Laparoscopic excision of endometriosis is the treatment of choice. British Journal of Obstetrics and Gynaecology 104:513–515

Guerrieo S, Ajossa S, Mais V, Risalvato A, Lai M, Melis G 1998 The diagnosis of endometriomas using colour Doppler energy imaging. Human Reproduction 13(6) 1691–1695

Halme J, Hammond MG, Hulka JF, Raj SG, Talbert LM 1984 Retrograde menstruation in healthy women and in patients with endometriosis. Obstetrics and Gynecology 64:151–154

Haney AF 1991 The pathogenesis and aetiology of endometriosis. In: Thomas EJ, Rock J (eds) Modern approaches to endometriosis. Kluwer Academic, Lancaster, ch 3, pp 3–19

Healy DL, Rogers PAW, Hii L, Wingfield M 1999 Angiogenesis for endometriosis. Human Reproduction Update 4(5): 736–740

Henderson AF, Studd JWW 1991 The role of definitive surgery and hormone replacement therapy in the treatment of endometriosis. In: Thomas EJ, Rock J (eds) Modern approaches to endometriosis. Kluwer Academic, Lancaster, ch 15, pp 275–290

Jiang X, Hitchcock A, Bryan EJ, Watson RW, Engelfield P, Thomas EJ 1996 Microsatellite analysis of endometriosis reveals loss of heterozygosity at candidate tumour suppressor gene loci. Cancer Research 56(15):3534–3539

Jiang X, Morland SJ, Hitchcock A, Thomas EJ, Campbell IG 1998 Allelotyping of endometriosis with adjacent ovarian carcinoma reveals evidence of a common lineage. Cancer Research 58

Lim YT 1996 New insights into adolescent endometriosis. In: Minagh H, Sugimoto O (eds) Endometriosis today – advances in research and practice. Parthenon, Carnforth, Lancashire, vol 13, ch 3, pp 21–27

Lindsay PC 1995 Medical and endocrine modulatory treatments. In: Shaw RW (ed) Endometriosis – current understanding and management. Blackwell Science, Oxford, ch 10, pp 187–205

McLaren J, Prentice A, Charnock Jones DS, Smith SK 1996a Vascular endothelial growth factor (VEGF) concentrations are elevated in peritoneal fluid of women with endometriosis. Human Reproduction 11(1):220–223

McLaren J, Prentice A, Charnock Jones DS, Millican SA 1996b Vascular endothelial growth factor is produced by peritoneal fluid macrophages in endometriosis and is regulated by ovarian steroids. Journal of Clinical Investigation 98(2):482–489

McLaren J, Dealtry G, Prentice A, Chadwick Jones DS, Smith SK 1997 Decreased levels of the potent regulator of monocyte/macrophage activation, interleukin-13, in the peritoneal fluid of patients with endometriosis. Human Reproduction 12(6):1307–1410

McMeekin DS, Burger RA, Manetta A, Disaia P, Berman ML 1995 Endometrioid adenocarcinoma of the ovary and its relationship to endometriosis. Gynecologic Oncology 59:81–86

Mangtani P, Booth M 1993 Epidemiology of endometriosis. Epidemiology and Community Health 47:84–89

Markham SM 1991 Extrapelvic endometriosis. In: Thomas EJ, Rock J (eds) Modern approaches to endometriosis. Kluwer Academic, Lancaster, ch 9, pp 151–182

Mellor SJ, Thomas EJ 1994 The action of oestradiol and epidermal growth factor in endometrial and endometriotic stroma in vitro. Fertility and Sterility 62:507–513

Miyazawa K 1976 Incidence of endometriosis among Japanese women. Obstetrics and Gynecology 48(4):407–409

Muyldermans M, Cornillie FJ, Koninckx PR 1995 Ca125 and endometriosis. Human Reproduction 11(2):173–187

Oliker AJ, Harris AE 1971 Endometriosis of the bladder in a male patient. Journal of Urology 106:858–861

Outwater EK, Siegelman ES, Van Deerlin V 1998 Adenomyosis: current concepts and imaging considerations. American Journal of Roentgenology 170(2):437–441

Peveler R, Edwards J, Daddow J, Thomas EJ 1996 Psychosocial factors and chronic pelvic pain: a comparison of women with endometriosis and with unexplained pain. Journal of Psychosomatic Research 40(3):305–315

Pinkert TC, Catlow CE, Strauss R 1979 Endometriosis of the urinary bladder in man with prostate cancer. Cancer 43:1562–1567

Prentice A, Randall BJ, Weddell A, McGill A, Henry L, Horne CHW, Thomas EJ 1992 Ovarian steroid receptor expression in endometriosis and in two peritoneal parent epithelia: endometrium and peritoneal mesothelium. Human Reproduction 7(9):1318–1325

Redwine DB 1987a The distribution of endometriosis in the pelvis by age-group and fertility. Fertility and Sterility 47:173–175

Redwine DB 1987b Age related evolution in colour appearance of endometriosis. Fertility and Sterility 48:1062–1063

Rock JA, Truglia JA, Caplan RJ and the Zoladex Endometriosis Study Group 1993 Zoladex (goserelin acetate implant) in the treatment of endometriosis: a randomised comparison with danazol. Obstetrics and Gynecology 82:198–205

Sampson JA 1921 Perforating haemorraghic chocolate cysts of the ovary. Archives of Surgery 3:245–323

Sampson JA 1927 Peritoneal endometriosis due to the menstrual dissemination of endometrial tissue into the peritoneal cavity. American Journal of Obstetrics and Gynecology 14:422–690

Shaw RW 1992a An open randomised study of the effect of goserelin depot and danazol in the treatment of endometriosis. Fertility and Sterility 58(2):265–272

Shaw RW 1992b An atlas of endometriosis. The Parthenon Publishing Group, Carnforth, Lancashire

Smith SK 1991 The endometrium and endometriosis. In: Thomas EJ, Rock J (eds) Modern approaches to endometriosis. Kluwer Academic, Lancaster, ch 4, pp 57–77

Stones RW, Thomas EJ 1995 Cost effective medical treatment of endometriosis. In: Bonnar J (ed) Recent advances in obstetrics and gynaecology. Kluwer Academic, Lancaster, ch 10, pp 39–152

Sutton CJG, Pooley AS, Ewens SP, Haines P 1997 Follow-up report on a randomised controlled trial of laser laparoscopy in the treatment of pelvic pain associated with minimal to moderate endometriosis. Fertility and Sterility 68(6):1070–1077

Thomas EJ 1991 Endometriosis and fertility. In: Thomas EJ, Rock J (eds) Modern approaches to endometriosis. Kluwer Academic, Lancaster, ch 7, pp 113–128

Thomas EJ 1993 Endometriosis: should not be treated just because it is there. British Medical Journal 306:158–159

Thomas EJ 1995 Endometriosis 1995 – confusion or sense. International Journal of Gynecology and Obstetrics 48(2):149–155

Thomas EJ, Cooke I 1987 Impact of gestrinone on the course of asymptomatic endometriosis. British Journal of Obstetrics and Gynaecology 294:272–274

Vercellini P, Trespidi L, De Glorgi O, Cortesi I, Parazzini F, Crosignani P 1996 Endometriosis and pelvic pain: relation to stage and disease. Fertility and Sterility 65(2):299–304

Vercellini P, Aimi G, Panazza S, De Giorgi O, Pesole A, Crosignani P 1999 A levonorgestrel-releasing intrauterine system for the treatment of dysmenorrhea associated with endometriosis: a pilot study. Fertility and Sterility 72(3):505–508

Vessey MP, Villard Mackintosh L, Painter R 1993 Epidemiology of endometriosis in women attending family planning clinics. British Medical Journal 306:182–187

Waller KG, Shaw RW 1995 Endometriosis, pelvic pain and psychological functioning. Fertility and Sterility 63(4):796–800

Wingfield MB, Wood C, Henderson LS, Wood RM 1997 Treatment of endometriosis involving a self-help group positively affects patients' perception of care. Journal of Psychosomatic Obstetrics and Gynecology 18(4):225–258

FURTHER READING

Hawkridge C 1989 Understanding endometriosis. Macdonald Optima division of Macdonald & Co (Publishers Ltd)

Shaw RW (ed) 1995 Endometriosis – current understanding. Blackwell Scientific, Oxford

USEFUL ADDRESSES

National Endometriosis Society
50 Westminster Palace Gardens, 1–7 Artillery Row, London SW1P 1RL
Tel: 020 7222 2781 (open 10.00 a.m. – 5.00 p.m.)
National Helpline: 020 7222 2776 (7.00 p.m. – 10.00 p.m.)
Information officer: Ros Rosenblatt
Tel: 020 722227 86

Royal College of Obstetricians and Gynaecologists
27 Sussex Place, Regents Park, London NW1 4RG
Tel: 020 7262 5425

12

Chronic pelvic pain

Vera Rogers

Chronic pelvic pain (CPP) is the most common condition for which a gynaecologist is consulted. All family doctors are familiar with the problems of diagnosing and treating pelvic pain in premenopausal women. This complaint is responsible for many days absence from work, loss of income and serious breakdown in relationships with increasing stress and unhappiness. Referral to the gynaecological department for investigation of pelvic pain often fails to demonstrate treatable pathology. In 1978 the Royal College of Obstetricians and Gynaecologists conducted a survey of indications for diagnostic laparoscopy. They found that out of a total number of 21 000 women, 52% were complaining of chronic pelvic pain but only 9% had identifiable pathology such as endometriosis, pelvic inflammatory disease or adhesions (Chamberlain and Brown 1978). It is estimated that 350 000 women in Britain suffer from CPP with 13 000 new cases presenting each year (Davis et al 1992). The economic and human cost in terms of time off work, investigations and breakdown of relationships is considerable. It has been established that over 80% of women with unexplained pelvic pain who have had a negative laparoscopy, have demonstrable **pelvic venous congestion** (PVC) (Beard et al 1984).

It is well known that people's perception of pain varies according to many factors, such as age, sex, previous experience, culture, state of health (both mental and physical), fatigue, fear and stress. Many of the women with CPP condition have also been found to have a history of anxiety and depression, and in particular to have experienced severe emotional deprivation either during their childhood years or in adult life. Some have suffered from poor parental bonding, a feeling of insecurity as a result of parental separation or divorce, bereavement or a fear of repeated physical or sexual abuse. The pain may have developed after a termination of pregnancy or miscarriage and can be aggravated by feelings of regret or guilt. The pressures

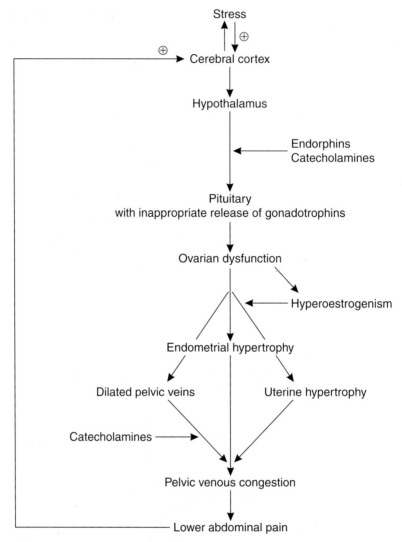

Figure 12.1 Aetiology of lower abdominal pain due to pelvic venous congestion – a hypothesis. From Beard et al 1986, with permission.

of modern living on these women add to the stress in their present relationship, which may well be deteriorating as a direct result of the CPP. They often look unhappy and may resent being questioned about their early childhood memories or difficulties in their current relationships. They say that they take large quantities of analgesics – often without any good effect

– and have more hospital referrals than patients with proven disease.

DEFINITION

Chronic pelvic pain of unknown origin occurs particularly during a woman's reproductive years. It is described as a chronic ache of more than 6 months duration with acute exacerbations, predominantly on one side but occasionally on the other.

AETIOLOGY

The aetiology of CPP remains a subject of continued research and discussion. It can be described under two headings.

Pain of known aetiology

- Endometriosis.
- Pelvic inflammatory disease.
- Adhesions.

Pain of unknown aetiology

- Pelvic venous congestion (PVC).
- Irritable bowel syndrome.
- Undetected endometriosis.
- Ovarian pathology (residual or trapped ovary; or ovarian remnants).
- Ilio-inguinal nerve entrapment in Pfannenstiel scar tissue.
- Lower abdominal pelvic pain.
- Vulvodynia.

PELVIC VENOUS CONGESTION

Pelvic venous congestion is the result of chronic dilatation of the pelvic veins leading to the delayed clearance of venous blood, which causes increasing pelvic congestion and pain. The pain is made worse by stand-

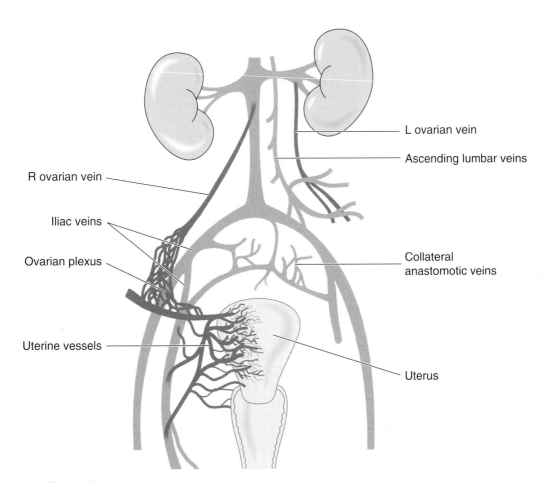

Figure 12.2 The pelvic veins.

ing, walking, bending, exercise and sexual intercourse. **Postcoital ache** after orgasm is frequently described and is unique to this condition.

Any stressful factors, such as working under pressure or relationship problems, may aggravate the problem, which in turn increases the stress response (Fig. 12.1).

One hypothesis to account for pelvic venous congestion was put forward by Hassan et al in 1992: 'The chronic state of dilatation of the pelvic veins of women with PVC is due to ovarian dysfunction resulting in a loss of normal vascular tone. This phenomenon occurs transiently in normal women in the luteal phase of the menstrual cycle'.

THE PELVIC CIRCULATION (Fig. 12.2)

The pelvic vasculature is controlled by the autonomic nervous system. It accommodates the changing increases in volume of venous blood resulting from:

- vascular responses during sexual excitement and orgasm
- the regulation of the menstrual cycle, ovulation and conception
- the provision of an adequate blood supply to the developing fetus, placenta and uterus throughout pregnancy.

The absence of valves in the pelvic veins enables them to dilate in response to these demands but interferes with the venous return when in the upright position, thus causing pooling of the venous blood in the pelvis. The high concentration of both oestrogens and progesterones in the ovarian veins interferes with the regulation by the autonomic nervous system, resulting in loss of vascular tone. However, Forbes and Kapadia in 1976 stated that oestradiol and testosterone induce uterine enlargement, bladder distension and selective dilatation of ovarian and uterine veins, but that progesterone did not have this effect.

The 'stress response' through the autonomic nervous system accentuates this condition via the hypothalamus and pituitary gland in the brain (see Fig. 12.1). This produces an inappropriate release of the follicle stimulating hormone (FSH) and luteinizing hormone (LH) gonadotrophins. Approximately 60% of women complaining of CPP caused by pelvic venous congestion have polycystic changes in their ovaries, which may well be a stress-related response (Figs 12.3 and 12.4).

IRRITABLE BOWEL SYNDROME

This is frequently suggested as a diagnosis for CPP when no gynaecological cause can be found. The symptoms may include colicky, abdominal pain and frequent loose motions alternating with constipation. There is a tendency for sufferers to be overanxious, very easily stressed and have many minor ailments.

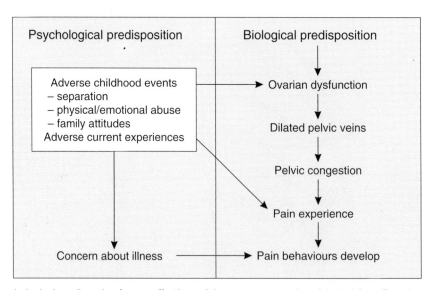

Figure 12.3 Psychological predisposing factors affecting pelvic venous congestion. Adapted from Beard et al 1994, with permission.

Relationship between stress and the menstrual cycle

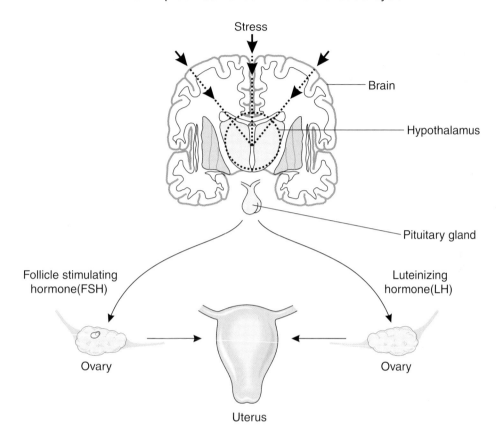

Cyclical influences of FSH and LH release on ovulation

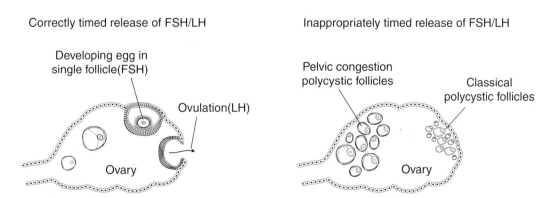

Figure 12.4 The relationship between stress and the menstrual cycle. Adapted from an original drawing by Professor R W Beard, with permission.

Case study: Maggie

Maggie is a 30-year-old married woman who was referred by her GP with a history of lower abdominal pain for 3 years. She has two children aged 4 and 6 years and felt that the pain started after the second pregnancy. She did not enjoy this pregnancy and delivery was more difficult than for her first child.

During the following year Maggie became exhausted by her constant pain and having to cope with an active toddler during the day and a baby who left her awake most of the night. They moved house during this time and her husband's new job involved him being away a lot. Eventually, the pain became more acute and she could no longer carry on a normal life. It was impossible to plan family holidays, family outings or have visitors. Standing and walking made the pain worse and this meant that Maggie needed help with shopping, housework and looking after the children.

Some relief was felt by applying heat or lying down but it never lasted long. Maggie's marriage started to deteriorate and she became severely depressed. Her GP, who was very understanding, referred her to her local hospital but no cause could be found. It was suggested that she was overreacting. Eventually she was referred to the Pelvic Pain Clinic where, after a series of investigations, she was found to have pelvic congestion. Treatment by ovarian downregulation with Provera plus relaxation therapy was started. Maggie's periods stopped after 2 months and gradually the pain lessened to the extent that she could start to lead a normal life.

Discussion with the pain counsellor revealed that many aspects of Maggie's daily life, which she had previously considered normal, were unsatisfactory and the result of compromises that she had had to make to adapt to the pain. After she had practised the relaxation, she found that the pain could be controlled. She was able to talk more freely with her husband and sort out many problems that she had suppressed over the years.

Gradually, in response to medical treatment, Maggie found that she was able to go shopping and eventually, as she gained confidence, she was able to start her sex life again. She continued with the medication while continuing to practice the pain management and relaxation and after 8 months she felt confident enough to stop the medication. To her surprise even though the pain did come back to some extent, she was not frightened by it, and by using the relaxation and avoiding stressful events that she had come to recognize brought on the pain, she 'got on top of it'. In time she found that she no longer feared the pain and it slowly disappeared. Two years later she felt she was cured because, despite getting the occasional twinge of pain, she knew that by reducing her daily stress it soon passed.

Clinical features of irritable bowel syndrome

- Change of bowel habit.
- Association with food, flatus and defecation.
- Lack of cyclicity.
- Bloating (also occurs in patients who have pelvic venous congestion).

Patients need referral to a gastroenterologist for investigation, treatment and stress management by a psychotherapist.

ILIO-INGUINAL NERVE ENTRAPMENT

This nerve may have been damaged by previous operations, particularly appendicectomy, herniorrhaphy

---

Case study: Joyce

Joyce is 48 years old and has been complaining of chronic pelvic pain for 19 years. It started after she had a coil inserted following the birth of her second child. Despite being treated for pelvic inflammatory disease, she described a dragging pain in the lower abdomen becoming worse in the last year. She scored the pain as 9 on the visual analogue scale of 0–10 and found it was made worse by exercise, standing, bending, stress and intercourse, but improved on lying down. She also complained of dypareunia and postcoital ache. She had an appendicectomy at 22 years of age and three exploratory laparotomies at 18, 30 and 31 years for pelvic adhesions. On the last occasion, she also had the right tube and ovary removed. At 32 years, she had a total abdominal hysterectomy and left salpingo-oophorectomy but the pain did not disappear after surgery. At 47 years she had another exploratory operation and a cystoscopy, both of which were normal.

Joyce could not work because of the pain and it interfered with her marital, social and family life, often waking her at night. Her early family life as a child was uneventful. Ultrasound scan revealed no abnormality.

On examination Joyce had multiple scars from her previous surgery with moderate tenderness over the right **ovarian point**. The pain was markedly tender over the right of the hysterectomy scar. Bupivacaine hydrochloride 0.25% × 10 ml was injected into the sites of the right and left ilio-inguinal nerves. She kept a pain diary for the next 24 h and this showed that the pain disappeared completely for the first 6 h and slowly returned to the previous intensity during the following 18 h. This confirmed the diagnosis of entrapment in scar tissue of both right and left ilio-inguinal nerves. Excision of both nerves resulted in complete absence of pain at follow-up 6 weeks later. Joyce said she felt like a new woman and wished she could have been diagnosed years ago.

and the Pfannenstiel incision. The main symptom is described as a stabbing pain, often colicky in nature and made worse by exercise but relieved by rest. Diagnosis is confirmed by injection of local anaesthetic into the aponeurosis over the site of maximum tenderness. The pain disappears for 4–6 hours and slowly returns as the effect of the local anaesthetic wears off. Treatment is by surgical division of the nerve.

LOWER ABDOMINAL PELVIC PAIN

Myofascial and 'trigger point' pain of the lower abdominal wall can be distinguished from that originating within the abdomen by asking the patient to raise her head and shoulders off the couch, thereby tensing her abdominal muscles. If pressure over the site of the pain persists in reproducing the tenderness, then the abdominal wall may well be the site primarily causing the pain. These trigger points can be identified by the doctor by introducing a 22 gauge needle into the fat-pad above the abdominal fascia. Movement of the needle tip will reproduce the pain and subsequent injections of local anaesthetic will temporarily remove the pain.

Treatment is by massaging the skin surface by ice cubes or cold spray, stretching the tissues by exercising the muscle and repeated injections of local anaesthetic at regular intervals.

VULVODYNIA

This condition is more common in the postmenopausal woman. It may be described as CPP but, on taking a careful history and examination, the site of the pain is confined to the perineal or vaginal areas. The pain may be worse on lying down. To date, no treatment has been found to be effective.

CHRONIC PELVIC PAIN OF UNKNOWN ORIGIN – DIFFERENTIAL DIAGNOSES

Pelvic venous congestion

This condition affects nulliparous women and parous women.

Age. Reproductive years (18–50).

Symptoms. Chronic ache with acute exacerbations, predominantly on one side but occasionally on the other (66%). Exacerbated by standing and by exercise (86%). Congestive dysmenorrhoea (68%) and postcoital ache (66%).

Signs. Tender over ovaries (86%). Tender ovarian points (77%) (Fig. 12.5).

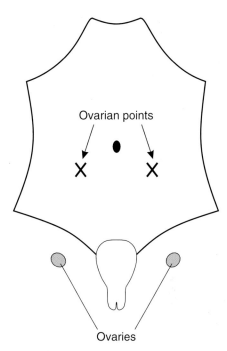

Figure 12.5   Sites of tenderness – the ovaries and ovarian points.

Undetected endometriosis

This condition affects nulliparous women and parous women.

A histological diagnosis is made from a surgical specimen.

Age. Reproductive years.

Symptoms. Local tenderness of affected organ (uterus/ovary). Dyspareunia and cyclical pelvic discomfort/pain.

Sites. Within the myometrium (adenomyosis) and the ovary.

Symptomatic residual and trapped ovary and ovarian remnant

These conditions present with continuous lower abdominal ache, often with cyclical exacerbation. There is usually deep dyspareunia or postcoital ache.

Results of investigations

- Ultrasound scan – cystic ovaries (residual). Tiny fragment (remnant)
- Gonadotrophins – pre- or perimenopausal.
- Laparoscopy – adhesions, which may be mild to severe, with a fixed (trapped) ovary.

Pathological ovary – investigations

Vaginal examination. Location of ovarian tissue corresponds with point of maximum tenderness.

Ultrasound scan.

● Locates the ovarian tissue. May be cystic in the case of trapped residual ovary.

● Volume may be less than 1 cm in an ovarian remnant.

Gonadotrophins. These can be pre- or perimenopausal.

Laparoscopy. Trapped or residual ovaries visualized.

Investigations

Pelvic ultrasound scan

Fifty-six per cent of women complaining of chronic pelvic pain have polycystic ovaries (the incidence in the general population is 23%). The pelvic pain cystic ovaries have large peripheral cysts, which are characteristic of PVC, and evidence of ovarian dysfunction (Adams et al 1990) (see Plate 20). The distribution is different from the ovarian cysts seen in polycystic ovary syndrome. The uterus is larger than normal and the endometrium is thicker (Figs 12.6 & 12.7). Dilated pelvic veins are measured by high resolution ultrasound scanning. The request form should indicate that the patient is complaining of pelvic pain and ask '? Venous congestion and/or pathology'. It is usual now for these scans to be done vaginally, which saves the patient having to drink the two pints of water that are necessary for an abdominal scan.

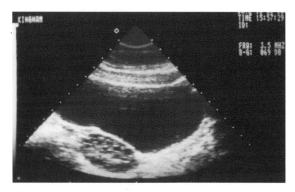

Figure 12.7 Ultrasound scan of a pelvic congestion cystic ovary.

Pelvic venography

These venograms are now performed as a day case procedure. The patient is admitted and prepared for X-ray, with the ward nurse checking the date of the last menstrual period, any allergies, any regular medications taken or pre-existing medical conditions and whether she took any pain killers the previous day or has had any unprotected intercourse since her last period. If there is any question that the patient might be pregnant the procedure would be delayed until after the next period. When the patient signs the consent form in the X-ray Department she takes the responsibility for acknowledging that she is not pregnant, that she does not have any allergies and that she has not taken any other medication. A tablet of Ponstan (mefenamic acid) 500 mg is given to the patient orally so that it can become active before the end of the procedure. As these patients are usually very nervous it is important to explain the procedure to them in detail when they are in position on the X-ray table, so that they know what to expect. An intravenous injection of Hypnovel (midazolam) 10 mg is given intravenously and this helps the patient to be completely relaxed with the additional benefit that she does not remember the procedure once it is finished. Eighty-two per cent of these patients have a venogram showing dilated veins and delayed clearance of the dye. A scoring system from 3 to 9 indicates the degree of congestion demonstrable 40 s after the end of the injection of the dye. A score of 3 to 5 means 'no congestion', score of 5 is considered borderline and a score of 6 to 9 indicates the degree of congestion seen at X-ray is from 'moderate' to 'severe'.

Prior to the procedure the nurses should confirm the following information has been obtained:

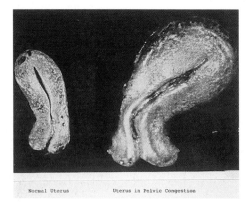

Figure 12.6 Comparison of normal uterus and uterus in pelvic congestion.

- That the patient has not had unprotected intercourse since her last period.
- Date of the last menstrual period.
- Any allergies or other medical conditions
- An informed consent is signed
- Time of administration of:

  Mefanamic acid 500 mg
  i.v. Hypnovel 10 mg
  i.v Buscopan 20 mg (to relax uterine muscle spasm if necessary).

This is a sterile procedure and the nurse attending the patient for the venogram will have previously laid-up the trolley wearing sterile gloves (Figure 12.8). The doctor performing the venogram will also wear sterile gloves and draw up the Omnipaque 350 mg I/ml contrast medium, which has been pre-warmed to enable it to be injected more freely. It is helpful to place a radio-opaque measure under the pelvis before commencing the procedure to assist the measurements of the veins. A series of three X-rays are taken: the first at the end of the injection, the second after 20 s and the third after a further 20 s. In a normal study the dye would have all disappeared 40 s after the injection. When there is severe congestion the circulation may not have moved the dye through the pelvis very quickly and 40 s after the injection there is often a lot of dye remaining in the pelvic veins. This can be assessed (Figure 12.10). Occasionally, the uterus may go into spasm, making injection of the dye very difficult. If this should happen it is helpful to give an intravenous injection of Buscopan 20 mg; this relaxes smooth muscle. Great care must be taken not to perforate the uterus. Should this inadvertently happen it is essential to give an antibiotic cover and observe the patient by taking

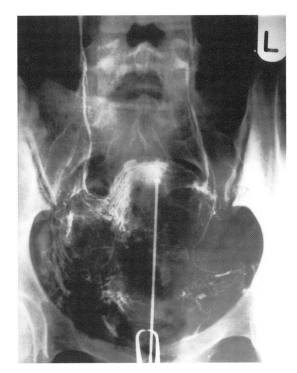

Figure 12.9 Normal study – pelvic venogram.

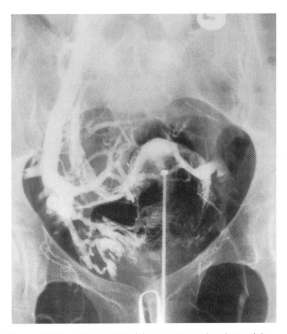

Figure 12.10 Abnormal pelvic venogram showing pelvic venous congestion.

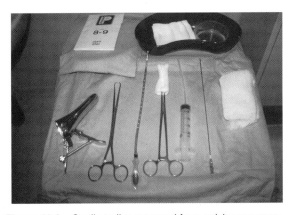

Figure 12.8 Sterile trolley prepared for a pelvic venogram.

pulse and blood pressure recordings at half-hourly intervals. If all goes well and no change is seen, the patient may go home later that day. A doctor must check that the patient is fit enough for discharge before she is allowed to go home. She should always be accompanied by a friend or relative and taken home by car. When booking a date for a pelvic venogram the patient must be told that this cannot be performed if she is menstruating or thinks she might be pregnant. She may have a light breakfast on the day of the procedure but it is not advisable to take any liquids less than 2 hours before the time of her venogram.

Laparoscopy (see Plates 21 and 22)

These patients may already have had one or more laparoscopies performed elsewhere for pelvic pain. However, unless the surgeon was specifically looking for congested veins this condition may have been ignored and a normal pelvis may have been observed, i.e. clear of endometriosis, PID and adhesions. A repeat laparoscopy is therefore advisable and may show large veins in the broad ligament and ovarian hilum with a very congested-looking uterus. It is helpful for the patient to be given an early follow-up appointment after the date of the last investigation, if possible within 2–3 weeks, so that the results of all the investigations can be explained and the treatment options discussed.

Medical treatment

To reduce the inappropriate levels of oestrogen that are causing the pelvic venous dilatation, ovarian suppression is achieved by prescribing medroxy progesterone acetate (MPA) 50 mg daily, for at least 6 months. In some patients this may stimulate their appetite and so dietary advice is also given. The addition of Premarin 0.625 mg daily is recommended for long term use in order to maintain bone density and offset side-effects such as mood changes, depression, tiredness or breakthrough bleeding. Farquhar et al 1989 showed the value of combined psychotherapy and treatment with MPA.

The reduction of pain by inducing amenorrhoea and regular practising of stress management greatly improves the quality of life and relationships of these patients. They can continue on this regime for some considerable time providing regular checks are made to ensure bone density is maintained. When their lifestyle is more stable, the patient will be prepared to

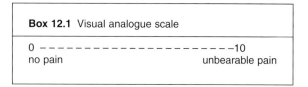

Box 12.1 Visual analogue scale

0 —10
no pain   unbearable pain

try without medication, knowing that they are now more in control of the pain. They should be encouraged to continue stress management techniques and regular relaxation. It is particularly helpful if they can have the telephone number of a specialist nurse in the clinic who is available to discuss relapses or concern over side-effects or new personal problems. It is important to adopt a positive, optimistic approach to these patients and look for signs of returning self-confidence as the pain reduces.

If a follow-up appointment is given in 3 to 6 months time for assessment of improvement, the patient should be given a pain chart to complete in the interim using the Visual analogue scale (see Box 12.1) of 0–10 whereby 0 is 'no pain' and 10 is 'unbearable pain'. She will quickly get used to assessing her pain daily and encouraged with the improvement in her quality of life, relationships and ability to socialize, work and look after her family.

A recent study by Gilling-Smith (personal communication) has shown that the use of gonadotrophin-releasing hormone analogue (GnRHa) is also very effective in producing pain relief through ovarian suppression. Add-back hormone replacement is essential to avoid menopausal symptoms (Premarin 0.625 mg daily) and endometrial hypertrophy (MPA 5 mg daily).

The injections of Prostap SR 3.75 mg (or Zoladex implant) are given at 4-weekly intervals for 6 months and should be started on day 5 of the menstrual cycle. As it takes approximately 3 weeks to achieve ovarian suppression, the HRT can be started after 3 weeks. The GnRHa acts by downregulating GnRH receptors in the pituitary. This results in the suppression of serum oestrogens to postmenopausal levels within 3 weeks. This effect is reversible with cessation of therapy. Zoladex implants are usually into the fat layer of the abdominal wall just above the hairline, whilst the Prostap injections can be given into the arm muscle or the abdominal fat. The nurse can use these occasions to encourage the patient to enquire about her pain and discuss any possible side-effects.

Possible side-effects.
- Break through bleeding.
- Mood changes.

- Depression.
- Loss of energy.
- Joint pains.
- Hot flushes and/or night sweats.
- Vaginal dryness.

Before adjusting the dose of HRT it is important to ask the patient if they have been under any new stresses or have any new problems that might account for the change in their emotional reactions. Breakthrough bleeding may be improved by increasing the dose of Provera from 5 mg to 10 mg a day whereas hot flushes, night sweats, vaginal dryness, etc. can be improved by increasing the level of Premarin to 1.25 mg a day. If there is no great improvement on these increases, it is worth considering changing the HRT to an oestrogen patch combined with a progestogen. It is important to remind the patient to continue with the HRT until at least 1 month after the last injection. At about 6 weeks after the last injection, the ovaries gradually return to activity and at this time the patient should be reminded about the need to use contraception if she does not want to become pregnant. If the pain has substantially reduced during this time and the patient is on a calm plateau in her life, she can stop the injections. She should continue practising relaxation therapy as appropriate, knowing that if the pain does return to some small extent she can keep it under control by practising all she has learnt from her counsellor.

If, for personal reasons, she is not ready to stop the injections, these may be continued, with the proviso that her bone mineral density (BMD) is ascertained. If the medication is continued for more than 1 year her BMD should be repeated at regular intervals (perhaps yearly). The patient's improvement should be assessed at 6-monthly intervals whilst on ovarian downregulation.

Prostap and Zoladex are fully reimbursable by non-dispensing GPs in England and Wales according to Section 44 of the Statement of Fees and Allowances. The medication is supplied in a convenient package and should be stored at room temperature (below 25°C). The makers of these two medications will provide guidelines for their administration in a convenient leaflet for the nurse and the patient.

Surgical treatment

Patients who respond to medical and psychological treatment, have completed their family and feel that their quality of life is intolerable, may be desperate for a permanent cure in order to enjoy a normal family life once more.

Total abdominal hysterectomy and bilateral salpingo-oophorectomy (TAH & BSO). As a last resort, TAH & BSO can be very successful. If there are dilated veins in the pelvis, the surgeon may prefer to perform a subtotal hysterectomy. This should reduce the blood loss and make the excision of the uterus an easier procedure. Alternatively, a GnRH analogue may be prescribed for 3 months prior to surgery to shrink the veins. If the cervix is not removed at the time of surgery, the woman must be reminded about the need for regular 3-yearly cervical smear checks. Beard et al followed-up 36 women for almost 5 years after surgery and found that their pain had resolved almost completely with a return to a normal life and increased frequency of sexual intercourse. The patient is normally seen for follow-up postoperatively at 6 weeks and at this time she should be well healed and possibly starting to try sexual intercourse. She may have noticed that she has loss of libido and if this is still present 3 months postoperatively, a testosterone implant may be useful. Most patients are so pleased to be able to enjoy intercourse again without pain that their relationships improve and usually loss of libido is no longer a problem.

Ovarian vein ligation or embolization of ovarian veins. For women who have completed their family but who do not wish to undergo a hysterectomy, an alternative operation is an ovarian vein ligation or embolization of the ovarian veins. Counselling needs to be given to patients before any decision is taken that may affect their long-term fertility.

In the case of ovarian vein ligation the patient is admitted for a general anaesthetic and is usually able to go home a day or two later. Ovarian vein embolization is performed in the X-ray department. The patient is admitted via day care and on arrival is offered a tablet of Ponstan (mefenamic acid) 500 mg orally, which can become active during the procedure. She will also have sedation in the form of intravenous Hypnoval 10 mg. A catheter is passed into the femoral vein and up into the ovarian vein under direct vision control and a coil is pushed through into the ovarian vein, which will cause a clot to form and block the vein. This is done on both sides and has the effect of diminishing the amount of oestrogen circulating throughout the pelvis so that the veins can subsequently shrink. At this moment in time the long-term effect on the function of the ovaries is not known. It is important that the woman has completed her family if this procedure is to be performed. The advantages are:

- it is quick and effective
- the woman can continue with her daily activities with minimal interruption.

The disadvantages are:

- the pain is not removed immediately
- it takes varying lengths of time for the veins to shrink and the pain to reduce.

Counselling is important to reassure the patient that she is going to be successful. The doctor and the nurse, and indeed the pain counsellor/psychologist, all have a role to play in reinforcing their expectancy of a complete cure so that the patient approaches the results in a positive, optimistic way.

Psychological assessment

Prior to attending a specialist Pelvic Pain Clinic, many women have had numerous investigations over the years without any definite cause of the pain being found. Many have been diagnosed unjustifiably of having repeated attacks of pelvic inflammatory disease. Emotional disturbances due to the pain are common and many women are labelled 'neurotic'. They can often relate the onset of the pain to a stressful life event, and it is important to help them understand the relationship between stress and the acute exacerbations of pain that may follow. A good history will identify these events and enable the pain counsellor to teach coping mechanisms and stress and pain management by deep relaxation techniques (Farquhar et al 1989).

What is stress and pain management? Assessment, education and short-term counselling of women with pelvic venous congestion (PVC) and pain involves one to four sessions of stress and pain counselling (50 minutes each) with the Pain Management Counsellor. There is the option to recontract for a further four to eight sessions if necessary.

First session. This involves assessment and education including:

- When the pain started?
- What was happening at the time in their life to bring on the PVC? It has been found that it usually develops:
  - During or after a particularly stressful time in their life.
  - If it starts at onset or soon after the menarche there is usually a history of stress and conflict in their family upbringing.
  - After a difficult and/or stressful childbirth.
  - Occasionally after a clip sterilization.

- What triggers or exacerbates the PVC pain now? This is usually:
  - Emotional stresses, e.g. if they get upset or angry at someone or something, including the pain, or if there are too many pressures in their life at any one time such as, family, work, health, etc. These activate the body's 'stress response' or 'arousal response' through the autonomic nervous system and causes an increase in blood supply, which pools in the slack veins and causes pain. There may be unresolved issues causing ongoing upset and conflict, such as bereavement or relationship issues. These factors also keep the body's arousal response activated. It is these issues that sometimes give the need to contract for extra sessions to help them identify the issues, work through them and hopefully resolve most of the difficult feelings.
  - Physical stressors such as lifting, exercise and sexual intercourse.
  - Gravitational factors such as standing or sitting for long periods of time, which causes pooling of blood in the slack veins.
- What coping mechanisms they are using, including medical, physical and psychological? They are assessed for both effective and ineffective coping

---

Box 12.2 Stress chart (from Holmes and Rahe, with permission.)

Events	Stress points
Death of a spouse	100
Divorce	73
Marital separation	65
Jail term	63
Death of a close family member	63
Personal injury or illness	53
Marriage	50
Loss of job	47
Retirement	45
Change in health of family member	44
Pregnancy	39
Sex difficulties	39
Change of financial state	38
Death of a close friend	37
Large mortgage	31
Foreclosure of mortgage or loan	30
Son or daughter leaving home	29
Trouble with boss	23
Change in work hours or conditions	20
Change in residence	20
Holidays	13
Christmas	12
Minor violations of the law	11

assessed for both effective and ineffective coping mechanisms, for example:

- Ineffective coping – carrying on with the physical stressors, such as lifting, or the emotional stressors, such as an argument. When the pain gets so bad they may lie down, which can help, but instead of relaxing physically and mentally they become more upset and angry about the pain and worry about what it is. This keeps the body's arousal and stress response activated and hence exacerbates the condition.
- Effective coping – understanding what PVC is and the factors that exacerbate it. Making the link between stress and PVC. Learning to manage the factors and issues differently. Learning effective relaxation techniques for physical and mental relaxation.

Subsequent sessions. Once these issues have been identified and an assessment made of the woman's level of understanding of PVC and how to control these stress factors, then the ongoing management can be planned. This includes:

- help with learning to manage the triggers and PVC more effectively
- counselling the identified or unresolved emotional issues, including coming to terms with PVC
- teaching relaxation skills
- further education with PVC if necessary
- further education about the body's stress response and how stress impacts on the condition if necessary.

Some patients find that the first session is enough for them and helps to answer their questions of 'What is PVC'? 'What causes it to develop'? 'How can I learn to manage it'? For many women, making the connection between stress and PVC gives them the significant information they needed. They are able to manage their pain much more effectively themselves without any ongoing help. Others may need a further four to eight follow-up sessions.

The role of the nurse

The nurse has a valuable role in reassuring the patient that she has come to the right place to have her chronic pelvic pain investigated; and that diagnosis, treatment and cure by medical and surgical intervention, plus counselling in stress and pain management, are also possible. The Clinical Agorithm (Fig. 12.11) is a useful tool in assisting the nurse identify factors responsible for chronic pelvic pain, standardize the investigations

and determine the factors leading to stress. There should be a team approach to patient care, with regular meetings to discuss difficult, medical, social or psychological problems of certain patients to encourage maximum cooperation within the team. This also enables the discussions of papers and ongoing research to keep the team up-to-date with new developments. The nurse is the ideal person to provide the patient with continuity of care and be the nucleus of the team. Patients need to understand that the team is concerned to treat the whole person, often involving the partner or other members of the family. It is important that the patient knows that she is believed, that her pain is real and 'not all in her mind'. A positive, optimistic approach will give hope of improvement in quality of life, general mental and physical health and relationships. It is helpful for all patients to have access, by telephone, to the same person, i.e. the clinic nurse, who knows them personally and understands their situation, and the cause of their pain. In addition, the clinic nurse is someone who knows the dates of their investigations; normal medical therapy and pos-

---

Box 12.3 Key points 1 – pelvic pain of unidentified origin

- It is essential to have a good history in order to make a diagnosis.
- Of all patients laparoscoped for chronic pelvic pain, 65% will have a normal pelvis, 20% adhesions and 12% endometriosis.
- Trapped or residual ovary syndrome occurs in 1–3% of cases after hysterectomy.
- Chronic pelvic pain can be caused by entrapment of the ilio-inguinal nerve in a Pfannenstiel scar.

Box 12.4 Key points 2 – pelvic pain of unidentified origin

- Pelvic congestion occurs almost only in women of reproductive age, whether nulliparous or parous.
- Pelvic congestion can be diagnosed by vaginal or abdominal ultrasonography, pelvic venography and laparoscopy.
- Pelvic congestion can be treated medically by: (i) medroxyprogesterone acetate 50 mg daily for 6 months with Premarin 0.625 mg daily for side-effects or (ii) 6-monthly injections of GnRH analogue with Premarin 0.625 mg daily to prevent menopausal symptoms and Provera 5 mg daily to prevent endometrial hyperplasia.

Clinical algorithm
Pelvic pain in women

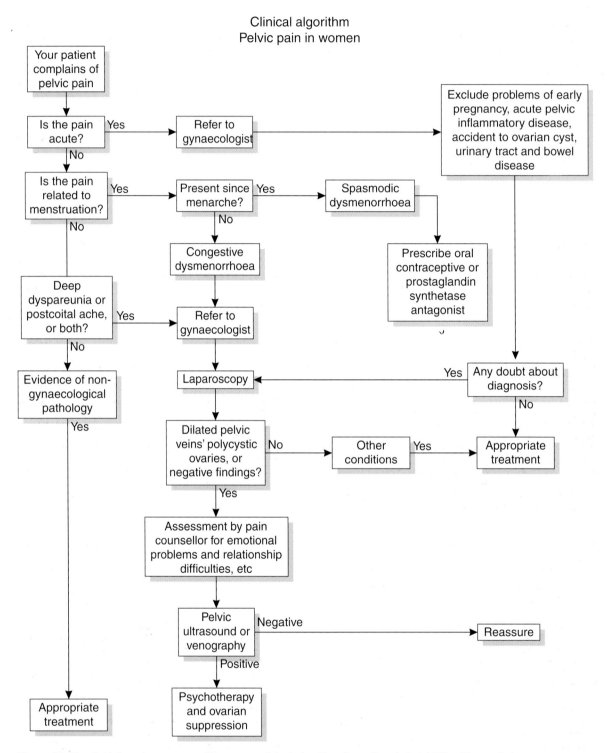

Figure 12.11   Guidelines for nurse practitioners – a clinical algorithm. From Beard et al 1986, with permission.

CONCLUSION

Women suffering with chronic pelvic pain need to be treated in a holistic manner and with an increased understanding of their psyche in addition to their soma. This will help to eliminate the assumption that a cure depends solely on the treatment of somatic pathology diagnosed by a clinician. The above-mentioned method of management of chronic pelvic pain involving the patient, doctor, nurse and counsellor, and which accepts the interdependence of the body and the emotions, will achieve a more effective and longer-term result.

ACKNOWLEDGEMENT

I should like to thank Professor R W Beard and colleagues in the Pelvic Pain Clinic for allowing me to use material and diagrams to illustrate the causes, investigations and treatment of chronic Pelvic Venous Congestion.

Box 12.5 Key points 3 – pelvic pain of unidentified origin

- Psychological assessment by a pain counsellor is helpful to identify trigger factors of pain and to teach alternative methods of coping with these stresses including relaxation techniques.
- As a last resort, pelvic congestion can be treated surgically by total abdominal hysterectomy and bilateral salpingo-oophorectomy followed by hormone replacement therapy if all more conservative methods have failed.

---

sible side-effects or complications arising from ovarian suppression; what is likely to happen next; and can reiterate what the doctors have told the patient. This reassurance enables the patient to feel supported and cared for individually.

GLOSSARY

Chronic pelvic pain: a history of lower abdominal pain lasting for more than 6 months.
Congested cervix: bluing of the cervix, often spreading to the vagina, similar to that seen in pregnancy.
'Ovarian point': an anatomical landmark situated at the junction of the upper and middle thirds of a line drawn between the umbilicus and the anterior superior iliac spine.
Pelvic venous congestion: this can be diagnosed at pelvic venography by the presence of ovarian vein dilatation, stasis (as evident by slow clearance of dye from the uterus and dilated pelvic veins) and visual evidence of vascular conges-

tion in the pelvis. These are assessed objectively by a scoring system (Beard et al 1984). A score of greater than 5 is abnormal and indicates the presence of CPP.
Postcoital ache: a persistent pain starting after intercourse and lasting for a variable time up to 24 hours
Regular sexual intercourse: a stated frequency of intercourse of at least once a week.
Tachyphylaxis: a falling off in the effect produced by a drug during continuous use or constantly repeated administration (common in drugs that act on the nervous system).

REFERENCES

Adams J, Reginald RW, Franks S, Wadsworth J, Beard RW 1990 Uterine size and endometrial thickness and the significance of cystic ovaries in women with pelvic pain due to congestion. British Journal of Obstetrics and Gynaecology 97(7):583–587

Beard RW, Higham JE, Pearce SM, Reginald RW 1984 Diagnosis of pelvic varicosities in women with chronic pelvic pain. Lancet ii:946–949

Beard RW, Reginald PW, Pearce S 1986 Pelvic pain in women: Clinical Algorithm. British Journal of Obstetrics and Gynaecology 293:1160–1162

Beard RW, Reginald RW, Wadsworth J 1988 Clinical features of women with chronic lower abdominal pain and pelvic congestion. British Journal of Obstetrics and Gynaecology 95:153–161

Beard RW, Kennedy R, Gangar KF 1991 Bilateral oophorectomy and hysterectomy in the treatment of intractable pelvic pain with pelvic congestion. British Journal of Obstetrics and Gynaecology 98:988–992

Beard RW, Gangar KF, Pearce S 1994 Chronic gynaecological pain. In Wall PD, Melzack R (eds) Textbook of pain. Churchill Livingstone, Edinburgh, pp 597–614

Chamberlain G, Brown JC 1978 Gynaecological laparoscopy. Report of the working party of the confidential enquiry into gynaecological laparoscopy of the Royal College of Obstetricians and Gynaecologists, London.

Davies L, Gangar KF, Drummond MS, Beard RW 1992 The economic burden of intractable gynaecological pain. Journal of Obstetrics and Gynaecology 12(suppl 2): 54–56

Duncan CH, Taylor HC 1952 A psychosomatic study of pelvic congestion. American Journal of Obstetrics and Gynecology 64:1–12

Farquhar CM, Rogers V, Franks S, Wadsworth J, Beard RW 1989 A randomised controlled trial of Medroxyprogesterone acetate and psychotherapy for the treatment of pelvic congestion. British Journal of Obstetrics and Gynaecology 96:1153–1162

Fry RPW, Crisp AH, Beard RW 1991 Patient's illness models in chronic pelvic pain. Psychotherapy and Psychosomatics 55:158–163

Gangar KF, Siddall-Allum J, Reid BA, Beard RW 1992 The aetiology and medical treatment of pelvic pain. Journal of Obstetrics and Gynaecology 12(suppl 2) S46–49

GillingSmith C, Rogers V, Foong C, Beard RW 1996 Comparison of GnRH analogue with Medroxyprogesterone acetate for the treatment of pelvic venous congestion. American Journal of Obstetrics and Gynecology.

Hassan et al 1992

Holmes and Rahe 1967 Social readjustment rating scale. Journal of Psychometric Research 11(2):213–218

FURTHER READING

Jones H. (1997) I am too busy to be stressed. Hodder & Stoughton, Sevenoaks (How to recognize and relieve the symptoms of stress)

Wells C, Newn G (1993) The pain relief handbook. Vermillian, London (Self-help methods for managing pain)

Relaxation tapes:
- Coping with Pain by Dr Bill Wiles. Recommended for anyone with chronic pain – strategies for effective pain relief and a relaxation programme.
- The Relaxation Kit – four different and highly effective relaxation programmes covering coping with depression, coping with anxiety, feeling good and coping with stress at work. From Wendy Lloyd Audio Productions Ltd, PO Box 1, Liverpool L47 7DD.

USEFUL ADDRESSES

The Pain Foundation
Rice Lane, Liverpool L9 1AE
Tel: 0151 523 1486

The Pelvic Pain Clinic
Northwick Park & St Mark's NHS Trust, Watford Road, Harrow, Middlesex HA1 3UJ
Tel: 020 8869 2919

13

Cancer of the uterine cervix

Cathryn Hughes

Cancer of the uterine cervix directly affects about 4200 women in the UK every year. Worldwide, it is a significant cause of **morbidity** and **mortality**, with about 437 000 new cases and over 200 000 deaths annually. Cervical cancer is the second most common female cancer after breast cancer, and its incidence internationally exceeds that of either cancer of the endometrium or cancer of the ovary. Cervical cancer is the most common female cancer in many developing countries.

Most cervical cancer has a recognized preinvasive state, which can be screened for using the Pap smear. The incidence of cervical cancer is falling in the majority of developed countries, thought largely to be due to the introduction of national cervical screening programmes. However, there is evidence to suggest that the mortality from the disease is increasing in younger women, in whom the less common **adenocarcinomas** may go undetected within the screening programmes. The peak incidence of preinvasive lesions, cervical intraepithelial neoplasia (CIN), occurs between the ages of 25 and 35 years. The peak incidence for cervical cancer is in the 40 to 50 age group.

ANATOMY

The cervix is one of the two major parts of the uterus or womb, located in the female pelvis. It forms the lower part of the uterus and is sometimes called the neck of the womb. It lies partly in the vagina and partly in the retroperitoneal space, behind the bladder and in front of the rectum. The cervix projects into the vaginal vault and can easily be seen when a speculum is passed into the vagina. Anteriorly, the cervix is separated from the bladder by fatty tissue and, posteriorly, lie the rectosigmoid and rectum. Lymphatic drainage occurs to the parametrial glands and to the obturator, internal, external and common iliac lymph nodes.

The stratified squamous epithelium that lines the vagina and outer part of the cervix (ectocervix) meets

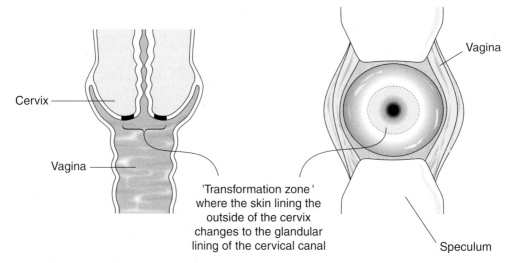

Figure 13.1 Normal anatomical position of the cervix indicating the transformation zone. From Health Press Ltd 1997, with permission.

the columnar epithelium of the uterine cavity at the squamocolumnar junction. This junction is just inside the external cervical os in young women, rising up the inner part of the cervix (endocervical canal) following the menopause. With puberty, the cervix grows and exposes the thin glandular epithelium of the endocervical canal, which is gradually replaced by squamous epithelium, a process known as squamous metaplasia. This part of the cervix is known as the transformation zone (Fig. 13.1) and is the site of most cervical **neoplasms**.

AETIOLOGY

As with many cancers, the exact **aetiology** of cancer of the cervix remains unknown. It is important to remember that cervical cancer can occur in any woman but epidemiological studies have suggested several associated risk factors.

Infective agents

Viral infections increasingly appear to play a significant role in the development of cervical neoplasia, preinvasive and invasive. Human papilloma viruses (HPV) are most commonly associated with the disease. There are over 70 different types of HPV and about 20 have been found in the genital tract and linked to high-grade CIN lesions or invasive cancer. HPV 16 has been shown to be present in over 90% of invasive squamous

cell **carcinomas** and HPV 18 has been associated with adenocarcinoma of the cervix.

The exact role of the papilloma virus in the genesis of cervical neoplasia is not understood. The prevalence of the virus in the normal population varies between age groups. It is not always acquired sexually and infection may be transient. Not all women who are HPV positive will go on to develop cervical cancer. It is possible that some women are able to eradicate the virus, those who cannot being at greater risk of developing the disease. Research into the use of a vaccine against HPV is currently underway. The exact benefit of such a vaccine remains unknown.

The herpes virus (specifically herpes simplex virus type 2) was once considered to be strongly linked to cervical cancer but this opinion is generally no longer held. The presence of the herpes virus appears to be related to sexual activity rather than cervical neoplasia but may be a contributory factor in the development of the disease.

Immunosuppression

Suppression of the immune system appears to increase the risk of developing cervical cellular abnormality. Women who are taking immunosuppressive medication following organ transplantation and women who are human immunodeficiency virus (HIV) positive have been shown to be at a greater risk of developing CIN and cervical cancer. Cervical cancer, in the presence of the HIV virus, has been designated an AIDS-defining illness. The increased incidence of the disease in the HIV-positive patient may be due to the immuno-suppression caused by the virus or could be linked to the increased risk of coexisting infections.

Sexual history

The age at which a woman becomes sexually active, and the number of sexual partners she has, appear to be significant risk factors. There is a higher incidence of CIN and invasive cancer in women who commence sexual intercourse before their 20th birthday. The total number of sexual partners is thought to be an even more significant factor. Harris et al (1980) showed an increased risk of developing severe dysplasia with a past history of six or more sexual partners and Brinton et al (1987) describe women with ten or more sexual partners as having a three times greater risk of developing cervical cancer than women with one partner or less.

Associations have been made with the sexual activity of the male partner. In Latin America the incidence of cervical cancer is high despite female sexual monogamy. Studies of risk factors in sexually monogamous women have shown an association with the sexual behaviours of the husband, where the use of prostitutes is not uncommon. It has also been suggested that the relative risk of developing cervical neoplasia is increased in a woman if her partner's previous wife had cervical cancer.

Oral contraceptives and multiparity have also been shown to increase the risk of cervical cancer but are often disputed in the literature and difficult to separate from other risk factors. A lower incidence of cervical cancer has been found in women who use barrier methods of contraception.

Smoking

An epidemiological link has been shown between cigarette smoking and cervical neoplasia. For smokers, a two to four times greater risk of developing the disease has been reported (Winkelstein 1990). The products of smoking are found in high concentrations in the cervical mucosa of women with CIN. Smoking can cause direct changes in the DNA of cervical cells. It can also lead to a reduction in Langerhan's cells, which form part of the cervical immune system, thus potentially leading to a degree of immunosuppression.

PATHOLOGY

About 80% to 90% of cervical cancers are squamous cell in origin. Of the remainder, 10% to 20% are adeno-carcinomas. Less common **tumours** include adeno-squamous, glassy cell, small cell, sarcomas and melanomas. With a change in staining techniques in histopathology, it is thought that the detection rates of adenosquamous lesions will increase. Squamous cell cancer of the cervix is often expressed as a continuum from normal cells through the degrees of abnormal changes to invasive cancer. The abnormal development of cells and tissue is graded cytologically and histologically.

Preinvasive disease

In preinvasive disease, the degree of abnormality is based upon the proportion of the squamous epithelium replaced by atypical or dysplastic cells. CIN I, CIN II and CIN III are histological terms that describe increasing degrees of abnormality or dysplasia, from mild, to moderate, to severe. CIN III, the most severe preinvasive abnormality, now includes what was previously called carcinoma *in situ*. In **cytology**, the terms mild, moderate and severe dyskariosis are used to suggest an underlying pathology.

It has been estimated that about one-third of CIN III lesions will go on to develop into cervical cancer in about 10–20 years if left untreated. Similarly, about one-third of all CIN I lesions will revert back to normal. Treatment decisions are based upon the **malignant** potential of the lesion and the views of the patient.

Adenocarcinoma *in situ* can sometimes be found by cytological recognition of abnormal glandular cells or simply because of an association with CIN. It is often not detected until a cone biopsy or hysterectomy is performed to treat the CIN.

Superficial or microinvasive disease

Once the disease has progressed beyond the basement membrane of the epithelium and starts to invade the tissue beyond, it is considered invasive or malignant. When this invasion is only visible microscopically into the cervical stroma, it is termed superficially invasive or microinvasive. This is the first stage in the International Federation of Gynaecology and Obstetrics (FIGO) staging for cervical cancer (Box 13.1). The depth of invasion is measured for accurate subdivision

Box 13.1 FIGO (International Federation of Gynaecology and Obstetrics) staging of cancer of the cervix

Stage	Description
0	Preinvasive carcinoma (CIN)
I	Carcinoma strictly confined to the cervix
Ia	Invasive cancer identified only microscopically. All gross lesions, even with superficial invasion, are stage Ib cancers. Measured stromal depth should not be greater than 5 mm and no wider than 7 mm
Ia1	Measured invasion no greater than 3 mm in depth no wider than 7 mm
Ia2	Measured depth of invasion greater than 3 mm and no greater than 7 mm
Ib	Lesions of greater dimensions than stage Ia2, whether seen clinically or not
Ib1	Clinical lesions confined to the cervix or preclinical lesions greater than Ia
Ib2	Clinical lesions greater than 4 cm
II	Involvement of the vagina but not the lower third, and/or infiltration of the parametria but not out to side wall
IIa	Involvement of the vagina but no evidence of parametrial involvement
IIb	Infiltration of the parametria but not out to side wall
III	Involvement of the lower third of the vagina, and/or extension to the pelvic side wall
IIIa	Involvement of the lower third of the vagina but not out to pelvic side wall if the parametria are involved
IIIb	Extension into the pelvic side wall and/or hydronephrosis or non-functional kidney
IV	Extension outside the reproductive tract
IVa	Involvement of the mucosa of the bladder or rectum and/or extending beyond the true pelvis
IVb	Distant metastasis

(based on FIGO 1995, Shepherd 1995)

staging, which is important in planning the degree of treatment.

Invasive disease

Most squamous carcinomas involve the ectocervix and can therefore often be seen on speculum examination. Adenocarcinomas generally occur in younger women and appear to be increasing in frequency. Adenocarcinomas were once talked about as being more aggressive in nature than squamous carcinomas but prognosis seems to be related to tumour volume and nodal status in the same way as with squamous

lesions. The risk factors for adenocarcinoma are different from those cited for squamous cell carcinoma. Sexual behaviour does not appear to be related to the development of this disease. Adenocarcinoma arises from the endocervical glandular cells. Delays in diagnosis can result because of the location of these lesions in the endocervical canal. The use of the endocervical brush when taking a smear has possibly improved detection rates.

Cancers are often classified according to the degree of differentiation. Cells assume features that distinguish them from other cells; they are considered to be differentiated. Cancer cells tend to be less differentiated than normal cells from the surrounding tissue. Tumours can be well differentiated (grade 1), moderately differentiated (grade 2) and poorly differentiated (grade 3). The differentiation or grade of the cervical tumour can act as a prognostic indicator.

CERVICAL SCREENING

Screening for a disease is a costly and complicated process. For screening to take place there should be a recognized preinvasive state or proven advantages to early treatment, an effective test (both specific and sensitive), readily available treatment and, essentially, the screening programme should be cost effective. The object of cervical screening is to reduce the incidence of, and mortality from, cervical cancer.

Preinvasive lesions of the cervix have been recognized for over 100 years and were described by Williams (1886) as presenting with no distinct symptoms. Papanicolaou and Traut (1943) described the routine use of cytology in the management of this disease. The cervical smear, or Pap smear, involves taking a sample of cells from the cervix and vagina. It is used to detect preinvasive lesions for early treatment or surveillance. Screening in the UK is recommended for women aged between 20 and 60 years, every 3 to 5 years. It is important to remember that cervical and vaginal smears can be taken at any time as an investigation: symptomatic women may need cervical smears outside the national screening programme. Uptake of screening was initially a problem but with the introduction of recall systems, GP incentives and increased public awareness, the UK is finally seeing a reduction in incidence and mortality.

Taking a cervical smear

A sample of the cells on the cervix needs to be removed, fixed, labelled and sent to the laboratory for microscopic examination. The nurse should:

- Explain the procedure and rationale.
- Make the woman comfortable in the lithotomy position. Observe the external genitalia while inserting the speculum into the vagina. A speculum is used to separate the vaginal walls and allows visualization of the cervix. A clear view of the cervix is necessary to exclude gross abnormality and facilitate effective sampling.
- Use a wooden or plastic spatula to scrape the ectocervical and endocervical exfoliated cells (Aylesbury or Ayers spatulas are commonly used). The pointed end of the Aylesbury spatula is inserted into the cervical canal and rotated through 720 degrees. An endocervical brush can be used to sample the endocervical canal.
- Spread the cells, in one direction, onto a labelled microscope slide and fix them immediately with alcohol to prevent air-drying.
- Remove the speculum observing the vagina.
- Inform the woman that light spotting and/or mild cramping pains may occur. Give an expected time for the results to be available. Explain how the woman will be made aware of her results and who to contact should that system fail.
- Send the labelled slide and patient details to the cytology laboratory for staining and examination.

Participation in the national screening programme requires the repeated compliance of the women to be screened. Time in explanation and reassurance, especially for the first smear, are vital as this will encourage the woman to feel safe and confident to return regularly.

There has been some recent media debate about the psychological cost to women of cervical screening. Some feel that the idea of taking healthy young women and introducing an intimate procedure, which may cause significant anxiety, is unnecessary, even harmful. The number of lives saved, it is argued, is debatable and does not justify the level of medical 'intrusion'. This is generally an unconventional view.

Colposcopy

Colposcopy is a method of magnifying the cervix for closer examination and was first described in the 1920s. Abnormal cervical cytology suggests an underlying pathology, which needs to be assessed. All grades of dyskaryosis are now referred for colposcopic examination. Inflammatory smears are often repeated, following treatment for any infection, but persistent inflammatory smears will probably also need colpo-

scopic assessment. Any cervix that looks suspicious or any woman with worrying symptoms should be referred for colposcopy even if her smear is normal.

Using the colposcope, the clinician can examine the cervix more closely with well-illuminated, low-power, binocular microscopy. Staining the cervix and upper vagina with acetic acid and then iodine allows any abnormal epithelium to be visualized for assessment and directed biopsy for histological diagnosis (see Plate 23).

In the UK, the British Society for Colposcopy and Cervical Pathology (BSCCP) regulates colposcopy and colposcopists. Unsupervised colposcopy should be performed only by those accredited by the BSCCP. Nurses can become accredited if they complete the accreditation training and maintain practice as stipulated by the BSCCP. There are an increasing number of nurse colposcopists developing and maintaining their own clinical practice.

Photographs of the cervix can be taken – cervicography – following the application of acetic acid and the pictures can be assessed at high speed by trained personnel (see Plates 23 and 24). Cervicography provides a reliable, permanent and objective record, which can be performed without the need for specialist colposcopy training and accreditation. The sensitivity of the test is high but specificity may be low. It is not in widespread use, at present, but may prove useful in the future.

CIN does not, in itself, cause any major problems; it is the potential to become malignant that gives rise to treatment plans.

TREATMENT OF PREINVASIVE DISEASE

Treatment involving removal or ablation of the abnormal tissue will, in most cases, provide a cure. CIN I has the potential to go on and develop into cancer but can also revert back to normal. CIN I can be treated or can be reassessed at regular intervals – kept under surveillance. Persistent CIN I is often treated. CIN II and CIN III are usually treated either on the first visit to the colposcopy department (based upon smear and clinical appearance, so-called 'see and treat') or upon histological confirmation of the disease.

Local ablation can be used to treat CIN, including cryotherapy, laser vaporization and cold coagulation. Even the most experienced colposcopist will not always identify an early invasive lesion. Ablation does not allow for the histological assessment of the whole lesion and may 'hide' a cancer. Treatment involving excision allows for histological assessment of the tissue and, therefore, avoids undertreating any invasive disease. This excision biopsy can be taken with a surgical knife, using a laser or loop diathermy, and is usually removed in the shape of a cone, hence the term cone biopsy. Knife cones are rarely performed any more because of the complications associated with the procedure, such as haemorrhage, infection and cervical stenosis. Laser cone biopsy is associated with fewer complications and can be performed under local anaesthesia. Large loop electrodiathermy of the transformation zone (LLETZ) has made excision treatment quicker and easier to tolerate for the patient. Hysterectomy should be performed only once invasive disease has been excluded.

Adenocarcinoma *in situ* can also be treated with a cone biopsy. A knife cone or laser cone is usually recommended to sample high enough into the endocervical canal to clear the glandular abnormality.

Colposcopic follow-up of women varies. UK guidelines recommend a follow-up colposcopy at 6 months then 1 year. After 3 years of negative cytology the woman may return to the national screening programme.

Case study: Margaret

Margaret is a 43-year-old married nurse with two children. She was contacted by her GP to attend the surgery following a routine cervical smear. The GP told Margaret that her smear suggested CIN III with evidence of glandular abnormality. She was referred urgently to the local colposcopy department. Colposcopic assessment of the cervix showed probable CIN III but no other obvious abnormality. A biopsy and repeat smear was taken. The biopsy confirmed CIN III.

The local colposcopist did not perform large treatments and so Margaret was referred to a specialist centre. Cone biopsy was performed in theatre under general anaesthesia using the laser, due to the possibility of a glandular abnormality, which could be high in the endocervical canal.

Histology of the cone biopsy showed CIN III with no evidence of invasion. Margaret returned for follow-up after 6 months and again after 1 year. Follow-up smears and colposcopy were, and have remained, normal.

Her main concern at the time of diagnosis was the smear report, which read 'suggestive of glandular invasion', which she took to mean lymphatic gland spread. The other factor that particularly upset her was the initial biopsy, which showed evidence of HPV infection. Margaret felt this was a sexually transmitted disease that suggested promiscuity or infidelity.

NATURAL HISTORY

Carcinoma of the cervix spreads primarily by direct invasion of local tissue and by lymphatic permeation. As the tumour spreads it can begin to involve the vaginal mucosa or extend into the uterine cavity. Laterally, the parametrial tissues may be involved, extending to the pelvic side wall. The ureters may be invaded or constricted by tumour. Involvement of the bladder and/or rectum can occur with disease progression. The risk of pelvic lymph node involvement is increased with the stage of the disease, lymphatic vessel involvement within the tumour, poor differentiation and large tumour volume. Lymph node involvement in stage Ib is about 16%, in stage II is about 30%, in stage III about 44%; and in stage IV about 55% (Anderson et al 1997). Metastatic spread via the bloodstream is not common but lung, bone and liver can be involved especially in the presence of locally advanced disease. Most women who die from cervical cancer will die with uncontrolled pelvic disease.

DIAGNOSIS

Once a woman presents with symptoms or via the national screening programme the diagnosis of cervical cancer is relatively easy to make.

SIGNS AND SYMPTOMS

Early stage cancer of the cervix can be without symptoms. The most common presenting complaint is abnormal vaginal bleeding: postcoital, intermenstrual or postmenopausal. Offensive vaginal discharge is the second most common symptom. As the disease progresses, pain can be experienced as a dragging sensation or in the lower back. Nerve involvement can lead to severe and referred pain. Spread into the bladder can lead to urinary symptoms, such as frequency and haematuria. Spread of the tumour into the rectum can lead to tenesmus and rectal bleeding. Fistula formation may occur into either the bowel or the bladder. Heavy vaginal bleeding can lead to anaemia.

Example of presentation

Ms Smith is a 40-year-old woman with four children. She is divorced from her husband and works part-time in her local supermarket. She smokes an average of ten cigarettes per day. She has been bleeding following sexual intercourse with a new partner for several months. This bleeding has become increasingly heavy.

She finally presented to her GP, who on examination, felt a hard 'mass' in the cervix. An urgent referral was made to a specialist gynaecologist. She has never had a cervical smear.

INVESTIGATIONS

The process of investigation and diagnosis begins with history taking and clinical examination. Examination under anaesthetic (EUA) is an essential requirement for the accurate staging of the disease for treatment planning. The staging of cervical cancer is done clinically rather than surgically. Pretreatment staging is necessary because if the tumour appears more advanced, then the treatment involves radiotherapy alone, with no surgical removal. Without the surgical removal of the uterus, nodes and surrounding tissue, full histological assessment of the disease cannot be made. It is important to adhere to standardized methods of staging in order to communicate treatment results from one institution to another and from one country to another.

Staging is based upon clinical examination, using chest X-ray, renal tract imaging, colposcopy, cystoscopy, sigmoidoscopy and barium studies of the colon and rectum. Cervical tissue needs to be obtained for a histological diagnosis. A cervical punch biopsy may be taken, or a larger cone biopsy. Some women may not have a visible lesion on the cervix and the disease may be detectable only upon cytological and histological assessment. Renal tract imaging is used to exclude ureteric obstruction or stenosis, which defines stage III disease. Chest X-ray excludes lung **metastasis**, studies of the bowel and bladder exclude infiltration and, therefore, stage IV disease.

Magnetic resonance imaging (MRI) and computerized tomography (CT) findings can influence treatment decisions but should not influence the initial staging. The use of MRI is becoming increasingly popular in specialist centres to help treatment decisions, especially where there may be some poor prognostic feature or a large tumour. The use of a vaginal coil and MRI may prove to be the way forward (Da Souza et al 1998) but even this technique cannot accurately predict lymph node involvement. Unfortunately, there are no tests to consistently establish lymph node metastasis. Histological assessment of the lymph nodes, following removal, is the only reliable way of determining disease involvement.

Initial accurate staging is important because treatment varies according to the stage and substage of the disease. The initial staging remains unchanged once the treatment has begun despite later evidence of

---

Box 13.2 Approximate average 5-year survival rates for cancer of the cervix

FIGO stage	5-year survival
Stage I	80%
Stage II	50%
Stage III	30%
Stage IV	10%

---

disease spread. This would obviously affect morbidity and mortality. Survival rates are generally dependent upon stage (Box 13.2) but do differ slightly from unit to unit and study to study.

Tumour markers

Studies in Poland and the Netherlands have suggested the value of using the squamous cell carcinoma antigen (SCC-ag) as a prognostic indicator for cervical cancer. Raised serum SCC-ag was associated with high risk disease, especially the presence of lymph node metastasis. Other tumour markers – CA 125, CA 19-9 and carcinoembryonic antigen (CEA) – have also been shown to be raised in poor-prognosis cervical cancer. Currently, tumour markers are not routinely used in the clinical setting.

TREATMENT

Treatment decisions in cervical cancer are based upon the stage of the disease as assessed by EUA, the histopathology of the tumour and the radiological findings, together with the general fitness, health and preference of the patient. On completion of pretreatment evaluation the patient will be discussed at the tumour board meeting to make the final recommendations for treatment. Members of the tumour board can include gynaecologists, oncologists, surgeons, pathologists, radiologists, nurses and social workers or counsellors. All investigations can be reviewed and discussed by this multidisciplinary team. The nurse specialist or nurse counsellor will be able to represent the fears and concerns of the patient, as well as any expressed preferences or perceived problems.

Microinvasion or superficial carcinoma

Identification of women with superficially invasive cancer who are at minimal risk of metastatic spread and disease recurrence allows for less radical treatment to be performed, with conservation of the uterus and therefore potential fertility. If a cone biopsy completely excises the lesion and there are no other significant poor prognostic indicators, then no further treatment is required in younger women. These women would be followed up carefully. Hysterectomy is often performed in women who have completed their family.

Invasive carcinoma

The treatment for invasive cancer of the cervix currently involves surgery, radiotherapy (with or without chemotherapy) or a combination of the two. Surgery is only a curative option in early stage disease. As the tumour progresses, treatments using radiotherapy are the only potentially curative options.

Surgery

There has long been a debate regarding the treatment of stage I and stage IIa cancer of the cervix. Comparable survival rates have been seen with both treatment modalities in clinical research. Surgery is generally the treatment of choice in women who have stage Ib or IIa cancer of the cervix, in whom the risk of nodal involvement is low. Compared to radiotherapy, surgery has the advantages of shorter treatment time, preservation of ovarian function, higher patient acceptance and limited sexual morbidity. Psychologically, patients often express a preference for removing the tumour, physically 'taking it away', even 'throwing it away'.

Radical hysterectomy

The surgical procedure generally undertaken is a radical hysterectomy or Wertheim's hysterectomy (see Plate 25). In a radical hysterectomy the whole uterus is removed together with the upper third of the vagina, the parametria and the pelvic lymph nodes with or without the para-aortic nodes. The ovaries are generally conserved in younger women thus avoiding an immediate menopause. The operation can be performed using a midline incision, a transverse incision or a laparoscope. A laparoscopically assisted Wertheim's hysterectomy can remove the same amount of tissue as an open procedure. The advantages of using the laparoscope include shorter hospitalization and reduced surgical morbidity.

The removal of the lymph nodes (lymphadenectomy) can be seen as therapeutic or as a means of establishing prognosis. Women who have histological disease in the lymph nodes have a higher risk of treatment failure. Identification of nodal disease allows for the consideration of postoperative treatment, usually pelvic radiotherapy. Any large, fixed or suspicious pelvic or para-aortic nodes can be **frozen sectioned** during the operation. If positive for disease, the surgeon may modify or abandon the procedure in favour of radical radiotherapy.

Removal of the ovaries is not an integral part of radical hysterectomy. The incidence of ovarian metastasis in premenopausal women with a stage Ib squamous lesion is minimal. Ovaries that look grossly normal at the time of the operation are not generally removed in premenopausal women. Some surgeons prefer to remove the ovaries when treating all women with adenocarcinoma but Brown et al (1990) showed that, where the ovaries looked normal, ovarian involvement was seen only in patients who were postmenopausal or who had positive lymph nodes. Some surgeons transpose the ovaries out of the radiation field. This is an attempt to preserve ovarian function in the event of postoperative radiotherapy.

Radical trachelectomy

Radical hysterectomy and radical radiotherapy have been the traditional approaches to the management of invasive cervical cancer greater than microinvasion. Both forms of treatment result in the loss of fertility and associated morbidity. In 1994 Dargent et al described the use of a less radical, fertility-sparing procedure for the management of carefully selected patients. Radical trachelectomy involves the surgical removal of the cervix, upper vagina and parametriom together with the pelvic lymph nodes. Women who wish to preserve their fertility and have a small, early invasive lesion may be offered this procedure. Careful selection and follow-up of these patients is vital. This remains an essentially experimental procedure.

Adjuvant treatment

Following surgery, full histological assessment of the tumour can be made. Postoperative pelvic radiotherapy is often recommended for women found to be lymph-node-positive. This has been shown to reduce the incidence of central pelvic disease recurrence; as most recurrences occur centrally the implication would be an associated improvement in survival.

There is, however, little research evidence to support this. Uncontrolled pelvic disease causes many difficult symptom control problems. Pelvic radiotherapy following surgery in the high-risk patient, at the very least, will help to control such disease.

Preoperative care

Once all the pretreatment investigations have been carried out the patient can be given a date to organize her admission. A common reaction is to request surgery immediately but some time taken in preparation can prove invaluable postoperatively. The woman needs to feel in control of the situation but also needs to be guided by the healthcare professionals. On the day prior to the operation, routine bloods to assess fitness for surgery can be taken. The patient needs to know it is possible she will require a blood transfusion following or during the surgery. Any objections to blood or blood products that the patient may have could result in the tumour being treated with radiotherapy as a safer option. Prophylactic antibiotics and antithrombotic therapy should be given: cervical cancer patients are at high risk of developing a deep vein thrombosis (DVT) because of the length of the surgical procedure and the presence of a pelvic malignancy.

Postoperative care

The usual postoperative observations need to be maintained, with careful observation of urinary output. Drains may be left *in situ* for bleeding. The surgery is reasonably extensive in gynaecological terms and postoperative pain management needs to be a priority. A urethral catheter is left draining immediately postoperatively and, once removed, the patient needs to void with the residual bladder volume being recorded. A suprapubic catheter (clamped until postvoid), intermittent catheterization or ultrasound can be used to measure residual volume. Once the residual volume is lower than 100 ml the suprapubic catheter may be removed or the intermittent catheterization or ultrasound ceased. If the tissue dissection around the bladder is reduced or modified, then the risk of bladder dysfunction is minimal and no such measurements need to be made. Some patients are discharged home with a suprapubic catheter or practising self-catheterization, to allow more time for the bladder to settle.

Complications of surgery

Acute complications of radical hysterectomy are not common but include infection, haemorrhage, damage to the urinary or intestinal tract and pulmonary embolus. Wound infections are rare, especially with the use of prophylactic antibiotics.

Subacute complications include bladder dysfunction, formation of lymphocysts and lower limb **lymphoedema**. Extensive dissection involved in identifying and isolating the ureters and mobilizing the bladder can lead to postoperative bladder dysfunction. This dysfunction is usually displayed by a loss of the sense of urgency to void and the inability of the bladder to empty completely. Long-term bladder dysfunction can be avoided by preventing overdistension of the bladder in the postoperative period. Information on how to recognize a bladder infection should be given to the patient.

Lymphocysts are usually small and asymptomatic. They generally resolve in time by reabsorption. Occasionally, lymphocysts require formal drainage.

Lymphoedema of the lower extremities can follow radical hysterectomy alone, although the incidence increases with the addition of postoperative radiotherapy. Women should be given advice on the prevention of lymphoedema, being advised to:

- take general care of their legs, i.e. protect them from injury, especially when cutting toe nails and during leg shaving (high-risk patients may be advised to avoid shaving their legs)
- walk regularly
- walk or exercise their legs during extended travelling
- take antibiotics (commonly erythromycin) for wounds or insect bites that are slow to heal
- wear support hosiery for work, etc.

Should lymphoedema become a problem, then the use of custom-fitted stockings and an exercise plan can help. Referral to a specialist lymphoedema clinic, where available, would be recommended. Injections into the affected leg should be avoided. The possibility of deep vein thrombosis (DVT) or recurrent disease should be excluded in a woman who suddenly develops lymphoedema.

The surgical complication rate is thought to be significantly reduced in cases where the operation is performed by a surgeon familiar with the surgery, i.e. those practising the procedure on a regular basis.

Radiotherapy

Radiotherapy is the therapeutic use of ionizing radiation. The biological effects of ionizing radiation were not recognized until the late 1890s. Following extensive experimentation, the first reported patient cure appeared in 1899, after which radiation therapy became popular. Radiation has an effect at three levels:

- molecular: the production of free radicals and DNA damage
- cellular: inhibition of proliferation
- tissue: damage/necrosis.

Radiation therapy works by the process of ionization: the breakdown of atoms or molecules into ions (when electrons are removed or added, an ion is formed). The result is the formation of free radical ions, which are extremely unstable and quickly form neutral free radicals that are uncharged atoms or molecules. Both free radical ions and the resultant neutral free radicals disrupt normal molecular structures and damage the biological target. Cell damage occurs. Most cells do not die immediately, a doomed cell can usually function until mitosis. Some non-proliferating cells die in interphase by a process of programmed cell death or apoptosis.

The problem of devising a clinically acceptable therapeutic ratio between normal tissue damage and tumour damage has been addressed. With experimentation, the early radiotherapists learnt that the dose needed to destroy cancer cells would also damage healthy tissue, sometimes irreversibly. In general, normal cells can repair more effectively than cancer cells but neither can repair damage totally. The total dose needed to kill the cancer is too great to be given in one dose and is therefore fractioned in order to cause as little normal cell damage as possible. Cell damage can be 'passed on' in normal tissue and the resulting mutation can potentially lead to cancer development, perhaps 10–20 years later.

Radiotherapy for carcinoma of the cervix involves a combination of external treatment and intracavitary treatment or brachytherapy. In early disease, the shift in treatment has been towards surgery, as mentioned, but even in early disease radiotherapy has the advantage of being given as an outpatient. Radiotherapy is the treatment of choice for women with more advanced disease, generally greater than Ib–IIa. Such patients are unlikely to be cured by surgery alone. Women who are not suitable for major surgery, or where other prognostic factors point to a high risk of nodal disease, are also treated with radiotherapy. It would be fair to say that some of the conditions that preclude a patient from surgery also make radiotherapy difficult and increase treatment morbidity. External radiotherapy is given to the whole pelvis, followed by intracavitary treatment, where a radioactive source is placed into the uterine cavity and upper vagina. External beam radiotherapy is used to control disease spread within the pelvis, in particular the pelvic lymph nodes. It is possible to control early disease with intracavitary treatment alone but most treatment involves a combination of the two.

External beam radiotherapy

External beam therapy using a linear accelerator is normally given first, to reduce the tumour mass. The pelvic field of radiation can be extended, in early stage disease, where there is evidence or suspicion of para-aortic nodal involvement. There is no evidence to support the use of extended fields in patients with locally advanced disease.

The ovaries are very sensitive to radiation and relatively low doses (in cancer treatment terms) will render a woman infertile. Ovaries that are moved or transposed during surgery will still suffer radiation scatter, even when shielded, and fail in up to 50% of cases. Attempts have been made to preserve ovarian function but none have been successful so far. Recent trials, however, are looking at storing ovarian tissue, to be used at a later date. Frozen embryos and eggs can be stored. The destruction of ovarian function will render the premenopausal woman menopausal. Young women need information and advice to consider hormone replacement therapy (HRT). There is no contraindication to the use of HRT post-treatment for cervical cancer.

Intracavitary radiotherapy

Intracavitary treatment involves giving a dose of radiation from a source close to the tumour. A uterine tube and vaginal applicators are inserted to deliver a high dose of radiation to the cervix and immediate surrounding tissue. These applicators are usually inserted in the operating theatre and loaded with the radioactive source at a later time, termed afterloading. The afterloading of the radioactive source can be done manually or by using remote systems such as selectron. High or low energy sources may be used. Typical treatment time for low-dose treatment using selectron may be 20 h, while high-dose selectron may be given over a few minutes.

Case study: Bethany

Bethany, a 28-year-old, single, shop assistant presented to her GP for a routine cervical smear within the national screening programme. The cervix looked normal on speculum examination and a smear was taken. The smear report suggested CIN I/II. Bethany was referred to the colposcopy department for routine assessment of her cervix, in the light of a mildly abnormal smear. She was seen in 6 weeks.

Colposcopic appearance of the cervix suggested CIN I and a biopsy confirmed this level of abnormality. A second routine follow-up colposcopy 6 months later failed to show any significant abnormality but the smear report suggested CIN III. A cone biopsy of the cervix diagnosed a poorly differentiated squamous cell carcinoma with a greater than 5 mm depth of invasion.

Bethany was then contacted and asked to attend the clinic to discuss her result. She attended with her boyfriend and was informed she had cervical cancer and would require major surgery, providing a formal examination under anaesthetic (EUA) confirmed the disease to be stage I. She was given the choice of having the EUA and Wertheim's hysterectomy as a joint or separate procedure. She was told about the operation and possible follow-up treatments, together with the fact that she would no longer be able to bear children but that her ovaries would be conserved enabling her to use her own eggs (ova) for any surrogate pregnancy.

She and her partner were seen by the consultant, specialist nurse and the associate specialist who had first colposcoped her. She decided to have a two-stage

procedure and underwent an EUA. The tumour was staged as an Ib. An MRI was also booked prior to surgery, which was normal. Renal ultrasound and chest X-ray were also normal.

Bethany was admitted for a Wertheim's hysterectomy. There were no surgical complications and she recovered well. Unfortunately, on histological examination, two of the removed pelvic lymph nodes contained metastatic tumour. It was then recommended that she attend for a course of external beam radiotherapy to the pelvis. She was informed of the rationale for this planned treatment and the fact that her ovaries would be irradiated and therefore ovarian function would be destroyed, along with any possibility of using her own ova. She was offered the facility of freezing embryos or the experimental option of storing ovarian tissue. After due consideration she declined.

Bethany felt that she shouldn't have got this cancer if she was under the surveillance of the colposcopy department. All results, specimen slides and management decisions were reviewed with no cause for concern. She felt that every time she was reassured by a doctor something worse happened: cone biopsy, fine → cancer → operation, went well, retain ovaries → positive nodes → radiotherapy, destroy ovarian function.

Bethany is now 3 years post-treatment. She and her boyfriend have split up and she has no new relationship in her life. She has had sporadic bowel problems necessitating hospital admission and investigation. No recurrent disease or significant pathology has been found.

Complications of radiotherapy

The complications of radiotherapy can be classified as early or acute and late or delayed. Acute complications are often associated with effects upon the bowel or bladder. The intestinal mucosa is particularly sensitive to radiation and most patients experience diarrhoea during treatment. If the diarrhoea is severe or associated with pain or nausea there is a possibility of significant bowel damage and treatment may be stopped or doses reduced. Antidiarrhoeal medication is successful in most cases. Acute reaction cystitis or haematurea can occur; any urinary tract infection should be excluded. Most acute reactions will settle down 2–3 weeks following completion of the treatment.

Long term complications will be suffered by 5–10% of women. These complications may develop any time following treatment but most commonly occur 1–2 years after completion. Symptomatic patients should be investigated for the presence of recurrent disease but radiation complications also need to be

recognized and treated appropriately, without the need for constant biopsy and EUA.

Late complications include bowel obstruction, radiation cystitis and bleeding, fistulae formation and vaginal stenosis. Bowel obstruction may respond to conservative treatment, primarily resting the bowel. Teaching patients to recognize and manage bouts of subacute obstruction and cystitis will help them to cope. Surgical correction is possible where other options have failed. Radiation necrosis can result in fistulae formation and perforation. Surgery may be the only management option, necrotic fistulae rarely heal spontaneously. Patients can become very ill, and even die, from such complications. Prompt and appropriate treatment by doctors and nurses familiar with managing radiation complications is vital.

Trauma to the vaginal epithelium caused by radiotherapy can lead to reduced lubrication and dyspareunia. As the vagina heals, scar tissue forms, with a loss of the ability to stretch during sexual intercourse, more specifically penetrative sex. Women postpelvic radio-therapy, especially brachytherapy, need to be sexually active or use a vaginal dilator to keep the vagina satis-factorily patent. In women with severe vaginal steno-sis, surgical reconstruction or release may be possible but the risk of fistulae formation is high. Following the procedure, these women then need to maintain the patency of the vagina by having regular sexual inter-course or using vaginal dilators. Some gynaecological oncologists recommend the use of vaginal dilators in women who are not sexually active to facilitate follow-up examinations of the vaginal vault. Vaginal douch-ing is also recommended by some specialist units but there seems to be little conclusive evidence to support this form of management.

Any surgery in the postradiotherapy patient is diffi-cult, especially where the problems are treatment related. Such surgery should be considered carefully and undertaken by a surgeon familiar with operating in such circumstances. The success rates and possible further complications needs to be explored with the patient.

Chemotherapy

To date, only surgery and radiotherapy have the potential to provide a cure in cervical cancer. Improving survival rates and acceptability of treat-ment is a constant aim of researchers. Chemotherapy has been used in many clinical trials, prior to surgery or radiotherapy, during radiotherapy, and after surgery and/or radiotherapy. Many different chemo-therapy agents have been used including cisplatin, ifosfamide, methotrexate, bleomycin and etoposide.

The ability of radiotherapy to cure locally advanced tumours is, in part, dependent upon the size of the tumour. Cisplatin-based chemotherapy has been used successfully as a radiosensitizer in locally advanced cervical cancer (Rose et al 1999). Cisplatin appears to enhance the effects of radiation, inhibiting the repair of cancer cell damage, sensitizing hypoxic cells, reducing the bulk of the tumour and encouraging reoxygenation. Many units have now adopted the recommendations of this research and cisplatin-based chemotherapy is routinely being given concomitantly with radiotherapy.

Advanced disease and disease recurrence

Despite the success of primary treatment for cervical cancer, there remain a number of women for whom treatment will not provide a cure. Recurrence or persist-ence of cervical cancer is disheartening. The clinical pre-sentation is varied and often insidious. Vaginal bleeding, vaginal discharge, pain, lymphoedema, weight loss, per-sistent cough are all signs to be investigated. Potentially curative and palliative treatment can be offered.

Radiation therapy

In women who present with disease outside the pelvis (stage IVb), radiation therapy can be effective in reliev-ing symptoms: controlling bleeding, discharge and pain. Pelvic recurrence following surgery alone can be treated effectively with radiotherapy in patients where the disease recurs centrally. It is not possible to retreat the pelvis with radiotherapy once a radical dose has been given and radiation therapy is therefore not an option in women who have had primary radiotherapy. When the disease occurs outside a previously irradi-ated field then radiation may be successful in provid-ing local control and symptom relief.

Surgery

Surgery can be performed when disease recurs despite previous treatment with radiotherapy, with or without surgery. Pelvic exenteration is a surgical option when the disease recurs centrally, is mobile and there is no evidence of disease spread outside the pelvis or to the pelvic side wall. The patient is assessed very carefully preoperatively for any disease spread. Biopsies can be taken during the operation and **frozen-sectioned**. If the frozen sections are positive then the operation is abandoned or modified for symptom control. Total pelvic exenteration involves the removal of the uterus, tubes and ovaries (if not previously removed) together with the vagina, bladder and rectum. Anterior exenter-ation involves removal of the uterus, anterior vagina and the bladder with preservation of the rectum. A posterior exenteration involves the removal of the uterus, posterior vagina and rectum with preservation of the bladder. There will be resultant single or double stoma formation depending upon the procedure. The operation has huge implications for the patient physi-cally, socially and psychologically and should be undertaken only after full counselling has been given.

Chemotherapy

Response rates of up to 48% have been seen in patients given chemotherapy for advanced or recurrent disease but this is rarely curative. In general, the response is limited to between 4 and 10 months but may provide good symptom control during that time. Cisplatin and ifosfamide are the two drugs most commonly used.

PAIN

Pain is one of the most feared aspects of **terminal** cancer. In cervical cancer over 70% of women with advanced disease will experience unrelieved cancer pain. The pain picture may be a complex one and involve many and multiple types of pain:

- sacral, aching low back pain, which may indicate bony infiltration
- lumbar and sacral plexopathy, which may reflect nerve infiltration
- direct pressure or distension or fistulae development with excoriation from bodily fluids
- treatment-related pain from surgery, radiotherapy or chemotherapy.

A good assessment is fundamental in the management of pain. The assessment will facilitate the use of the most appropriate medication or strategy. It is very easy to attribute any pain in advanced disease to the cancer but there are many other causes of pain, e.g. constipation, urinary tract infection, chest infection, pressure sores, position, haemorrhoids and, most importantly, fear and anxiety.

The treatment of pain is completely dependent upon the cause but good nursing care can replace, or significantly enhance, medication. Intervention for pain control should always be monitored for effect. Pain caused by advanced cervical cancer can sometimes be very difficult to treat and may need referral to a specialist pain team.

NURSING MANAGEMENT

Nursing has a large and extending role to play in the management of women with cervical cancer.

Health education

Involvement in primary health education gives nurses the opportunity to inform women about the disease, the risk factors and protective measures, together with the role and effectiveness of the national screening programme.

Cervical screening

The national screening programme is being run by nurses in many areas. Practice nurses, family planning nurses, genitourinary nurses and acute care nurses are taking cervical smears within the programme and for women with specific complaints. The introduction of nurse colposcopists has allowed women to be seen with the continuity and support that nurses provide. Luesely (1996) has shown that nurses can achieve the same levels of skill and competence as medical personnel and that the addition of nurse colposcopists to the team greatly enhances the efficiency and quality of the service. It is now recognized that nurses can reduce waiting times and lists, are more cost-effective than doctors and provide better access (Paniagua 1997). Patient surveys have indicated the need for more information and support within the colposcopy department and nurses are in the best position to create a less formal relationship during colposcopy and to maintain that relationship as a permanent member of staff.

Nurse specialist

Clinical nurse specialists in gynaecological cancer are working closely with their medical colleagues to provide a more rounded, patient-centred approach to care. Rapid assessment clinics and follow-up clinics are being run independently by specialist nurses and nurse practitioners. Nurse specialists are well placed to support their patients through the cancer journey. Corney et al (1993), in a study of women postgynaecological cancer treatment, recommend the use of a nurse specialist/counsellor in the management of women with gynaecological cancer to reduce the level of psychological and sexual morbidity. Chemotherapy is increasingly being given by nurses, and specialist nurses in radiotherapy departments are also providing expert advice and support to patients, other nurses and healthcare professionals.

Palliative care

Palliative care has long been a nursing stronghold. Expert palliative care is now available for most patients in the UK, both in the acute and primary settings.

The nursing management of a woman with cancer of the cervix begins at the time of diagnosis. The impact of the disease upon the life of the woman and her family can not be overestimated.

Psychological care

A woman with cervical cancer has to deal with the emotional problems relating to a cancer diagnosis and the fear of death and disease. She has to face the prospect of infertility, loss of sexual function and the concept of a having a potentially sexually transmitted disease. She may suffer a sense of loss of control – control of what is happening within her body and control of her life in the face of medical intervention.

When planning treatment the multidisciplinary teams need to consider how best to enable the woman to cope with her disease, her treatment and the implications of both. The psychological support of patients comes in a variety of ways from a variety of people. Providing information enables patients to regain control. The British Association of Cancer United Patients (BACUP) provides a series of booklets that explain the nature of specific cancers, the various treatments, the medications, how to find support and how to cope. The 'Patient Picture' series of booklets provides a good visual aid to the anatomy, disease and treatment involved, which can be invaluable during a consultation. Nurses often have more time to spend with the patient to allow open discussion to take place where fears can be exposed and myths dispelled.

Sexuality

Sexuality is a fundamental part of the personality. The majority of women with cervical cancer will survive but over 90% have been reported as suffering some degree of sexual dysfunction (Anderson 1985). There are three main ways in which cancer influences sexuality and fertility: (i) the actual biological disease process; (ii) the physiological effects of treatment; and (iii) the overall psychological effects. Women need to be made aware of the sexual and reproductive implications of their disease and treatment. There are still many misconceptions around sex and fertility following disease or treatment. It is not uncommon to come across women who have not had sex since their operation because they thought they couldn't/shouldn't. Being comfortable to discuss sex and recognize sexual dysfunction as a potential problem gives the patient permission to tackle a traditionally taboo subject. Information or access to information should be offered to all patients. Patients can always refuse the information but may find it difficult to seek advice. Accurate information can reduce anxiety and allow the patient to make informed decisions.

Quality of life

Cure or prolongation of life was once considered the ultimate aim of healthcare professionals. Today, with an increasing elderly population and the control of disease with high technology, the notion of chronic illness, prolonged remission and maximal quality of life are key topics in cancer care. Hawthorn in 1993 describes a lack of consensus on the definition of quality of life but suggests the defining theme in the literature could be expressed as 'the degree of satisfaction with perceived life circumstances'. Quality of life has to be defined by the life in question whenever possible. Too often, healthcare professionals are overly concerned with outcome measures such as survival and disease-free intervals, while the patient and/or the family are afraid to speak out, or feel confused and powerless to make any significant decisions. All disrupted aspects of the patient's life can affect the quality of that life. Cancer, however, is not always a negative experience. Some women feel that it gives them a new direction in life – a positive way forward.

CONCLUSION

Cancer of the uterine cervix is on the decline. In its early stages, the disease is a very 'curable' cancer, although it presents the women it affects with a multitude of complex problems. Nurses are key players in screening, diagnosis, treatment and support and can significantly contribute to the management and care of these women and their families.

GLOSSARY

Adenocarcinoma: a cancer arising in glandular tissue.
Adjuvant treatment: a secondary treatment.
Aetiology: the study or science of the causes of disease, the cause of a specific disease.
Carcinoma: a cancer that develops from epithelial cells, the most common form of cancer.
Cytology: the study of cells.
Frozen section: a rapid way of examining tissue for urgent diagnosis.
Histology: the study of tissue.
Lymphoedema: swelling of a part of the body because the normal lymphatics have been blocked or destroyed.

Malignant: a tumour that is cancerous.
Metastasis: the spread of cancer from one part of the body to another.
Morbidity: the symptoms of effects of a disease or its treatment.
Mortality: death.
Neoplasm: new growth.
Pathology: the study of disease.
Terminal: the end, leading to death.
Tumour: a mass of swelling of tissue, may be malignant or benign (non-cancerous)

REFERENCES

Anderson BL 1985 Sexual function and psychological morbidity and improving quality of life for women with gynaecological cancer. Cancer 55(8):1835–1842

Anderson MC, Coulter CAE, Mason WP, Soutter WP 1997 Malignant disease of the cervix. In: Shaw RW, Soutter WP, Stanton SL (eds) Gynaecology, 2nd edn. Churchill Livingston, New York, ch 35, p 546

Brinton LA, Hammon RF, Huggins GR et al 1987 Sexual and reproductive risk factors for invasive squamous cell cervical cancer. Journal of the National Cancer Institute 79:23–31

Brown JV, Fu YS, Berek JS 1990 Ovarian metastases are rare in stage I adencarcinoma of the cervix. Obstetrics and Gynaecology 76:623

Corney RH, Crowther ME, Everett H, Howells A, Shepherd J 1993 Psychosexual dysfunction in women with gynaecological cancer following radical pelvic surgery. British Journal of Obstetrics and Gynaecology 100(1):73–78

Dargent D, Brun JL, Roy M, Mathevert P, Remy I 1994 La Trachelectomie elargie (T.E), une alternative a l'hysterectomie radicale dans le traitement des cancers infiltrants developpes sur la face externe du col uterin. Journal of Obstetrics and Gynaecology 2:285–292

Da Souza N, McIndoe A, Soutter WP, Krausz T, Chui KM, Hughes C, Mason WP 1998 The value of magnetic resonance imaging with an endocervical receiver coil in the preoperative assessment of stage I and IIa cervical neoplasia. British Journal of Obstetrics and Gynaecology 105(5):500–507

Harris RWC, Brinton LA, Cordwell RH et al 1980 Characteristics of women with dysplasia or carcinoma in situ of the cervix. British Journal of Cancer 42:359–369

Hawthorn H 1993 Measuring quality of life. European Journal of Cancer Care 2:77–81

Health Press Ltd 1997 Patient Pictures Gynaecological Oncology, Oxford

Luesely D 1996 A structured programme for colposcopy training. City Hospital NHS Trust, Birmingham

Paniagua H 1997 Are nurse practitioners a viable option? British Journal of Nursing 6(5):245

Papanicolaou GN and Traut HF 1943 Diagnosis of uterine cancer by the vaginal smear. Commonwealth Fund, New York

Rose PG, Bundy BN, Watkins EB, et al 1999 Concurrent cisplatin-based radiotherapy and chemotherapy for locally advanced cervical cancer. New England Journal of Medicine 340(15):1144–1153

Shepherd JH 1995 Staging announcement. FIGO staging of gynaecological cancers; cervical and vulval. International Journal of Gynaecological Cancer 5:319

Williams J 1886 Cancer of the uterus. Harveian Lectures for 1886. H K Lewis, London

Winkelstein W Jr 1990 Smoking and cervical cancer – current status. A review. American Journal of Epidemiology 131:945–957

FURTHER READING

Groenwald S, Frogge Hansen M, Goodman M, Yarbro Henkie C (eds) Cancer nursing: principles and practice, 5th edn. Jones and Bartlett, Massachusetts

Moore G (ed) Women and cancer: a gynecologic oncology nursing prospective, 1st edn. Jones and Bartlett, Massachusetts

Tschudin V (ed) Nursing the patient with cancer, 2nd edn. Prentice Hall, London

USEFUL ADDRESSES

CancerBACUP
  3 Bath Place, Rivington Street, London EC2A 3JR
  Tel: 020 7696 9003
Cancerlink
  11–21 Northdown Street, London N1 9BN
  Tel: 020 7883 2818 and
  9 Castle Street, Edinburgh EH1 2DP
  Tel: 0131 228 5557 and
  Asian Cancer Information Helpline
  0800 590415
Cancer Relief Macmillan Fund (CRMF)
  15–19 Britten Street, London SW3 3TZ
  Tel: 020 7351 7811
Cancer Support UK
  Diana PWMF Project, Royal Marsden Hospital,
  FREEPOST 14022, London SW3 6YT

COU-RAGE UK (Coalition for Unity in Radiotherapy Advice and Guidance)
  24 Lockett Gardens, Trinity, Manchester M3 6BJ
  Tel: 0161 839 4256
Hospice Information Service
  St. Christopher's Hospice, 51–59 Lawrie Park Road,
  Sydenham, London SE26 6DZ
  Tel: 020 8778 9252
Lympheodema Support Network
  St Luke's Crypt, Sydney Street, London SW3 6NH
  Tel: 020 7351 4480
Marie Curie Cancer Care
  89 Albert Embankment, London SE1 7TP
  Tel: 020 7599 7777
National Cancer Alliance
  PO Box 579, Oxford OX4 1LB
  Tel: 01865 793566

Institute of Psychosexual Medicine
11 Chandos Street, Cavendish Square, London W1M 9DE
Tel: 020 7580 0631
Relate
Herbert Gray College, Little Church Street, Rugby
CV21 3AP
Tel: 01788 573241

Women's Nationwide Cancer Control Campaign
Suna House, 128–130 Curtain Road, London EC2A 3AR
Tel: 020 7729 4688
Urostomy Association
Beaumont Park, Danbury, Essex CM3 4DE
Tel: 01245 224294

14

Cancer of the ovary

Hilary Hollis

Ovarian cancer is the most common and most lethal gynaecological cancer, with over 5000 women being diagnosed and 4000 dying each year in the UK (Cancer Research Campaign (CRC) 1991). Unfortunately, cancer of the ovary often goes unrecognized until it is at an advanced stage, consequently many women go on to die from their cancer; 72% of women with cancer of the ovary die within 5 years of diagnosis. With such poor long-term survival it is essential that an effective method for the early detection of ovarian cancer is identified and that more effective treatments are found. Research continues to focus on these areas to enable a better outcome for women with ovarian cancer in the future.

EPIDEMIOLOGY

Ovarian cancer is the seventh most common cancer in women in the world (Parkin et al 1988). The incidence of ovarian cancer is highest in industrialized countries, in particular Northern and Western Europe and North America, and lowest in India, Japan and China (CRC 1991). However, the incidence of ovarian cancer in second-generation Japanese women in North America has risen to match that of American women, suggesting that environmental factors play a part in its development. Within Europe, the UK has the highest incidence of ovarian cancer and Denmark the highest death rate, followed by the UK (CRC 1991).

Ovarian cancer is predominantly a disease of the older postmenopausal women, with 90% of cases occurring in women over the age of 45. The incidence rate for ovarian cancer shows a sharp increase from the age of 45, after which it steadily increases up to the age of 70 years when the rate begins to slightly decline, indicating that although the ovaries may no longer be functional they can still become cancerous (CRC 1991).

RISK FACTORS

A number of risk factors have been identified in the development of ovarian cancer and are summarised in Box 14.1. Reproductive factors associated with ovarian cancer risk are all linked to the issue of ovulation. Risk appears to be inversely related to the cumulative time that ovulation is suppressed during childbearing years, thus pregnancy, lactation and the use of oral contraceptives, which all prevent ovulation, protect against ovarian cancer. Conversely, there is an increased risk of ovarian cancer for the nulliparous woman and in early menarche and late menopause. Infertile women who have received fertility drugs may have an increased risk of ovarian cancer, but this link has yet to be firmly established (Whittmore et al 1992). Hysterectomy without oophorectomy or with unilateral oophorectomy and tubal ligation have been reported to reduce the risk of ovarian cancer (Neijt et al 1995).

With the incidence of ovarian cancer being higher in industrialized environments, a number of possible risk factors have been investigated including talcum powder, asbestos and diet. Women exposed to talcum powder and asbestos may have an increased risk of ovarian cancer as it appears that these substances can migrate up the genital tract to the ovaries and act as co-carcinogens. However, the association between these products and ovarian cancer remains controversial (Shoham 1994, Tzonau et al 1993). The link between diet and ovarian cancer is also not confirmed, with some supporting a link between a diet high in meat animal fats and protein, milk and eggs while others have failed to demonstrate this association (Yoder 1990).

Family history and the genetic predisposition to ovarian cancer is the single most significant risk factor. Three hereditary syndromes have been identified as:

- site-specific ovarian cancer syndrome: where women are only at risk of developing ovarian cancer
- breast ovarian syndrome: associated with a first degree relative who has breast and/or ovarian cancer
- the cancer family syndrome (Lynch II Syndrome): associated with ovarian, breast and colon cancer.

These syndromes may account for up to 10% of all cases of ovarian cancer. The transmission of these syndromes is via an autosomal dominant gene, which can be passed through either the female or male parent (Lynch et al 1991). Mutations in the BRAC1 gene are thought to be responsible for approximately 50% of familial ovarian cancer cases, but only 2 or 3% of all ovarian cancer, with a second gene BRAC2 also being linked with breast ovarian syndrome. As a result of the increased risk of developing ovarian cancer in such families, a Familial Ovarian Register was established in the UK in 1989, in close cooperation with a European registry founded at the same time. Registration of such families will provide more information on the familial distribution of ovarian cancer, provide greater understanding of the genetic basis of this disease and provide advice to women at high risk of ovarian cancer on the need for annual screening or prophylactic oophorectomy (CRC 1991).

An association between ovarian cancer and blood group A has been suggested due to reports of an excess of cases among blood group A women.

Ovarian cancer is more common in white Caucasian women from higher social classes and this may be related to delaying childbearing and having fewer children.

PATHOLOGY

The three major histological types of ovarian cancer are:

- epithelial tumours
- sex cord or stromal tumours
- germ cell tumours.

Box 14.1   Risk factors in cancer of the ovary

- Reproductive and endocrine factors:
  - oral contraceptive
  - pregnancy
  - infertility
  - late menopause
  - hysterectomy.

- Environmental and dietary factors:
  - talc in genital area
  - exposure to radiation
  - obesity.

- Genetic factors:
  - family history of ovarian cancer
  - breast cancer
  - cancer family syndrome
  - blood group.

- Demographic factors:
  - age
  - social class
  - ethnic origin.

Box 14.2 Classification of epithelial ovarian cancer

- Serous tumours
- Mucinous tumours
- Endometrioid tumours
- Clear cell (mesonephroid) tumours
- Brenner (transitional cell) tumours
- Mixed tumours
- Undifferentiated tumours
- Unclassified/miscellaneous tumours

Table 14.1 Survival rates for ovarian cancer by stage of disease at diagnosis

Stage	% surviving 3 years	% surviving 5 years
Stage I Growth limited to ovaries	80	73
Stage II Growth limited to pelvis	60	46
Stage III Growth extending to abdominal cavity	27	19
Stage IV Metastases to distant sites	10	<5

The most common histological type are epithelial tumours, which constitute 80–90% of all ovarian cancers. Sex cord tumours account for 6% and germ cell tumours account for the remaining 4% and occur most commonly in children and premenopausal women (Walczak et al 1997). Epithelial tumours can be further classified according to cell type (see Box 14.2). Epithelial tumours will be the main focus of this chapter, with the treatment of sex cord and germ cell ovarian cancers discussed at the end of the chapter. Each of these tumour types can be subdivided according to their malignant potential into benign tumours, borderline malignancy or low malignant potential (LMP) and malignant tumours. Epithelial ovarian tumours of LMP account for 15% of such tumours, carrying with them a more favourable prognosis whatever the stage at presentation (Walczak et al 1997). Malignant epithelial ovarian cancers are graded histologically into three groups:

- grade 1: well differentiated
- grade 2: moderately differentiated
- grade 3: poorly differentiated.

Well differentiated epithelial ovarian cancers are more often associated with an earlier stage of the disease (Blake et al 1998).

SCREENING

Five-year survival rates and stage at diagnosis suggest that early detection may improve survival (Table 14.1), however less than 20% of women present with a tumour confined to the ovaries (stage Ia or Ib). In order to diagnose ovarian cancer at an early stage a suitable screening test that can be incorporated into a comprehensive screening programme needs to be identified. Whilst several screening tests for ovarian cancer are available, to date, no screening programme has been established (Box 14.3).

Box 14.3 Problems in screening in ovarian cancer (adapted from Austoker 1994)

- Lack of evidence that early detection through screening reduces mortality.
- Lack of understanding of how ovarian cancer develops.
- No one test has high enough sensitivity and specificity to screen for early ovarian cancer, but current research indicates combining tests as the way forward.
- Lack of evidence demonstrating the benefits of screening against possible harm.
- Lack of evidence of the acceptability of the current tests to the general population.
- Inability at present to determine a high-risk population suitable for screening.

A suitable screening test for ovarian cancer needs to be acceptable to the women being tested, sensitive, specific, cost-effective and lead to a reduction in mortality. In addition, an effective treatment for the cancer, if detected, needs to available. A number of screening tests have been considered over the last 10 years for ovarian screening, including bimanual pelvic examination, antigen marker CA 125 (normal < 35 U/ml), abdominal ultrasonography and transvaginal ultrasonography. However, studies considering these methods have been uncontrolled and composed of small, self-selected samples (Austoker 1994). More recently, Doppler colour flow imaging has been used with transvaginal ultrasonography to attempt to distinguish between benign and malignant ovarian tumours (Bourne et al 1993), new serum antigen markers such as OVX 1 (Woolas et al 1993) have been identified and genetic markers are being investigated.

Evidence indicates that screening by bimanual pelvic examination should not be routinely performed in general practice on asymptomatic women because it has low sensitivity and specificity when used alone (Austoker 1994). Transvaginal ultrasonography has advantages over abdominal ultrasonography in that a full bladder is not required and a more precise picture is produced due to the proximity to the ovary, with the possibility of improved sensitivity. However, it is a more invasive procedure. Doppler colour flow imaging appears to be a useful secondary procedure in women found to have enlarged ovaries at ultrasound screening, improving specificity (Bourne et al 1993).

Whilst no single screening test is either specific or sensitive enough to detect ovarian cancer, combining tests may prove to be the way forward. The screening tests that currently show the most promise are serum CA 125 and new markers such as OVX 1, ultrasound scanning and colour Doppler flow imaging. Currently, clinical trials are combining tests to improve detection with the National Cancer Institute in their Prostate Lung Colorectal and Ovarian (PLCO) study combining clinical examination, CA 125 and ultrasound (Kramer et al 1993); a randomized trial by the European Randomized Trial of Ovarian Cancer Screening (ERTOCS) in which patients are randomized to either a control group or transvaginal ultrasound at intervals of 1.5 or 3 years followed by Doppler colour flow if abnormalities are

detected at ultrasound; and the Ovarian Cancer Screening Unit at the Royal Hospitals Trust testing initially for CA 125 and OVX 1 followed by ultrasound if abnormalities are detected (Jacobs et al 1991, Study Protocol 1995). It is hoped that these trials will demonstrate reductions in mortality at acceptable cost levels to enable early detection through screening to be offered to asymptomatic women in the future.

CLINICAL PRESENTATION

There may be minimal or no symptoms at presentation in early ovarian cancer and symptoms are often non-specific in advanced ovarian cancer. The commonly cited symptoms are abnormal vaginal bleeding, abdominal distension, abdominal pain, urinary frequency, constipation, nausea, loss of appetite and dyspepsia. These non-specific complaints can be attributed to other causes, such as stress and midlife changes, so may not be investigated or attributed initially to ovarian cancer. Macmillan Cancer Relief have produced a leaflet entitled *Staying well*, which highlights the symptoms that can indicate ovarian cancer, provides useful contact numbers and can be used to provide easy-to-understand information for women on gynaecological health.

Case study: Pam

Pam, a 56-year-old junior school teacher, had been experiencing abdominal discomfort, weight gain, indigestion, fatigue and occasional nausea for 2 months. She believed her symptoms were related to stress at work and her increasing age and only went to her GP when the pain became so bad that she could no longer go to work. Pam explained that she had also been badly constipated. She did not want to make a fuss and felt very embarrassed. Her GP suggested that the constipation could account for her discomfort and prescribed some laxatives and discussed her diet. However, the pain persisted despite the constipation resolving so she returned to the GP, who then performed a rectal examination and discovered a pelvic mass. Pam was referred to her District General Hospital where further tests, including a CA 125, CT (computed tomography) scan, full blood count and serum biochemistry were carried out. The CT scan showed two large masses and her CA 125 was raised to 904 units/ml (normal <35 units/ml). Pam's care was then taken over by the gynaecologist at the hospital, who had a special interest in gynaecological cancers and a laparotomy was performed. During her laparotomy, Pam underwent a hysterectomy, salpingo-oophorectomy, omentectomy and

removal of other masses outside these organs. Peritoneal washings were obtained and a thorough examination of pelvis and its contents were made, with biopsies when necessary. Pam was diagnosed with stage IIIc ovarian cancer and, following this debulking surgery, was referred to the clinical oncologist for chemotherapy treatment. Pam did not want to enter a clinical trial so, following a GFR, was treated with six courses of carboplatin to an AUC of 6 every 4 weeks. She received granisetron 2 mg orally to prevent nausea and vomiting and dexamethasone 8 mg intravenously, with further oral antiemetics when required. She experienced one episode of neutropenia on course 5, when her treatment had to be delayed by 1 week, was severely fatigued and so did not return to work whilst receiving treatment, but otherwise tolerated her treatment well. She was, however, very concerned about resuming sexual intercourse following her surgery and was seen by the gynaecology nurse specialist to help her discuss and attempt to resolve the issues of sexuality that concerned her. By the end of her treatment her CA 125 had returned to normal and she was followed-up in a combined outpatient clinic by the gynaecologist and oncologist.

Women with suspected ovarian cancer should undergo the following investigations prior to laparotomy:

- haematological and biochemical blood tests, including a full blood count and liver and renal function
- clinical examination
- CA 125 tumour markers, which is elevated in 80–85% of epithelial ovarian cancers
- chest X-ray, to observe for pleural effusions or parenchymal metastases.

Other investigations that may be performed if indicated include barium enemas to exclude a gastrointestinal primary and liver, lung, bone and brain X-rays or scans if metastases are suggested, although spread to these sites normally occurs late, with most women dying whilst the disease is still confined to the peritoneal cavity. Metastatic spread in epithelial ovarian cancer normally occurs in the following sequence in the contralateral ovary, small bowel, large bowel, omentum, diaphragm, liver capsule, pleural cavity, bone or brain.

Staging

The staging of ovarian cancer is based upon the findings at laparotomy, which requires the surgeon, using a midline abdominal excision extending above the umbilicus, to:

- evaluate by palpation and inspection all intra-abdominal surfaces and organs, taking biopsies where necessary
- explore the retroperitoneal spaces to evaluate lymph nodes and resect when required
- aspirate ascites or collect peritoneal washings
- remove the ovarian tumour and, in most cases, perform a total abdominal hysterectomy, bilateral salpingo-oophorectomy and omentectomy.

The disease is staged from the surgical findings using the International Federation of Gynaecology and Obstetrics (FIGO) system (Box 14.4), a surgical system that makes accurate laparotomy findings essential, as future treatment is based on the stage of disease. Young et al (1983) identified that understaging is a common problem, which highlights the need for specialist gynaecological oncology surgeons to undertake such procedures to ensure that adequate and accurate staging occurs.

SURGICAL TREATMENT

Surgery remains the primary diagnostic and therapeutic procedure for ovarian cancer. Surgery for epithelial

---

Box 14.4 Cancer of the ovary stages using the International Federation of Gynaecology and Obstetrics (FIGO) system

Stage I	Growth limited to the ovaries
Stage Ia	Growth limited to one ovary; no ascites; no tumour on the external surfaces; capsule intact
Stage Ib	Growth limited to both ovaries; no ascites; no tumour on the external surfaces; capsule intact
Stage Ic*	Tumour either stage Ia or stage Ib, but with tumour on the surface of one or both ovaries, or with capsule ruptured, or with ascites present containing malignant cells, or with positive peritoneal washings
Stage II	Growth involving one or both ovaries with pelvic extension
Stage IIa	Extension and/or metastases to the uterus and/or tubes
Stage IIb*	Tumour either stage IIa or IIb but with tumour on the surface of one or both ovaries, or with capsule(s) ruptured, or with ascites present containing malignant cells, or with positive peritoneal washings
Stage III	Tumour involving one or both ovaries with peritoneal implants outside the pelvis and/or retroperitoneal or inguinal nodes; superficial liver metastasis equals stage III; tumour is limited to the true pelvis but with histologically proven malignant extension to small bowel or omentum
Stage IIIa	Tumour grossly limited to the true pelvis with negative nodes but with histologically confirmed microscopic seeding of abdominal peritoneal surfaces
Stage IIIb	Tumour involving one or both ovaries with histologically confirmed implants of peritoneal surfaces; none exceeding 2 cm in diameter; nodes are negative
Stage IIIc	Abdominal implants greater than 2 cm in diameter and/or positive retroperitoneal or inguinal nodes
Stage IV	Growth involving one or both ovaries with distant metastases; if pleural effusion present, there must be positive cytology to allot a case to stage IV; parenchymal liver metastases equals stage IV

*To assess the impact of prognosis of the different criteria for allotting cases to stage Ic or stage IIb it is of value to know whether the source of malignant cells was (i) peritoneal washings or (ii) ascites and whether rupture of the capsule was spontaneous or caused by the surgeon.

---

ovarian cancer falls into two categories – primary surgery and secondary surgery, which are further subdivided (Box 14.5).

> **Box 14.5** The categories of surgery for epithelial ovarian cancer. (Adapted from Neijt et al 1995.)
>
> - Primary surgery
>   - staging laparotomy
>   - cytoreductive or debulking surgery
>   - conservative surgery.
>
> - Secondary surgery
>   - intervention or interval debulking surgery
>   - second-look laparotomy
>   - secondary cytoreduction
>   - palliative surgery.

Primary surgery

Staging laparotomy

This was described on page 233, when considering staging for ovarian cancer

Cytoreductive or debulking surgery

Cytoreductive surgery is undertaken to reduce the tumour burden prior to treatment with chemotherapy or radiotherapy and aims to remove all the primary tumour and, when possible, all metastatic disease. If complete resection is not possible individual tumour sites should be reduced to the smallest possible, since the size of the remaining mass influences survival. Survival is increased if the remaining tumour masses are less than 1 cm in diameter (Griffths 1975) and further increased if they are less than 5 mm (Hacker et al 1983). During cytoreduction, bowel resection may become necessary to remove tumour but should be reserved for women in whom nearly all other tumour can be removed.

Conservative surgery

In some early stage ovarian cancers, unilateral salpingo-oophorectomy, partial omentectomy and peritoneal washings are possible, thus preserving fertility. Trimbos et al (1991) demonstrated that disease-free survival in stage I and IIa grade 1 women was 100% after careful staging and 88% without complete surgical staging.

Nevertheless, these women should be advised to have the remaining ovary and uterus removed on completion of their family and, if this is not done, close follow-up is necessary.

Secondary surgery

Intervention or interval cytoreductive/debulking surgery

Residual irresectable tumour may remain after primary cytoreductive surgery. If the residual tumour responds to chemotherapy, further surgery can be attempted to improve survival. This is called intervention or interval cytoreduction/debulking surgery. The survival benefits of such surgery have yet to be firmly established but some unexpected results from a prospective randomized trial carried out by the European Organization on Research and the Treatment of Cancer (EORTC) has led to further studies considering this type of surgical management for ovarian cancer. Whereas earlier studies (Jacobs et al 1991, Redman et al 1994) suggest that interval cytoreductive/debulking surgery does not improve survival, the EORTC trial demonstrated a median survival benefit of 5–6 months and survival at 3 years increased by up to 20% in those undergoing interval cytoreduction/debulking surgery (Van der Berg et al 1995). Following from this, a new trial has been proposed by the Medical Research Council (MRC) Gynaecological Cancer Working Party OVO6, which hopes to confirm or refute the findings from the EORTC study by randomizing women with residual ovarian cancer of > 1 cm to have either chemotherapy alone or chemotherapy and interval cytoreduction/debulking surgery by a surgeon with specialist expertise in gynaecological oncological surgery after the third cycle of chemotherapy. The future of this treatment option depends on this and any similar studies which are undertaken.

Second-look laparotomy

First described in 1957, this is a laparotomy that is undertaken to determine whether a woman who appears to have a complete clinical response following treatment is surgically and pathologically free from disease. During this procedure, multiple biopsies and cytological samples are taken in an attempt to detect any residual disease remaining and, if the primary surgery was not complete, hysterectomy, salpingo-oophorectomy and omentectomy should be undertaken. Unfortunately, persistent disease is detected during 60% of second-look laparotomies and, even with a negative second-look laparotomy, up to 40% of ovarian cancers recur within 5 years (Podratz & Kinney 1993). This treatment therefore remains controversial, although some suggest that further prospective clinical trials are required in relation to salvage and consolidation therapy and overall survival.

Secondary cytoreduction

Secondary cytoreduction is undertaken on women with clinical evidence of recurrent ovarian cancer to reduce tumour bulk prior to salvage therapy. Like other surgical procedures it remains controversial, although evidence suggests that survival improves if only microscopic disease remains following secondary cytoreduction, but this is also dependent upon the effectiveness of second-line treatments (Hoskins 1993).

Palliative surgery

Palliative surgery usually involves surgery to relieve bowel obstruction and should aim to improve the patient's quality of life. The decision to undertake such surgery should follow careful consideration of the woman's condition and possible outcomes on the woman's quality and quantity of life.

CHEMOTHERAPY

Chemotherapy plays an important role in the treatment of ovarian cancer following surgery. The role of adjuvant chemotherapy in early stage ovarian cancer is being explored. While the role of chemotherapy in advanced ovarian cancer is accepted, what constitutes optimal chemotherapy for advanced ovarian cancer has yet to be established, with chemotherapy schedules varying both nationally and internationally. The chemotherapy agents

---

Box 14.6 Chemotherapeutic drugs active in the treatment of ovarian cancer

Alkylating drugs
Melphalan
Chlorambucil
Cyclophosphamide
Ifosfamide
Treosulfan

Antimetabolites
5-Fluorouracil
Methotrexate

Cytotoxic antibiotics
Doxorubicin

Plant alkaloids
Etoposide
Paclitaxel
Doxetaxol
Topotecan

Others
Hexamethylmelamine
Cisplatin
Carboplatin

Table 14.2 Selected chemotherapy regimens used in the treatment of epithelial and germ cell ovarian cancer

Regimen	Schedule
Epithelial ovarian cancers	
Carboplatin	AUC factor of 5–9 i.v., repeat every 3 weeks
Taxol	175 mg/m^2 i.v., repeat every 3 weeks
CAP	
cyclophosphamide	500 mg/m^2 i.v.
doxorubicin	50 mg/m^2 i.v.
cisplatin	50 mg/m^2 i.v., repeat every 3 weeks
CP	
carboplatin	AUC 5 i.v.
paclitaxel	175 mg/m^2 i.v., repeat every 3 weeks
PC	
cisplatin	75 mg/m^2 i.v.
cyclophosphamide	750 mg/m^2 i.v., repeat every 3 weeks
Germ cell tumours	
BEP	
bleomycin	30 units i.v. days 1, 8 and 15
etoposide	120 mg/m^2 i.v. days 1–5
cisplatin	20 mg/m^2 i.v. days 1–5, repeat every 3 weeks

active in the treatment of ovarian cancer and regimens commonly used in the UK to treat ovarian cancer can be found in Box 14.6 and Table 14.2.

Adjuvant chemotherapy

Whether adjuvant chemotherapy provides a survival advantage over surgery alone as an initial treatment for early stage ovarian cancer has yet to be determined. In order to answer this the International Collaborative Ovarian Neoplasm (ICON) 1 trial has been designed and in the UK is coordinated by the MRC Gynaecological Cancer Working Party. By randomizing women diagnosed with ovarian cancer and in whom the need for chemotherapy is uncertain to receive either immediate platinum-based chemotherapy or to delay treatment until indicated, may resolve this question. This trial is ongoing and, as more patients are recruited, data will be available to provide a definitive answer to this important question.

Advanced ovarian cancer

First-line treatment

The treatment of advanced ovarian cancer in the UK prior to the introduction of platinum agents (cisplatin and carboplatin) was by a single alkylating agent, for example melphalan, cyclophosphamide or treosulfan. The use of single alkylating agent therapy today would be regarded as suboptimal treatment, with a response rate of only 20–30%, except in the treatment of occasional elderly patients with ovarian cancer who are not fit enough to be treated with platinum agents.

Since the introduction of platinum agents there has been a tendency in the UK to use single agent platinum and the most widely used first-line treatment is single agent carboplatin. In Europe and the USA platinum agents are more commonly combined initially with cyclophosphamide or/and doxorubicin and, more recently, with paclitaxel (Taxol). Whilst it is generally believed that platinum is the most active single agent, evidence to support the addition of other chemotherapeutic agents continues to be gathered (see Case Study 14.1).

In an overview analysis of 45 trials, the Advanced Ovarian Cancer Trialist Group (1991) suggested that there was a small but significant survival advantage in platinum combination therapy over single agent therapy, and the Ovarian Cancer Meta-Analysis Project (1991) suggested that the addition of doxorubicin to cisplatin and cyclophosphamide may result in a further survival advantage. However, the recent MRC ICON 2 study comparing single agent carboplatin versus CAP (cyclophosphamide, doxorubicin and cisplatin) showed no evidence of a difference between these two treatments in terms of progression-free or overall survival (MRC Trials Office, Cancer Meeting Report 1997).

More recently, the role of paclitaxel as first-line treatment in advanced ovarian cancer has been investigated. The Gynaecologic Oncology Group reported on a randomized trial (GOG#111) of approximately 400 women with advanced ovarian cancer and residual disease larger than 1 cm after initial surgery, who received either paclitaxel and cisplatin or cyclophosphamide and cisplatin. The results demonstrated that while the occurrence of surgically verified complete responses was similar in the two groups, improved progression-free survival (median 18 versus 13 months) and overall survival (median 38 versus 13 months) was seen in women receiving paclitaxel and cisplatin (McGuire et al 1996). It should be noted that paclitaxel was administered as a 24-h infusion rather than the 3-h infusion commonly used in the UK. More recent results presented at the American Society of Clinical Oncology (ASCO) in 1998 by a collective of European and Canadian investigators appear to support the findings of GOG#111, showing

that 680 women treated with cisplatin plus paclitaxel survived for a median of 35 months compared to 25 months for women treated with cisplatin and cyclophosphamide (Stuart et al, abstract from ASCO, 1998). The length of time over which the paclitaxel was administered was not identified. In addition, the data on quality of life and cost-effectiveness of these two regimens has yet to be ascertained, but is essential if the most active regimens with the least toxicity are to be used for large populations on a cost-effective basis (Blake et al 1998).

The MRC Gynaecological Cancer Working Party has set up the ICON 3 study to compare paclitaxel plus carboplatin with single agent carboplatin or CAP, to determine whether the addition of paclitaxel offers any benefit over current UK standard treatment. As more studies are undertaken, the role of paclitaxel in the management of ovarian cancer will become clearer.

Second-line treatment

Despite improvements in the treatment of advanced ovarian cancer with surgery and chemotherapy, the majority of these women relapse and die of their cancer. At present there is no agreed second-line treatment for women relapsing with advanced ovarian cancer. With many women in the UK receiving carboplatin as first-line treatment, the options on relapse are either to retreat with carboplatin or use a cisplatin-based treatment provided there was an interval of 6 months from the last treatment. Overall response rates to second-line platinum-based treatments of ovarian cancer is 20–30% (Gershenson et al 1989), with the probability of a second response being greater the longer the relapse-free period. The benefits of using paclitaxel rather than re-treating with platinum-based chemotherapy in women who relapse 6 or more months after their initial treatment remains unclear, although the MRC Gynaecological Cancer Working Party in the ICON 4 study aims to clarify this by comparing paclitaxel and platinum with conventional platinum-based chemotherapy for women with relapsed ovarian cancer. However, for women relapsing within 6 months of first-line platinum-based treatments, or with disease progressing whilst receiving platinum-based treatments (that is, resistant to platinum), an alternative chemotherapeutic agent is required and paclitaxel is active in these circumstances, with response rates of 20–30%.

With the increased use of paclitaxel in combination with platinum, other chemotherapeutic agents are being identified for use as second-line treatment in advanced ovarian cancer. One such drug is topotecan, which is now licensed for use after failure of first-line or subsequent treatment.

Chemotherapy administration

Much of the administration of chemotherapy in specialist cancer centres is undertaken by nursing staff in both daycare units and wards. The administration of platinum agents and taxanes will be described, together with the side-effects nurses need to be aware of when caring for women receiving chemotherapy.

Cisplatin. This was the first platinum compound to be developed and was found to be the most active drug for the treatment of ovarian cancer. However, it causes a number of side-effects, including severe nausea and vomiting, nephrotoxicity, electrolyte imbalance, ototoxicity, neurotoxicity, allergic reactions and mild myelosuppresion, which has led to its less frequent use since the development of carboplatin with its superior toxicity profile.

Within the UK, cisplatin is found in the CAP regimen, which consists of cyclophosphamide, adriamycin and cisplatin, or in combination with paclitaxel. The cisplatin dose usually used is $50–100 \ mg/m^2$.

The administration of cisplatin reflects it toxicities, with renal function requiring monitoring throughout the treatment period. Prehydration with normal saline is required and mannitol should be administered prior to the cisplatin to force diuresis and ensure a urine output of at least 100 ml/h. As it causes severe nausea and vomiting, a serotonin (5-hydroxytryptamine; 5-HT_3) antagonist – granisetron, ondansetron or tropisetron together with dexamethasone – needs to be administered. Following the administration of the cisplatin as an infusion over 2 h, further posthydration with normal saline is required. Electrolytes, including potassium chloride and magnesium sulphate, need to be added to the hydration to prevent imbalances occurring. Box 14.7 outlines a typical administration schedule. Further antiemetics will be required to control cisplatin-induced nausea and vomiting, which can continue for 24–48 h after administration.

Carboplatin. This is an analogue of cisplatin that was developed in an attempt to find an equally active but less toxic drug. Unlike most chemotherapy agents, where dose is calculated according to surface area of the patient, carboplatin dosage is calculated on the basis of glomerular filtration rate because it is excreted predominantly unchanged by the kidneys, with very little being metabolized. The glomerular filtration rate (GFR) can be calculated most accurately by ethylene-diaminetetraacetic acid (EDTA) clearance and renogram, but can also be calculated using measured creatinine clearance or the Cockcroft formula (see Box 14.8). The dose of carboplatin is calculated using the area under the curve (AUC) method described by Calvert et al (1989), where AUC refers to the area under the concentration versus time curve for carboplatin clearance. Thus:

$$\text{Dose in mg} = \text{Target AUC} \times (\text{GFR} + 25)$$

Box 14.8 The Cockcroft formula

$$\text{GFR based on calculated clearance} = \frac{1.05 \times (140 - \text{age}) \times \text{weight (kg)}}{\text{serum creatinine (mol/l)}}$$

For patients who have not received prior chemotherapy, the target AUC would be 7, with treatments every 4 weeks, and for patients receiving chemotherapy every 3 weeks the target AUC would be 5 to 6. In more elderly patients receiving 4-weekly treatment, the target AUC should be reduced intially to 5 to 6 and increased if well tolerated. Carboplatin is less nephrotoxic than cisplatin and the patient does not need to receive intravenous hydration pre- and post administration. Consequently, carboplatin can be administered as an outpatient treatment, being given as an intravenous infusion of 250–500 ml of 5% dextrose over 1 h. Although more expensive than cisplatin administration, costs are reduced because hospital admission is not required.

Side-effects described by a small sample of women receiving carboplatin for ovarian cancer include

---

Box 14.7 Administration schedule for Cisplatin

Prehydration
  1 litre of normal saline plus 10 mmol of magnesium sulphate, over 2 h
  1 litre of normal saline plus 40 mmol of potassium chloride, over 200 ml 2 h of mannitol 20% over 20 min (to ensure a urine output of >100 ml/h before starting cisplatin)

Chemotherapy
  1 litre of normal saline plus cisplatin $50–100 \ mg/m^2$, over 2 h

Posthydration
  1 litre of normal saline plus 10 mmol magnesium sulphate, over 2 h
  1 litre of normal saline plus 40 mmol potassium chloride, over 2 h

fatigue as the most common and troublesome, with nausea, difficulty sleeping, taste change and constipation also being severe (Buckingham et al 1997). Carboplatin is noted for its myelosuppression, in particular thrombocytopenia and leucopenia, however, it causes less vomiting, nausea and nephrotoxicity than cisplatin. Although uncommon, allergic reactions to carboplatin do occur. They include symptoms such as rashes, facial flushing, urticaria and bronchospasm, although they can be more severe and occasionally lead to anaphylaxis (Hendrick et al 1992). Mild to moderate reactions can be managed by the administration of corticosteroids and antihistamines.

Paclitaxel (Taxol). Paclitaxel originates from the bark of the Pacific Yew tree, although today it is produced synthetically from renewable resources. A number of administration schedules have been used, with a 24-h infusion being more common in the USA whilst in Europe a 3-h infusion is the norm. It is licensed for metastatic ovarian cancer where standard platinum-containing treatment has failed and the recommended dose is 175 mg/m^2. Its use is also being explored as first-line treatment in combination with carboplatin (ICON 3), as a single agent in women with stage IV ovarian cancer (Gore et al 1997) and in ovarian cancer that has relapsed after initial chemotherapy (ICON 4).

Paclitaxel has its own unique administration problems (Preston 1996). The main complications arise from the solution in which paclitaxel is made up, Cremorhor EL (polyethoxylated castor oil) being incompatible with PVC and causing leaching of plasticizers and the potential for hypersensitivity reactions. To overcome the first of these problems paclitaxel should be made up in the glass bottle supplied and administered via a non-PVC-containing giving set. In addition, a 0.22 micron filter must be incorporated in the line because a small number of fibres have been observed in the dissolved paclitaxel and an air inlet (either incorporated into the giving set chamber or a vent needle inserted into the bottle) is required to enable the bottle to empty (Preston 1996).

Hypersensitivity reactions, characterized by dyspnoea, hypotension, bronchospasm, urticaria and erythematous rashes, were found to occur in 41% of patients (Weiss et al 1990) treated with paclitaxel. Adequate premedication with corticosteroids, antihistamines and histamine receptor (H$_2$) antagonists reduces the risk of such reactions to approximately 2%, nevertheless, appropriate supportive equipment should be available and vital sign monitoring, particularly during the first hour, is recommended. Table 14.3 shows a premedication schedule for use with paclitaxel.

Table 14.3 Premedication for paclitaxel chemotherapy

Time before paclitaxel	Drug	Dose (mg)	Route
12 h	Dexamethasone	20	Oral
6 h	Dexamethasone	20	Oral
30 min	Chlorpheniramine	10	Intravenous
	Ranitidine	50	Intravenous
	or cimetidine	300	Intravenous

The side-effects most commonly observed in patients receiving paclitaxel are neutropenia, peripheral neuropathy and alopecia. Cardiac disturbances occur occasionally, and include conduction abnormalities, bradycardia, mild gastrointestinal upset, taste change, anorexia and mild fatigue.

New chemotherapeutic treatment

New chemotherapeutic agents, drug combinations, intraperitoneal administration and high-dose chemotherapy are all being explored in an attempt to improve survival for women with epithelial ovarian cancer. New chemotherapeutic agents being explored include gemcitabine, a pyramidine antimetabolite that has been found to have some activity in platinum-resistant disease: docetaxel (taxotere), a taxane drug that seems to have similar activity to paclitaxel, although whether it is as active as paclitaxel has yet to be established; and marimastat, which inhabits matrix metallaproteinases, enzymes that promote the spread and dissemination of solid tumours (Blake et al 1998). Preliminary clinical trials are currently investigating combining these new chemotherapy agents with more established drugs, such as carboplatin, cisplatin, cyclophosphamide and paclitaxel.

Intraperitoneal chemotherapy has been investigated as a method of treating ovarian cancer because it allows absorption of the chemotherapy agent locally and ovarian cancer can result in peritoneal disease without more widespread metastasis. Whilst further study is needed, Alberts et al (1996), in a randomized trial, demonstrated improved response and survival with intraperitoneal cisplatin and intravenous cyclophosphamide in stage III disease that had been optimally debulked. Interest is also being shown in administering paclitaxel as an intraperitoneal drug.

High-dose chemotherapy of cyclophosphamide, carboplatin and paclitaxel with peripheral stem cell infusion and granulocyte colony stimulating factor (GCSF) support to rescue the bone marrow from the haematological toxicity is also being explored in the

USA. Studies to date have not demonstrated any advantages, although this may be because patients with advanced disease were selected and the required dose intensity is not being achieved.

RADIOTHERAPY

Radiotherapy has limited use in women with ovarian cancer. Trials have been undertaken to determine the role of whole abdominal radiotherapy in both early stage and advanced disease and have concluded that, at present, there is no role for radiotherapy as part of any curative treatment. Intraperitoneal radioactive phosphorus (IP) has also been used to treat ovarian cancer, although clinical trials indicate no survival benefits to the patients (Young et al 1990). The side-effects of both whole abdominal radiotherapy and intraperitoneal radiotherapy include severe acute and chronic bowel problems.

Radiotherapy is used in palliative care, for example, to reduce a pelvic mass that is causing pressure symptoms and at sites of metastatic spread such as the bone or brain.

FURTHER TREATMENTS

In addition to chemotherapy and radiotherapy, other treatments that are being explored in relapsed ovarian cancer are hormonal therapy and immunotherapy.

Hormone treatments include the use of tamoxifen and goserelin (Zoladex), because oestrogen and progesterone receptors have been detected on ovarian tumours.

Immunotherapeutic approaches include the use of BCG (Bacille Calmette–Guerin) and alpha-interferon following chemotherapy to prolong response. Further clinical trials are needed to define the role of these treatments in ovarian cancer.

OVARIAN CANCER FOLLOW-UP

When complete remission has been achieved at the end of treatment, women with ovarian cancer require a period of follow-up to enable any relapse to be detected as early as possible and further treatment commenced. Ideally, women should be seen in joint clinics with the surgeon and oncologist. They should be followed up every 3 months for the first 2 years, every 4 months for the third year and every 6 months for the fourth and fifth years, with pelvic examinations and CA 125 at each visit. During follow-up, a rising CA 125 is thought to be the first indication of a relapse

and this rise may predate any other clinical evidence by several months. The knowledge that a women has a rising CA 125 but is otherwise well presents a treatment dilemma for the medical team, as at present there is no evidence that identification of the relapse site or early treatment increases survival. To try and resolve this question, the MRC has set up OVO5, a randomized trial in relapsed ovarian cancer. The aim is to identify whether early treatment with chemotherapy based on raised CA 125 alone, rather than chemotherapy based upon conventional clinical indicators, will improve symptom-free and overall survival and quality of life. Should this trial indicate no advantages, the use of CA 125 during follow-up will need to be reviewed.

PALLIATIVE CARE IN ADVANCED OVARIAN CANCER

The symptoms commonly associated with advanced ovarian cancer can be attributed to local disease in the pelvis and abdomen; to disease spread with the development of metastases, mainly in the liver and lungs and, more rarely, in the bone and brain; or to the treatment itself. The more common symptoms experienced by women with ovarian cancer include bowel obstruction, nausea and vomiting, ascites, renal failure resulting from obstruction of the ureters, anorexia and weight loss, dyspnoea, lymphoedema and, as in most advanced cancers, pain, with many of these symptoms being interrelated. The symptoms that will be considered further are bowel obstruction and ascites.

Bowel obstruction

Bowel obstruction is a well recognized and common complication of ovarian cancer, with presenting symptoms of nausea and vomiting, abdominal distension, constipation, colicky abdominal pain and anorexia. The onset of obstruction is usually by gradual insidious worsening of symptoms until they become continuous, but they can sometimes present as an acute event (Beattie et al 1989, Ripamonti 1994). The management of obstruction can be by surgical treatment or more conservative medical management.

Surgical management

Surgical management of bowel obstruction should always be considered, although in many cases it will be inappropriate. The decision to operate on a woman with advanced ovarian cancer should be carefully and individually assessed, taking into account poor prognostic factors including age and nutritional status, ascites, serum albumen, multiple partial bowel obstructions, previous radiotherapy to the pelvis, distant metastases and poor performance status. The most suitable candidate is the woman with limited disease, one point of obstruction and the option of further anticancer treatment in the future. Beattie et al (1989), in a retrospective study of bowel obstruction in 105 women with ovarian cancer, showed mean survival times of 211.4 days following surgery compared to 92.7 days following conservative management. Although this indicates improved survival following surgery, the authors do not address quality of life for these women. Overall survival following surgical intervention is usually months, operative mortality is high and complications are common, including wound infection and dehiscence, fistulae formation, sepsis, gastrointestinal bleeding, pulmonary embolism and deep vein thrombosis. Other surgically related treatment options include the use of nasogastric tube suction and intravenous fluids to maintain hydration prior to surgery while investigations are undertaken and treatment decisions are considered (Baines 1993). Prolonged use of such treatment is controversial as the placement of a nasogastric tube can often be distressing, with the tube causing discomfort and irritation for the patient, and symptoms can be managed using other measures such as gastrostomy tubes or pharmacological measures. The venting gastrostomy can be introduced by endoscope or percutaneously under ultrasound guidance and allows the stomach contents to be drained, thus relieving nausea and vomiting (Ashby et al 1991).

Medical management

The medical management of bowel obstruction centres around the symptoms of nausea, vomiting and pain.

Case study: Jean

Jean, a 68-year-old married woman with no children was admitted to hospital with recurrent abdominal ascites, severe nausea and vomiting. She had not opened her bowels for over 3 weeks. She had recommenced carboplatin chemotherapy treatment 3 months before but had unfortunately not responded to this course of treatment. Following discussion with the clinical oncologist, her husband and the clinical nurse specialist she decided that she did not want to receive any further treatment as she had felt extremely unwell whilst receiving her recent chemotherapy treatment. However, she wanted to have any medication that would relieve the symptoms that she was experiencing. She found having such a distended abdomen both uncomfortable and distressing, as she could no longer wear her normal clothes and felt very self-conscious that, as a mature woman, she looked as if she was 9 months pregnant. She was unable to keep any food or fluids down as she had a partially obstructed bowel. Her husband was extremely distressed at his wife's decision to stop treatment as he could not contemplate life without her after nearly 50 years of married life. Jean was referred to the palliative care consultant and seen by the palliative care nurse specialist. Her ascites was drained, although diuretics were not commenced at this stage as her vomiting made it impossible for her to tolerate them. A subcutaneous syringe driver containing cyclizine and diamorphine was commenced and her episodes of vomiting began to reduce. After 6 days in hospital she was transferred to the local hospice for continuation of her care.

Table 14.4 Antiemetic drugs used in bowel obstruction in ovarian cancer

Drug	Dose and route	Dose over 24 h subcutaneously
Cyclizine	50 mg t.d.s., p.o., s.c. or i.v.	150 mg/24 h
Methotrimeprazine	6.25–12.5 mg o.d. or b.d., p.o. or s.c.	25–150 mg/24 h
Hyoscine butylbromide (Buscopan)	20–40 mg t.d.s., s.c.	60–120 mg/24 h
Metoclopramide (in high obstruction)	10 mg t.d.s., p.o., s.c., or i.v.	60–240 mg/24 h

b.d., twice daily; i.v., intravenous; o.d., once a day; p.o., per os ; s.c., subcutaneous; t.d.s., three times a da

The use of a syringe driver to administer continuous subcutaneous analgesia and antiemetics has been found to be the most appropriate method for controlling these symptoms. The continuous abdominal pain of bowel obstruction will generally respond to diamorphine, whilst the colicky pain will require the addition of antispasmodics, usually hyoscine butylbromide and the cessation of use of metoclopramide, as it may cause or increase colic. Drugs with antiemetics effects used in bowel obstruction include cyclizine, methotrimeprazine and hyoscine; Table 14.4 indicates the typical doses and routes of administration. The use of octreotide, an analogue of somatostatin, is becoming more widespread in bowel obstruction where vomiting is difficult to control by standard drug treatment. It acts by decreasing the volume of gastrointestinal secretion and promotes the absorption of fluids and electrolytes from the bowel. It is administered subcutaneously, either as a bolus or by continuous infusion, with a starting dose of 0.3 mg over 24 h. This can be increased until the desired effect is obtained. Studies by Mercadante et al (1993) and Riley and Fallon (1994) both report the effectiveness of octreotide in controlling vomiting and improving quality of life for many patients.

Ascites

Ascites, which is defined as exudate into the peritoneal space due to malignancy, is present in up to 30% of women with ovarian cancer at diagnosis and up to 60% of women with ovarian cancer at death. The symptoms that commonly accompany ascites include abdominal distension and discomfort, dyspnoea, loss of appetite, nausea and vomiting, indigestion and ankle oedema (Regnard & Mannix 1989). The effects of these symptoms on the woman's daily activities and lifestyle, and the alteration of body image from abdominal distension, require treatment. The treatments available to control ascites include diuretic therapy, intraperitoneal therapy, repeated paracentesis and peritoneovenous shunts, with new strategies using breathing exercises and external pressure from an abdominal binder being investigated (Preston 1995).

The drainage of ascitic fluid under local anaesthetic can offer fast relief from the symptoms of ascites, although it can be uncomfortable for the patient and is only a temporary measure, with the fluid reaccumulating and successive paracentesis becoming more difficult to perform. Paracentesis carries the risk of bowel perforation and is most safely performed under ultrasound guidance. Repeated drainage of ascitic fluid may lead to protein depletion, hypotension and infection (Kehoe 1991). To control ascites and prevent reaccumulation, chemotherapy aimed at the active treatment of ovarian cancer can be employed, being administered systemically or into the peritoneal cavity. Intraperitoneal chemotherapy should be used only within the remit of clinical trials, as its benefits have yet to be proven and can lead to infection, chemical peritonitis, and side-effects from the chemotherapy drug used (Young et al 1996). The use of diuretics, commonly spironolactone with frusemide, may be effective in preventing reaccumulation of ascites but can result in dehydration with serum electrolyte imbalance and should be discontinued if no benefit occurs. The benefits of peritoneovenous shunts remain controversial and the potential risk of such devices are numerous, including fluid overload resulting in pulmonary oedema or heart failure, disseminated intravascular coagulation, infection and tumour cell infusion (Kehoe 1991) and complications of shunt malfunction are not uncommon. Its use in ovarian cancer when the prognosis is poor should be avoided.

Further research is required to find more effective methods of preventing reaccumulation of ascites. Also, both currently available treatments (and those under investigation, such as breathing exercises and abdominal binders) need to be evaluated to determine if they improve wellbeing and lifestyle (Preston 1995).

QUALITY OF LIFE AND CANCER TREATMENT

The diagnosis and subsequent treatment of ovarian cancer can result in distressing physical side-effects, sexuality problems and psychosocial difficulties such as anxiety, depression and fear of dying (Stegina & Dunn 1997). Whilst little is known about the quality of life (QOL) experienced by women with gynaecological cancers (Zacharias et al 1994) clinical trials such as the MRC's ICON trials are now increasingly incorporating QOL measures in their studies. To assess the degree to which a woman's QOL is changed as a result of her experience of cancer, a number of scales of performance status have been developed and QOL measurement instruments have been designed. Commonly used scales of performance status include those devised by Karnofsky and the World Health Organization (WHO; Box 14.9) and toxicity scales have been produced by the WHO and the Eastern Cooperative Oncology Group (ECOG) to assess the gravity of side-effects of treatment. QOL instruments commonly used in cancer care

---

Box 14.9 World Health Organization Performance Status

Grade	Performance status
0	Able to perform all normal activity without restriction
1	Restricted in physically strenuous activity but ambulatory, able to carry out light work
2	Ambulatory and capable of all self-care but unable to carry out work; up and about more than 50% of the waking hours
3	Capable of only limited self-care; confined to bed or chair more than 50% of waking hours.
4	Completely disabled; cannot carry out any self-care; totally confined to bed or chair

---

include the Rotterdam Symptom Distress scale, the Hospital Anxiety and Depression scale (HAD) and the EORTC Quality of Life questionnaire (Fallowfield 1990). Within the MRC ICON trials the WHO toxicity scales, HADS, Rotterdam or EORTC-QLQ are completed by the patient before, during and after treatment in an attempt to evaluate QOL before treatment, in addition to QOL following treatment. As yet, the data on QOL for women entering these trials has not been published.

PSYCHOSEXUAL IMPLICATIONS OF OVARIAN CANCER

Sexual dysfunction is common in women with gynaecological cancer, including ovarian cancer. Both the disease itself and the treatments required affect sexuality and may make sexual intercourse difficult – fatigue, nausea, diarrhoea, shortening of the vagina, tender scars, pain, alopecia and infertility, to name but a few, being common in women with ovarian cancer (Crowther et al 1994). Women need information, support and counselling on the effects of their treatment on physical, sexual and emotional aspects of their life and partners should be included in such discussions (Corney et al 1992). Research to date suggests that nurses find approaching and dealing with these sensitive and private issues difficult (Matacha & Waterhouse 1993, Webb 1988) and, although nurses identify sexuality as part of nursing practice, few address sexual concerns with their patients.

Whilst education for all healthcare professionals in relation to psychosexual issues is required in an attempt to meet women's needs in relation to issues of sexuality, specialist nurses with counselling training should be available in gynaecological oncology units. While the numbers of such specialist nurses are increasing, at present the level of support for women with gynaecological cancers may vary (Whyte 1997).

PATIENT INFORMATION

In *A Policy Framework for Commissioning Cancer Services* the Department of Health (DOH) (1995) identifies that patients, families and carers should be provided with clear information about treatment choices and outcomes at all stages of the cancer journey from diagnosis to palliative care. To meet this objective, the multidisciplinary team caring for the patient will need excellent communication skills to impart information in an easy-to-understand manner at a time when the patient may face fears and anxiety from their diagnosis of cancer and perceptions of cancer treatments. Ideally, verbal information should be supported in written form, and some centres will tape-record consultations and allow the patient to take the tape with them to listen to again. Written information is available at a local and national level, with departmental information packs and publications by organizations such as Cancer BACUP and Cancerlink on cancer of the ovary, cancer treatments and symptoms resulting both from the disease and the side-effects of treatment. Written information for patients entering clinical trials is required by ethics committees and many cancer centres will have a clinical trials nurse who coordinates research studies and spends time helping patients to decide whether they want to participate in clinical trials. A further source of information for patients is the internet, and organizations such as Cancer BACUP have a web site containing their publications. Medical centres such as the National Cancer Institute and Oncolink (from the University of Pennsylvania Cancer Center) providing easy internet access to much medical information. However, the wide availability of information on the internet can raise expectations and lead patients to seek treatments that may not be appropriate. Further information can be found in the list of useful addresses.

HEALTHCARE POLICY AND OVARIAN CANCER

Although the diagnosis of ovarian cancer may be made by a doctor who is not a cancer specialist, women with ovarian cancer should be managed in specialist cancer centres by a team with expertise in this area to ensure that they receive high quality, safe and effective treatment in line with the recommendations made by the DOH (1995). Studies conducted by a number of groups have show that care delivered by a gynaecologist resulted in better outcomes than care delivered by a general surgeon, and surgeons and physicians with special skills in gynaecological cancer should be available (DOH 1995). Likewise, nursing care for women with ovarian cancer should be planned and delivered by nurses with a postregistration cancer qualification. An English National Board course, ENB R16, Current Issues and Practice for Women with Gynaecological Cancer is available, plus allied courses such as the ENB 225, Gynaecological Nursing and the ENB 237, Cancer Nursing to provide specialist education for nurses in this field.

To enable women to gain access to such treatment, Cancer Relief Macmillan Fund have produced a leaflet *Gynaecological Cancers – How to help yourself*, which provides information on how to get the best care when diagnosed with a gynaecological cancer and outlines the six standards of care that have been agreed by the British Gynaecological Cancer Society and can be found in Box 14.10. These standards emphasise the need for a multidisciplinary approach to care, the availability of specialists for each treatment modality and the importance of information to enable the woman to participate in treatment decisions. In future, the NHS Executive plans to produce guidelines for purchasers for gynaecological cancers, as it has done for breast, colorectal and lung cancers. This will enable purchasers of health care to select services that provide care based on current clinical effectiveness.

Box 14.10 Standards of care for women with gynaecological cancer

Six key questions a women with gynaecological cancer should ask. 'Will I have…'
1. The opportunity of a prompt referral to a consultant-led team specializing in the diagnosis and treatment of gynaecological cancer?
2. Full discussion about the options, such as surgery, radiotherapy and chemotherapy, before treatment starts?
3. Surgery performed by a gynaecologist who has a special interest in gynaecological cancer?
4. Radiotherapy and chemotherapy undertaken by staff with a special interest in gynaecological cancer?
5. Access to a specialist nurse or counsellor and a symptom control (palliative care) team?
6. Information on support services for myself and my partner?

A further principle proposed by the DOH in their Policy Framework (1995) is that all patients should have access to uniformly high quality of care, wherever they live, to ensure the best possible cure rates. There is concern that as the evidence for the wider use of paclitaxel to improve quantity and quality of life mounts, it will not be funded by all purchasers. This situation already exists, with women in some areas having access to paclitaxel whilst in other areas this drug is not available. Mossman (1998) estimates that it would cost the average health authority only £250 000 to target every appropriate ovarian cancer patient.

NON-EPITHELIAL TUMOURS

Ten per cent of all ovarian tumours are non-epithelial, the most common being germ cell tumours and sex cord stromal tumours.

Germ cell tumours

Germ cell tumours can be divided into two main types – dysgerminomas and embryonal carcinomas which can form teratomas from embryonic cells or endodermal sinus tumours and choriocarcinomas from extra-embryonic cells. Germ cell tumours occur in young women and are rare, but need to be recognized at surgery so that conservative surgery can be undertaken to retain fertility. Further treatment with chemotherapy can be used to cure many of these women without affecting their chances of pregnancy. Surgical management consists of unilateral oophorectomy when possible, with further surgery if needed once the diagnosis is confirmed histologically. With bilateral tumours, some normal ovary should be preserved if possible to maintain hormone production and fertility.

These tumours are sensitive to both radiotherapy and chemotherapy; chemotherapy is the treatment of choice because it preserves fertility. Chemotherapy should be given to all patients except those with stage I teratoma, where follow-up with clinical examination, serum tumour markers and radiological review is required as the majority will not relapse. The chemotherapy of choice for all other stages is bleomycin, etoposide and cisplatin (BEP; Table 14.2). The tumour markers alpha-fetoprotein, beta-hCG (human chorionic gonadotrophin), lactate dehydrogenase and placental alkaline phosphatase should be measured (Blake et al 1998).

Sex cord stromal tumours

The most common sex cord stromal tumours are granulosa and theca cell tumours, which occur at any age but more often in postmenopausal women. The tumour produces hormones – mainly oestrogen – which can lead to endometrial hyperplasia or endometrial cancer. Staging and surgical treatment is the same as for epithelial ovarian cancer with chemotherapy being used to treat advanced or recurrent disease using regimens as for epithelial adenocarcinomas (Blake et al 1998).

Sertoli–Leydig cell tumours are the other type of sex cord stromal tumours but are extremely rare.

CONCLUSION

Most women with ovarian cancer are diagnosed with advanced disease as no effective method of screening is available to detect this cancer at an early stage. Further research is essential to identify a suitable screening test to help decrease the deaths from ovarian cancer. Treatment by surgery and chemotherapy using a platinum-based regimen has become standard although newer chemotherapy agents such as paclitaxel may improve survival in the future. However, it remains essential to identify the most effective treatment for ovarian cancer through clinical trials where both survival and quality of life are considered. When treatment does fail then palliative care with good management of the symptoms experienced is essential. Care by specialists in gynaecological oncology will ensure the highest quality of care, the maximum possible cure rates and the best quality of life.

REFERENCES

Advanced Ovarian Cancer Trialist Group 1991 Chemotherapy in advanced ovarian cancer: an overview of randomised clinical trials. British Medical Journal 303:884–893

Alberts DS, Liu PY, Hannigan EV et al 1996 Intraperitoneal cisplatin plus intravenous cyclophosphamide versus intravenous cisplatin plus intravenous cyclophosphamide for stage III ovarian cancer. New England Journal of Medicine 335,1950–1955

Ashby MA, Game PA, Devitt P et al 1991 Percutaneous gastrostomy as a venting procedure in palliative care. Palliative Medicine 5:147–150

Austoker J 1994 Screening for ovarian, prostatic, and testicular cancers. British Medical Journal 309:315–320

Baines M 1993 The pathophysiology and management of malignant intestinal obstruction. In: Doyle D, Hanks GWC & Macdonald N (eds) The Oxford textbook of palliative medicine. Oxford University Press, Oxford, ch 4.3.4, pp 311–316

Beattie GJ, Leonard RCF, Smyth JF 1989 Bowel obstruction in ovarian carcinoma: a retrospective review of the literature. Palliative Medicine 3:275–280

Blake P, Lambert H, Crawford R 1998 Gynaecological oncology: a guide to clinical management. Oxford University Press, New York, ch 2, pp 12–44

Bourne TH, Campbell S, Reynolds KM et al 1993 Screening for early familial ovarian cancer with transvaginal ultrasonography and colour blood flow imaging. British Medical Journal 306:1025–1029

Buckingham R, Fitt J, Sitzia J 1997 Patients' experiences of chemotherapy: side-effects of carboplatin in the treatment of carcinoma of the ovary. European Journal of Cancer Care 6:59–71

Calvert AH, Newell DR, Gumbrell LA et al (1989) Carboplatin dosage: prospective evaluation of a simple formula based on renal function. Journal of Clinical Oncology 7:1748–1756

Cancer Research Campaign 1991 Ovarian cancer – UK Factsheet 17.1. CRC, London

Corney R, Everett H, Howells A, Crowther M 1992 The care of patients undergoing surgery for gynaecological cancer: the need for information, emotional support and counselling. Journal of Advanced Nursing 17:667–671

Crowther ME, Corney RH, Shepherd JH 1994 Psychosocial implications of gynaecological cancer. British Medical Journal 308:869–870

Department of Health 1995 A policy framework commissioning cancer services. HMSO, London

Fallowfield L 1990 The quality of life: the missing measurement in healthcare. Souvenir Press, London

Gershenson DM, Kavanagh JJ, Copeland LJ, Stringer CA, Morris M, Wharton JT 1989 Retreatment of patients with recurrent epithelial ovarian cancer with cisplatin-based chemotherapy. Obstetrics & Gynaecology 73:798–802

Gore ME, Rustin G, Slevin M et al 1997 Single-agent paclitaxel in patients with previously untreated stage IV epithelial ovarian cancer. British Journal of Cancer 75(5):710–714

Griffiths CT 1975 Surgical resection of tumour bulk in the primary treatment of ovarian carcinoma. National Cancer Institute Monographs 42:101

Hacker NF, Berek JS, Lagasse LD, Nieberg RK, Elashoff RM 1983 Primary cytoreductive surgery for epithelial ovarian cancer. Obstetrics and Gynaecology 61:413–420

Hendrick AM, Simmons D, Cantwell BMJ 1992 Allergic reactions to carboplatin. Annals of Oncology 3:238–240

Hoskins WJ 1993 Surgical staging and cytoreductive surgery of epithelial ovarian cancer. Cancer 71(4):1534–1540

Jacobs I, Oram D, Jeyarayah A et al 1995 Randomised trial of screening for ovarian cancer. Ovarian Cancer Screening Unit, St Bartholomews Hospital, London

Jacobs JH, Gepshenson DM, Morris M et al 1991 Neoadjuvant chemotherapy and interval debulking for advanced epithelial ovarian cancer. Gynaecologic Oncology 42(2):146–150

Kehoe C 1991 Malignant ascites: etiology, diagnosis and treatment. Oncology Nursing Forum 18:523–530

Kramer BS, Gohagan J, Prorok PC, Smart CA 1993 A National Cancer Institute sponsored screening trial for prostatic, lung, colorectal and ovarian cancers. Cancer 71:589–593

Lynch HT, Watson P, Bewtra C et al 1991 Hereditary ovarian cancer. Cancer 67:1460–1466

McGuire WP, Hoskins WJ, Brafy MF et al 1996 Cyclophosphamide and cisplatin compared with paclitaxel and cisplatin in patients with stage III and stage IV ovarian cancer. The New England Journal of Medicine 34(1):1–6

Matocha LK, Waterhouse JK 1993 Current nursing practice in relation to sexuality. Research in Nursing & Health 16:371–378

Mercadante S, Spoldi E, Caraceni A, Maddaloni S, Simonetti MT 1993 Octreotide in relieving gastrointestinal symptoms due to bowel obstruction. Palliative Medicine 7:295–299

Mossman J 1998 Tide is turning on inequality of care: new evidence leads to a consensus on ovarian cancer treatment. Nursing Standard 12(36):14–15

MRC Cancer Trials Office 1997 International open meeting on gynaecological cancer – meeting report. Medical Research Committee, London

Neijt JP, Allen DG, Colombo N, Verorken JB 1995 Carcinoma of the ovary. In: Peckham M, Pinedo H, Veronesi U (eds) Oxford textbook of oncology, Vol 2. Oxford University Press, Oxford, ch 9.1, pp 1293–1308

Ovarian Cancer Meta-analysis Project 1991 Cyclophosphamide, doxorubicin and cisplatin chemotherapy of ovarian cancer: a meta-analysis. Journal of Clinical Oncology 9:1668–1674

Parkin DM, Laarke, Muir CS 1988 Estimates of the worldwide frequency of sixteen major cancers in 1980. International Journal of Cancer 41:184–187

Podratz KC, Kinney WK 1993 Second-look operation in ovarian cancer. Cancer 71(4):1551–1558

Preston N 1995 New strategies for the management of malignant ascites. European Journal of Cancer Care 4:178–183

Preston NJ 1996 Paclitaxel (Taxol) – a guide to administration. European Journal of Cancer Care 5:147–152

Redman CWE, Warwick J, Luesley DM, Varma R, Lawton FG, Blackledge GRP 1994 Intervention debulking surgery in advanced epithelial ovarian cancer. British Journal of Obstetrics and Gynaecology 101:142–146

Regnard C, Mannix K 1989 Management of ascites in advanced cancer – a flow diagram. Palliative Medicine 4:45–47

Riley J, Fallon M 1994 Octreotide in terminal malignant obstruction of the gastrointestinal tract. European Journal of Palliative Care 1(1):23–25

Ripamonti C 1994 Malignant bowel obstruction in advanced and terminal cancer patients. European Journal of Palliative Care 1(1):16–19

Shoham Z 1994 Epidemiology, etiology and fertility drugs in ovarian epithelial carcinoma: where are we today? Fertility and Sterility 62(3):433–448

Steginga SK, Dunn J 1997 Women's experience following treatment for gynaecologic cancer. Oncology Nursing Forum 24(8):1403–1408

Stuart S, Bertelsen K, Mangioni et al 1998 Updated analysis shows a highly significant improved overall survival (OS) for cisplatin-paclitaxel as first line treatment of advanced ovarian cancer: mature results of the EORTC-GCCG. Proceedings of the American Society of Clinical Oncologists, Conifer Information System, Amsterdam

Trimbos JB et al 1991 Watch and wait after careful surgical treatment and staging in well-differentiated early ovarian cancer. Cancer 67:597–602

Tzonou A, Polychronopoulou A, Hsieh C et al 1993 Hair dyes, analgesia tranquillizers and perineal talc application as risk factors for ovarian cancer. International Journal of Cancer 55(3):408–410

Van der Berg MEL et al 1995 The effects of debulking surgery after induction chemotherapy on the prognosis in advanced epithelial ovarian cancer. The New England Journal of Medicine 332:629–634

Walczak JR, Klemm PR, Guarnieri C 1997 Gynaecologic cancers. In: Groenwald SL, Hansen Frogge M, Goodman M, Henke Yarbro C (eds) Cancer nursing: principles and practice. Jones and Bartlett, Boston

Webb C 1988 A study of nurse's knowledge and attitudes about sexuality in health care. International Journal of Nursing Studies 25(3):235–244

Weiss RB, Donehow RC, Wiernik PH et al 1990 Hypersensitivity reactions from taxol. Journal of Clinical Oncology 8:1263–1268

Whittemore AS et al 1992 Characteristics relating to ovarian cancer risk: collaborative analysis on 12 case control studies. II Invasive epithelial ovarian cancers in white women. American Journal of Epidemiology 136:1184–1203

Whyte A 1997 Out of Darkness. Nursing Times 93(40):30

Woolas RP, Xu FJ, Jacobs IJ et al 1993 Elevation of multiple serum markers in patients with stage I ovarian cancer. Journal of the National Cancer Institute 85:1748

Yoder LH 1990 The epidemiology of ovarian cancer: a review. Oncology Nursing Forum 17(3):411–415

Young RC, Decker DG, Wharton JT et al 1983 Staging laparotomy in early ovarian cancer. Journal of the American Medical Association 250:3072–3076

Young RC, Walton LA, Ellenberg SS et al 1990 Adjuvant therapy in stage I and stage II epithelial ovarian cancer: results of two prospective randomized trials. New England Journal of Medicine 322:1021–1027

Young A, Gilbert J, Sherman M, Chatwin D, Budden J 1996 Intraperitoneal chemotherapy: a prolonged infusion of 5-fluorouracil using a novel carrier solution. British Journal of Nursing 5(9):539–543

Zacharias DR, Gilg CA, Foxall MJ 1994 Quality of life and coping in patients with gynaecological cancer and their spouses. Oncology Nursing Forum 22(10):1699–1706

FURTHER READING

Blake P, Lambert H, Crawford R 1998 Gynaecological oncology: a guide to clinical management. Oxford University Press, New York

Bloch B, Dehaeck K, Soeters R 1995 Manual of practical gynaecological oncology. Chapman and Hall, London

Lambert HE, Blake PR 1992 Gynaecological oncology. Oxford University Press, New York

Shepherd JH, Monaghan JM (eds) 1990 Clinical gynaecological oncology, 2nd edn. Blackwell Scientific Publications, London

USEFUL ADDRESSES:

Cancer BACUP
3 Bath Place, Rivington Street, London, EC2A 3JR
Tel: 020 7696 9003
Freephone: 0800 181199
Web site: www.cancerbacup.org.uk.
Cancer nurses provide information, support and advice by telephone or letter

Macmillan Cancer Relief
Anchor House, 15–19 Britten Street, London, SW3 3TZ
Tel: 020 7351 7811
Supports and develops services to provide specialist care for people with cancer at every stage of their illness. Funds gynaecological cancer nurse specialist posts.

Cancerlink
11–21 Northdown Street, London, N1 9BN
Freephone: 0800 132905
Provides support and information to people with cancer, their families, friends, carers and health professionals on all aspects of cancer care. Have a Asian cancer information helpline in Bengali, Hindi, Punjabi and Urdu.

Marie Curie Cancer Care
28 Belgrave Square, London, SW1X 8QG
Tel: 020 7235 3325

Provides hands-on care for patients in their own home both day and night

Ovacom
191A South Croxted Road, Dulwich, London, SE21 8AY
Tel: 020 8244 9226
Support organization for women with ovarian cancer

Hysterectomy Support Network
3 Lynne Close, Green Street, Orpington, Kent, BR6 6BS
Informal encouragement, advice and support to women, family and partners concerned about hysterectomy

Women's Nationwide Cancer Control Campaign
Suna House, 128–130 Curtain Road, London EC2A 3AR
Tel: 020 7719 2229
Supports and encourages the provision of facilities for the early diagnosis of cancer in women

Oncolink
Web site: www.oncolink.upenn.edu/
Provided by the University of Pennsylvania Cancer Centre. Helps to disseminate information and promotes education for health professionals, patients and carers

Oncology Forum
Web site: www.oncology-forum.org/
Provided by SmithKline Beecham. Reliable information for patients and professionals

15

Cancer of the vulva

Cathryn Hughes, Karen Handscomb

Cancer of the vulva remains a relatively rare cancer. It affects about 900 British women per year; approximately 4% of all gynaecological cancers. Cancer of the vulva is primarily a disease of the elderly, with the greatest occurrence in women over the age of 70 years. It is rarely seen in women under the age of 40 years. The incidence of the disease has remained relatively stable but it is thought that the incidence will rise with the increase in life expectancy.

The relationship between vulval intraepithelial neoplasia (VIN), a premalignant condition of the vulva, and invasive cancer remains unclear and does not appear to have the strength of association as that seen with cervical intraepithelial neoplasia (CIN) and cervical cancer. The reported incidence of VIN has increased since the 1970s, particularly in women under the age of 40 years. There has not, as yet, been a corresponding increase in the number of women presenting with vulval cancer.

ANATOMY

The vulva consists of those parts of the female genital tract that are externally visible in the perineal area: the vulvar vestibule, the clitoris, the labia minora, labia majora and the mons pubis. The vulval labia provide a split covering (vulva means covering) for the entrance to the vagina and the urethra, and is in close proximity to the anus (Fig. 15.1). These structures are covered by squamous epithelium. Lymphatic drainage of the vulva, lower vagina and perineum occurs to the inguinal and femoral lymph nodes in the groin.

AETIOLOGY

The way in which cancers are generated is thought to be a multistep process resulting from errors in the regulation of normal cells. As with many other cancers, the exact **aetiology** of cancer of the vulva remains

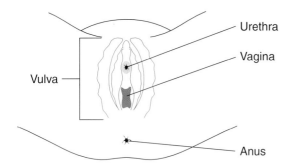

Figure 15.1 The position of the vulva. From Health Press Ltd 1997, with permission.

unknown, but is likely to be the result of a combination of factors.

The role of the human papilloma virus (HPV) in the development of vulval neoplasia is not fully understood. There are over 70 different types of HPV and around 20 have been found in the genital tract. HPV types 16 and 18 have been detected in VIN and invasive cancer. About 50% of vulval **carcinomas** have been shown to be linked to the presence of HPV infection and HPV has been found in up to 80% of VIN III lesions. However, where there is no history of VIN III, only about 15% of vulval cancers will be HPV positive. Such conflicting results have led to the view that vulval cancer may be more than one distinct disease; that which is generally seen in the older woman with chronic inflammation and that which is generally seen in the younger woman with VIN.

The herpes virus (specifically herpes simplex virus type 2) has also been associated with the disease. The exact relationship is not understood and often disputed in the literature, but it may represent a cofactor.

Lichen sclerosis is a **benign** inflammatory disease that causes pruritus and usually occurs in postmenopausal women. It has been reported as being associated with vulval cancer in anything up to 60% of cases but only about 5% of women with lichen sclerosis will go on to develop vulval cancer (Kaufman et al 1974).

Suppression of the immune system due to disease or immunosuppressive medication appears to increase the risk of developing vulval cellular abnormality, especially in younger women. Other possible factors include multiple sexual partners, cigarette smoking and a previous abnormal Pap smear or genital tract malignancy (Brinton et al 1990).

Vulval cancer is associated with older age groups, obesity, diabetes and chronic vulval irritation. Obesity and diabetes are linked together, as are age and dia-

betes. In the elderly obese it may be difficult to maintain vulval hygiene, which may also lead to vulval irritation. As seen, it can be difficult to separate these risk factors and as such their significance is often disputed.

PATHOLOGY

Over 80% of vulval cancers are squamous cell in origin (see Plates 26 and 27) the remainder are made up of basal cell carcinomas, **malignant** melanomas (see Plate 28), **adenocarcinomas**, sarcomas and various others.

In 1987 the International Society for the Study of Vulvar Disease (ISSVD) defined VIN as a condition in which the cellular abnormality of the vulva is confined to the epithelium and is described as squamous and non-squamous. The histological features of squamous VIN are similar to those of CIN. In preinvasive disease, the degree of abnormality is based upon the proportion of the epithelium replaced by atypical or dysplastic cells. VIN I, VIN II and VIN III are histological terms that describe increasing degrees of abnormality or dysplasia, from mild, to moderate, to severe. VIN III, or carcinoma in situ, being the most severe preinvasive abnormality suggesting full thickness changes of the epithelium. In **cytology**, the terms mild, moderate and severe dyskariosis are used to suggest an underlying pathology. VIN often presents as multifocal disease.

Non-squamous VIN comprises Paget's disease of the vulva and melanoma in situ. Paget's disease of the vulva is rare but can be associated with an underlying adenocarcinoma in up to 30% of cases.

Cancers are often classified according to the degree of differentiation. Cells assume features that distinguish them from other cells; they are considered to be differentiated. Cancer cells tend to be less differentiated than normal cells from the surrounding tissue. **Tumours** can be well differentiated (grade 1), moderately differentiated (grade 2) and poorly differentiated (grade 3). Most vulval cancers are well or moderately well differentiated. The grade of vulval cancer has not consistently been shown to affect the prognosis.

NATURAL HISTORY

Vulval cancer tends to be a slow growing condition, which enlarges locally retaining well defined margins. Most vulval cancers involve the labia; most commonly the labia majora. Carcinoma of the vulva spreads primarily by direct invasion of local tissue, by lymphatic permeation or, less commonly, via the bloodstream. Infiltration of local tissue usually occurs before

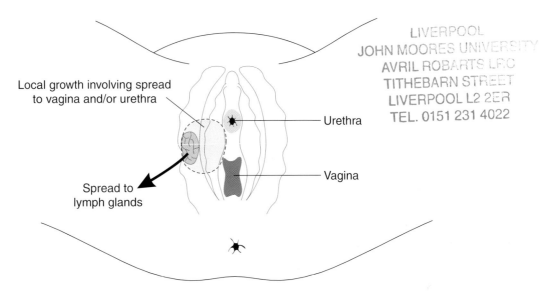

Local growth involving spread
to vagina and/or urethra

Urethra

Vagina

Spread to
lymph glands

LIVERPOOL
JOHN MOORES UNIVERSITY
AVRIL ROBARTS LRC
TITHEBARN STREET
LIVERPOOL L2 2ER
TEL. 0151 231 4022

Figure 15.2   Vulval cancer spread. From Health Press Ltd 1997, with permission.

lymph node metastasis. This local spread can extend to involve the vagina, urethra, anus and rectum (Fig. 15.2).

Lymphatic spread increasingly occurs with the increase in the size of the **primary tumour**. Lymph node **metastasis** is found in about 30% of all cases.

Hacker (1990) showed that where a lesion is on one side (unilateral), away from the midline, and no larger than 2 cm, there is little chance of lymphatic spread to the nodes on the other side. Defining patterns of cancer spread is important for treatment planning.

Uncontrolled vulval disease is unpleasant and painful. Because the disease increases locally and primarily affects only local structures, death can be a long, degrading and miserable process. This is why most women with resectable lesions are offered surgery, regardless of age and general medical condition. Women with vulval cancer can often be managed badly in non-specialist hospitals.

Signs and symptoms

Over 136 years ago Meigs (1854) observed a reluctance for women with vulval irritation or lesions to seek medical advice, thus causing a significant delay in diagnosis. Today there remains, all too often, a delay in the diagnosis of this disease. This may in part be due to a reluctance of the elderly woman to present to her doctor and in part due to the failure of the doctor to recognize the symptoms as being due to vulval cancer.

It is possible that women in the future, who have been involved in the cervical and breast screening programmes, may be less reticent in performing self-examination of the vulva and seeking medical advice.

VIN often presents with pruritus vulvae but in up to 50% of cases it can be asymptomatic. Women with vulval cancer most commonly present with pruritus or irritation. A vulval lesion is found in about half of all cases. Other symptoms include pain, bleeding and discharge.

Example of presentation

Mrs Jones is a 73-year-old widow. She lives alone but has two daughters living away from home in other parts of the country. She finally presented, after 2 years of vulval irritation, to her GP. Mrs Jones was reluctant to be examined and 'just wanted some cream'. Her GP convinced her of the need for examination and reassured her she was not wasting his time. On examination, he could clearly see a lesion on the vulva, which was hard and immobile. An urgent referral was made to a specialist gynaecologist.

DIAGNOSIS

Women with VIN need careful examination to assess the full extent of the disease bearing in mind the multifocal or 'field' change nature of the condition. Invasive cancer needs to be diagnosed or excluded. It is important to examine all the genital tract, taking a cervical smear and performing colposcopy as necessary. VIN lesions can be raised, with a rough surface and appear red, white or brown. The application of acetic acid can reveal the full extent of the disease, staining the affected tissue white. A colposcope can be used to examine the vulva. With the colposcope the clinician can see the vulval tissue more closely with well-illuminated, low-power, binocular microscopy. Any areas of abnormality seen and revealed with acetic acid can then be biopsied for histological diagnosis. The diagnosis of VIN can only be made histologically.

Vulval cancer, also, can only be diagnosed on histo-logical assessment of biopsied tissue. Benign vulval conditions can appear clinically malignant. An exami-nation under anaesthetic (EUA) allows for full assess-ment of the genital tract to exclude any other malignant and/or premalignant disease, as well as allowing for assessment of vulval cancer spread. A cystoscopy and proctosigmoidoscopy may be performed at the same time. A cervical and vaginal smear should also be taken. A chest X-ray will exclude lung metastasis as well as being required in the older patient prior to anaesthesia. Magnetic resonance imagining (MRI) can provide assistance in the assessment of local spread whilst computerized tomography (CT) will assess pelvic, abdominal, para-aortic node and liver disease, if required. Any suspicious groin nodes found on palpa-tion can be sampled with fine needle aspiration (FNA) and sent for cytological assessment.

Table 15.1 Staging – FIGO 1995 International Federation of Gynaecology and Obstetrics (based on Shepherd 1995)

Stage	Description
0	Preinvasive carcinoma (VIN)
Ia	Confined to the vulva and/or perineum, 2 cm or less maximum diameter. Groin nodes not palpable. Stromal invasion no greater than 1 mm
Ib	As for Ia but stromal invasion greater than 1 mm
II	Confined to vulva and/or perineum, more than 2 cm maximum diameter. Groin nodes not palpable
III	Extends beyond the vulva, vagina, lower urethra or anus; or unilateral regional lymph node metastasis
IVa	Involves the mucosa of rectum or bladder; upper urethra or pelvic bone and/or bilateral regional lymph node metastases
IVb	Any distant metastasis, including pelvic lymph node

Staging

Cancer staging is designed to describe the tumour location, local and regional spread and metastasis. The staging allows for treatment planning and provides an international language for clinicians and scientists to communicate about the given disease, treatment and prognosis. In gynaecology the staging system most commonly used is the International Federation of Gynaecology and Obstetrics (FIGO) system revised in 1995 (Table 15.1).

TREATMENT
Preinvasive disease

Treatment of preinvasive disease can be difficult because of the uncertainty about the malignant poten-tial, the multifocal nature of the disease and the poten-tial mutilation caused by treatment. Currently, surgery is the main form of treatment. If women are asympto-matic then careful follow-up, with biopsy as necessary, may be sufficient, especially in younger women. For symptomatic women, where malignancy has been excluded, topical steroid cream can provide relief but prolonged use should be avoided and monitored care-fully. Wide local excision of the lesion provides treat-ment and allows for full histological assessment of the lesion and excision margins. **Primary closure** is usually possible. If the disease is extensive or multi-focal then a skinning vulvectomy with skin graft can be performed. A skinning vulvectomy involves the removal of the epidermal layer of the vulva. Surgery may be the only option for symptomatic relief.

Ablation of the abnormal tissue has been used as a method of treatment but this does not allow for the histological assessment of the tissue and has also resulted in painful, slow-healing **ulcers**.

Paget's disease is usually treated with a wide local excision or simple vulvectomy (without removal of the regional lymph nodes) to exclude an underlying malignancy and because of the possibility of recur-rence in remaining tissue.

Invasive disease

Vulvectomy, along with the surgical excision of the bilateral regional lymph nodes, was first described by Basset (1912) and is considered standard treatment for cancer of the vulva. It is important to remember that the prognosis for this disease improved dramatically once radical resection of the tumour together with

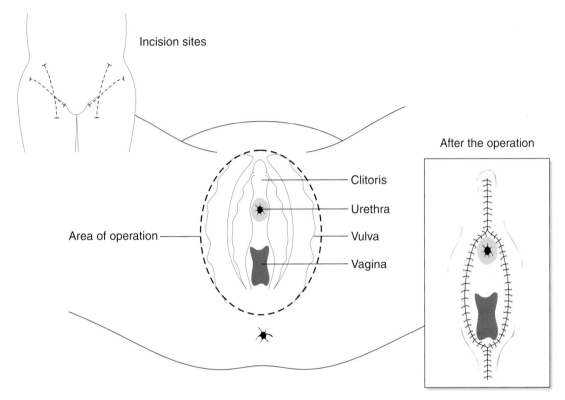

Figure 15.3   Radical vulvectomy. From Heatth Press Ltd 1997, with permission.

lymph node dissection was accepted and practised as described by Way (1948). The vulval tissue was originally removed en bloc (removing the tissue in one piece), which created a large defect, usually left to heal by **secondary intention**.

Surgery continues to be the main form of treatment for cancer of the vulva. Hacker et al (1981) moved away from the en bloc method of vulvectomy and recommended the use of the triple incision technique. Radical vulvectomy involves the dissection of the invasive primary lesion, contiguous skin, subcutaneous fat, regional inguinal and femoral nodes and the vulva (Fig. 15.3). The principles of treatment are evolving, driven by the need to reduce treatment **morbidity**.

DiSaia et al (1979) suggested the use of 'wide local excision' (on lesions no greater than 1 cm with a depth of stromal invasion less than 5 mm) together with bilateral inguinal lymph node dissection. Others have successfully followed this practice and modified the surgery further. Not all patients need bilateral lymph node dissection.

The choice of surgical technique offered depends upon the location and extent of the primary tumour, the **histology** and estimated risk of lymph node involvement and the presence of metastasis.

Grafts may be used to close large surgical defects where primary closure is not possible or advisable. Skin grafts are most commonly used following skinning vulvectomy where there is little loss of subcutaneous tissue. Musculocutaneous grafts are used to cover severe defects in the vulva.

Preoperative care

Once the patient is aware of the diagnosis and the planned treatment she can be given a date to organize her admission and plan convalescence. A common reaction is to request surgery immediately but some time taken in preparation can prove invaluable postoperatively. The woman needs to feel in control of the situation but also needs guidance from the healthcare professionals in order to make decisions. Preoperative counselling should include preparation for the sexual and psychosexual impact of the disease and the surgery. Prophylactic antibiotics and antithrombotic therapy should be given: vulval cancer patients are at high risk of developing a deep vein thrombosis (DVT) because of the length of the surgical procedure, the general age of the patient and the presence of malignancy.

Postoperative care

The usual postoperative observations need to be maintained remembering that the elderly patient may be slower in the physiological response to the complications of surgery. Drains are usually left in the groins until drainage is minimal, to avoid lympho cysts. Pain control is important but many patients find the pain associated with this type of surgery is minimal and responds well to moderate analgesia, taking into account the age of the patient, the probability of polypharmacy and drug side-effects. A urethral catheter is left draining immediately postoperatively and removed once the patient is mobile and the wound is stable. The woman needs to be able to void comfortably 'through' the surgical site. This does not appear to hamper wound healing or cause a significant amount of pain. Women may find they spray urine instead of the previous flow.

Recommendations for vulval wound care following vulvectomy vary and there seems to be little research on the subject. The medical emphasis on improving the rates of wound breakdown and infection has veered towards the reduction in surgery and modification of surgical technique. Nurses have a vital role to play in the postoperative management of vulvectomy wounds. Hughes (2000) looked at current practice in the UK regarding the management of these wounds and found practice to be varied, based primarily upon individual preference. It is common practice in some units to dry the vulval area with a hair dryer following a bath or shower in the belief that it is more comfortable for the patient, avoiding the potential trauma and discomfort caused by rubbing the delicate tissue (for further information see p. 257).

Complications of surgery

Wound breakdown is the most commonly listed complication of all the types of surgical procedures but obviously varies with the extent of the dissection and the general condition of the patient. Other complications include infection, pulmonary embolism, lymphocyst formation and leg oedema. Commonly, patients will complain about paraesthesia on the front of the thigh due to nerve damage. Long-term complications may include chronic leg oedema, urinary incontinence and pelvic floor prolapse. Vulvectomy is associated with significant body image problems and sexual dysfunction.

Radiotherapy

Radiotherapy is the therapeutic use of ionizing radiation. Radiotherapy is not generally used in the primary treatment of vulval cancer because of the morbidity associated with the treatment and the success of surgery. Radiation therapy can be used in conjunction with surgery; preoperatively to reduce tumour size and postoperatively in poor prognosis disease. Preoperative radiotherapy and/or chemotherapy can be used to try and reduce the size of advanced tumours and allow for less radical surgery avoiding stoma formation. Postoperative radiotherapy to the nodes can be given when there is histological or clinical evidence of disease spread to the nodes and/or close or positive surgical excision margins (Thomas et al 1991).

Complications of radiotherapy

Acute reactions following radiotherapy include vulval erythema and swelling. The vulva can become extremely uncomfortable. Radiation cystitis can also be seen. Long-term complications include **lymphoedema**. Lymphoedema of the lower extremities can follow radical vulvectomy alone, although the incidence increases with the addition of postoperative radiotherapy.

Chemotherapy

Chemotherapy has a limited role in the management of vulval cancer. The general age and medical fitness of women with vulval cancer makes multitreatment modality problematic. The use of chemotherapy as a radiotherapy sensitizer has been used but not yet effectively evaluated. Several drugs have been tried in a combination with radiotherapy and surgery and continue to be investigated.

Advanced disease and disease recurrence

A primary vulval cancer lesion may become very large, causing considerable distress and discomfort.

Case study: Pat
Pat was a 63-year-old divorcee who lived with her son and helped out in his security company, which she loved. Her main support was her daughter, who accompanied her on all her hospital visits.
Pat had lived for many months with a lump in her vulval area, which she had first felt when she wiped herself and which was now getting bigger and becoming irritated. She had stopped wearing knickers as she felt relief from the air getting to this area, but this also meant that she had stopped many of her usual social activities.
One evening Pat bled very heavily from this area and her daughter took her to casualty. She was seen by the specialist gynaecological oncology consultant who could see an obvious vulval cancer.
A radical vulvectomy was performed and the inguinal nodes were found to be involved. Pat and her family were told that she would need radiotherapy, which would start when it was felt she was fit enough after surgery, usually about 6 weeks. She was given the opportunity to ask questions and was also given printed information.
After 10 days Pat was discharged from hospital into the care of her daughter. The specialist gynaecological oncology Macmillan nurse kept in telephone contact and visited Pat at home. Pat refused all help at home but gradually seemed to be doing more, her appetite had improved and she was back wearing knickers!
Pat had 5 weeks of radiotherapy treatment, which proved very difficult. She had diarrhoea, which made keeping the perineal area clean a problem and she became very sore. Aperients helped and a low fibre diet was suggested. The radiotherapy team were concerned that Pat was looking very tired and they felt the travelling was too difficult. Pat spent a week in hospital but became increasingly depressed – she missed her cable television and MacDonalds. Reluctantly, the doctors let her go home with increased support from social services and weekly visits from the District nurses and the specialist Macmillan nurse.
Pat never seemed to fully recover after her surgery and radiotherapy. Her consultations showed no further problems and yet her energy levels did not return and her appetite remained very poor, despite supplements suggested by the dietician. Her legs began to swell and lymphoedema advice was given. All this was increasingly frustrating for Pat, who talked of travelling to Australia, the haggis she was going to enjoy and the small business she was going to set up when she was well.
One day Pat's daughter telephoned the specialist Macmillan nurse and said that they had found another lump. Pat was rushed to the hospital where her condition quickly began to deteriorate and it was decided not to undertake any further treatment. Pat and her daughter visited her local hospice. She died there very peacefully later that week.

Despite the size of the lesion surgery is still considered, even radical surgery. Complete excision of the tumour is needed for a reasonable chance of cure. Extensive local surgery with reconstruction may be required. When removing extensive areas of tissue of the mons, groin, perineum and down to the thigh, skin flaps are often used to fill the defect. Skin flaps vary from small transposition flaps to myocutaneous flaps.

If the tumour involves the urethra and/or anus then consideration will be given to the extent of the dissection required and the chances of maintaining continence. If the tumour extensively involves the vagina, upper urethra, bladder and rectum, or if clear margins cannot be obtained with preservation of these structures, then a total or partial exenteration can be performed. Vaginal reconstruction will be considered for women who wish to be, or remain, sexually active. Where the pubic bones are involved the surgery may include removal of the diseased bone but this is a poor prognostic indicator and such patients will require further treatment.

Despite the success of primary treatment for vulval cancer, there remain a number of women for whom treatment will not provide a cure. The clinical presentation of recurrence is varied. Recurrence on the vulva is usually re-excised, some patients have more than one recurrence and excision is often associated with recurrence of preinvasive disease. Distant or groin recurrence is often a bad sign, with 5-year survival in these patients at about 10% (Podratz et al 1982). Chemotherapy and radiotherapy can be used to try to control disease but the results are generally poor.

The overall 5-year survival rate for women with vulval cancer is approximately 70%. For stage I disease the survival rate is around 90% but drops to about 50% when metastatic disease is present (Table 15.2).

NURSING MANAGEMENT

Health education and screening

Involvement in primary health education gives nurses the opportunity to inform women about the disease.

Table 15.2   Five-year survival for vulval cancer (based on Homesley et al 1991)

Stage	5-year survival (%)
I	98
II	85
III	74
IV	3

The national cervical screening programme allows for large numbers of women to be examined and educated. During the cervical-smear-taking process the vulva should be examined visually and the history taking should include any vulval symptoms. Encouragement of vulva self-examination can form part of the consultation. Within the community, nurses can participate in the education of other healthcare professionals, particularly those caring for the elderly.

Specialist nursing

There are an increasing number of specialist nurses in all fields of nursing; gynaecological **oncology** is no exception. The role of the gynaecological oncology nurse varies from centre to centre but, fundamentally, the role involves informing and supporting the woman with vulval cancer and her family. The diagnosis of cancer provokes feelings of fear and uncertainty and begins the 'cancer journey'. Specialist nurses can accompany patients along part of their cancer journey, leading the way when necessary, and linking with other professionals to make the journey as smooth and straightforward as possible. The Cancer Relief Macmillan Fund produces leaflets to give women guidance on gynaecological health and advice on the minimum that a woman with gynaecological cancer should expect from the healthcare system. Access to a specialist nurse or counsellor is considered a fundamental requirement for these women. The Government has also recommended that all gynaecological cancer centres should have a specialist nurse in post. Corney et al (1993), in a study of women post gynaecological cancer treatment, recommend the use of a nurse specialist/nurse counsellor in the management of women with gynaecological cancer to reduce the level of psychological and sexual morbidity, especially in relation to vulval cancer.

Sexuality

Anderson & Hacker (1983) were the first to study the psychosocial and sexual impact of surgery for vulval cancer. Their study of 15 patients showed a significant disruption in body image, with body image scores lower than those for healthy women and comparable to women following pelvic exenteration. It also showed very low sexual arousal levels. In the largest published British study Corney et al (1993) discuss the feelings of 105 women post gynaecological cancer treatment. These women express feelings of embarrassment and unattractiveness. The study attempts to

assess pretreatment feelings but the data is collected retrospectively. Steginga & Dunn (1997), investigating 82 women post gynaecological cancer treatment, reported anxiety and depression, reflecting a sense of vulnerability.

There are three main ways in which cancer influences sexuality and fertility: (i) the actual biological disease process; (ii) the physiological effects of treatment; and (iii) the overall psychological effects. Women need to be aware of the sexual and reproductive implications of their disease and treatment. There are still many misconceptions concerning sex and fertility following cancer or treatment for cancer. It is not uncommon to come across women who have not had sex since their operation because they thought they couldn't or shouldn't. Being comfortable to discuss sex and recognize sexual dysfunction as a potential problem gives the woman permission to tackle a traditionally taboo subject. Information or access to information should be offered to all women, and partners where possible. Patients can always chose to ignore the information but may find it difficult to seek advice. Accurate information can reduce anxiety and allow the woman or couple to make informed decisions. Considering the sexual needs of women in a single-sex relationship is also important, there may be different implications and solutions.

Cancer of the vulva and radical vulvectomy can affect a woman's sexuality by affecting her body image and her sexual function. Fertility is not commonly an issue because of the age group usually affected by the disease and the nature of the surgery, which generally leaves the vagina, uterus and ovaries intact. Fertility obviously needs to be considered when an exenteration is performed in a younger woman and when radiotherapy and chemotherapy are used in treatment. Following vulvectomy or wide local excision, the pulling together of the surgical edges can cause tension, which may affect movement and positioning for sexual intercourse. Removal of the clitoris does not necessarily mean that a woman will be unable to achieve orgasm although orgasm from clitoral stimulation, especially masturbation, will be lost.

Women who are experiencing severe or long-lasting sexual problems following treatment for vulval cancer should be offered referral to a psychosexual counsellor, preferably with an interest in gynaecological cancer.

Lymphoedema

The lymphatic system parallels the circulatory system and is responsible for the balance of interstitial fluid.

When swelling occurs as a response to surgery, radiotherapy or infection, new routes of lymph flow can be found to compensate. When the demand for drainage cannot be compensated for, fluid accumulates in the interstitial tissue, resulting in swelling or oedema. If this oedema persists then fibrosis occurs in the subcutaneous tissue that further hinders lymphatic drainage. Removal of, or radiotherapy to, the lymph glands potentially weakens the lymphatic drainage, especially when put under stress. Radiotherapy combined with surgery compounds that risk. Advice is generally given to women following surgery and/or radiotherapy for vulval cancer to prevent added stress to the lymphatic system in order to prevent lymphoedema:

- taking general care of the legs, protection from injury, especially when cutting toe nails and during leg shaving (high-risk patients may be advised to avoid shaving the legs), gardening, etc.
- regular walking
- walking or leg exercise during extended travelling
- taking antibiotics (commonly erythromycin) for wounds or insect bites that are slow to heal or obviously infected
- wearing support hosiery for work, etc.

The advice given to women for prevention of lymphoedema varies from centre to centre. There is little research into the specifics of such advice. The general principle should be to teach the woman about the role of the lymphatic system, how to avoid infection, how to recognize infection, how to treat it and who to report it to.

Lymphoedema is usually characterized as mild, moderate or severe:

- Mild – 2–3 cm difference in circumference from one limb to the other. There may be no obvious swelling but the woman may complain of pain or heaviness in the limb.
- Moderate – 3–5 cm difference from one limb to the other. The difference is visible. The skin may be stretched and shiny with oedema.
- Severe – 5 cm or more difference. The swelling is obvious. The skin may be discoloured and stretched. The leg may feel hard and the oedema non-pitting. The woman will probably find the leg uncomfortable and it will limit mobility.

Should lymphoedema become a problem, then the use of custom-fitted stockings and an exercise plan can help. Referral to a specialist lymphoedema clinic, where available, would be recommended. Injections into the affected leg should be avoided whenever possible. The possibility of deep vein thrombosis (DVT) or recurrent disease should be excluded in a woman who suddenly develops lymphoedema.

Wound care

Wound breakdown is considered a major complication of vulval surgery. As mentioned above, there appears to be little research on the subject. The groin and vulval excision wounds, because of the anatomy, are difficult to immobilize and dress adequately. The surgery involved in removing the lymph nodes creates pockets of dead space in which fluid can collect, resulting in the use of drains. Wound care strategies are generally based upon the fundamentals of wound healing and adapted to suit the specific problems associated with the vulval area.

When tissue injury occurs, in the case of radical vulvectomy surgical injury, it stimulates the body's inflammatory and immune responses. The process of wound healing can be divided into four main phases (Morison 1993):

1. Acute inflammatory response – involves haemostats, the release of histamine and other mediators from damaged cells and the migration of white blood cells to the damaged site.
2. Destructive phase – involves the clearance of dead and devitalized tissues by polymorphs and macrophages.
3. Proliferative phase – during which new blood vessels infiltrate the wound.
4. Maturation phase – involves re-epithelialization, wound contraction and connective tissue reorganization.

The surgical removal of the vulval and groin tissue will instigate the inflammatory response. The damaged tissue and mast cells release histamine and other mediators, causing vasodilatation of surrounding intact blood vessels and increased blood supply to the area (which becomes warm and red). Permeability of blood capillaries increases and protein-rich fluid passes into the interstitial spaces, causing local oedema. Structures in the locality may suffer loss of function; a urinary catheter will enable the free and comfortable passage of urine. Polymorphs and macrophages migrate out of the capillaries into the damaged area in response to the chemotactic agents triggered by the injury. The estimated duration of this inflammatory response phase is 0–3 days. This is an important phase, which can be hampered by foreign bodies or infection. In a surgical wound, the site is considered sterile and free from contamination until the first dressing change. Some units therefore recommend leaving the surgical dressing intact for at least 3 days. A pressure dressing may be applied. Regular observation of the wound dressing for signs of haemorrhage and 'wetness' are carried out. 'Wet' dressings enable microorganisms to track through the dressing using the exudate/blood as a channel for infection to the wound site.

As most vulvectomy defects are closed healing occurs by first intention – full thickness surgical incisions are sutured together. Maintaining the primary closure is the aim of wound care at this stage. An infected wound will open and often reveal a significant defect, which will then need to heal by **secondary intention**. Dehiscence of the wound will also usually be left to heal in this manner. If the wound remains intact, then keeping the wound clean and comfortable forms the basis of nursing care. It is not uncommon for women with intact vulvectomy wounds to bath (even hydrotherapy bath) or shower daily followed by careful drying of the area with gauze, towel, hairdryer or exposure for air drying. This wound care/vulval hygiene is often maintained by the patient at home.

Collagen fibres continue to repair the wound with the formation of scar tissue. Scar tissue contracts; if the wound remains closed then there is less scarring and contraction. Vitamin C and amino acids, which are present in proteins, are required for collagen synthesis. Elderly women may experience a delay in the healing process as a phenomenon of the natural ageing process. Diabetes is also known to delay the healing process and increases the chances of infection. Mobility is also an important factor, exercise is used to increase blood flow and perfusion to the area and to improve lymphatic drainage of excess fluid and debris. Nursing care plans should reflect the need for good nutrition, blood sugar control in the diabetic patient and the need for exercise.

There is a progressive decrease in the vascularity of the scar tissue, which changes in appearance from dusky red to white. The collagen fibres are reorganized and the wound's tensile strength increases. This phase can take between 24 and 365 days and it should be remembered that the wound remains vulnerable.

If wound breakdown or dehiscence occurs then wound management can prove a difficult task, mostly in maintaining the moist environment for normal healing to take place. Advice from the tissue viability team can be sought but the general principles at this time are: cleaning of the wound, debridement of the wound and providing an optimal environment for healing. Each wound will need to be assessed for the appropriate dressing, bearing in mind the difficult anatomy, the relief of pain and discomfort and the prevention of complications. Even the largest of wounds will generally heal well given time.

Case study: Mary

Mary is 71, she presented to the gynaecologists 8 years ago. She had been experiencing irritation in her vulval area for the previous 6 years but it wasn't until she found a small lump that she went to her GP. She is married with five children and had not been sexually active since the irritation had begun.

The gynaecological oncology surgeon performed a wide local excision of the vulva and bilateral groin dissections. There was no spread to the inguinal lymph nodes. Her main problem after the surgery was stress incontinence on coughing, this was resolved by pelvic floor exercises and Mary and her husband resumed sexual activity.

Mary was taught to be increasingly vigilant and to examine her vulval area regularly. A year later she presented with a lesion on her scar – again a wide local incision was undertaken. Six months later she noticed discoloration of the skin close to the previous excision margin. This was felt to be due to the return of the stress incontinence – the use of tampons, 2-hourly voiding, scrupulous hygiene and barrier creams resolved this within a month.

A year later Mary noticed further irritation and soreness, which was thought to be candida infection and antifungal creams were used with good effect. However, a year and a half later Mary telephoned the hospital as she had spotted another lesion near to her labia. Another wide local excision was undertaken and the lesion completely excised. At the same time a fine needle aspiration was taken of the lymph nodes – this was negative.

A year and a half later Mary noticed a red area and soreness below her clitoris. The doctors noted some vulval dystrophy and **leucoplakia**, which was treated with steroid cream and an analgesic gel, which was not helpful. Again a wide local excision was undertaken and VIN I was found on histology.

Nearly a year later Mary came to the outpatients department with another area of soreness, which was treated with a further local excision.

Living with the threat of cancer and what that may bring is very real to Mary. She manages to enjoy life and her outpatient department visits are organized around family commitments and long holidays abroad. She is reassured by the hospital's open access policy and her strong links with the multiprofessional team. She knows that she has to remain vigilant and that if a lump, soreness or anything she is worried about develops she needs to be in contact almost immediately.

Psychological care

Any woman with cancer has to deal with the emotional problems relating to a cancer diagnosis and the fear of death and disease. With vulval cancer she has to face the prospect of mutilating surgery and reduced sexual function. She has to consider the affect upon her family and her family has also to come to terms with the disease and treatment. They may suffer a sense of loss of control; for the woman a loss of control of what is happening within her body, and the general loss of control in the face of medical intervention. When planning treatment, the multidisciplinary team needs to consider how best to enable the woman and her family to cope with the disease, the treatment and the implications of both. The psychological support can come in a variety of ways from a variety of people. Providing information enables the patient and the family to begin regain control; information is power. The British Association of Cancer United Patients (BACUP) provides a series of booklets to explain the nature of site-specific cancers, the various treatments, the medications, how to find support and how to cope. The 'Patient Picture' series of booklets provides a good visual aid to the anatomy, disease and treatment involved, which can be invaluable during a consultation. Cancer Support UK provides a free directory of services available to people with cancer. Nurses often have more time to spend with the patient and the family to allow open discussion to take place where fears can be exposed and myths dispelled.

Quality of life

Cure or prolongation of life were once considered the primary aims of medical treatment. Today, with an increasing elderly population and the control of disease with medication and technology, the notion of chronic illness, prolonged remission and maximal quality of life are key topics in cancer care. Hawthorn (1993) discusses the lack of consensus on the definition of quality of life but suggests the defining theme in the literature could be expressed as 'the degree of satisfaction with perceived life circumstances'. Quality of life should be defined by the life in question whenever possible. All too often healthcare professionals are concerned only with outcome measures such as survival and disease-free intervals, whilst the patient and/or the family are afraid to speak out, or feel confused and powerless to make any significant decisions to 'buck the system'. Cancer is not always seen as a negative experience. Some women feel that the cancer experience has given them a new direction in life, a positive way forward.

CONCLUSION

Cancer of the vulva is a rare but unpleasant genital malignancy. It is most commonly found in older women and in the early stages there is a high overall survival rate. There may be an increase in the incidence of vulval cancer in the future with the increase in the elderly population. The surgical management of the disease is increasingly being tailored to the individual. Cancer of the vulva presents many challenges to the nursing profession, especially in the early detection of the disease and in the reduction of disease and treatment morbidity.

GLOSSARY

Adenocarcinoma: a cancer arising in glandular tissue
Aetiology: the study or science of the causes of disease, the cause of a specific disease
Benign: a term used to describe tissue which is not cancer
Carcinoma: a cancer that develops from epithelial cells, the most common form of cancer
Cytology: the study of cells
Histology: the study of tissue
Leucoplakia: thickened white patches on membranes
Lymphoedema: swelling of a part of the body because the normal lymphatics have been blocked or destroyed
Malignant: a cancerous tumour
Metastasis: the spread of cancer from one part of the body to another

Morbidity: the symptoms or effects of a disease or its treatment
Oncology: the study of tumours
Pathology: the study of disease
Primary closure: healing by the union of two closely opposing wound edges
Primary tumour: the site of the origin of the cancer
Secondary intention: healing where the wound bed is left open
Tumour: a mass or swelling of tissue, may be malignant or benign
Ulcer: an erosion in a surface membrane, may be benign or malignant

REFERENCES

Anderson BL, Hacker NF 1983 Psychosexual adjustment after vulval surgery. Obstetrics and Gynaecology 62(4):457–462

Anderson BL 1985 Sexual function and psychological morbidity and improving quality of life for women with gynaecological cancer. Cancer 55(8):1835–1842

Basset A 1912 Traitement chiurgical operatoire de l'epithelioma primitif du cliotoris indications – technique – resultats. Review Chiurgical 46:546

Brinton LA, Nasca PC, Mallin K et al 1990 Case-control study of cancer of the vulva. Obstetrics and Gynaecology 75(5):859–866

Corney RH, Crowther ME, Everett H, Howells A, Shepherd J 1993 Psychosexual dysfunction in women with gynaecological cancer following radical pelvic surgery. British Journal of Obstetrics and Gynaecology 100(1):73–78

DiSaia PJ, Creasman WT, Rich WM 1979 An alternative approach to early cancer of the vulva. American Journal of Obstetrics and Gynecology 133:825–832

Hacker NF, Leuchter RS, Berek JS et al 1981 Radical vulvectomy and bilateral inguinal lymphadenectomy through separate groin incisions. Obstetrics and Gynaecology 58:479–574

Hacker N 1990 Current treatment of small vulval cancers. Oncology 4:21–25

Hawthorn H 1993 Measuring quality of life. European Journal of Cancer Care 2:77–81

Health Press Ltd 1997 Patient Pictures Gynaecological Oncology, Oxford

Homesley HD, Bundy BN, Sedlis A et al 1991 Assessment of current International Federation of Gynaecology and Obstetrics staging of vulval cancer relative prognostic factors for survival. American Journal of Obstetrics and Gynecology 164:997–1004

Hughes C 2000 Attitudes, beliefs and behaviours regarding the post operative management of radical vulvectomy wounds (MSc thesis). University of Surrey, Guildford

Kaufman RH, Gardner HL, Brown D, Berth Y 1974 Vulval dystrophies: an evaluation. American Journal of Obstetrics and Gynecology 120:363–367

Meigs CD 1854 Woman: her diseases and remedies (pp. 35) Letter I11

Morison MJ 1993 A colour guide to the nursing management of wounds. Mosby, London, ch 1, pp 2–3

Podratz KC, Symmonds RE, Taylor WF, Williams TJ 1983 Carcinoma of the vulva: analysis of treatment and survival. Obstetrics and Gynaecology 61:63

Shepherd JH 1995 Staging announcement FIGO staging of gynaecological cancers: cervical and vulval. International Journal of Gynaecological Cancer 5:319

Steginga SK, Dunn J 1997 Women's experience following treatment for gynaecological cancer. Oncology Nursing Forum 24(8):1403–140

Thomas G, Dembo A, Bryson SCP et al 1991 Changing concepts in the management of vulval cancer. Gynaecologic Oncology 42:9–21

Way S 1948 The anatomy of the lymphatic drainage of the vulva and its influence on the radical operation for carcinoma. Annals of the Royal College of Surgeons England 3:187–209

FURTHER READING

Groenwald S, Frogge Hansen M, Goodman M, Yarbro Henkie C (eds) Cancer nursing: principle and practice, 5th edn. Jones and Bartlett, Massachusetts

Moore G (ed) Women and cancer: a gynecologic oncology nursing prospective, 1st edn. Jones and Bartlett, Massachusetts

Tschudin V (ed) Nursing the patient with cancer, 2nd edn. Prentice Hall, London

USEFUL ADDRESSES

CancerBACUP
3 Bath Place, Rivington Street, London EC2A 3JR
Tel: 020 7696 9003

Cancerlink
11–21 Northdown Street, London N1 9BN
Tel: 020 7883 2818 and
9 Castle Street, Edinburgh EH1 2DP
Tel: 0131 228 5557 and
Asian Cancer Information Helpline
0800 590415

Cancer Relief Macmillan Fund (CRMF)
15–19 Britten Street, London SW3 3TZ
Tel: 020 7351 7811

Cancer Support UK
Diana PWMF Project, Royal Marsden Hospital, FREEPOST 14022, London SW3 6YT

COU-RAGE UK (Coalition for Unity in Radiotherapy Advice and Guidance)
24 Lockett Gardens, Trinity, Manchester M3 6BJ
Tel: 0161 839 4256

Hospice Information Service
St. Christopher's Hospice, 51–59 Lawrie Park Road,
Sydenham, London SE26 6DZ
Tel: 020 8778 9252

Lympheodema Support Network
St Luke's Crypt, Sydney Street, London SW3 6NH
Tel: 020 7351 4480

Marie Curie Cancer Care
89 Albert Embankment, London SE1 7TP
Tel: 020 7599 7777

National Cancer Alliance
PO Box 579, Oxford OX4 1LB
Tel: 01865 793566

Institute of Psychosexual Medicine
11 Chandos Street, Cavendish Square, London W1M 9DE
Tel: 020 7580 0631

Relate
Herbert Gray College,
Little Church Street, Rugby CV21 3AP
Tel: 01788 573241

Vulval Pain Society
PO Box 514
Slough
Berks SL12BP

Women's Nationwide Cancer Control Campaign
Suna House, 128–130 Curtain Road, London EC2A 3AR
Tel: 020 7729 4688

Urostomy Association
Beaumont Park, Danbury, Essex CM3 4DE
Tel: 01245 224294

16

Problems of the lower urogenital tract in the postreproductive years, with associated psychosexual experiences

Joy Hall

The aim of this chapter is to explore the common problems of the lower urogenital tract experienced by women in their postreproductive years. As will be seen in this chapter and the others in this section, many of these problems are often directly or indirectly linked to the women's postmenopausal hormone status, together with their possible childbearing history. Many of the problems encountered have serious consequences for the women's physical and mental wellbeing, reflected in terms of their psychosocial and sexual morbidity. The chapter will, therefore, also discuss these effects, focusing specifically on the psychosexual consequences and concerns for and of these women. Further to this, it is intended to explore the role of psychosexual nursing in the field of gynaecological nursing with this group of patients.

PHYSIOLOGY OF THE LOWER UROGENITAL TRACT IN THE POSTREPRODUCTIVE YEARS

When considering the common problems affecting the urogenital tract in older women, it is necessary to be cognisant with both the systemic and urogenital-specific effects of reduced levels of circulating oestrogen, which is the most important hormonal change to occur as a woman passes through the menopause. Prior to the menopause, the ovary produces significant amounts of oestrogen (oestradiol and oestrone) as a result of the stimulating action of follicle stimulating hormone (FSH), secreted by the anterior lobe of the pituitary gland. With approach of the menopause, the ovary becomes progressively resistant to the stimulating effect of FSH, with a resultant reduction in oestrogen production (Riley 1991).

Changes in the urogenital tract

When considering the changes in the urogenital tract that occur as the result of the postmenopausal fall in circulating oestrogens, it is important to remember that the upper bladder, lower urethra and vagina have a shared embryological origin (Cardozo et al 1993, Cardozo 1996). The cells of the urethra and vagina are oestrogen dependent, containing oestrogen receptors that bind to oestrogen to keep the tissues healthy. The postmenopausal decrease in oestrogen levels results in a decreased blood supply to these tissues, together with a lowering of cellular start, which results in an alteration in the vaginal pH (becoming more alkaline), thus the vagina becomes more prone to infections. Plate 29 illustrates the changes in the vulva and vagina across the female lifecycle.

Additionally, as the epithelium lining the base of the bladder and urethra is oestrogen responsive, oestrogen defiency is related to the atrophic changes in these structures, which makes them vulnerable, predisposing to urinary problems and trauma during sexual intercourse. The common urinary symptoms experienced collectively known as the urethral syndrome, comprising dysuria, frequency, urgency and nocturia, occur in up to 67% of postmenopausal women (Brown & Hammon 1987, Riley 1991, Nazareth & King 1993).

Dolman & Chase (1996) discuss the role of the **pubococcygeal muscle** in a satisfying sexual experience. They suggest that as the vagina has relatively few sensations, most of the sensations experienced come from the pelvic floor muscles that loop around behind the vagina. The nerve endings in these muscles respond to stretching, therefore good muscle tone means that muscle is more able to respond to an erect penis during vaginal penetration, thus heightening sensations and sexual pleasure. Furthermore Heiman & LoPiccolo (1988) state that improving the strength of the pelvic floor muscles leads to increased blood flow, which is related to a greater ease of arousal (and thus vaginal lubrication) and orgasm. As the pelvic floor muscle tone is affected by the fall in oestrogen in the postmenopausal woman, it can be seen that this may have an important part to play in postmenopausal sexual dysfunction. In addition, male sexual arousal is also influenced by the degree of sexual sensation produced by the 'vaginal tightness' of his partner. Therefore, postmenopausal reduction in muscular tone coupled with vaginal dryness can contribute to the development of erectile dysfunction in some male partners (Bancroft 1989).

PROBLEMS OF THE UROGENITAL TRACT IN LATER LIFE

Atrophic vaginitis

Secondary to the lack of oestrogens postmenopausally, the vaginal epithelium becomes thin, smooth and shiny with subepithelial haemorrhages (see Plates 30 & 31). This presents as vulval soreness, superficial **dyspareunia**, persistent discharge and introital shrinkage – a condition known as **atrophic vaginitis**. These alterations have several possible physical consequences for the postmenopausal woman, namely persistent vaginal discharge, potential postmenopausal bleeding and sexual difficulties such as dyspareunia and reduced sexual desire. The first two of these problems will be discussed below; the sexual difficulties will be addressed later in the chapter. What should also be remembered is that although these are physical problems they have the potential to cause considerable psychological and social distress for the woman.

Persistent vaginal discharge

Vaginal discharge is one of the most common gynaecological complaints. According to Emens (1995), 37% of GP referrals made to the outpatient department of Birmingham Women's Hospital made reference to vaginal discharge or vaginitis. Atrophic vaginitis is an aspect of intractable vaginal discharge that is poorly understood, often trivialized by the medical profession and carelessly treated. For the woman, their vaginitis is a cause of considerable distress and should therefore be managed sympathetically. Women may present with intractable discharge as a result of: (i) cervicitis; (ii) recurrent vulvovaginal candidiasis; and (iii) atrophic vaginitis. Although the first two of these conditions are important, this chapter will deal only with the effects of atrophic vaginitis.

Diagnosis of a patient with atrophic vaginitis should be fairly straightforward, that is, she will be either postmenopausal or be receiving therapy that renders her hypo-oestrogenic. However, patients are often given an assortment of anti-infective agents before being referred for investigation. It is important to distinguish between the symptomatic patient with an inflamed atrophic vagina and the patient with a simple atrophy who has no symptoms and significant inflammation.

Symptoms include vaginal soreness, dyspareunia and occasional spotting. Diagnosis is made by careful inspection of the vagina. When compared to a well oestrogenated vagina, the inflamed atrophic vagina is frequently smooth with mural haemorrhages. Microscopic examination of the vaginal secretions classically shows a great number of intermediate and parabasal cells with a virtual absence of mature squames (Emens 1995).

The symptoms of spotting and postmenopausal bleeding are ominous, therefore, despite apparent bleeding from the vaginal epithelium, an endometrial biopsy should be taken before any treatment is started to rule out endometrial carcinoma. Treatment of atrophic vaginitis is with systemic or topical oestrogens, via tablets creams, pessaries or a silastic ring. Topical therapies are the first-line mainstay treatments. The length of treatment is important, local oestrogen is initially poorly absorbed by the atrophic vaginal mucosa, so treatment should be continued for 4–6 weeks.

Postmenopausal bleeding

This is bleeding from the genital tract occurring 6 months or more after the menopause. As stated above, it can be caused by atrophic vaginitis, however it is a serious symptom that may indicate the presence of malignant disease in the genitourinary tract. Every woman with postmenopausal bleeding should therefore be assumed to have a malignancy until full investigation, including cytology, curettage and biopsy, has proved to the contrary. Box 16.1 lists the main causes of postmenopausal bleeding.

Following investigation, treatment is dependent on the cause, each of which is explored elsewhere in this book.

Urinary problems

As stated earlier, the epithelium lining the base of the bladder and urethra is oestrogen responsive. Oestrogen deficiency is related to atrophic changes in these structures leading to the problems collectively known as the urethral syndrome; that is dysuria, urinary frequency, urgency and nocturia.

Whilst these urinary symptoms are unpleasant, painful and socially restricting, another result of oestrogen deficiency and often childbearing urinary incontinence is especially distressing. It is estimated that between 35 and 57% of postmenopausal women suffer from urinary incontinence (Brocklehurst et al 1972,

---

> **Box 16.1** The main causes of postmenopausal bleeding (adapted from Chamberlain & Malvern 1996)
>
> - The vulva:
>   - carcinoma
>   - urethral caruncle.
>   - rectal bleeding and haematuria must be excluded.
>
> - The vagina:
>   - carcinoma
>   - vaginitis, especially atrophic vaginitis
>   - foreign bodies, especially pessaries.
>
> - The cervix:
>   - carcinoma of the ectocervix
>   - carcinoma of the cervical canal.
>
> - The endometrium:
>   - carcinoma
>   - sarcoma
>   - mixed mesodermal tumours
>   - polyps
>   - atrophic endometritis.
>
> - The fallopian tubes:
>   - carcinoma.
>
> - The ovary:
>   - feminizing tumours
>   - granulosa cell tumour
>   - theca cell tumour.
>
> Withdrawal bleeding may follow administration of oestrogens for menopausal symptoms. This should not be assumed to be the cause of any postmenopausal bleeding until full investigation has excluded more sinister causes.

Jolleys 1988). It is therefore a problem faced by a large section of the population, and clearly poses a great potential threat in terms of physical, psychological and social wellbeing. It is not intended to discuss these urinary problems further, as they are well covered in Chapter 18.

Non-neoplastic disorders of the vulva

These are dermatological conditions of the vulval skin of uncertain aetiology, and were previously known as vulval dystrophies. Some are most commonly seen in postmenopausal women, often accompanied by a history of chronic candidal vulvovaginitis. These disorders are classified by the International Society for the Study of Vulvar Disease (Ridley et al 1989) as:

- squamous cell hyperplasia (formerly hyperplastic dystrophy)

- lichen sclerosus (formerly hypoplastic dystrophy)
- other dermatoses, e.g. psoriasis, lichen planus and condyloma acuminata.

Clinical presentation and diagnosis

Chronic itching, burning/vulval dysuria, pain and superficial dyspareunia. The pruritus is often worst at night and can lead to insomnia if severe. Vulval discharge or bleeding suggest the presence of concomitant infection or malignant ulceration.

Inspection of the vulva, perianal area, vagina and cervix should be thorough and performed gently, as the vulva can be extremely sensitive. The examination includes assessment of the mobility of the clitoral hood and introitus, together with mobility and thickness of the vulval tissues, noting any vulval lesions. The examination should include a speculum examination of the vagina and cervix (as intraepithelial neoplastic lesions of the lower genital tract may be multifocal), together with a bimanual examination (although if the vulva is very sensitive this can be deferred).

Lichen sclerosus has the appearance of a white, shrunken vulva with shiny papery skin extending to encircle the anus in a figure of eight fashion, involutional adhesions of the labia minora to the labia majora, burying the clitoris and shrinkage of the introitus.

Extensive squamous cell hyperplasia makes the vulval skin rubbery and redness may show through the white plaques. Differential diagnosis from vulval intraepithelial neoplasia (VIN) is made by vulval biopsy, this taking place after the application of the toluidine

blue test (application of 1% aqueous toluidine, washed off with 1% acetic acid after 1 min), the sky blue areas being biopsied. The nurse needs to be aware of the possibility of false negatives associated with hyperkeratosis and false positives due to excoriation (Gleeson 1995).

A thorough systemic review is also required to exclude:

- generalized dermatological conditions, e.g. lichen planus, eczema, psoriasis, allergic dermatitis
- multisystem disease, e.g. Behçet's syndrome, Crohn's disease, ulcerative colitis, sarcoidosis and amyloidosis
- autoimmune diseases, e.g. thyroid disease, pernicious anaemia and diabetes
- tumour, e.g. glucagonoma.

Treatment

The preliminary treatment is focused on the alleviation of symptoms, and further management on the risk of malignant progression and associated medical conditions (Box 16.2).

Histologically proven dystrophy is no longer an indication for aggressive surgery, i.e. simple vulvectomy. Meyrich-Thomas et al (1988) estimate that 4% of women with lichen sclerosus develop invasive carcinoma. Squamous cell hyperplasia and mixed dystrophy are more likely to be associated with atypia and invasive carcinoma (Elliott 1988). Long-term follow-up is required because of the small risk of malignant progression and the need to review symptoms and provide psychological support (as these problems can have tremendous impact on the quality of life of the women suffering from them).

Box 16.2 Preliminary treatments for squamous cell hyperplasia and lichen sclerosus

- Changes in personal hygiene methods, e.g. avoiding deodorants, talcum powder, perfumed soaps and detergents.
- Wearing cotton underwear and avoiding synthetic tights, to reduce vulval moisture.
- Treating any concomitant infections, e.g. candida.
- Itching managed by 1% hydrocortisone aqueous cream/ointment and/or oral antihistamine, e.g. chlorpheniramine 4 mg at bedtime (to break the itch–stratch cycle). Local anaesthetic gel, e.g. 2% lignocaine, for intense itching.

Squamous cell hyperplasia: topical corticosteroids.

Lichen sclerosus: 2% testosterone propionate ointment twice daily for 3–6 weeks, then 1–2 times per week **or** 0.05% clobetasol propionate topically.

SEXUAL BEHAVIOUR IN THE POSTMENOPAUSAL YEARS AND SEXUAL DYSFUNCTION ASSOCIATED WITH GYNAECOLOGICAL PROBLEMS

Sexuality forms an integral part of every person's life. Consequently, serious change in a person's life influences their sexuality. The inverse is also true, disturbance in a person's sexual life can lead to problems in their daily life (Woods 1987). The postmenopausal hormonal changes, common gynaecological conditions and/or their treatments are examples of the serious changes that may affect sexual and general functioning. It is intended to explore how an older woman's sexuality is potentially compromised in this way, together with the role of psychosexual nursing with this patient group.

Classification of sexual dysfunction in women is related to Kaplan's (1974) triphasic model of the female sexual response cycle. Therefore, the major manifestations of female sexual dysfunction are:

1. inhibited/hypoactive sexual desire
2. inhibited/hypoactive sexual arousal
3. orgasmic dysfunction
4. dyspareunia
5. problems with resolution of sexual arousal.
   (Anderson & Lachenbach 1986).

Hyposexual desire disorder is the term used to describe those individuals who report that they are generally uninterested in sexual activity. It can manifest itself behaviourally by avoidance of sexual contexts or refusal of sexual activity. Emotionally, women with hypoactive desire describe themselves as not feeling 'sexy' or feminine, and not being interested in initiating or responding to sexual activity. Furthermore, these women report an absence or low frequency of sexual fantasy or other pleasant, arousing cognitions. Weeks (1987) describes hypoactive desire disorder as being one of the most difficult and resistant sexual dysfunctions to treat. When the dysfunction arises in an established relationship it presents a severe threat to existing relationship dynamics and the couple's happiness.

Inhibited/hypoactive sexual arousal disorder pertains to difficulties experienced during the arousal phase of the sexual response. This leads to inhibition or disruption of the vasocongestive response, which in turn leads to insufficient vaginal engorgement and/or lubrication (making vaginal penetration difficult). Psychologically, the woman may report that she is not feeling aroused and/or that her body does not respond. Indeed, Riley (1991) states that the production of genital lubricating fluid is not only necessary to facilitate penile–vaginal penetration, but that it also appears to be an important factor upon which a woman perceives her own level of sexual arousal; so that when a poor lubrication response occurs she may not feel sexually aroused. Furthermore, one of the benefits of the localized vasocongestive response is to cushion penile thrusting, thereby preventing trauma to the perivaginal tissues, the urethra and base of the bladder. Thus, the postmenopausal alterations in response increase the potential for women experiencing dyspareunia.

As is also the case with the desire phase difficulties, subsequent orgasmic disruption can easily occur due to lowered levels of arousal.

As with any of the sexual dysfunctions, orgasmic dysfunction can be either primary (having always been absent) or secondary. When related to the post-

menopausal woman and/or gynaecological disorder, the complaint more commonly comprises a dramatic decline in orgasm frequency or complete failure to orgasm (secondary). In these circumstances, the problem is typically associated with a lack of arousal, with the woman feeling that she does not become sufficiently aroused to get close to experiencing orgasm, with a subsequent impairment of sexual interest.

Dyspareunia refers to pain during sexual intercourse. Sometimes this pain is localized at the vaginal entrance, in which case it may be the result of one of several factors, including mild **vaginismus**, lack of sexual arousal, a vaginal infection or a Bartholin's cyst. Pain resulting from lack of arousal usually eases as intercourse proceeds because vaginal lubrication increases and the vaginal muscles relax. Therefore, in the older postmenopausal woman, dyspareunia can be secondary to the poor vasocongestive response outlined previously.

Dyspareunia on deep penetration often has a physical basis, for example vaginal infection such as candida or herpes, pelvic infection or ovarian pathology. The pain worsens with thrusting and does not usually diminish during intercourse. However, deep dyspareunia sometimes results from impaired sexual arousal, when the ballooning of the inner part of the vagina and elevation of the uterus do not occur. Therefore, the cervix is subjected to intense buffeting by the penis, which causes the woman pain and may lead to further inhibition of her arousal. It is always important to suspect a physical cause for the dyspareunia until ruled out by detailed assessment and gynaecological examination.

Actual sexual dysfunction during the resolution phase of the female sexual response has not been demonstrated. However, women who experience difficulties with sexual arousal or orgasm report dissatisfaction with the resolution period associated with continued vasocongestion, residual sexual tension and/or concern that their sexual responsiveness has altered permanently. In addition, those women who experience dyspareunia often suffer from residual discomfort immediately after intercourse.

Postmenopausal alterations in sexual function

Several studies have reported a decline in sexual interest and coital frequency with increasing age. Pfeiffer et al (1972) found the largest decline in sexual activity was between 40 and 50 years (58% reduction) and 51 and 55 years (78% reduction). Hallstrom (1973) demonstrated a progressive decrease in sexual desire across menopausal status, with 52% of women aged 54 years reporting reduced desire compared to 20% aged 38 years. Sarrel and Bajulaya (1984) showed an increase in loss of desire from 13% in premenopausal women to 47% 1–3 years postmenopause; indeed by 9 years postmenopause 70% of the women had become sexually inactive. Although these studies highlighted that a significant factor associated with loss of desire was dyspareunia, it would seem that there is a complex relationship between the bio-psychosocial aspects of the postmenopausal situation, not least of these are society's and the individual woman's views and expectations of sex after the menopause (Rix 1998).

As stated previously, the formation of genital lubrication by transudation through the vaginal epithelium is dependent upon sufficient oestrogen production and adequate vasocongestive response. Both of these processes are changed in postmenopausal women, affecting their experience of sexual arousal. Another factor associated with postmenopausal arousal difficulties is the problem of generalized tactile impairment. Indeed, changes in tactile sensitivity may cause the woman to perceive touch by a loved one as unpleasant and painful, leading to avoidance and relationship conflict. Fortunately, altered tactile sensitivity generally responds well to oestrogen replacement.

Secondary orgasmic dysfunction is also seen in postmenopausal women. This is partly explained by the difficulties experienced with both sexual desire and arousal discussed above. In addition, decreased clitoral sensitivity may result from changes in nerve function, with the possible consequences of delayed or absent orgasm. Some women, however, experience a clitoral hyperaesthesia, which can be unpleasant or even painful (Riley 1991).

As discussed earlier, dyspareunia is a problem frequently associated with postmenopausal alterations in sexual activity. In addition to the problems caused by reduced vaginal lubrication, as the postmenopausal years advance the occurrence of atrophic changes in the genitalia contribute to the problem. These changes include shortening and narrowing of the vagina, shrinkage of the vaginal introitus, loss of fat from the mons pubis and labia, together with loss of elasticity of all the genital organs. These atrophic changes can be effectively prevented by prophylactic oestrogen replacement therapy or by continuing sexual activity (Leiblum et al 1986). Dyspareunia may also act as a trigger for the development of vaginismus. Postmenopausal dyspareunia usually responds well to oestrogen replacement

therapy, therefore the persistence of pain after restoration of good vaginal lubrication may suggest the presence of vaginismus.

Sexual dysfunction associated with gynaecological problems

The effects of undergoing a non-oncological or vaginal hysterectomy on sexual function are somewhat controversial, with many people suggesting that the perceived alterations in the sexual response are mainly of a psychological origin, that is that the women expect to feel different and are 'defeminized' by the removal of their uterus. There is, however, some evidence of physiological changes, which may help to explain the perceived alterations. Zussman et al (1981) and Rubin (1980) found that there is a decrease in the vasocongestive response, together with no vaginal ballooning/tenting with arousal (possibly due to vaginal scarring), furthermore, some women experience purely uterine orgasms, which will obviously be absent.

The effects of ovarian failure have been covered previously, suffice to say here that the natural menopause leads to a gradual reduction in oestrogen levels coupled with the ability to still produce androgens for some time, therefore there is little alteration initially in desire, arousal and fantasy. This is clearly not the case with surgically induced menopausal women, these women may therefore require more information and support in adapting to the changes in their function/behaviour.

Women undergoing vaginal repair and colposuspension may experience changes sexually. Anterior repair has the potential for interfering with the sensitivity of the anterior vaginal wall and the controversial G spot. Posterior repair sometimes leads to narrowing of the introitus and vagina, whilst colposuspension should have positive affects by decreasing dysuria, nocturnal enuresis and incontinence during sexual activity.

Anderson & Lachenbrach (1986) found that 75% of women with gynaecological malignancy had altered sexual function prior to diagnosis. It was postulated that this was due to fatigue, postcoital bleeding, discharge and dyspareunia. At the time of diagnosis and throughout treatment, each woman will obviously respond to her illness in different ways, each potentially impacting on her self-esteem and relationships. At this time sexual activity may very well be low on the woman's agenda, however, the need for affection and intimacy may be very strong. For some couples, this may present a problem, if their traditional behaviour is to show affection only through sexual contact.

The woman is likely to experience fatigue and perhaps continuing debilitation leading to problems with social isolation, again affecting her self-esteem negatively.

Following radical hysterectomy there is possible damage to the pelvic plexus leading to decreased vasocongestion, lubrication, vaginal expansion and sensory perception during arousal and coitus. Furthermore, removal of the vaginal cuff will lead to vaginal shortening and this, together with the possibility that the bladder trigone and sigmoid colon may be adherent to the vagina, may result in pain on penile thrusting and reduced arousal. The effect of lymph node clearance is unclear.

As would be expected, the sexual affects of a radical vulvectomy appear to be extensive. The physical alterations, due to removal of sexual tissue together with scarring, stenosis, sensory alterations and numbness, reduced tissue mobility and cushioning can all contribute to pain or discomfort and lack of arousal. Furthermore, the psychological affects of such genitally 'mutilating' surgery should never be underestimated. These women and their partners will require extensive counselling and psychological support to help them adapt to the situation. Even a previously close and supportive relationship can be 'rocked' by the illness and surgery; the situation may be worse when the pre-illness relationship was distressed.

In addition to the effects of surgery, the adjunctive treatments of radiotherapy and chemotherapy can also drastically alter sexual function. Radiotherapy can lead to narrowing and obliteration of small blood vessels and increases fibrosis, causing decreased vasodilatation/congestion, lubrication difficulties, sensory perception and vaginal expansion, furthermore, 80% of women receiving radiotherapy experience vaginal stenosis, which can cause dyspareunia.

The effects of chemotherapy are those of ovarian failure, coupled with the effects of altered body image from hair loss, weight gain, etc.

THE ROLE OF PSYCHOSEXUAL NURSING

It is obvious from the discussions throughout the chapter that a woman's sexuality is potentially altered or compromised by changes in the urogenital and reproductive systems, which result from normal biological processes, diseases and/or their adjunctive treatments. This area poses a challenge to a lot of nurses, especially as sexuality is regarded by many as a very sensitive and personal area of the patient's life, perhaps not to be intruded upon. And yet many patients look to the nurse as a professional to give help, support and empowerment in this area. Indeed, given the intensive therapeutic relationship that often exists between patient and nurse it is very likely that it is to the nurse that the patient will first voice their concerns, including their sexual concerns. The degree of practitioner effectiveness will largely depend on their depth of knowledge and their degree of comfort in talking about sexuality issues. As a nurse, it is important to be aware that patients do not often voluntarily ask sex-related questions, possibly because of modesty or embarrassment. Nurses therefore need to create a comfortable, open, non-judgemental atmosphere of communication to facilitate the exchange of the patient's concerns. This can be achieved by ensuring privacy, patient confidentiality, appropriate timing and providing written/reading material specifically related to the patient's problem, together with the utilization of existing counselling skills. It is important to give the patient 'permission' to discuss her concerns by conveying a sense that sexuality is a suitable topic for discussion. This could be achieved by normalizing comments/questions, such as those adapted from Woods (1987) below:

- How, if at all, has your illness and/or treatment changed the way you feel about yourself as a woman?
- How, if at all, has your illness and/or treatment altered your role as a woman/wife/partner/mother, etc?
- Other women who have had the same physical problem (illness/surgery, etc.) have told me that they have concerns about their sexual lives. Is this something you would like to discuss?
- If you could choose, what would you like to be different?

The answers to these questions help to determine baseline coping mechanisms, patient expectations and the learning needs of the patient and/or her significant others.

The nurse needs to be aware that some women would find such a discussion unacceptable in their husband's/partner's presence. Furthermore, for other women the discussion per se would be unacceptable, for personal, religious or cultural reasons. The nurse therefore needs to be sensitive to these and other variables, they also need to acknowledge the patient's right not to disclose or discuss these areas of their lives.

A very useful counselling tool, which offers nurses direction when dealing with patient's sexuality concerns, is the PLISSIT model (Anon 1971):

Permission.
Limited Information.
Specific Suggestions.
Intensive Therapy.

When adopting this framework, increasing knowledge and clinical skills are required as the intervention levels increase in complexity. However, using the four levels of involvement means that the nurse engages in counselling at her/his own level of comfort and expertise. As the levels increase the nurse continues to be free to make referrals at any time.

Permission

The nurse can give the patient 'permission' to discuss concerns and problems related to sexuality – as outlined previously. The willingness of the nurse to discuss any area will help relieve anxiety and tension on the part of the patient. The nurse can give professional 'permission' and reassurance that the patient's current sexual practices are appropriate and healthy. It is important, however, that activities that are potentially harmful to the individual are not condoned. 'Permission' can also be given to experiment with new forms of sexual expression. It is important to recognize that 'permission' can also be given not to be sexual, if this is appropriate for the patient and her partner. 'Permission' giving can be seen as preventive because it can resolve concerns that may otherwise grow into problems. This level of intervention is the least complex of the levels in the PLISSIT model and requires minimal preparation on the part of the nurse. Furthermore, the simple reassurance that behaviour is normal is often enough to alleviate the patient's concerns.

Limited information

Giving limited information provides patients with specific facts that are directly related to their areas of concern (having established these via the previous level of intervention). This information may relate to how their age, ill health and/or medical interventions affect their sexual abilities. Providing directly related information can be helpful in changing potentially negative thoughts and attitudes about particular aspects of sexuality, for example postmenopausal sexual behaviour. Furthermore, giving information that is of immediate relevance and limited scope can also effect behavioural change. As with permission giving, helping patients to increase their knowledge about sexuality and answering questions about sexual

> **Box 16.3** Common sexual myths and concerns
>
> - Myths regarding the characteristics of male and female sexual experiences and roles.
> - Notions of what constitutes the body, e.g. 'normal' genital size, body shape and size, disability, etc.
> - Body image changes or sexual functional ability changes related to age, ill health or surgery.
> - Myths about masturbation, oral–genital contact, sexual experimentation and fantasy.

concerns can be viewed as preventive, as these interventions can prevent or limit dysfunctional behaviour.

The information may revolve around dispelling of the myths that still abound in society in regard to sex, especially for the older person. A list of common sexual myths and concerns is given in Box 16.3.

Providing limited information takes more time and requires more knowledge than permission giving, and frequently the two levels of intervention are utilized simultaneously. Patients are often concerned about what is 'normal' or acceptable behaviour, and are struggling to place sexual behaviour in the context of 'normality'. Therefore, there is the need for both permission giving and information to clarify misinformation, dispel myths or provide specific information. Information giving can be anticipatory or at the patient's direct request. Careful assessment of the need and readiness for learning, the nature and extent of knowledge deficit and the most appropriate teaching method should be carried out before actual content is shared. Information giving is only helpful when a patient has a knowledge deficit. Here, the nurse's skills as a health educator are brought into play.

As stated earlier helping couples to adapt to ageing, illness or surgery that may affect sexual functioning is an important preventive and therapeutic measure. For instance, consider a 50-year-old perimenopausal woman. Such a woman would probably benefit from the following limited information-giving interventions: explaining to her and her partner how the menopause will affect her reproductive capacity; explaining how it may affect sexual functioning; clarifying misinformation and dispelling myths that may contribute to her negative feelings and fears about this natural process; discussing the treatment options available as appropriate and discussing with her and her partner ideas about anticipated changes in physical self-concept or role as a sexual being after the menopause.

Case study: Sarah

Sarah was a 54-year-old woman who had been married to Pete for 30 years. Sarah's history included a mastectomy for breast cancer and a hysterectomy with adjunctive radiotherapy for uterine cancer. She was referred by the practice nurse at her GP surgery, who had identified that Sarah had mild depression, possibly secondary to her generalized loss of sexual desire.

In addition to taking a detailed sexual and relationship history, Sarah was investigated via a gynaecological examination and an endocrine blood screen to exclude any organic basis for her problems.

It was identified that Sarah's loss of desire and depression were multifaceted in origin:
- severe superficial and deep dyspareunia, secondary to atrophic vaginitis, severe vaginal shrinkage and scarring from the previous radiotherapy
- the above had led to secondary vaginismus
- altered body image and low self-esteem – Sarah felt 'less of a woman' since her cancer, especially as both of these threatened the 'root' of her femininity
- relationship distress, possibly due to both the sexual dysfunction and the couple's fears about the cancer returning.

Both Sarah and Pete held stereotyped and myth-ridden ideas about sexual contact–very much male superior, missionary position intercourse following very limited foreplay.

Sarah and Pete were seen as a couple and were given both individual and couple home-based exercises to complete. Overall, the interventions used with the couple were as follows:
- Increased sexual education, that is, anatomy and physiology of the sexual response, and how these are changed by age, surgery and radiotherapy. Exploration

of sexual myths and alternative forms of expressing sexual intimacy.
- For Sarah, individual body self-focusing together with pelvic floor exercises, leading to the graduated use of vaginal trainers (inserted with the ample quantities of a water-based lubricating gel). In addition, appropriate erotic reading – initially individually, but eventually with Pete. Sarah was also offered individual self-esteem work.
- A modified sensate focus programme for the couple, leading eventually to full sexual intercourse when Sarah was comfortable with the insertion of the vaginal trainers without noticeable vaginismus or dyspareunia and again using a lubricant. These non-sexual but sensual exercises helped the couple to communicate their needs, likes and dislikes more freely and shifted the emphasis from vaginal penetrative sexual contact. In addition, the couple was advised to 'court' each other again, leading to better general communication.
- The couple was provided with some general counselling pertaining to their fears about Sarah's cancer returning. This allowed them to voice those fears they had previously been hesitant to share with each other.

Working with Sarah and Pete took place over a period of months, with several sessions to feed back and process the home-based work. Eventually, Sarah and Pete were able to have full intercourse at least once or twice a fortnight, together with a lot of close sexual and sensual intimate contact, all of which was satisfactory for both of them. Furthermore, they were communicating much better, both sexually and non-sexually, thus their previous relationship distress regressed and they said that they were closer now than they had been for many years.

Specific suggestions

This level of intervention involves directing efforts to assist the patient to change behaviour in order to attain stated goals by providing specific suggestions directly related to the particular problem. These involve direct problem-solving strategies or referral for specific medical interventions. The suggestions made may help the patient rethink the problem and make changes to alleviate the concern. Furthermore, the suggestions may involve giving practical advice, for example, the use of lubrication, changing sexual positioning, emptying the bladder prior to sexual intercourse, or the exploration of alternative methods of sexual expression. Fogel & Lauver (1990) suggest that in some situations giving a patient direct behavioural suggestions can help relieve a sexual problem. They

further state that this level of intervention is time- and problem-limited, with the nature of the problem treated at this level also being limited in scope. Problems of sudden onset and/or short duration are the most responsive to this form of brief treatment (perhaps one or two 30-min sessions). Sexual dysfunction that is generated by interpersonal conflict or of a long duration cannot be treated by this approach.

Intensive therapy

Here the concern may be a long standing sexual problem that requires highly individualized therapy. This final level of intervention is the most complex and is used when the patient's problems have not been resolved after the three earlier levels and/or where the problems are ones in which personal and emotional difficulties are interfering with sexual expression. The therapeutic processes at this final level are longer and more involved and should only be undertaken by a suitably trained therapist. Poorman (1988) suggests that nurses should be able to work to level 3 of the PLISSIT model, but only within their own boundaries of comfort, knowledge and skills.

The nurse's role in the provision of psychosexual healthcare includes education together with the use of counselling skills and techniques. A nurse's abilities to develop an open, genuine therapeutic relationship with their patients will ultimately allow the patients the 'freedom' to discuss concerns related broadly to their sexuality. As stated earlier, a woman's sexuality is potentially altered or compromised by changes in the urogenital and reproductive systems. By adopting the framework proposed by Woods (1987) – of assessing and addressing the women's concerns about their sexual self-concept, sexual role relationships and sexual function – the nurse can guide discussion to cover all the biopsychosocial elements of the woman's life. In this way the nurse can begin to give truly holistic care.

CONCLUSION

A woman in her postmenopausal, later years can experience many changes and problems related to her lower urogenital tract. This chapter has explored many of these, together with some of the difficulties posed by some of the therapeutic interventions aimed at rectifying the problems. The physical alterations in the urogenital tract experienced can clearly have negative effects on the woman's psychosocial wellbeing. The nurse working with patients in this age group needs to be sensitive to these potential difficulties and give holistic care accordingly. The chapter appears to have painted a rather gloomy picture of life after the menopause, perhaps reflecting the way in which some patients, and indeed, society, view these years. A woman's experience of these years is clearly bound up with her expectations of what life should or will be like in later life. For many women these later years are the most positive and liberating ones they experience. Therefore let us not end on a gloomy note – *viva* the older woman' and let us hope we will all experience many positive, happy and enriching years well into old age!

GLOSSARY

Atrophic vaginitis: thinning, dryness and inflammation of the vaginal tissues, resulting from the depletion of circulating oestrogen
Dyspareunia: recurrent and persistent genital pain experienced before, during and after sexual intercourse

Pubococcygeal (PC) muscle: the muscle surrounding the outermost vaginal canal
Vaginismus: a tendency involuntarily to contract the muscles surrounding the vaginal entrance, making penetration for intercourse tight and painful

REFERENCES

Anderson BL, Lachenbrach PA 1986 Sexual dysfunction and signs of gynaecological cancer. In: Weijmar Schultz WCM, De Wiel HBM, Bouma J, Lappohn RE 1991 Journal of Sexual and Marital Therapy 6(2):177–194
Anon J 1971 The PLISSIT model: a proposed conceptual scheme for the behavioural treatment of sexual problems. Journal of Sex Education and Therapy 2:1–15
Bancroft J 1989 Human sexuality and its problems, 2nd edn. Churchill Livingstone, Edinburgh
Brocklehurst JC, Try J et al 1972 Urinary infection and symptoms of dysuria in women aged 45–65 years: their relevance to similar findings in the elderly. Age and Ageing 1:41–47
Brown KH, Hammon CB 1987 Urogenital atrophy. Obstetric and Gynaecological Clinics of North America 15:13–32
Cardozo L, Cutner A, Wise B 1993 Basic urogynaecology. Oxford Medical, Oxford

Cardozo L, Hill S 1996 Urinary incontinence. The Royal College of Obstetricians and Gynaecologists, London
Chamberlain G, Malvern J 1996 Lecture notes on gynaecology, 7th edn. Blackwell, Oxford
Dolman L, Chase J 1996 Comparison between the health belief model and subjective expected utility theory: predicting incontinence prevention behaviour in post partum women. Journal of Evaluation Clinical Practice 2(3):217–222
Elliott P 1988 Vulvar cancer after treatment of microinvasive lesions. Journal of Reproductive Medicine 33:717
Emens MJ 1995 Intractable vaginal discharge. The Royal College of Obstetricians and Gynaecologists, London
Fogel CI, Lauver D 1990 Sexual health promotion. WB Saunders, Philadelphia
Gleeson NC 1995 The management of vulval dystrophy. In: Bonnar J (ed) Recent advances in obstetrics and gynaecology. Churchill Livingstone, Edinburgh

Hallstrom T 1973 Mental disorder and sexuality. Scandinavian University Press, Gotenberg

Heiman JR, LoPiccolo J 1988 Becoming orgasmic. Piatkus, London

Jolleys JV 1988 Reported prevalence of urinary incontinence in women in a general practice. British Medical Journal 296:1300–1302

Kaplan HS 1974 The new sex therapy: active treatment of sexual dysfunction. Brunner, New York

Leiblum SR, Swartzman LS 1986 Women's attitudes about the menopause: an update. Maturitas 7:47–56

Meyrick-Thomas RH, Ridley CM, McGibbon DH, Black MM 1988 Lichen sclerosus and autoimmunity – a study of 350 women. British Journal of Dermatology 118:41–46

Nazareth I, King MB 1993 The urethral syndrome: a controlled evaluation. Journal of Psychosomatic Research, October 37(7):737–743

Poorman SG 1988 Human sexuality and the nursing process. Norwalk, Appleton & Lange

Pfeiffer E, Verwoerdt A, Davis GC 1972 Sexual behaviour in middle life. American Journal of Psychiatry 128:1262–1267

Ridley CM, Frankman O, Jones IS et al 1989 New nomenclature in vulvar disease: International Society for the Study of Vulvar Disease. Human Pathology 20:495–496

Riley AJ 1991 Sexuality and the menopause. Journal of Sexual and Marital Therapy 6(2):135–146

Rix S 1998 Inhibition of sexual desire and the menopause. BASMT Bulletin 15:6–10

Rubin L 1980 Psychological and physiological concepts in female sexuality. In: Weijmar-Schultz WCM, De Wiel HBM, Bouma J, Lappohn RE 1991 Journal of Sexual and Marital Therapy 6(2):177–194

Sarrel PM, Bajulaiya P 1984 A survey of menopause related symptoms in Nigeria. In: Riley AJ, 1991 Sexuality and menopause. Journal of Sexual and Marital Therapy 6(2):135–146

Weeks GR 1987 Systematic treatment of inhibited sexual desire. In: Weeks GR, Hof L (eds) Integrating sex and marital therapy: a clinical guide. Brunner, New York

Woods NF 1987 Towards a holistic perspective of human sexuality: alternatives in sexual health and nursing diagnosis. Holistic Nursing Practice 1(4):1–11

Zussman LZ, Zusman S, Sunley R, Bjornson E 1981 Sexual response after hysterectomy–oophorectomy: recent studies and reconsideration of psychogenesis. American Journal of Obstetrics and Gynaecology 140:725–729

FURTHER READING

Comfort A 1990 A good age. Pan Books, London

Gibson HB 1992 The emotional and sexual lives of older people: a manual for professionals. Chapman & Hall, London

Greengross W, Greengross S 1989 Living, loving and ageing. Age Concern, London

Nelson-Jones R 1988 Practical counselling and helping skills. Cassell, London

Nissim R 1984 Natural healing in gynaecology. A manual for women. Pandora, London

RCN 2000 Sexuality and Sexual Health in Nursing Practice. RCN, London

Schover LR 1997 Sexuality and fertility after cancer. John Wiley, New York

Stoppard M 1994 Menopause. Harper Collins, London

Tschudin V 1991 Counselling skills for nurses, 3rd edn. Baillière Tindall, London

USEFUL ADDRESSES

British Association for Sexual and Marital Therapy
P.O. Box 13686, London SW20 9ZH.
Website: http:www.basmt.org.uk
RELATE
Herbert Gray College, Little Church Street, Rugby, Warwickshire CV21 3AP
Tel: 01788 573241

Women's Nutritional Advisory Service
PO Box 268, Lewes East, Sussex BN7 2QN
Tel: 01273 487366
Association to aid the sexual and personal relationships of people with disability (SPOD)
286 Camden Road, London N7 0BJ

17

Uterine displacement/prolapse

Sandra Brown

Uterine displacement and uterovaginal **prolapse** is experienced by many women, many of whom accept the inconvenience of the symptoms that occur and never seek medical help. Millions of pounds are spent each year within and outside of the NHS 'mopping up' the result of uterovaginal prolapse.

Many gynaecology units all over the UK admit women every day for treatment of this condition. It is a common occurrence to see a woman in a gynaecology outpatient department, who has been referred by her GP for a consultation for this problem.

Although many women do seek the help and advice of their GP when they first become concerned that they may have a problem, there is still a vast number of women who never seek help at all. These women cope with the symptoms themselves at home, and therefore a true figure of how many women are affected is not known.

Many women are too embarrassed to be examined vaginally. Gynaecology nurses are skilled at providing support at this time to enable a full examination to be carried out, in order for a diagnosis to be obtained, and this is a very important part of their role within any gynaecology unit.

UTERINE DISPLACEMENT
Definition

A uterovaginal prolapse is defined as 'the descent of the uterus/and or vagina'. The word prolapse means 'to slip out of place'. The uterus and the front and back walls of the vagina 'slide down' and bulge out of the vagina or vulva (Rhodes 1996). There are three main classifications of uterovaginal prolapse (Box 17.1).

Uterine displacement or **retroversion** occurs in 10% of the female population (Llewellyn-Jones 1994). In the other 90% the uterus is anteverted and anteflexed (Fig. 17.1) – the normal anatomical position.

Box 17.1 Classification of uterine prolapse – the three stages of uterine prolapse

- First degree prolapse – not yet descended below the introitus.
- Second degree prolapse – cervix descending to or beyond introitus.
- Third degree prolapse (**procidentia**) – whole of the uterus is outside of the vagina.

In most cases, a retroverted uterus is a developmental occurrence (Llewellyn-Jones 1994) and should not be considered as abnormal; however, in some cases it can be acquired, usually after childbirth (Rhodes 1996). At the time of childbirth the uterus is very large and, as it tries to return to its normal position during the first few weeks, it can fall backwards into the retroverted position.

For many decades a retroverted uterus was wrongly blamed for many gynaecological symptoms, such as dysmenorrhoea, backaches, menorrhagia and subfertility (Rhodes 1996). Much was done to try to correct the displacement, ranging from non-surgical to surgical techniques.

Non-surgical techniques

A vaginal examination would be carried out on the woman, the uterus would be manipulated into the anteverted position and a surgical ring pessary would be inserted and left in position for a number of weeks. This ring pessary had little effect, as the uterus would invariably fall back into the retroverted position, even with the pessary in situ and, if this didn't happen, then it would fall back again as soon as the pessary was removed a few weeks later.

Surgical techniques

Following the unsuccessful pessary insertion an operation would be considered. This operation was called a '**ventrosuspension**' and was carried out either laporo-

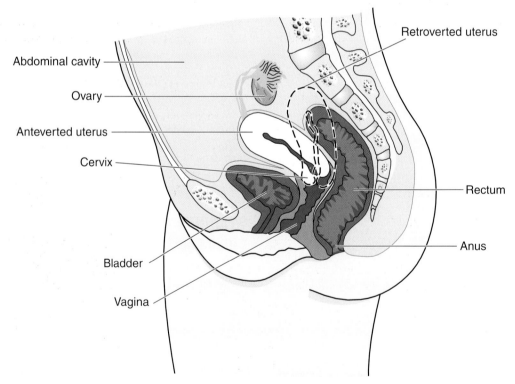

Figure 17.1 Normal position of the uterus. Reproduced with permission from Patients Pictures Gynaecology, Stafford Michael MRCOG, Health Press 1997.

scopically or by laparotomy. The round ligaments were shortened and sutured to the rectus sheath.

This operation would usually be performed for the symptoms of deep dyspareunia. This symptom is caused by the position of the ovaries when the uterus is in the retroverted position. When sexual intercourse takes place the ovaries are repeatedly hit by the penis, which can be very painful.

Very often, even after surgery, the woman still complained of deep dyspareunia, and it was therefore assumed that a wrong diagnosis had been made and that the dyspareunia was being caused by other factors, such as chronic lumbar backache (Rhodes 1996).

Treatment

In many cases, reassurance for the woman is needed, to help her understand that the retroverted uterus may not be the cause of her symptoms and that to operate may not be the answer (Llewellyn-Jones 1994). Manipulation may be carried out if it is felt it may relieve some of the pain.

UTEROVAGINAL PROLAPSE

There are other types of prolapse, such as those listed below. Many women assume that when they feel a 'lumpy swelling down below' that it is the uterus that is prolapsed (Fig. 17.2) but this is not always the case.

Types of prolapse

The most common types of prolapse are:

- cystocele
- **rectocele**
- **enterocele**
- **urethrocele**.

Cystocele

A cystocele is prolapse of the bladder and the anterior vaginal wall (Fig. 17.3).

Cystocele is fairly common and can be completely symptom free, although problems can occur if the cystocele becomes large. These are usually bladder irritation and the presence of a lump.

Residual urine is the cause of irritation due to infection. Dysuria and frequency of micturition will be experienced.

Rectocele

A rectocele is a prolapse of the rectum and posterior wall. The perineal body separates the lower third of

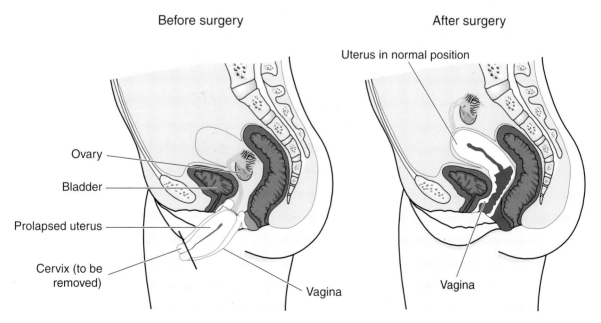

Figure 17.2 Procidentia – before and after surgery. Reproduced with permission from Patients Pictures Gynaecology, Stafford Michael MRCOG, Health Press 1997.

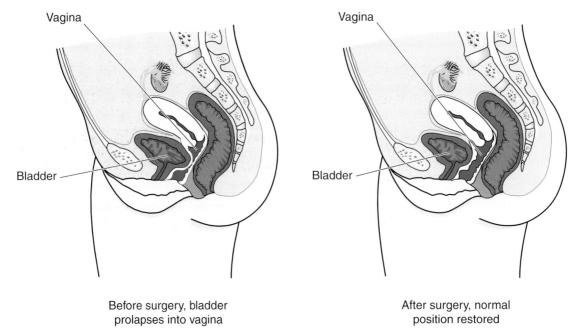

Before surgery, bladder
prolapses into vagina

After surgery, normal
position restored

Figure 17.3 Cystocele – before and after surgery. Reproduced with permission from Patients Pictures Gynaecology, Stafford Michael MRCOG, Health Press 1997.

the vagina from the rectum and a 'bulge' protrudes over the vulva.

Symptoms will occur if the rectocele becomes large. Problems with defecation are the most common symptom and can be very distressing; the woman has to use digital pressure to empty the rectum.

Enterocele

An enterocele is a prolapse of the pouch of Douglas through the posterior vaginal fornix. Small amounts of intestine are found in this type of prolapse, which is why it is known as enterocele. A large enterocele may cause deep pelvic discomfort.

Urethrocele

A urethrocele may occur if vaginal laxity occurs at the lower part of the anterior vaginal wall. The urethra is displaced downwards and rotates backwards at the junction with the bladder. The woman can develop stress incontinence.

All the above types of prolapse are graded into three main categories:

- slight
- moderate
- severe.

Aetiological factors

There are four aetiological factors for a prolapsed uterus:

- obstetric
- postmenopausal
- intra-abdominal pressure
- postoperative.

Obstetric factors

One of the most common causes of prolapse is childbirth (Chamberlain 1995). The supporting structures of the uterus can be damaged during this time. Problems do not always occur immediately after the birth, or in fact for many years to come. The time of the menopause can be the point at which women start to have symptoms due to atrophic changes.

Prolapse is not common in women who have not given birth, but it can occur in nulliparous women due

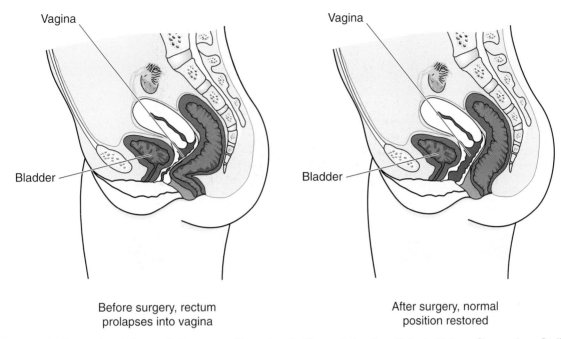

Before surgery, rectum
prolapses into vagina

After surgery, normal
position restored

Figure 17.4 Rectocele – before and after surgery. Reproduced with permission from Patients Pictures Gynaecology, Stafford Michael MRCOG, Health Press 1997.

to a congenital weakness of the supporting structures (Chamberlain 1995).

A prolonged labour and use of instruments at the birth can all contribute to a damaged pelvic floor.

Post-menopausal factors

Atrophic changes due to decreased secretion of oestrogen in the postmenopausal woman can contribute to the cause of uterovaginal prolapse. Women who present with procidentia (see Fig. 17.2) are mainly these who have atrophic changes. Muscles gradually become lax and muscle tone decreases.

Intra-abdominal pressure factors

Chronic constipation can be a contributing factor in the cause of prolapse. Strain on passing hard stools puts pressure on the intra-abdominal muscles. Heavy smoking resulting in persistent coughing is also a factor to be considered.

Postoperative factor

Prolapse can occur after a total abdominal hysterectomy, which involves surgery to the supporting ligaments, although this is not common (Chamberlain 1995).

To understand more fully about uterovaginal prolapse it is necessary to know more about the supporting structures of the pelvic floor. Anatomical considerations must be given, especially when one of the major causes of uterovaginal prolapse is childbirth.

Anatomical factors

As described earlier, the pelvic floor is under considerable strain during labour. In the first stage of labour the cervix is greatly stretched to allow the baby's head to pass through. The head is then driven down into the pelvic floor, and the ligaments are stretched downwards.

During the second stage of labour the baby's head may move up and down within the vagina, and this can cause shearing of the skin, causing damage. At the end of the second stage of labour massive distension of the pubovaginalis muscle may occur, to such an extent that some backward tearing into the perineal body may be a result. This tearing could extend into the rectum and damage the muscles that control defecation and flatus.

All of this activity of the ligaments and muscles during childbirth can have lasting effects on the pelvic floor. The stretched ligaments are left to recover naturally, but can be strengthened again by pelvic floor exercises. These exercises can be taught by physiotherapists and midwives. To be of any value, however, they must be continued by the woman after discharge home.

The ligaments are partly dependent on oestrogen to maintain their supporting role of the pelvic organs. At the time of the menopause oestrogen secretion is reduced and therefore atrophic changes occur and can contribute to a uterovaginal prolapse.

Signs and symptoms of uterovaginal prolapse

Various signs and symptoms associated with uterovaginal prolapse are experienced by women.

The most common symptom of uterovaginal prolapse is a 'feeling of something coming down'. Ninety-nine per cent of women will describe this when discussing their problems This can be a very distressing symptom because the 'lump' can be mistaken for something more sinister than it is.

Urinary symptoms are very common for women with a cystocele prolapse. This is due to the bladder being displaced to some degree and causing frequency of micturition. Infection of the urinary tract must always be ruled out in the first instance, by a laboratory examination of a specimen of urine.

Stress incontinence is also a frequent symptom of cystocele/urethrocele. This occurs when the woman laughs, coughs, runs, sneezes or does any strenuous exercises such as aerobics. It is caused by the raised intra-abdominal pressure that occurs with uterovaginal prolapse. This incontinence must not be confused with genuine stress incontinence, which is diagnosed when the woman is wet most of the time and constantly dribbles urine (see Chapter 18).

Constipation can be a symptom of rectocele prolapse but is more likely to be the cause, due to the constant strain of trying to pass hard stools.

Urge incontinence of urine can be present in the absence of a prolapse, and can be helped by a system of bladder retraining. The woman is asked to pass urine on the hour every hour until she feels she is improving, with the urge to pass urine decreasing as she retrains her bladder. She then extends the time to one and a half hours and so on until she feels the problem is greatly improved.

Backache is another symptom frequently described by women with prolapse, although it may not be the only cause and should always be investigated separately (Chamberlain 1995).

Ulceration and bleeding can occur with a procidentia and is very distressing to the woman.

The use of ring pessaries in uterovaginal prolapse

Prior to effective surgical treatment of prolapse, vaginal pessaries were the treatment of choice (Wood 1992). Since the 1960s, the use of these pessaries has decreased amongst providers of healthcare. An article published in 1961 discussed how 13 women were admitted to an infirmary because of complications attributed to vaginal pessaries (Russell 1971). The major factor cited in these women's cases was lack of follow-up following fitting of the pessary. Pessaries are still fitted in women but much stricter follow-up is required to ensure that no complications of this therapy are occurring.

Some women are not suitably fit for surgery and may be considered high anaesthetic risks and therefore a pessary can help symptoms, although it is not a cure for uterovaginal prolapse (Wood 1992).

Vaginal pessaries date back to ancient times and have been made of wood, plastic, rubber, metal, ivory, whalebone and sponge. Modern pessaries are made primarily of plastic or rubber. Some specialists believe that plastic pessaries are less irritating and are therefore preferable; shape is not seen as a deciding factor when fitting a pessary (Wood 1992; Fig. 17.5).

After selecting the type of pessary the size is then decided upon. The largest pessary that can fit comfortably admitted through the vaginal orifice should be tried first. Before inserting the pessary the prolapse should be manually reduced to allow for examination of the vaginal mucosa. Any lesions that might be suspicious or pre-existing infection should be treated first. A woman with atrophic vaginitis should insert oestrogen cream nightly for 2–3 weeks prior to insertion of the pessary to strengthen the vaginal walls.

The nurse in the clinic must reassure the patient throughout the procedure and support her whilst the pessary is fitted. If discomfort is felt by the woman

---

Case study: Sarah

Sarah is an active 65-year-old who works part-time in the local school cafeteria and has just started attending weekly line dancing sessions with her husband Dennis.

For about 6 months now, Sarah has been troubled by a 'lump', which feels it is 'coming down' into her vagina. Sarah is a smoker, usually smoking between 15 and 20 cigarettes per day and has a troublesome 'tickly' cough. She is also overweight, weighing 11 ½ stone.

Sarah has recently had some episodes of incontinence whilst at work, which have been particularly embarrassing. She feels it is worse when lifting heavy objects at work, but she had also noticed it occurring at the line dancing sessions, and she has been making excuses to sit out of some of the dances.

Sarah has been using pads to minimize the wet patches on her clothes. Eventually, she plucked up courage to see her GP and booked an evening appointment. Sarah did not often visit her GP as she had been reasonably fit apart from the usual coughs and colds that everyone gets. She had brought up a family of four children and just got on with things.

After listening to Sarah's problem her GP did a gentle vaginal examination and told Sarah that he thought she had a prolapse but he would need the opinion of a gynaecologist. He gave Sarah a letter and asked her to take it with her on the day the appointment was due.

Sarah asked if the 'lump' could be something serious and her doctor assured her that in his opinion it wasn't, that it could mean that she needed an operation, but it could all be sorted out quite soon.

Sarah attended the gynaecology outpatients department and once again described her symptoms, which had got slightly worse whilst waiting for the appointment. The gynaecologist listened whilst she described the way that urine leaked when she exerted herself. He then took a full medical history and obstetric history, noting that Sarah had one forceps delivery and that her babies had all been quite big. He questioned her about her smoking and also weighed her. He asked if he could carry out a vaginal examination and she agreed. The Consultant told Sarah that he could feel a prolapse (cystocele) and this was the cause of her symptoms, although they were being aggravated by her smoking and increased weight.

He explained to Sarah about the wear and tear on the pelvic floor after four babies and especially after forceps delivery.

He advised Sarah to stop smoking because the constant coughing was contributing to the problem by raising the abdominal pressure. He also advised her to lose weight and referred her to the dietician in the outpatient department for advice.

The Consultant then gave Sarah his advice as to how she might best be treated. She was told that it would be best to have the prolapse repaired by a surgical operation and this would mean coming into hospital for 5–7 days. He told her she would have a general anaesthetic and that this was another important reason for giving up smoking.

Sarah was shocked to find out that she needed an operation but was willing to take the advice from the Consultant. The Consultant told her that the prolapse would not get better without an operation, but he could make her feel more comfortable in the meantime with a ring pessary. This would just be a temporary treatment until she came into hospital in the future.

Sarah agreed to have a pessary and a 77 mm ring pessary was selected and fitted. Sarah was told that the pessary would need changing in 3 months time if the operation date had not come through. After fitting of the pessary Sarah did feel more comfortable and asked if it might fall out. She was told that sometimes they do and if that happened she would need to contact her GP for advice.

The Consultant added Sarah's name to his waiting list for a date to come into hospital and also to attend the preadmission assessment clinic.

---

after fitting the pessary then a smaller one may be necessary.

The nurse should discuss the pessary aftercare with the woman and a referral to the community nurse may be applicable if the woman is elderly or does not understand how to care for the appliance afterwards. Initial follow-up should be 2–4 weeks after insertion and the nurse must make sure an appointment is given. At each visit the nurse should question the woman about any problems she has had with the pessary. Signs such as vaginal bleeding, odour, discomfort or urinary problems should be discussed. The pessary should be removed by the doctor and a pelvic examination carried out. The pessary can then be changed and a subsequent appointment booked.

Vaginal pessaries may not be a popular treatment for uterovaginal prolapse but for those women for whom an operation is not feasible it is one way of providing palliative treatment to reduce discomfort and symptoms.

Nursing management and symptom control

Throughout the chapter reference has been made to patients' feeling of embarrassment and invasion of privacy due to the very personal problems.

The majority of patients with uterovaginal prolapse will have similar symptoms, the most common being urinary incontinence. Incontinence, no matter how

Before insertion

After insertion

Ovary

Bladder

Prolapsed
uterus

Vagina

Ring
supporting
bladder and
uterus

Vagina

Figure 17.5 Relieving a prolapsed uterus by inserting a ring pessary. Reproduced with permission from Patients Pictures Gynaecology, Stafford Michael MRCOG, Health Press 1997.

mild, can have a devastating effect on the sufferer, who feels isolated and embarrassed because of the incontinence. Even after diagnosis and agreeing to be operated on there can still be a considerable time to wait and therefore help may be needed to overcome the problem of incontinence to establish a better quality of life.

Managing the incontinence is a role that nurses are well equipped to do. Good nursing care can make all the difference providing the nurse can find out what is

needed (Ross 1994). A good assessment of the patient can be carried out by a nurse with knowledge and interest in women with incontinence problems. Unfortunately, a nurse specialist in women's continence is a luxury that not every gynaecology unit can afford.

A problem-solving cycle can be used (Box 17.2) to help both the patient and the nurse.

The key to assessment is communication and privacy. Questions should be put privately and sympathetically. Communicating with those with continence problems requires sensitivity and understanding.

The elderly patient in whom an operative procedure is not being considered, mainly because of the medical problems and high anaesthetic risk, will need an in-depth approach to assessment. Environmental factors will have to be included, whereas the woman waiting for an operation may need only appliance information. A prescription for pads or information on where to buy incontinence wear may be the only help she will need until her operation has been carried out.

An elderly woman living alone may require help from the primary care team. The continence assessment may need to take in the factors listed in Box 17.3.

Helping the patient who is incontinent is a valuable part of nursing a patient with prolapse and should not be overlooked when a woman presents with this

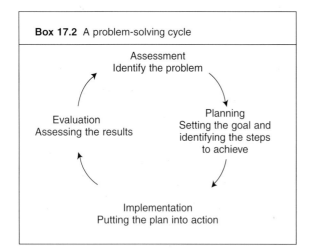

Box 17.2 A problem-solving cycle

Assessment
Identify the problem

Planning
Setting the goal and
identifying the steps
to achieve

Implementation
Putting the plan into action

Evaluation
Assessing the results

Box 17.3 Environmental factors to look at when making an assessment

- Are there adequate toilet facilities that are easily accessible to the patient – commode, downstairs toilet?
- Is clothing easily removed?
- Has the patient adequate washing facilities?
- Is the patient on diuretic therapy and is it being taken at the right time of day?
- Has medication been assessed recently?
- Are adequate fluids being taken throughout the day?

Box 17.4 Surgical approach for anterior colporrhaphy and repair of cystocele

1st step	Opening up the anterior vaginal wall.
2nd step	Mobilizing the cystocele from vaginal walls.
3rd step	Mobilizing the cystocele from the cervix.
4th step	Placing the tightening suture as far laterally as possible.
5th step	Obliterating the cystocele completely.
6th step	Removing the redundant vaginal wall with a continuous catgut suture.

---

problem. Information on support groups and associations aligned to incontinence sufferers can be given to these women to enable good support at all times.

Ideally, a nurse specialist within the gynaecology unit with an interest in incontinence issues is the best person for this work. Her continuous visits and support, both in the hospital and at home, is a very valuable service. The patient who will be admitted to the gynaecology unit for an operation will already have a familiar face to recognize and a relationship will already have been established.

Likewise, the patient who is not waiting for an operation will know that the continence nurse advisor is always available when problems occur or appliances need re-assessing and this kind of nursing support is to be recommended in all gynaecology services.

Helping the patient to stop smoking and reduce weight is part of the nurse management for the patient with uterovaginal prolapse. Stressing the importance of both the effect on the pelvic floor and the postoperative benefits should be explained by the nurse.

Many patients will find it extremely difficult to achieve even one of these healthier options and therefore will need help and advice from the nurse. Here the patient's GP can help by providing support in the community. Information can be given about self-help groups in the area.

The advice and help from the dietician can also be sought in order for a healthier diet to be established. Health education from nurses should be given on a daily basis to patients and not be seen as a luxury at critical times (McCleod & Latter, 1990). If patients with problems of obesity and smoking can be encouraged to modify their lifestyles, they themselves would soon reap the benefits. Troublesome coughing would improve and in return less incontinence of urine and with that an increase in self-image. No-one wants to be

wet if it can be avoided and nurses can play a major part in a successful health education plan for a woman who is eager to help herself.

Surgical restoration of the normal anatomy is an option which may be considered by the woman with a prolapse.

Anterior *colporrhaphy* and repair of cystocele

The shortening of the cardinal and uterosacral ligaments is called for, and each operation is adapted according to the extent of the prolapse. The operation is classed as a major procedure and is carried out using the six steps outlined in Box 17.4.

Preoperative preparation of the patient is vital and must include a full medical and anaesthetic assessment. Patients recover very quickly and within 48 h

---

Box 17.5 Surgical approach for Manchester repair/Fothergill's procedure.

1st stage	Repairing the cystocele and stripping the cervix from the vaginal walls.
2nd stage	Stripping back the posterior vaginal wall.
3rd stage	Suturing and dividing the elongated transverse cervical and uterosacral ligaments.
4th stage	Amputating the cervical stump.
5th stage	Covering the posterior stump with vaginal wall.
6th stage	Typing of the transverse ligaments in front of the cervix and so shortening them and raising the uterus (this is the so-called Fothergill's suture).
7th stage	Covering the cervical stump and closing the vaginal wall. On release of the cervical stump the uterus returns to the pelvis.

should be carrying out some aspects of self-care. Details of preoperative assessment and postoperative care are covered fully in Chapter 20.

Manchester repair/Fothergill's procedure

Named after the surgeon who first carried out this particular operation, it is individualized by the amputation of the elongated supravaginal cervix. It is often done in conjunction with anterior and posterior repairs.

A **Manchester repair** is the operation of choice when a uterine prolapse is present but is not prolapsing down enough to warrant a vaginal hysterectomy. It is carried out under a general anaesthetic and again can be staged (Box 17.5).

Posterior colpoperineorrhaphy and repair of rectocele

The operation of choice for a prolapse of the rectum into the posterior vaginal wall. Again, carried out under a general anaesthetic with relevant preoperative assessments. Operative procedures are carried out using four stages (Box 17.6).

Box 17.6 Surgical approach for colpoperineorrhaphy and repair of rectocele

1st stage	Mobilizing the posterior vaginal wall.
2nd stage	Separating the rectocele from the posterior vaginal wall.
3rd stage	Obliterating the rectocele by tightening the fascial layer.
4th stage	Removing excess vaginal skin. The perineal muscles are sutured over the obliterated rectocele. Catgut sutures are used to close the skin and vagina.

Box 17.7 Surgical approach for repair of enterocele

1st stage	Removing a section of the vaginal wall.
2nd stage	Identifying and opening the enterocele sac.
3rd stage	Mobilizing the sac and then suturing the neck as far as possible to obliterate the enterocele. The sac is then sutured to the neck of the cervix.
4th stage	Closing the vaginal wall in the usual way.

Box 17.8 Surgical approach for vaginal hysterectomy

1st stage	Mobilizing the bladder and stretching the uterine ligaments.
2nd stage	Entering the uterovesical pouch.
3rd stage	Removing the uterus and suturing the posterior peritoneal leaf to the peritoneum of the bladder.
4th stage	Suturing the lateral pedicles together to support the pouch of Douglas.
5th stage	Obliterating the cystocele in the usual way and closing the vaginal vault and anterior wall. Posterior colporrhaphy follows.

Repair of enterocele

Used to repair a prolapse of the pouch of Douglas peritoneum, in between the upper vagina and rectum (Box 17.7)

Repair by vaginal hysterectomy

Carried out when the uterus is prolapsed completely. Some patients find it confusing when referring to 'their prolapse'; they very often assume that it is the uterus that is bulging down but this is not always the problem. A full explanation to each woman about the type of prolapse she has is essential. A vaginal hysterectomy is not a more complicated operation than the 'repair' type of surgery, but more complications can occur, including haemorrhage, vault haematoma and ureteric distortion. This operation is carried out in five stages (Box 17.8).

Nursing management of the patient planning surgery for uterovaginal prolapse

Nursing management of women requiring surgery for uterovaginal prolapse has two main elements:

- pre-/postoperative counselling and information giving
- clinical care whilst in hospital.

The first element of nursing management is within the preadmission clinic assessment. Nursing research has demonstrated that patient anxiety levels, stress and pain can be reduced by good preoperative information (Hayward 1978). It can also reduce lengths of stay. Women who have elected to come into hospital have elevated anxiety levels and good nursing input at this

Case study: Doreen

Doreen Wilson, aged 72 years, lives in Manchester and has been a widow for the past 2 years. She lives alone but has good support from her family. She has two daughters who both live near by and call in regularly.

Doreen worked in the local factory all the time her family were growing up, and only gave up work 6 years ago to start her retirement.

Recently, Doreen has started to feel that she could feel something 'hanging down' and has been having problems controlling her bladder. She does not feel like going out because she is worried she may have to dash to the toilet, and therefore she has been isolating herself.

Doreen at first was too embarrassed to see her GP but now things are getting worse and she feels constant 'dragging pains'. Doreen booked an appointment to see her family GP.

Doreen's GP diagnosed a prolapsed uterus and a small cystocele that would need a surgical operation to restore anatomy. Doreen's GP gave her a letter for the local hospital and an appointment was sent to her home.

After a gentle examination Doreen was told that she would need to come into hospital for a vaginal hysterectomy and an anterior repair of the vaginal wall.

On admission to hospital Doreen was prepared for theatre. She had attended the preadmission assessment clinic the week before and was familiar with some of the nursing staff so she felt quite relaxed. All of the preanaesthetic tests had all been carried out and because everything was normal she came in fasting and was having her operation within 3 h of her admission.

The vaginal hysterectomy and anterior repair was completed without complications and Doreen returned to the ward once she was conscious and her vital signs were stable. She was connected to an intravenous infusion with dextrose–saline the fluid of choice. An indwelling urethral catheter was in situ and a vaginal tampon inside the vagina. The postoperative instructions were to remove the tampon after 24 h and the catheter was to be removed after 48 h.

Regular observations of Doreen's vital signs were carried out and a regular checking of vaginal bleeding was also noted.

Doreen made a very good recovery and the intravenous drip was taken down the day after surgery, when Doreen was able to eat and drink adequately. The catheter was removed on the second postoperative day and the urine output measured for a further 24 h. Four days after her operation Doreen was ready to go home. Her daughter took her home and arrangements were made for her family to call in every day and do the shopping and heavy housework as required.

Doreen was encouraged to have a daily bath and to carry out the postoperative exercises that she had been taught by the physiotherapist.

A follow-up appointment was given to Doreen for 6 weeks after her operation at the outpatients department for a routine medical check-up, which included a gentle vaginal examination.

Doreen was extremely relieved to have the operation over and, after 6 weeks convalescence, was back to her normal self. She now had finally got rid of the awful symptoms of the prolapse and felt a new woman.

stage can do much to alleviate a good proportion of this anxiety. It has been said that patients who are admitted electively have higher anxiety levels than those admitted as emergencies (Cochran 1984).

Patients awaiting admission have more time to think about the unknown and start experiencing symptoms such as insomnia, nausea and diarrhoea.

The nurse in the gynaecology preadmission assessment clinic is in a prime position to counsel the patient about her forthcoming surgery and allay any fears or apprehensions that she may have. Questions can be answered, problems addressed socially or medically, in privacy and away from the main busy ward area.

The woman may be concerned about pain, loss of independence, altered body image, ward routines or childcare or have any number of unanswered questions that have been churning around in her mind for months.

This is an ideal opportunity for the nurse to establish a rapport with the woman, which can be immensely satisfying to both patient and nurse.

Referrals to other agencies can be carried out during this assessment. The woman may be a carer for another member of the family and will need help over the next 6–8 weeks whilst she convalesces. She may need childcare or respite care for a dependent child or disabled partner and this can be organized well before admission.

The nurse can explain about pain and pain relief following surgery, helping the woman to understand what is available to alleviate the pain and therefore reduce her fears.

Ward routines can be explained and an opportunity to visit the ward should be given at this point.

A thorough explanation of the clinical care she will receive will do the woman an immense amount of good if a knowledgeable gynaecology nurse carries out the assessment. All questions should be answered, wherever possible, about what is expected of the woman pre- and postoperatively. Achievable goals can be set to give the woman some feeling of independence within her own care. Care plans can be written with the involvement of the woman to provide a sense of partnership between nurse and patient.

A full medical assessment can also be carried out to ensure the woman is fit to have major surgery and a general anaesthetic. Last minute cancellations of operations can be avoided by a good preassessment clinic nurse, checking blood results and communicating with the medical staff. Imbalances in blood can be corrected, anaemic patients can be transfused preoperatively to reduce the need to cancel an operation, which wastes valuable time to both patient and hospital.

Leaflets and information booklets should be given to patients during this clinic as it is well documented that patients only retain between 50% and 70% of verbal information (Ley 1967). The patient will be able to read the leaflets and booklets at home in their own time.

Physiotherapy education can be incorporated into the preassessment clinic session, therefore providing collaborative care at one point within the service. Women often enjoy their physiotherapy education alongside other women who are all experiencing similar problems.

The preadmission assessment clinic can become a very pleasant social gathering. From my own experience it has become a very focal point within our area. The input from nurses is a major contribution and its value is recognized throughout our service.

Physical and psychological preparation for surgery is the ultimate goal of the preadmission assessment clinic and is recommended for every gynaecology unit.

Nursing management in the clinical area for uterovaginal prolapse

Expert nursing care in the field of gynaecology should be the expectation of every woman entering hospital to have a repair of a uterovaginal prolapse.

Expertise of nursing staff, highly trained in this particular speciality, is a must if standards of care are to be maintained for women.

The nurse will not only have knowledge about the physical preparation of the patient, but also the psychological care that is necessary to get women well again and regain independence as soon as possible.

Privacy and dignity on a gynaecology ward are elements of care that must be given and should not be seen as something that is given when there is time. They should be incorporated into every gynaecology ward's 'philosophy of care'.

Women undergoing uterovaginal repair are often very apprehensive preoperatively and should be welcomed and settled into the ward as soon as possible. An explanation of what will happen should be given soon after arrival. The expertise of the nursing staff will soon be judged by the initial welcome and subsequent involvement of the patient and other new arrivals to the ward.

A calm, unhurried approach by nursing staff will help the anxiety of the woman being prepared for operation.

The woman should be prepared for theatre and a pre-med given if prescribed. The call bell should always be in reach to give reassurance.

It is good practice to allow the woman to empty her bladder before going to theatre, even though catheterization will be performed at the beginning of the operation. A good time to ask the woman to do this is when the 'check list' is completed.

Good nursing management at this point is vital because the woman can be very frightened of going to theatre and a calm nursing approach is needed. A swift handover to theatre staff with all relevant investigations and safety checks completed instills confidence into the woman and can really make a difference to her future recollection of having an operation.

Regular observations of blood pressure, pulse, respirations and vaginal loss need to be carried out on return to the ward. A vaginal tampon is sometimes placed inside the vagina but this is not routine procedure.

Most vaginal tampons are removed 24 h later and the nurse's role is to check any seeping or leakage through the tampon and report to the medical staff.

Intravenous fluids are given for the first 12–18 h, but some oral sips of water are allowed if nausea is not present. Strict fluid balance is required to maintain hydration of the patient until oral fluids are reintroduced, and urine output should be measured frequently in the first 48 h.

Catheterization is not used by all clinicians and care should be carried out accordingly. Offering a bed pan within 6 to 8 h after operation and monitoring output is required if a catheter is not in situ.

Women recover very quickly after this operation and, within 24 h, are able to start mobilizing independently, although individuals differ. Age does not seem to be a barrier for longer delays in recovery, and quite elderly women can be seen keeping up with their younger counterparts.

Postoperative retention of urine and haemorrhage are the main complications that may arise. Careful observation of both vaginal loss and urinary output is a vital part of the nursing management of these.

Urine infections can occur in the catheterized woman and specimen of urine should be obtained from the catheter to be sent for culture. Regular temperature taking should be carried out to detect any infection that may be arising. Antibiotics can be prescribed if a temperature is not settling, until microscopy of the urine is complete and a result has been obtained.

Constant reassuring and an informative approach by the nursing staff is a major contributing factor to a good postoperative recovery. Health education regarding personal hygiene, both in hospital and at home, will help the patient to understand how to care for the perineum, which can be sore and painful due to suturing. Good analgesia can reduce the pain but bathing regularly in plain water will alleviate much of the soreness.

By the fourth postoperative day a return to independence and normality should have been established. Urine output should be restored without complication and the patient should be thinking of discharge home.

Again, the role of the nurse should be aimed at arranging a problem-free discharge home. Postoperative advice and support should be offered in the form of leaflets, booklets and if necessary a visit from a community nurse if circumstances at home require it – some women may live alone and would be reassured by a visit from the local community nurse just to check that all is well.

Haemoglobin levels should be checked before discharge home and any medication prescribed in the form of a take-home prescription.

The woman should feel greatly relieved that the distressing 'lump' has now gone and the operation is safely over.

Some women do feel very emotional following an operation and this should be recognized as normal by nursing staff and reassurance and support given. A happy, relaxed atmosphere on the ward can help to make women feel cared for and can make their stay a positive experience.

CONCLUSION

Uterovaginal prolapse is not life threatening but it can bring about very distressing symptoms. With good nursing management these symptoms can be lessened to enable a quality of life that is tolerated until treatment can be carried out and a cure obtained.

If a cure is not possible, then good palliative care can be considered and, with good nursing assessment, achieved. Nurses working in the primary care setting have the unique opportunity to educate women with prolapse that incontinence need not simply be put up with. They can show that help is at hand and the expertise of nurses in this field should be sought out and used.

Case study: Rose

Rose is a 71-year-old woman who was admitted as an emergency, although her condition did not really require an emergency bed.

Rose lived with her son in a small cottage on the outskirts of a large city in the Midlands. Although Rose was only 71, she looked ten years older. She was admitted by her GP with a large **procidentia**, which was ulcerated and very sore. The GP did not know how long Rose had been suffering with this problem and had called to see her for another reason, but on finding the procidentia he rang the gynaecology on-call SHO, who thought she should be admitted.

Rose had had a very hard life, with the cottage she lived in never being modernized at all. Her husband had died and her son did little for her. She was very dirty, undernourished and was known to the local Social Services department. Some mobile meals were being delivered to her house but they were inadequate and her son cooked only occasionally.

According to her records Rose had had numerous medical problems and had recently had a thyroid operation, but she could not recollect this happening, and seemed surrounded by some degree of confusion.

The procidentia was protruding outside of her body and was indeed ulcerated, but Rose did not complain of pain. A saline-soaked dressing was put around the procidentia to prevent further ulceration.

Surgical intervention to remove the procidentia was ruled out due to Rose being a high anaesthetic risk. The consultant in charge of Rose's case thought that the best treatment would be to try a ring pessary.

The ring pessary was fitted and it was decided to keep Rose for a few days to give her some nursing care and attention and to see if the pessary stayed in place.

Rose was bathed daily and consumed large amounts of food, which she seemed to eat all day. Social services were alerted and her cottage was cleaned whilst she was in hospital. Five days after being admitted Rose was taken home by ambulance. Her son had been seen by social services and extra services were draughted in.

The ring pessary was still in place on discharge home and the community nurses in her area were contacted to call regularly to keep a check on things. Rose had an appointment for 2 weeks time in the gynaecology outpatient department and a regular follow-up plan was agreed. Rose has not returned to hospital with a further reoccurrence of the procidentia.

A true cure would be to operate and remove the prolapsed uterus but the consequences of this may be great and could put Rose's life in danger, therefore palliative treatment at this stage is recommended.

Gynaecology nurses with expertise and experience in women's care are also in the unique position to offer woman-centred care within their own gynaecology unit.

Symptom control and health education are the key elements in which nurses can contribute to women with uterovaginal prolapse.

GLOSSARY

Colporrhaphy: vaginal repair in which sutures are used
Enterocele: vaginal vault prolapse that contains intestine
Manchester repair: repair of anterior and posterior vaginal walls with amputation of the cervix. The perineal muscle is also repaired
Procidentia: downward displacement of the uterus, when the neck of the uterus lies outside the vagina
Prolapse: downward displacement of tissues or organs

Rectocele: prolapse and herniation of the rectum against a weakened vaginal wall
Retroversion: backward displacement of the uterus
Urethrocele: prolapse of the urethra against the anterior vaginal wall
Ventrosuspension: shortening of the round ligaments in order to correct retroversion of the uterus

REFERENCES

Chamberlain G 1995. Gynaecology by ten teachers. 16th Edition. Arnold, London.
Cochran RM 1984 Psychological preparation of patients for surgical procedures. Patient Education and Counselling 5:153–158
Hayward J 1978 Information: a prescription against pain. Royal College of Nursing, London
Ley P 1967 Communicating with the patient. London.
Llewellyn-Jones D 1994 Fundamentals of obstetrics and gynaecology, 6th edn. Mosby, London.

Macleod CJ, Latter S 1990 Working together. Nursing Times 86(48):28–30
Rhodes P 1996 Gynaecology for every woman, 1st edn. Haigh & Hochland, Cheshire
Ross J 1994 Continence assessment: a plan of action. 90(27):64–66
Russell JK 1971 The dangerous vaginal pessary. British Medical Journal 1595–1597
Wood N 1992 The use of vaginal pessaries for uterine prolapse. Nurse Practitioner 17(7):31–38

FURTHER READING

Laycock J 1987 Graded exercises for the pelvic floor muscle in the treatment of urinary incontinence. Physiotherapy 73(7):371–373

Laycock J 1989 Physiotherapy in the treatment of incontinence. Geriatric workshop on incontinence, Manchester. Geriatric Medicine, February 28–9.

USEFUL ADDRESSES

National Childbirth Trust
Alexandra House, Oldham Terrace, London, W3 6NH.
Tel: 020 8992 8637

The Chartered Society of Physiotherapists
14 Bedford Row, London WC1R LED
Tel: 020 7242 1941

18

Disorders of micturition

Kate Anders

INTRODUCTION

It is necessary to have a basic knowledge of how the lower urinary tract functions in order to understand how disorders of micturition occur.

Although many disorders of the lower urinary tract, particularly urinary incontinence, are not necessarily life threatening, they are an unpleasant disability that can have devastating adverse effects both psychologically and socially. Even in less severely affected women, urinary problems can have a profound effect on the day-to-day lives of most who suffer from them.

It is estimated that more than 3.5 million people have urinary incontinence in the UK (MORI 1991). Studies have produced figures to suggest that one in four women have some degree of loss in urinary control (Thomas et al 1980), and that 14% have suffered urinary incontinence at some point in their life (Brocklehurst 1993). The true extent of the problem may be much higher but is unknown. Urinary symptoms are very common in the healthy female population but the prevalence of incontinence of urine varies on the population being studied. In a survey of women who considered themselves 'normal', 32% admitted to having one or two episodes of incontinence a week (Glenning 1985).

Approximately 25% of women delay in seeking medical advice (Norton et al 1988) and 61% have a problem for 4 years or longer (Brocklehurst 1993) before they pursue help. Aside from the women who are too embarrassed to admit openly that they have a urinary problem, many women also believe that many urinary complaints are a natural progression in the ageing process. However, although urinary symptoms, and in particular incontinence, do show a gradual increase in prevalence with age, women of all ages can be effected (Thomas et al 1980).

DEFINITION

Voluntary control of the bladder is acquired at an early age. A young child learns to identify the signs of a full bladder before the reflex mechanism causes an involuntary contraction and empties the bladder inappropriately. This learning process towards continence depends on normal anatomical, physiological and neurological function as well as a social awareness to become dry.

CLINICAL SIGNS AND SYMPTOMS

In general terms, disorders of micturition can be broadly divided into three groups: (i) disorders that can result in incontinence; (ii) voiding difficulties; and (iii) disorders that present with irritative symptoms (Table 18.1). However, it is possible to present with a combination of urinary symptoms and disorders:

- **Stress incontinence** presents most commonly in incontinence. It is leakage that occurs during episodes of raised abdominal pressure, for example during coughing, sneezing and physical activity.
- **Urge incontinence** is urinary leakage associated with an intense desire to void.
- Giggle incontinence is generally seen only in young women up to the age of around 25 years; they tend to grow out of it as they become older.
- Dribble incontinence suggests a constant leakage of small volumes of urine.
- **Nocturnal enuresis**, commonly known as bed-wetting, may present as a sole complaint or in association with other urinary symptoms.
- Leakage during sexual intercourse, which can happen either at time of penetration or during orgasm, can be particularly distressing and embarrassing.
- Overflow incontinence can present with stress or dribble incontinence, and is often associated with small, frequent voids.

Women with voiding difficulties can present with:

- **hesitancy**
- poor urinary flow
- strained voiding
- a sense of incomplete emptying
- the need to double void.

They may also complain of the need to pass small frequent volumes both day and night.

Irritative urinary symptoms include diurnal **frequency** and **nocturia**, urgency and **dysuria**:

- Urinary frequency is generally considered to be the need to void more than seven times during the day.
- Nocturia is the need to wake up at night to pass urine two or more times.
- Urgency is the sudden desire to need to pass urine which may result in urge incontinence if they are unable to make it to the toilet in time.
- Dysuria is the involvement of pain on passing urine.

ASSESSMENT AND CLINICAL EXAMINATION

Assessment is a necessary preliminary step in planning appropriate intervention and management of presenting urinary problems (Duffin 1992). It is important to phrase questions carefully as many women, embarrassed by their problem, will deny 'incontinence' but might admit to the occasional 'leak'.

Aside from assessment of symptoms, a clinical examination needs to be performed. It is possible that other gynaecological factors will have an effect on urinary symptoms, such as the presence of prolapse or disturbances in menstruation. Although stress incontinence may be demonstrated on clinical examination, it only confirms a symptom and therefore requires further investigation. A large fibroid uterus can compress the bladder and will cause urinary frequency

Table 18.1 Urinary disorders and their common symptoms

Incontinence	Voiding difficulties	Irritative disorders
Stress	Poor flow	Frequency
Urge	Straining	Nocturia
Dribble	Incomplete emptying	Urgency
Nocturnal enuresis	Double voiding	Dysuria
Sexual intercourse	Frequent, small volumes	Suprapubic pain
Overflow	Hesitancy	

(Langer et al 1990). Similarly, pregnancy can cause frequency and urgency and, in some cases, stress incontinence.

Constipation or faecal impaction can considerably disturb bladder dysfunction in several ways. A loaded rectum can press on any part of the urinary tract causing 'outflow obstruction', possibly leading to urinary **retention** and overflow incontinence. An unstable bladder can be aggravated by constipation and the pressure on the **pelvic floor** can bring about stress incontinence.

Urinary tract infections cause dysuria, frequency and urgency, and can lead to incontinence even in fit people who normally have no bladder problems. If there is an underlying unstable **detrusor**, then an acute urinary infection can quite easily aggravate the problem, which can prove disastrous.

Common drugs can affect bladder function. The most obvious is diuretics. A swift diuresis can have catastrophic results. In the elderly or less mobile they may cause urge incontinence where only urgency existed previously. Other drugs affecting bladder function include tricyclic antidepressants, sedatives, caffeine and alcohol. Concomitant diseases that affect bladder function include endocrine disorders such as diabetes, which can affect peripheral nerves resulting in neuropathy of the bladder; oestrogen deficiency in women; and pituitary disorders. It is not unusual for urinary symptoms to be the first sign of a neurological disorder, such as multiple sclerosis, so it is important to ask about neurological symptoms (e.g. leg weakness and tingling sensations).

Associated factors can influence the ability to cope with urinary problems. These can possibly cross the line of suffering from a urinary complaint to actually being 'wet'. For the elderly and disabled this is all too true and therefore mobility, environment and mental awareness become of paramount importance in an assessment of urinary symptoms.

Unfortunately, the 'bladder is an unreliable witness' (Bates et al 1973) and the relation between clinical assumptions and diagnosis is usually poor. It is, therefore, difficult to make an accurate diagnosis based solely on history and clinical examination.

INVESTIGATIONS

Investigation techniques vary from simple frequency volume charts, pad testing, uroflowmetry, simple cystometry and ultrasound, to more sophisticated multichannel videocystourethrography, electromyography and ambulatory **urodynamics**. Urodynamic

---

Box 18.1 Investigations of the lower urinary tract

- *Non-specialist investigations*:
  - urinalysis
  - mid-stream sample of urine
  - frequency volume chart
  - pad testing.
- *Simple urodynamic investigations*:
  - uroflowmetry
  - cystometry.
- *Complex urodynamic and further investigations*:
  - videocystourethrography
  - ambulatory urodynamics
  - urethral pressure profilometry
  - ultrasonography and magnetic resonance imaging
  - urethral electrical conductance
  - electromyography
  - micturating cystography
  - intravenous urography
  - cystourethroscopy.

---

investigations are designed to assess the function rather than the structure of the lower urinary tract. The classification of investigations of the lower urinary tract are summarized in Box 18.1.

Not all women with voiding dysfunction need complex specialist investigation. Simple urodynamic investigations such as cystometry with uroflowmetry and postmicturition residual is often sufficient. However, women with complex neurological disorders, mixed symptoms or failed incontinence surgery will need more elaborate investigation.

Non-specialist investigations

Urinalysis and mid-stream sample of urine

Dipstick urine testing will give a relatively good indication of infection (nitrate, leukocytes, protein), although a sample of urine needs to be sent to the laboratory for culture and sensitivity. The presence of a urinary tract infection may invalidate results obtained from urodynamic testing and must therefore be excluded prior to investigation. Haematuria (blood), dehydration (high specific gravity), urine acidity (pH) and diabetes (glucose) can also be easily indicated. Any presence of these may require further investigation.

Frequency volume charts

A fluid input and output chart will provide information concerning frequency and the volume of urine

KING'S COLLEGE HOSPITAL

FREQUENCY VOLUME CHART

Time	Day 1 In	Day 1 Out	Day 1 W	Day 2 In	Day 2 Out	Day 2 W	Day 3 In	Day 3 Out	Day 3 W	Day 4 In	Day 4 Out	Day 4 W	Day In	Day Ou
6 am														
7 am /30		700 hrs	W											
8 am	200 hcg				900	W		700	w		850	w		70
9 am				200			200			200			200	
10 am /15	200 hcg			200		W							100	
11 am					200			100				v		30
12 pm			W				200							
1 pm /15		250 hcg		200	100			200		200	✓	W 200		
2 pm	200			200		W	200							
3 pm /50		100			200			400	W	200				30
4 pm	200			200										
5 pm /45	200		W		450		200							150
6 pm								200			200		200	
7 pm /5		200 hcg		200				200			200			
8 pm					100									✓
9 pm				200			200			200	✓			
10 pm	200			200						200		200		
11 pm		200			350		200							
12 am								350			✓			20
1 am														
2 am														
3 am														
4 am														
5 am														

Figure 18.1   Example of a frequency volume chart suggestive of genuine stress incontinence.

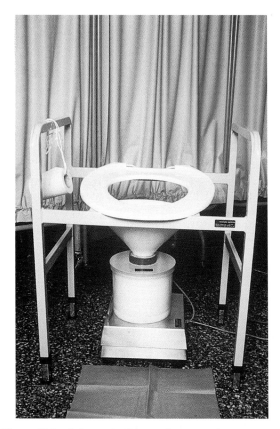

Figure 18.2   A flowmeter (Neomedix systems).

voided, which in turn will give an idea of functional bladder capacity and incontinent episodes (see Fig 18.1). A complete fluid balance can be assessed over a 24-h period if the chart is filled in accurately. An excessively low or high fluid intake will be quickly recognized. Frequency volume charts are also a simple objective tool in the assessment of treatment progress or cure.

Pad testing

Pad testing will verify and quantify the degree of urine loss, however, it does not give a diagnosis. It was first described by Sutherst et al, in 1981, and subsequently modified and accepted by the Standardization Committee of the International Continence Society (ICS) in 1989 (Abrams et al 1989). The recommendation is that the subject has a fluid load of 500 ml prior to the test, which lasts for 1 h. There are some variations, though, in test time and some investigators instil a standard volume (usually 250 ml) into the bladder.

The pad (or device) is weighed prior to the test and then again after the set time, which usually contains some standard provocative manoeuvres (e.g. coughing and hand washing). Anything below 1 g is considered insignificant, as this may be due to perspiration or vaginal discharge. Home pad testing is less controlled, lasting from 24 to 48 h, but generally has a better reproducibility (Lose & Versi 1992).

Simple urodynamic investigations

Uroflowmetry

Uroflowmetry is simple, non-invasive and provides an objective measurement of voiding ability (Fig. 18.2). It is particularly pertinent to women complaining of voiding dysfunction and was first described by von Garretts in 1956. It measures the volume of urine voided, maximum flow rate, acceleration to maximum flow, time to maximum flow, flow time and average flow time (Fig. 18.3).

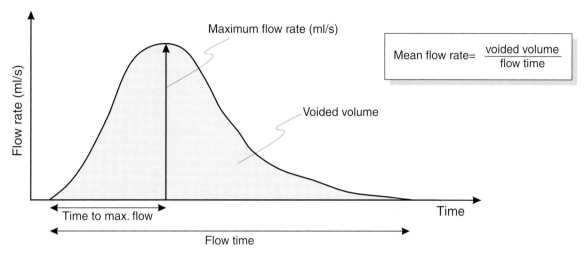

Figure 18.3 Information obtained from a urinary flow rate.

A normal flow rate is bell-shaped in appearance and, with a voided volume of greater than 150 ml, should have a maximum flow rate of greater than 15 ml/s. Urinary flow rate and voided volume does, however, vary significantly with age and sex (von Garretts 1956). Nomograms have been established to provide a normal reference range of volumes voided for both women and men (Haylen et al 1989).

The cause of voiding difficulties cannot be identified by uroflowmetry alone and simultaneous recording of detrusor pressure will be needed to differentiate a hypotonic detrusor or outflow obstruction.

It is usual to measure a postmicturition residual of urine following voiding, either by ultrasound or catheterization (less than 50 ml is normal). This is particularly important in women with symptoms suggestive of voiding difficulties and in those who require continence surgery or pharmacological therapy, which may exacerbate voiding difficulties.

Cystometry

The measurement of pressure–volume relationships within the bladder (**intravesical**) was first described in 1882 by Mosso and Pellacani. Intravesical pressure was measured using a water manometer at increasing volumes and recorded over a smoke drum. However, this type of measurement, commonly known as simple cystometry is not altogether accurate as it presumes intravesical pressure is detrusor pressure. It does not take into account that the bladder is situated intra-abdominally, which may lead to pressure rises that are not detrusor in origin. It was not until the early 1970s that this test became clinically useful, with the introduction of pressure transducers and accurate chart recorders that were able to electronically subtract abdominal pressure from intravesical pressure, thus giving a true detrusor pressure.

Subtracted cystometry (Fig. 18.4) measures the pressures within the bladder during filling and voiding. It involves passing a filling catheter (this is also used to measure postmicturition residual following initial uroflowmetry) and a pressure transducer into the bladder, and a pressure transducer into the rectum (or vagina) to measure intra-abdominal activity.

Intravesical and abdominal pressure can then be recorded simultaneously resulting in the subtracted detrusor pressure.

Physiological bladder filling is around 100 ml/h. During retrograde cystometry, the bladder is filled (filling phase) with saline, with the patient supine, sitting or both. A filling rate of 100 ml/min is common (fast fill cystometry). First bladder sensation and bladder capacity is recorded. A normal first bladder sensation is between 150 and 250 ml and a normal bladder capacity is between 400 and 600 ml. During filling (to 500 ml), the detrusor pressure should not normally rise above 15 cmH$_2$O (Fig. 18.5). A rise greater than this will indicate a non-compliant bladder. **Low compliance** (see Plate 32) is demonstrated only during fast filling of the bladder and can be associated with chronic inflammation and postradiotherapy fibrosis or following long-term catheterization, although many cases are idiopathic (Coolsaet 1985).

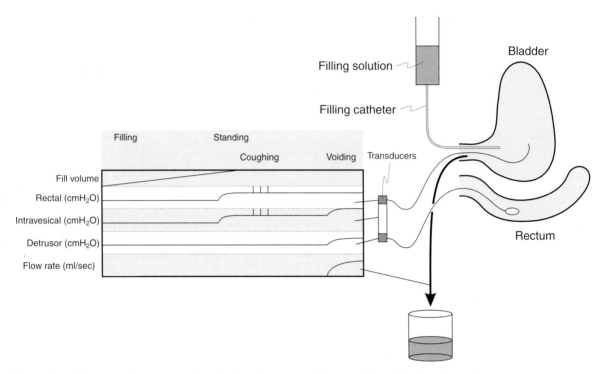

Figure 18.4 Diagrammatic representation of where the pressure lines are situated during subtracted cystometry.

Any uninhibited spontaneous detrusor contractions during the filling phase indicate systolic detrusor instability (see Plate 33). If detrusor contractions are demonstrated during provocation, such as hand washing, standing or coughing, they indicate provoked detrusor instability (see Plate 34).

Once the bladder is filled, the subject then stands up (if possible) and the filling catheter is removed. Whilst standing they are asked to perform a set of provocative manoeuvres, which may include coughing, hand washing or heel bouncing. Any detrusor rise or leakage is noted (diagnoses will be discussed later in the chapter). Once the required information is obtained they are asked to pass urine into the flow meter (voiding phase). Simultaneous detrusor pressure readings can then be recorded in relation to the urinary flow.

Videocystourethrography

Cystometry plays an essential role in the assessment of urinary tract disorders and can be aided by the use of a radio-opaque contrast rather than saline to fill the bladder. This allows visualization of the lower urinary

tract during cystometry. Following the filling phase, the patient is stood upright on an X-ray screening table. The provocative manoeuvres are then performed whilst the bladder is screened. Any bladder morphology can be noted during voiding (**trabeculation**, vesico-**ureteric reflux**, and diverticulae (see Fig. 18.6)). Rare conditions such as a vesicovaginal fistula or urethral **diverticulum** can also be identified.

Videocystourethrography is considered the 'gold standard' in urodynamic testing (Turner-Warwick 1979). However, although it is the optimum in urodynamic testing it is an expensive technique requiring specialist expertise and access to an X-ray department. Therefore, many centres perform only 'eyeball' cystometry, giving direct visualization of urinary leakage.

Ambulatory urodynamics

Ambulatory techniques are used frequently in many fields of diagnosis. Ambulatory urodynamics, first described by Bhatia et al 1981, was developed to assess bladder function under more physiological conditions. Rather than the retrograde filling used in static urodynamics, the bladder fills naturally. Solid state

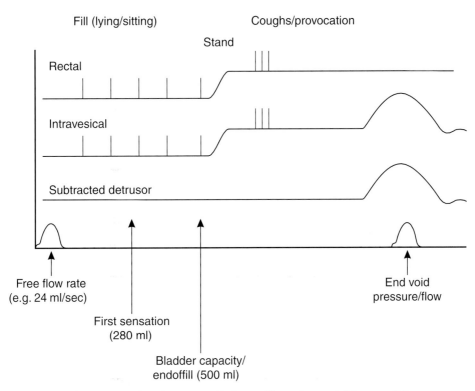

Fill (lying/sitting)

Stand

Coughs/provocation

Rectal

Intravesical

Subtracted detrusor

Free flow rate
(e.g. 24 ml/sec)

First sensation
(280 ml)

Bladder capacity/
endoffill (500 ml)

End void
pressure/flow

Figure 18.5 Diagrammatic representation of a cystometric trace with no abnormal detrusor activity.

microtipped pressure catheters are inserted into the bladder and rectum to measure detrusor activity. A urinary loss detector is also used to identify the exact time of urinary leakage. Due to the nature of a portable recording system, women are ambulant to perform normal activities over a period of time, e.g. 4 h. They are asked to keep a urinary symptom diary to record events such as urgency, episodes of leakage and voiding. They are instructed to pass urine into a flow meter so that pressure–flow studies are obtained.

The technique has been shown to be more sensitive in the detection of abnormal detrusor contractions in symptomatic women (Webb et al 1991). Although it has now been standardized many still question its sensitivity (Van Waalwijk van Doorn et al 2000), as detrusor overactivity has been identified in 'normal' volunteers. Interpretation, therefore, of any abnormal activity needs to be approached with caution.

Presently, the cost, inconvenience and limited availability precludes ambulatory urodynamics as a widely used investigation. It would be of use, however, in women with persistent urinary symptoms who have normal conventional cystometry.

Urethral pressure profilometry (UPP)

Urethral pressure measurement was first described in 1923, by Bonney, using a technique known as retrograde sphincterometry. Today, solid state microtransducers are used to obtain more accurate results. A catheter, with two transducers a set distance apart, is slowly pulled along the urethra at a constant rate. Simultaneous recordings of intravesical and intraurethral pressures are then recorded. Electronic subtraction allows measurement of true urethral pressure.

Parameters that can be measured vary; of particular interest is the maximum urethral closure pressure (MUCP) and functional urethral length (FUL) (Fig. 18.7). The profile can be assessed both at rest and during stress (i.e. with the patient repeatedly coughing). A normal pressure profile in a healthy woman, during a stress test, should remain positive.

Urethral pressure profilometry is helpful in the diagnosis of women with voiding difficulties or failed continence surgery. For example, women with urethral stricture or stenosis will have a high MUCP. Although it is not an accurate test for **genuine stress**

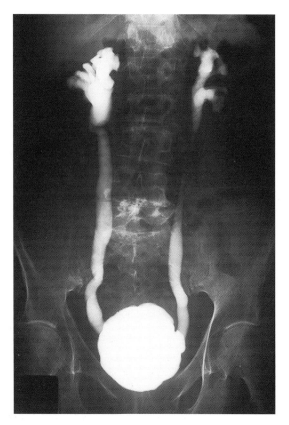

Figure 18.6 Grade IV ureteric reflux, with a trabeculated bladder, shown during videocystourethrography.

incontinence, it is useful for the understanding of the pathophysiology of genuine stress incontinence and its treatment.

Ultrasonography and magnetic resonance imaging

Transabdominal ultrasound is a non-invasive and relatively inexpensive tool, commonly used in the assessment of postmicturition residuals. Bladder wall thickness can also be measured, which has been reported as a possible indicator of an unstable bladder (Khullar et al 1994). Transvaginal and perineal ultrasound have become useful techniques in understanding the 'normal' pelvic floor musculature and in the detection of defects that may arise following trauma (e.g. before and after childbirth).

Although MRI provides good soft tissue differentiation it is extremely expensive and limited to static studies. At present, it is not a practical aid in the diagnosis of female urinary incontinence.

Urethral electrical conductance

Although this has been recommended screening test for urinary incontinence (Plevnik 1985), it is not widely used and has not been properly assessed. It works on the principle that the amplitude of a weak current passing between two electrodes placed in the urethra or at bladder neck, will change when urine enters the urethra from the bladder.

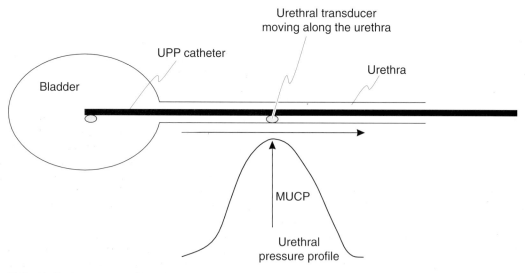

Figure 18.7 Urethral pressure profilometry.

Electromyography

Electromyography (EMG) is used to assess the integrity of a muscle and its nerve supply. During either spontaneous activity or following neural stimulation, electrical impulses in the muscle fibres are measured. In urinary tract disorders the two main types used are surface EMG and single fibre needle EMG. EMG is most useful if there is a suspected neurological abnormality.

Micturating cystography

As the morphological information is similar, micturating cystograms have been largely replaced by video-cystourethrography. It may be useful in the detection of anatomical abnormalities, such as urethral diverticulum and fistulae, when there is no other dysfunction within the lower urinary tract.

Intravenous urography

Intravenous urography (IVU) is primarily used to look at the upper urinary tract and is used in cases when there is haematuria, recurrent urinary tract infections, outflow obstruction, voiding difficulties or in vesico-ureteric reflux. Additionally, other pathology such as calculi, transitional cell carcinoma or ureteric fistula may be identified.

Cystourethroscopy

When there is a history of recurrent urinary tract infections or unexplained haematuria, and no abnormality can be found on other investigations, cystoscopy can be particularly useful. Usually performed under general anaesthetic, it may reveal abnormalities of the bladder epithelium, such as superficial ulcers due to interstitial **cystitis** or chronic inflammation suggestive of infection. Papillomas and other tumours may also be visible. Biopsies need to be taken to identify the underlying diagnosis.

The role of the nurse in urodynamics

There is no formal training for the nurse within urodynamics and many of their skills are acquired through time and experience. Due to the diversity of how urodynamic units are organized, the nurse's role can range from that of a highly skilled nurse specialist, who performs their own investigations and manages a complex workload, to that of a nurse whose main role is to assist the clinician and chaperon the patient.

However, a nursing input is always of paramount importance to the quality of care provided during any investigation, particularly invasive urodynamic tests.

One of the main advantages of having a nurse present during urodynamics is that she can act as the patient's advocate (UKCC 1992). The nurse needs to ensure that the patient has received enough information prior to the test and should have enough knowledge to answer any questions. The nurse should also ensure that all investigations are performed in an appropriate manner and by the appropriate person (i.e. a female in ethnic considerations); and ensure a chaperon is provided at all times. Infection control is of major importance and catheterization during tests must always be performed in an aseptic manner. Urinary tract infection following urodynamic studies is reported at 1.9% (Carter et al 1991) The nurse is responsible for the assessment of available resources and ensuring that all equipment is in good working order. Nurses thus need to have an understanding of the basic mechanics of the equipment used.

The experienced urodynamic nurse has a unique role and passing their knowledge on to other disciplines should be encouraged. The art of teaching in a clinical setting is a skilled one and care needs to be taken not to isolate the patient whilst explaining about the investigation to a visitor. For the patient, urodynamics is an intimidating investigation, hence it is not advantageous to have many visitors present during a study.

The nurse's managerial role will depend on their overall role within the department. However, they should have an input into how the service is run to ensure that it provides the best in quality of care.

CAUSES OF LOWER URINARY TRACT DISORDERS
INCONTINENCE

Urinary incontinence is a symptom, not a diagnosis, and therefore, although it suggests an abnormality, it does not give an explanation of the cause or whether it is treatable. The International Continence Society (ICS) defines urinary incontinence as 'a condition of involuntary urine loss that is a social or hygienic problem and is objectively demonstrable' (Abrams et al 1989).

Incontinence is frequently considered as inevitable, especially in the elderly, and is commonly managed rather than investigated. It was once considered very much a nursing issue to be controlled with pads and timed toileting, but today attitudes are changing and much research is being done on all aspects of urinary incontinence, its causes, treatments and its effect on quality of life. The causes of urinary incontinence are often multifactorial and it is therefore crucial to take a holistic approach to its management.

Causes of urinary incontinence

Urinary symptoms are common but the underlying causes are often complex. There are many types of urinary incontinence (Box 18.2) and these can be seen in isolation or in combination. To maintain continence, the maximal urethral pressure must exceed intravesical pressure (Enhorning 1961), (Fig. 18.8).

In the majority of cases, incontinence is caused either when the intravesical pressure exceeds the urethral pressure because of a weakness in the urethral sphincter mechanism (genuine stress incontinence), or when the detrusor pressure is exceptionally high in relation to the urethral pressure (detrusor instability/hyperreflexia).

Box 18.2 Causes of urinary incontinence

- Genuine stress incontinence
- Detrusor instability/hyperreflexia
- Retention causing overflow
- Fistulae
- Congenital abnormalities (e.g. ectopic ureter, epispadias)
- Transient (e.g. immobility, faecal impaction, urinary tract infection)
- Functional

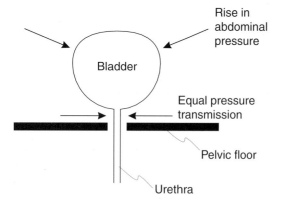

Figure 18.8 The mechanisms of continence.

Genuine stress incontinence

Genuine stress incontinence (GSI) is the most common form of incontinence found in women and some would suggest that over half of all women experience stress incontinence at some point in their life (Wolin 1969).

Definition

The International Continence Society (1990) defines GSI as the involuntary loss of urine when the intravesical pressure exceeds the maximum urethral pressure in the absence of detrusor activity.

Signs and symptoms

Leakage of urine occurs during episodes of raised intra-abdominal pressure. This includes coughing, sneezing, laughing and during exercise. It may also be demonstrable on clinical examination. Women may also complain of frequency, urgency and possibly urge incontinence (with or without prolapse) (Cardozo & Stanton 1980). Without conducting urodynamic studies it is impossible to determine whether these symptoms are caused by GSI or whether the stress incontinence is associated with a detrusor contraction.

Aetiology

The bladder neck and proximal urethra are supported by the pubourethral ligaments and normally situated above the pelvic floor musculature in an intra-abdominal position. Any rise in intra-abdominal pressure (e.g. coughing) will be transmitted equally to the bladder neck and proximal urethra, thus maintaining the positive pressure within the urethra needed to maintain continence. Damage to the pelvic floor or ligaments may result in descent of the bladder neck and proximal urethra, which results in the loss of the equal intra-abdominal pressure transmission to the proximal urethra. Leakage of urine occurs because the bladder pressure then exceeds the urethral closure pressure. The causes are summarized in Box 18.3.

GSI is more common in multiparous women due to the denervation and reinervation of the pelvic floor after vaginal delivery (Smith et al 1989). More recent studies have attempted to predict urinary incontinence following childbirth in previously nulliparous women. Toozs-Hobson et al (1998) found that ultrasound used to measure sphincter volumes demonstrated a high sensitivity in prediction.

> **Box 18.3** Causes of genuine stress incontinence
>
> - Pelvic floor muscle or nerve damage:
>   - childbirth
>   - pelvic surgery
>   - menopause.
> - Urethral scarring:
>   - vaginal (urethral) surgery
>   - incontinence surgery
>   - urethral dilation/urethotomy
>   - recurrent urinary tract infections
>   - radiotherapy.
> - Raised intra-abdominal pressure:
>   - pregnancy
>   - chronic cough (bronchitis)
>   - abdominal/pelvic mass
>   - faecal impaction
>   - obesity
>   - ascites.

Both prolapse and GSI can occur if there is damage to the supporting structures of the bladder and levator ani muscles, although both can also exist independently. Oestrogen plays an important role in the integrity of the urethral epithelium by maintaining vascularity and collagen content. It is therefore not surprising to see an increase in the prevalence of stress incontinence in postmenopausal women suffering from oestrogen deficiency.

Damage to the urethral sphincter may also occur from trauma, surgery or repeated or long-term catheterization. Fibrosis of the delicate urethral mucosa from chronic inflammation or radiotherapy can result in a non-functioning 'drainpipe urethra'. Genuine stress incontinence can also be caused or exacerbated by conditions that cause prolonged raised intra-abdominal pressure, such as chronic bronchitis, constipation, obesity, pregnancy, ascites or pelvic/ abdominal mass.

Treatment

Women who have GSI can be treated conservatively, which includes pelvic floor therapy, drug therapy and managing devices, or surgery will be offered if appropriate.

Conservative treatment. Conservative therapy should be an option for all women with GSI. It has few complications, is relatively inexpensive, readily available and does not compromise any future surgical outcomes. The main reasons for giving conservative therapy rather than surgery, are:

- if the patient is frail and elderly or very young
- during pregnancy or if the family is incomplete
- immediately postpartum
- if complicating factors are present, e.g. voiding difficulties, mixed incontinence
- if the patient is a poor anaesthetic risk
- if incontinence is occasional or subjectively not a major problem
- if the patient prefers not to have surgery
- long surgical waiting lists.

There are three main categories of conservative treatment, which can be used separately or conjunctively: physiotherapy, pharmacological therapy and devices (although these only contain urinary leakage rather than actively treat the complaint).

Physiotherapy usually involves pelvic floor exercise (PFE) with or without the additional aid of a mechanical (e.g. vaginal cone) or electrical (e.g. electrical stimulation) device. To maximize the benefits of this type of therapy, women need be instructed properly, but a successful outcome will depend on the patient. They need to be well motivated and sufficiently mentally aware to perform the exercises. The traditional type of exercise are the Kegal exercise, which involves contraction of the pelvic floor five times every hour, every hour of the day (Kegal 1949). However, in recent years there has been some modification on this type of instruction.

Women will have different 'starting points' (i.e. strength, hold time and repetition ability), which means an exercise programme must be tailored to the individual's abilities.

Women do need to be aware that, as with any muscle, regular exercise (increasing the strength, hold time and the number of repetitions) is the key to success. Explanation of the pelvic floor musculature is vital if the patient is to understand how increasing her pelvic floor muscle strength will help her urinary leakage, as this understanding will encourage compliance and continued motivation. Ideally, vaginal examination should be carried out, primarily to assess initial strength and to evaluate that the woman is managing the exercises correctly, but also to reassess the patient's progress.

The use of **biofeedback** (where the patient is able to visualize, hear (or sense) their progress) has become commonplace to aid progress assessment. A perineometer, which uses a vaginal probe, measures the pressure increase as the patient contracts her pelvic floor, although these meters are not selective to just the pelvic floor musculature. More complex systems,

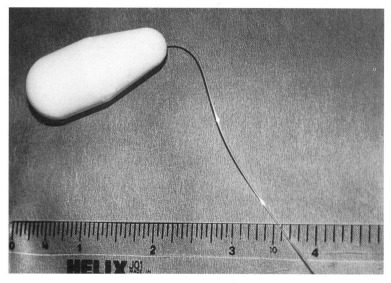

Figure 18.9 Vaginal weight.

which provide biofeedback and measure EMG activity, as well as abdominal activity, are now available, although expensive.

Vaginal cones, introduced by Plevnik (1985) help the patient to identify her pelvic floor, assess her initial pelvic floor strength and are an exercise guide (see Fig. 18.9). These are graded weights, which are used twice a day for 10–15 min at a time, by inserting them into the vagina. Once the patient has mastered 'holding on' to the 'starting' weight, they move onto the next weight, thus gradually increasing the pelvic floor strength. They are not useful, though, if the patient also has a significant vaginal prolapse.

Electrical stimulation takes the form of faradism or interferential therapy. Faradism is a technique where a vaginal probe is inserted into the vagina to apply a current directly to the pelvic floor. Interferential therapy uses two high frequency voltages directed at the pelvic floor from two different directions. At the point that the two currencies cross over, there will be a low frequency effect causing the pelvic floor to contract (Laycock 1988).

Although pelvic floor re-education rests traditionally with physiotherapists, there are many opportunities (e.g. cervical screening) for the nurse to teach the basic principles of PFE.

Pharmacological therapy. Although oestrogen improves the strength of collagen fibres and therefore should improve the ligaments that support the bladder neck, there is no evidence that oestrogen therapy given in isolation improves GSI (Cardozo 1990). Within the bladder and proximal urethra are α-adrenergic receptors, which, when stimulated, result in a smooth muscle contraction and an increase in the urethral closure pressure. Drugs like phenylpropanolamine, which is found in many cold remedies (e.g. Night Nurse), tend to be of little benefit for the treatment of GSI, but studies have shown that, given in combination with oestrogen, there is both subjective and objective improvement (Hilton et al 1990, Walter et al 1990).

Devices. There has been a recent explosion of continent devices on to the market varying from intravaginal (e.g. the Introl, which supports the bladder

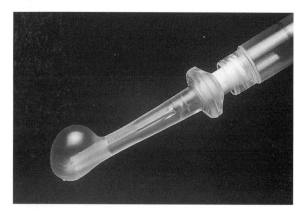

Figure 18.10 Urethral insert.

Table 18.2 Devices for incontinence

Urethral	Vaginal
Reliance insert	Tampons
Fem-assist	Smith Hodge Pessary
	Conveen Contiguard
	Vaginal Sponge

neck; Davila & Kondo 1997) to urethral devices (e.g. the urethral insert Reliance (see Fig. 18.10); Gallo et al 1997) (Table 18.2). They are particularly useful in women who have occasional leakage during certain physical activities, or have not responded to other forms of treatment. Women need to be instructed properly in their use and must be motivated to learn. Reassurance and encouragement plays an important role and the nurse is in a unique position to provide this.

Other coping strategies include pads, pants and other continence appliances. These should be used only as management of incontinence until suitable treatment can be instigated or in cases of intractable

---

Box 18.4 Surgical continence procedures

- Vaginal operations:
  - anterior colporrhaphy (repair)
  - urethrocliesis
  - Trans-vaginal tension free tape.

- Abdominal operations:
  - Marshall–Marchetti–Krantz operation
  - Burch colposuspension.

- Sling operations:
  - organic (e.g. rectus sheath)
  - synthetic (e.g. Gore-Tex, Vicryl, Mercilene).

- Bladder neck needle suspension (BNS):
  - Stamey
  - Raz
  - Pererya
  - Gittes

- Injectables (bulking agents)
  - natural – GAX collagen (bovine based)
  - man-made – macroplastique (silicone based).

- Laparoscopic procedures:
  - laparoscopic colposuspension
  - laparoscopic stamey.

- Other
  - artificial urinary sphincter
  - neo-urethra/bladder
  - urinary diversion (ideal conduit)
  - Mitroffanoff.

---

incontinence. Long-term catheters should not be used for incontinence until the woman has been fully investigated. Professionals and carers need to ensure that women are using the correct pad or appliance to allow maximum benefit.

Surgical treatment. Women with moderate to severe urinary leakage, with a large symptomatic prolapse, or in whom conservative therapy has failed, may require surgical intervention. The choice of operation will depend on the surgeon and the patient's condition, urodynamic results and medical and surgical history (Do they have a large prolapse? Have they had previous surgery?). A summary of continence procedures is shown in Box 18.4.

There are no absolute contraindications to performing surgery but the indications are similar to those of conservative therapy. Although older women have a slightly lower cure rate, age (as with obesity) should not be a contraindication. The ultimate choice lies with the patient, as it is unwise to persuade someone to have an operation if they do not want one. Complications of continence surgery include voiding difficulties, postoperative detrusor instability and the possibility of immediate and future failure. The aim of most surgical procedures is to support and elevate the bladder neck into an intra-abdominal position so that intra-abdominal pressure can then act as an additional closing mechanism. Comparisons with different types of surgery, as a primary procedure, can be seen in Table 18.3.

Although anterior colporrhaphy (with bladder buttress) used to be used as a primary procedure for GSI, it is best used for the repair of anterior vaginal wall prolapse, as its failure rate in treating GSI is high (Stanton 1984). The Marshall–Marchetti–Krantz has good objective cure rates but has generally been superseded by the colposuspension because of its reported 5–10% incidence of osteitis pubis. Hence, the Burch

Table 18.3 Objective cure rate comparisons (Fran Jarvis 1994)

Procedure	Mean (%)
Bladder buttress	67.8
Marshall–Marchetti–Krantz	89.5
Burch colposuspension	89.8
Non-endoscopic BNS	70.2
Endoscopic BNS	86.7
Sling	93.9
Injectables	45.5

Colposuspension (described by Burch in 1961) has become the operation of choice, as a primary procedure for GSI. The operation is performed through a transverse suprapubic incision. The bladder neck is mobilized and four sutures are inserted from the paravaginal fascia to the ileopectineal ligament. Long-term complications include voiding difficulties, detrusor instability and rectoenterocele formation. If there is much scarring from previous surgery, if the bladder neck is immobile or if the vagina too narrow, then an alternative surgical procedure may be used.

Slings are generally indicated where other surgical procedures have failed and are either organic or non-organic in material. The sling is inserted either through an abdominal or a vaginal incision, although commonly the approach is combined. Anchored either to the rectus sheath or the ileopectineal ligament, the sling is passed between the skin of the vagina and the bladder neck. Complications are high and include erosion of the sling onto the urethra, infections and severe voiding difficulties, often requiring long-term intermittent self-catheterization (ISC).

Tension Free Vaginal Tape (TVT). This is relatively new techniques which is similar to conventional sling techniques. However, the procedure uses a prolene mesh tape that is placed at the mid-urethra, unlike a conventional sling (Petros et al 1995). The tape is inserted via a small vaginal incision using two 6 mm trochars. Performed under local or regional anaesthesia it allows the tape to be adjusted during a series of coughs. The aim is to have the tape lying free at rest (hence 'tension free') and to only give sufficient pressure on the urethra during exertion. To date over 100 000 TVT tapes have been inserted world-wide. The most recent results from Ulmsten et al (1999) demonstrate a promising 86% objective cure after three years. Currently, large-scale randomised trials comparing the TVT and open colposuspension are underway in the UK and Europe. The initial six month data shows no difference between the two groups.

Bladder neck needle suspension (BNS) (e.g. Stamey, Raz) involves passing sutures, mounted on a long needle, either side of the bladder neck from the rectus sheath to the paravagina fascia or vice versa. BNS is more commonly used in the elderly and frail as a general anaesthetic is not necessarily needed and the cure rates are generally better than in younger, more active women who may put more strain on the sutures.

Various substances (injectables) have also been injected periurethrally around the bladder neck. They are used particularly in women who have had previous failed surgery with fixed, scarred 'drain-pipe' urethras.

Laparoscopic procedures require different surgical skills although laparoscopic colposuspensions are the same in their goals as their 'open' alternative. It is debatable whether the advantages of laparoscopic surgery (e.g. reduced hospital stay, absence of large incision) outweighs the high cure rates already achieved in 'open' surgery (Burton 1997).

For some women who have not achieved success in multiple previous operations there are other complex alternatives. These include the neourethra, artificial sphincters and urinary diversion.

Nursing issues in surgical procedures. The nurse looking after a patient who has undergone continence surgery should have a good understanding of the type of operation that is performed, the preoperative and postoperative care and the complications that may arise.

All women undergoing continence surgery must have an adequate explanation of the procedure, its cure rate and its associated complications. The nurse is in a unique position to ensure that informed consent is given before any surgical procedures are performed.

All major urogynaecological surgery has associated postoperative complications, which include:

- immediate complications:
  - haemorrhage and shock
  - bladder injury during surgery.
- early complications:
  - dysfunction to other systems, e.g. paralytic ileus, respiratory infection, urinary tract infection
  - secondary haemorrhage
  - deep vein thrombosis
  - pain
  - nausea and vomiting
  - dehydration.
- late complications:
  - constipation
  - urinary tract infection
  - voiding difficulties
- urinary urgency and **de novo detrusor instability**. Some women develop detrusor instability following surgery for genuine stress incontinence. These women need to be treated with **bladder drill** and anticholinergic therapy (see p. 303).

There is a high risk of immediate voiding difficulties following continence surgery (around 20%) and most major procedures require a suprapubic catheter to be in situ for 48 h to rest the bladder. A clamping regimen is then adopted and if the woman is unable to empty her bladder sufficiently, she is sent home with the catheter on free-drainage for a further 2 weeks. A second clamping regimen is adopted and if this proves to be unsuccessful (residuals greater than 100 ml) then intermittent self-catheterization (ISC) needs to be initiated. ISC greatly reduces the risk of infection (Moore 1995) but allows the woman to regain control over her bladder. Reassurance and support is vital if the woman is to be motivated to perform this. There is no set rule as to how long she will need to perform the catheterization, but residuals do tend to decrease with time, unless the woman had evidence of voiding difficulties preoperatively. In these cases, it may be necessary to teach her ISC before she undergoes any surgery, so that she is prepared and understands what to expect, should she need to self-catheterize following surgery.

It is the nurse's responsibility to provide the best pre- and postoperative care possible, including specific preoperative preparation and specific postoperative care. Following continence surgery, important issues include adequate pain control, strictly maintained fluid balance and quick mobilization of the patient. Advice must be given as to when women can resume normal activities, including sexual intercourse and returning to work, which will depend on the type of operation performed and how active the woman is.

Detrusor instability/hyperreflexia

An involuntary contraction in the bladder causing incontinence with little or no warning can be both extremely embarrassing and distressing. There is no time to 'brace' oneself in the way that is possible if one suffers stress incontinence alone. Detrusor instability occurs in up to 40% of women who present for urodynamics. The incidence increases as women grow older, although it is not a feature of old age. It is, though, the most common form of incontinence in the elderly (Castleden & Duffin 1985).

Definition

The ICS defines detrusor instability as a condition in which the detrusor is objectively shown to contract, either spontaneously or on provocation, during bladder filling whilst the subject is trying to inhibit micturition (ICS 1990).

Signs and symptoms

Most women present with a whole variety of urinary symptoms, including urgency, urge incontinence, stress incontinence, frequency, nocturia, enuresis and sometimes leakage during sexual activity, particularly orgasm (Hilton 1988). There are no specific clinical signs and diagnosis needs to be confirmed through urodynamic investigation.

Aetiology

The term idiopathic detrusor instability is used in most cases as there is no known underlying cause. It may be the result of poorly learnt control of the bladder as an infant, and in many cases one sees improvement when bladder re-education is adopted. More rarely, there is a neurological cause for an overactive bladder (for example multiple sclerosis or cerebral vascular accident), when the overactivity is termed detrusor hyperreflexia. In the overactive or unstable bladder the normal impulses from the cortical central control, which inhibit micturition, are not sent to prevent completion of the sacral reflex arc. Thus, the bladder starts to contract involuntarily. Detrusor instability cannot be 'cured', although the symptoms can be treated.

Treatment

Detrusor instability can be difficult to treat successfully. It tends to be a chronic condition creating fixed voiding and behavioural patterns. It is not clear whether psychological factors are significant in the development of idiopathic detrusor instability, but women who are anxious respond less well to treatment. The treatments employed can be seen in Box 18.5.

It is possible that women who complain of mild symptoms will need no more than general advice on fluid intake and the need to avoid caffeine-based drinks and alcohol as they have an irritant effect on the bladder (Creighton & Stanton 1990). However, women with high abnormal detrusor pressures will need to be treated pharmacologically to protect them from upper urinary tract damage. Ureteric reflux can be seen particularly in women with detrusor hyperreflexia.

Box 18.5 Therapeutic options for detrusor instability

- Bladder re-education
- Drug therapy
- Biofeedback
- Maximal electrical stimulation
- Acupuncture and hypnotherapy
- Denervation and surgery

Case study: Jo

Jo is a 35-year-old who suffers leakage when she coughs and does exercise. This apparently worsened after the birth of her first child who is now two. Her GP, assuming she had stress incontinence, referred her for pelvic floor exercises but these made no difference. She was then referred for further assessment.

On closer examination, and with the use of a frequency volume chart, it became apparent that Jo also had frequency and urgency, and that the leakage she complains of is actually associated with a strong desire to pass urine. She had also wet her bed up to the age of 12. In view of these findings, she was referred for urodynamic studies. These tests demonstrated provoked detrusor instability.

Treatment instigated for Jo was bladder retraining with the addition of anticholinergic therapy (in the form of oxybutynin – started at a low dose and increased according to her symptoms and tolerance of side-effects). Jo continued with the pelvic floor exercises (PFEs) she had learnt previously and, when she was seen 2 months later, her symptoms had improved significantly.

Jo was advised that her condition was not strictly curable, although her symptoms could be suppressed with the aid of bladder retraining, medication and PFEs. Some women find that after a period of time (perhaps 1 year), if they stop the medication, their symptoms are improved.

Note: Many women with detrusor instability suffer from stress incontinence. It is impossible to diagnose whether their symptoms are from a weak urethral sphincter or from a provoked bladder contraction, i.e. a cough or sudden movement may provoke the bladder into an abnormal contraction and thus force urine out.

It may be feasible to change medication given for concomitant medical disease and which influences bladder function, for example diuretics given for cardiac disease.

Other potential factors need to be excluded, such as a urinary tract infection and constipation, as these will certainly exacerbate existing symptoms and hinder success in any proposed treatment.

Bladder re-education. To regain the lost control of bladder function, a regimen of bladder re-education can be instigated. This is also described in the literature as bladder retraining, bladder drill or habit retraining. The techniques differ in detail, depending on the subject, her symptoms and the clinician's preferences. Nevertheless, the strategies are similar and are based on the need to overpower urinary urge and to extend intervals between passing urine. Observing voiding patterns at baseline and during a bladder re-education

programme is essential for success, and the use of a continence chart is widely acceptable.

A bladder retraining programme is commonly initiated at set voiding intervals and the patient is not allowed to pass urine between these predetermined times, even if she is incontinent. When she achieves continence, then the interval time is extended. This process will continue until a suitable duration between voids is achieved, usually around 3–4 h.

The literature on bladder retraining shows that it is effective in curing urinary frequency, urgency and urge incontinence, mainly in patients with detrusor instability, with cure rates of 44–90% in trials without any pharmacological assistance (Jarvis & Miller 1980, Pengally & Booth 1980).

Behavioural therapy is an attractive kind of treatment for urinary symptoms as it is generally simple, reversible and low-risk with minimal, if any, side-effects (Wilson & Herbison 1995). Unfortunately, successful voiding patterns can break down due to lack of staffing and a wish not to wake patients at night. Patients motivated to set alarms at night themselves when they are at home continue to receive the benefits, but sadly many carers or relatives are not so ready to have their sleep disturbed so that they can wake patients and help them to the toilet. As a result, a patient who has achieved continence by 2-hourly voids can become wet again once they go home (Castleden & Duffin 1981).

Drug therapy. Drug therapy remains the main line in treatment of detrusor instability in clinical practice (see Fig. 18.11), although the evidence suggests that the most effective form of treatment is pharmaceutical treatment in combination with bladder re-education. Jarvis (1981), compared outpatient drug therapy with inpatient

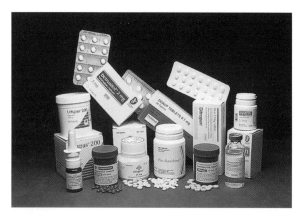

Figure 18.11 The wide range of drugs used for detrusor instability.

bladder retraining in 50 women over a 4-week period. He found a significant difference in success between the two groups. In the women who had bladder drill, there was an 84% cure rate compared to only 54% in those on drug therapy. He concluded that, with the advantage of fewer side-effects and an obviously better cure rate in the women studied, bladder drill was perhaps the treatment of choice. However, the long-term results are less clear. A number of therapeutic agents can be used; how they act and the side-effects they cause may not agree with everyone, therefore therapy needs to be tailored to suit the individual.

Drug therapy commonly used in the treatment of detrusor instability includes:

- anticholinergics
- tricyclic antidepressants
- oestrogens
- antidiuretics.

Anticholinergic drugs with antimuscarinic actions act to block transmission at the neuromuscular junction of the parasympathetic nerves activating the detrusor. This would, therefore, seem an ideal treatment in the use of detrusor instability. Unfortunately, their use is limited by their systemic side-effects: dry mouth, blurred vision, constipation, tachycardia, drowsiness and urinary retention.

Currently the most widely used drug available, and also the most effective, is oxybutynin hydrochloride (Ditropan, Cystrin); although a newly marketed drug, an M3-specific antimuscarinic, tolterodine (Detrusitol), has good clinical trial data, reporting good efficacy and fewer side-effects; this drug is yet to be evaluated long-term in clinical practice. Propantheline (Probanthine) is a synthetic quaternary ammonium compound with non-specific antimuscarinic actions. It is not in frequent use because of the high doses, and consequently unfavourable side-effects, needed to be effective.

Tricyclic antidepressants (for example imipramine and amitriptyline) act by inhibiting reuptake of noradrenaline and 5-hydroxytryptamine into the pre-synaptic membrane. They may, therefore, potentiate the bladder relaxant effect of the sympathetic system. They have similar side-effects as anticholinergics but also have sedative qualities and are therefore of most benefit for those troubled by nocturia.

Oestrogens. There is no evidence to suggest that hormone replacement therapy actively improves urinary incontinence due to detrusor instability (Fantl et al 1996). Deficiency of oestrogen causes changes in all layers of the urethra, which has abundant oestrogen receptors. The bladder, however, has fewer receptors.

Anti-diuretics. 1-Desamino-8-D arginine vasopressin (DDAVP) is a long-acting synthetic analogue of vasopressin. Like ADH (anti-diuretic hormone), it acts by increasing the permeability of the renal collecting ducts but it is without the systemic effects of ADH on blood pressure. It is a useful drug in the treatment of troublesome nocturia and nocturnal enuresis (Hilton & Stanton 1982). Because the total urine volume is reduced and the bladder fills more slowly, contractions within the bladder are less likely to occur. DDAVP can be supplied as both nasal spray and tablet.

Biofeedback. Alternative supplementary treatment includes the use of biofeedback (Cardozo et al 1978). Biofeedback in the treatment of detrusor instability is a method whereby the patient observes her own cystometric recording, or other measurement, and monitors the response of these indicators in order to control them. The disadvantage of this type of treatment is that it is time-consuming and invasive. Studies have proved that it is possible to inhibit a detrusor contraction by cystometry but, although initial results were promising, a 5-year review (Cardozo & Stanton 1984) found a high incidence of relapse.

Maximum urethral stimulation. Using a vaginal or rectal electrode, the pelvic floor musculature and pudendal nerve afferent fibres are stimulated. This results in inhibition of efferent motor impulses to the bladder with subsequent control of any spontaneous detrusor contractions. The objective success rates appear promising (77% cure at 1 year following short-term stimulation; Plevnik et al 1986). Recent studies, comparing vaginal electrical stimulation with a sham device, report 49% objective (stable on cystometric recordings) cure rates (Brubaker et al 1997).

Magnetic electrical stimulation has been used to stimulate the sacral (S3) nerve roots in patients with hyper-reflexia (neuromodulation), with some promising results (Marsh et al 1998).

Acupuncture and hypnotherapy. Other therapies include the use of hypnotherapy, which has been reported to have an 86% subjective and a 50% objective cure rate (Freeman & Baxby 1982), but this sees a high incidence of relapse.

Acupuncture has similarly shown some positive results. It is thought that the opiod release may block or reduce the autonomic innervation of the detrusor and urethral sphincter mechanisms (Murray & Feneley 1982). Some studies have demonstrated a 76% subjective improvement (Philp et al 1988), although there is a lack of controlled trials due to the difficulty of creating a placebo. One trial comparing acupuncture to drug therapy, oxybutinin 5 mg b.d., showed no significant differences in efficacy between the two treatments, but the women who received acupuncture reported fewer side-effects from their treatment (Keheller et al 1997).

Denervation and surgery. A number of surgical techniques have been used in an attempt to treat detrusor instability. These include:

- bladder distension
- augmentation or clam cystoplasty
- urethral dilation – this should be performed only if there is associated urethral obstruction
- phenol injections
- urinary diversion – a last resort, but will accomplish dryness in those who are desperate.

The poor long-term results and high incidence of complications have quashed much of the initial enthusiasm.

Mixed incontinence

Only around 5% of women have mixed detrusor instability and urethral sphincter incompetence, although many women complain of mixed symptoms. Unfortunately, they are a difficult group to manage. Most clinicians would advocate that the detrusor instability should be treated first. If the patient's main complaint is stress incontinence, and repeated urodynamics on anticholinergics demonstrate a stable bladder with sphincter weakness, then surgery may be an option. However, obstructive surgery may aggravate the bladder. Women must be warned of this, and of the possibility of having to take drug therapy long term.

Overflow incontinence

Incontinence due to overflow is caused when the bladder exceeds its functional capacity. It usually presents as stress incontinence in women who may also complain of the need to pass small, frequent amounts of urine, straining and recurrent urinary tract infections. It is caused either by a hypotonic detrusor or by obstruction, although the latter is less frequent in women. Voiding difficulties, its causes and treatment will be discussed further later.

Fistulae

A fistula is described as an abnormal link between two epithelial surfaces. In urinary fistulae the link is between the urothelium of bladder, urethra or ureter and the epithelium of the vagina or uterus.

Fistulae are uncommon but may occur in women following obstructed labour (although this is extremely rare in developed countries with good obstetric facilities). It is more common following surgery (e.g. hysterectomy, caesarean section, prolapse repair) or in women who have invasive gynaecological cancers, especially when radiotherapy treatment has been used. Women complain of constant urinary leakage, both day and night. The site of the fistula may be felt or seen on clinical examination, although further investigations may be needed to confirm the precise location. The treatment for urinary fistulae is surgical. A urinary fistula can cause much distress, especially when it is the result of routine pelvic surgery (e.g. posthysterectomy) and much explanation and reassurance is needed.

Congenital abnormalities

Congenital abnormalities of the lower urinary tract (e.g. ectopic ureter and epispadias) are usually diagnosed at birth or as an infant. They are relatively rare. The most obvious defect is ectopia vesicae (or exstrophy), where the bladder is openly exposed. Early surgical repair should obtain almost normal function as the child grows older. Epispadias is less obvious and may require reconstructive surgery in the form of a neourethra.

Transient factors

The many factors that may influence bladder function and affect a woman's ability to cope with her urinary problems (Box 18.6) were discussed in the section on Assessment and Clinical Examination (p. 290).

Functional causes

In a small minority of women, no organic cause can be found for urinary incontinence. In some cases, women

---

Box 18.6 Other factors influencing bladder function and the ability to cope.

Factors influencing bladder function	Factors influencing ability to cope
Urinary tract infection	Poor mobility
Faecal impaction	Poor manual dexterity
Drug therapy	Environmental factors
Endocrine disorders	Need for carers
Ageing	Mental awareness
	Psychological status

respond to psychotherapy or anxiety-reducing drugs like diazepam.

VOIDING DIFFICULTIES

Normal voiding requires almost simultaneous co-ordination between a contraction within the bladder and a relaxation of the bladder neck, urethra and pelvic floor musculature. The process to achieve this is complex and not completely understood. Therefore, problems with voiding and incomplete bladder emptying are not always treated most appropriately. This is apparent in the number of urethral dilatations and urethrotomies that are performed.

Prevalence studies from 600 women attending for urodynamic evaluation reported 32.5% complaining of voiding difficulties, although objective evidence was 14.5% (Stanton et al 1983). The true incidence is unknown.

Signs and symptoms

Women tend to complain of direct difficulties in micturating, symptoms of the underlying cause of the voiding difficulty or symptoms as a result of incomplete bladder emptying, such as urinary tract infections or incontinence. Voiding difficulties can be classified as follows;

- Asymptomatic voiding dysfunction, which may present with frequency and urgency associated with a urinary tract infection (UTI), or with no obvious symptoms at all.
- Symptomatic voiding dysfunction, commonly presenting with hesitancy, strained voiding, incomplete emptying, straining, prolonged voiding, the need to double void, frequency and nocturia, and possibly recurring UTIs.
- Acute retention – a sudden onset of the inability to void, which although it can cause considerable discomfort, can be quite painless when associated with a neurological disorder.
- Chronic retention, which often presents with a reduced sensation, hesitancy, frequency and nocturia, urgency, overflow incontinence, straining to void and recurrent UTIs. Chronic retention is generally associated with an enlarged, painless, palpable bladder, and it is interesting that some women are not even aware of their voiding dysfunction. Often, it is not until their condition starts to present with another symptom, such as stress incontinence, or continual dribbling, that they seek help. Chronic retention is

---

Box 18.7 Causes of voiding difficulties

- Neurological, e.g. multiple sclerosis, spinal injury
- Pharmacological, e.g. anticholinergic agents, tricyclic antidepressants, alpha-adrenergic agents, epidural anaesthesia
- Acute inflammation, e.g. urethritis/cystitis, vaginitis, vulvitis
- Obstruction, e.g. urethral stenosis/stricture, postsurgical oedema, fibrosis due to previous surgery/radiotherapy, calculus, pelvic mass (faecal impaction, fibroids, ovarian cyst, retroverted uterus), urethral distortion due to cystocele, pessary
- Endocrine, e.g. diabetic neuropathy, hypothyroidism
- Overdistension causing atonic detrusor
- Psychogenic, e.g. anxiety, depression, habit

---

difficult to define. One suggestion is that a diagnosis is made if the patient is unable to empty more than 50% of their bladder capacity on voiding (Stanton 1984).

Aetiology

There are several causes of voiding difficulties in the female. There may be a failure in the detrusor to contract, as in a hypotonic bladder; there may be an abnormality within the urethra, e.g. a stricture; or there may be a problem with the normal voiding reflex, which is present in neurological disease.

Normal voiding patterns can also be influenced by psychological disorders, habit and drug therapy. The causes are listed in Box 18.7.

It is imperative that women are investigated so the appropriate treatment and management can be instigated. Many symptoms do not correlate with urodynamic findings. A clinical examination can be performed to rule out many causes, e.g. a large cystocele or pelvic mass. A well-documented history will give evidence of any systemic disease, such as diabetes. Investigations that are particularly helpful and also non-invasive, are uroflowmetry and a postmicturition ultrasound. Cystometry will allow pressure–flow studies, which are perhaps the most clinically useful test in deciphering the cause. For example, a high detrusor pressure (during voiding) and a low flow rate will indicate an obstruction (see Plate 35). In these cases a cystourethroscopy may be required to establish the cause of the obstruction.

Neurological causes

There are many neurological causes for voiding dysfunction. The type of voiding abnormality will depend on where the lesion is situated, the severity and the presence of any concomitant medical disease. However, many patients may not fit exactly into distinct classifications, although they provide a good framework. They may also have a mixed lesion or secondary changes that further disrupt the normal pattern of voiding. Suprapontine lesions tend to result in detrusor hyperreflexia, but voiding difficulties may follow, if the area of lesion is affected by a cerebral vascular accident or brain tumour facilitatory to micturition. Trauma or demyelination (as in multiple sclerosis) in the central nervous system, distal to the pons but proximal to the parasympathetic outflow, may result in detrusor sphincter dyssynergia (DSD). DSD occurs when there is a loss in the co-ordination of urethral relaxation and detrusor contraction. What results is a bladder contraction against a closed sphincter.

Peripheral lesions at the sacral outflow (e.g. in polio or with a prolapsed intravertebral disc) result in a motor paralysis with some element of sensory loss and poor bladder sensation.

Pharmacological causes

Drugs that have anticholinergic properties may cause voiding dysfunction. Commonly used prescribed anticholinergic agents are atropine (used in premedication), probanthine, oxybutynin, imipramine and other tricyclic antidepressants. The power of detrusor contraction can be reduced by any one of these potent drugs. They are commonly used in the treatment of the overactive bladder (detrusor instability/hyperreflexia) to help reduce frequency and urgency, although they may cause incomplete bladder emptying and, in some, urinary retention.

Anticholinergics may be used in some cases where bladder instability and voiding difficulties are both present with the addition of assisted bladder drainage, usually in the form of intermittent catheterization.

Epidural anaesthesia, which interrupts the reflex arc, may produce temporary retention.

Acute inflammation

Any painful acute inflammation, whether pathological or surgical, may result in voiding inhibition. Local lesions include cystitis, urethritis, vulvovaginitis or a vulval abscess. Sacral sensory loss may occur in the presence of genital herpes.

Obstruction

An obstruction may be within the urethra or external to the urethra or bladder neck, as in the case of kinking created be a large cystocele or uterovaginal prolapse. Other extrinsic causes include pelvic mass and faecal impaction. Obstructions within the urethra are not common and usually occur secondary to fibrosis caused by surgery or previous radiotherapy. Urethral dilatation or 'recalibration' is appropriate only in women who have a proven intrinsic obstruction.

Endocrine causes

Endocrine disorders such as hypothyroidism and diabetes may result in peripheral neuropathy resulting in poor detrusor function. Damage to the afferent tracts results in poor bladder sensation, which may lead to overdistension and subsequent injury to the detrusor.

Case study: Elsie

Elsie is a 72-year-old, non-insulin controlled diabetic. She currently takes glicazide to control her diabetes. She has a 5-year history of frequency, nocturia, stress incontinence and recurrent urinary tract infections. She is otherwise fit and well, lives with her husband and leads a relatively active life. Her GP has managed her with antibiotics and has now referred her for further investigation.

Her first investigation is a flow rate. She is unable to pass more than 100 ml with a poor flow. Following this, she has a large postmicturition residual of 500 ml. A sample of her urine is sent for microscopy and culture. A cystometrogram demonstrates poor detrusor function with no obstruction. This explains the need for Elsie to pass urine frequently and explains the stress incontinence, which is in effect overflow incontinence.

In the first instance, Elsie is offered cholinergic medication to help facilitate bladder emptying, as well as treatment for her current urine infection. Although her urinary flow improved slighty and she was able to pass larger volumes, she continued to have a large residual of 200 ml.

Elsie was then taught intermittent self-catheterization (ISC) in a relaxed manner and she managed the technique well. She now continues on the medication and she performs ISC twice a day. She no longer has recurrent infections and her frequency is normal. She no longer has to get out of bed to pass urine at night and she no longer leaks urine when she moves suddenly or coughs.

Note: By removing the urinary residual the source of infection is eliminated. When the woman is no longer walking around with an overfilled bladder, she will no longer suffer an overflow incontinence.

Overdistension

Overdistension of the bladder can give rise to a hypotonic bladder. Many cases of overdistension, such as acute or chronic retention, can be avoided if noted and treated early. Unfortunately this is not always the case and many do not present until the bladder becomes hypotonic. Care needs to be taken, particularly in women who have had epidurals.

Psychogenic causes

Urinary retention in women has often been assumed to be psychogenic and caused by hysteria (Larson et al 1963, Margolis 1965). As urodynamic investigations became increasingly complex, many women have been excluded from this rather vague diagnosis. However, a study by Wheeler et al in 1990, implied that 25% of women did have psychosocial problems that seemed to relate to their voiding difficulties.

Treatment of voiding difficulties

Treatment of voiding difficulties can often be complex, especially if there are coexisting pathologies such as detrusor instability. The aims of treatment are to avoid further damage to the lower urinary tract as well as to treat the patient's current symptoms.

Acute urinary retention can quickly lead to chronic urinary retention due to the prolonged overdistension of the detrusor muscle resulting in a large acontractile bladder. Repeated UTIs caused by a postmicturition residual can lead to scarring and upper tract damage. Voiding difficulties are managed and treated by:

- drug therapy
- intermittent self-catheterization
- surgery.

Drug therapy

There seems to be little evidence that drugs with cholinomimetic agents such as bethanechol chloride (Barrett 1981) or carbachol, have adequate therapeutic actions in women with acontractile bladders with no obstruction. However, they may be helpful in a small group of women, although they have side-effects, including nausea and vomiting, headaches, gastrointestinal upsets and diarrhoea. These often dissuade women from using the drugs long term. Other types of pharmacological agents include striated muscle relaxants such as diazepam. These have been shown to be useful in women who are unable to initiate voiding

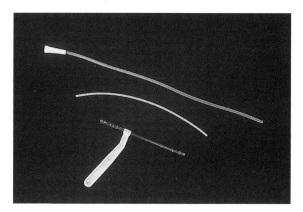

Figure 18.12 Example of catheters used for ISC.

following continence surgery (Stanton et al 1979). Drugs that act on the central nervous system, autonomic ganglia or cholinergic receptors, may be helpful in cases where there is a functional outlet obstruction.

Intermittent self-catheterization

Intermittent self-catheterization (ISC) (see Fig. 18.12) was first introduced by Lapides et al in 1972. It is a simple technique that can be easily taught. It enables women to take control of their own bladders, rather than their bladders controlling their lives, and greatly reduces the incidence of urinary tract infections and the complications associated with it. It does, however, need to be taught in a relaxed manner by professionals who have an adequate understanding of normal lower urinary tract function and bladder dysfunction. The main issues for patient selection in this technique are adequate manual dexterity, mental awareness and motivation.

ISC can be used in the following voiding disorders:

- neurogenic bladder
- hypotonic bladder
- obstruction
- postsurgically.

Neurogenic bladder. ISC is commonly used in women who have disorders of micturition due to neurological damage (either by trauma or disease, e.g. multiple sclerosis). Recurrent UTIs and upper tract damage (due to ureteric reflux from high intravesical pressures) are common and can become greatly reduced by the introduction of ISC. Many of these women will also have detrusor hyperreflexia and will need anticholinergics in addition to ISC. It is possible for this to be instilled intravesically via the catheter to reduce the side-effects of the drug.

Hypotonic bladder. Women who have little or no sensation in bladder filling or emptying will frequently have a build-up in postmicturition residual and, in some cases, will develop overflow incontinence.

Obstruction. Urethral stenosis or stricture may result in voiding difficulties requiring ISC. As a temporary measure, ISC may be useful in bladder emptying with obstructive prolapse or pelvic mass.

Postsurgically. Surgical continence procedures frequently result in short-term voiding difficulties. Many surgical techniques used, in their attempt to cure genuine stress incontinence, are obstructive in nature. If voiding difficulties do develop these can easily be managed by ISC. It is important that women are warned of this postoperative risk. Women who are identified preoperatively as 'high risk' should be taught ISC preoperatively (see p. 302).

Voiding difficulties may also follow other surgical procedures, including gynaecological surgery. The causes may include:

- Drugs – many drugs used in surgical procedures, such as atropine, have an anticholinergic effect. Many analgesics may delay the signals needed to void spontaneously.
- After surgery – the lack of mobility following major surgery, and postoperative pain, may hinder the perineal relaxation that is necessary to allow normal voiding.
- Surgery close to the bladder may cause localized inflammation or irritation to the bladder.
- Intravenous fluids – rapid filling of the bladder may occur, causing overdistension.
- Lack of privacy.

Treatment of postoperative voiding difficulties. Treatment aims to prevent further damage to the bladder and consequent permanent complications, including reducing the risk of urinary infection.

A general guide to postoperative care is that women should have voided within 6–8 h after any surgical procedure. Strict fluid balance must be maintained so that urinary retention can be avoided. If women are unable to void spontaneously then swift action needs to be taken.

Surgical treatment of voiding difficulties

If there is an obstruction from a large prolapse, for example, then after management of any acute symptoms, surgical correction of the primary cause should be performed. If there is an intrinsic urethral obstruction (and complete urodynamic investigations have demonstrated an obstruction) a urethral dilatation or an Otis urethrotomy may be appropriate. Urethral dilatation may see worsening urinary leakage if there is an incompetent sphincter already present. It is therefore vital that urethral dilatation is done for obstruction only.

Obstruction due to calculus is quickly treated by removal of the offending stone.

DISORDERS PRESENTING WITH IRRITATIVE SYMPTOMS

These are related to urinary frequency, nocturia, urgency, dysuria and bladder pain syndrome. The severity of these symptoms can vary from very mild to extremely distressing symptoms and are common to women of all ages.

Signs and symptoms

Diurnal frequency is defined as the need to pass urine 2-hourly or more than seven times during the day. Nocturnal frequency is defined as the need to get up to pass urine more than twice during the night. True nocturia does not include those who pass urine because of insomnia or a broken sleep pattern. Urgency is the strong desire to urinate, which can result in incontinence if a toilet is not reached. Women who have painful bladder syndrome complain of dysuria and sometimes suprapubic pain (either continuously or which is relieved by voiding) and other irritative symptoms but have negative urine cultures.

Causes and assessment

Common causes of urinary frequency and urgency are shown in Box 18.8. As many causes can be managed fairly easily it is important that assessment, clinical examination and history are detailed, so that complex, invasive investigations are not performed unnecessarily. Urinary tract infection is one of the most common causes of irritative symptoms and therefore a midstream sample of urine (MSU) should be sent for culture and sensitivity. If the woman has a history of sexually transmitted disease, or if she has vaginal discharge, urethral and vaginal swabs should also be taken. Investigations, including urodynamic investigation, can be performed in the absence of a UTI, or if symptoms continue when other contributing factors, such as excessive fluid intake and faecal impaction, have been dealt with.

> **Box 18.8** Causes of urinary frequency, urgency and painful bladder syndrome
>
> - Gynaecological
>   - prolapse (usually cystocele)
>   - pelvic mass, e.g. fibroids, ovarian cysts
>   - previous pelvic surgery
>   - vulvovaginitis
>   - genital atrophy (hypo-oestrogenism)
> - Urological
>   - urinary tract infection
>   - urethral syndrome
>   - detrusor instability
>   - sensory urgency
>   - bladder calculus/tumour
>   - chronic retention
>   - small capacity bladder
>   - interstitial cystitis
>   - radiation cystitis/fibrosis
>   - urethral diverticulum
>   - urethritis
>   - urethral caruncle
> - Medical
>   - diabetes mellitus/insipidus
>   - hypothyroidism
>   - upper motor neuron lesion
>   - impaired renal function
> - Other
>   - excessive fluid intake (with or without alcohol and caffeinated drinks)
>   - habit
>   - anxiety
>   - pregnancy
>   - faecal impaction
>   - medication, e.g. diuretics

Some women will have no obvious cause for their urinary frequency. Many acquire bad voiding habits, either residue from a previous urinary infection or possibly present since childhood. Interestingly, in this group, other family members suffer similar symptoms.

Prolapse and pelvic mass

A large cystocele may give rise to urinary frequency and urgency as it can drag on the trigone in the bladder. Voiding difficulties are also seen associated with prolapse due to kinking of the urethra. A sense of incomplete emptying can give rise to urinary frequency. A mass in the pelvis can press on the bladder resulting in similar symptoms. Women with fibroids, who undergo urodynamic studies, will frequently have a low compliant bladder.

Genital atrophy

The urethra is derived from the urogenital sinus and responds to female sex hormones in the same way as the genital organs. Oestrogen deficiency may lead to thinning of the lower urinary tract epithelium, thus predisposing to infection. Both oral and topical oestrogen has been shown to reduce the incidence of UTI in postmenopausal women, presumably by restoring normal flora and strengthening the corporal host defences.

Urinary tract infection

Urinary tract infections are common throughout the world. Up to the age of 1 year they are more prevalent in boys than in girls (Abbott 1972). In girls, the prevalence between the age of 1 year and 18 years is approximately 5%, and this increases dramatically when adulthood is reached; the prevalence in women being 50 times greater than in men. Between 20 and 30% of women will have at least one UTI per year (Sandford 1975). In the elderly, the prevalence can be much higher and is associated with incomplete bladder emptying, incontinence and confusion.

Recurrent UTIs are associated with residual urine, sexual intercourse and anatomical abnormalities. In women who suffer from frequent infections, long-term prophylaxis with continuous low-dose antibiotics is often used. If associated with sexual intercourse, then a single dose of antibiotic following intercourse is recommended (Stapleton et al 1990).

Signs and symptoms. Bacteria ascend from the urethra and produce an inflammatory response in the bladder lining. Classically, women complain of frequency, urgency, dysuria and suprapubic pain. They are often febrile and tender in the lower abdomen. If there is upper tract involvement, loin pain and tenderness around the kidneys are frequently present.

Treatment. This will depend on the rapid identification of which women have bacteriuria and therefore require antibiotic treatment. Dipstick testing is a useful first-line tool in the detection of bacteriuria, which results in the presence of nitrates. For culture and sensitivity an MSU must be analysed. Unfortunately, resistance is now a common problem, especially in hospital-acquired infection, and therefore, once bacteria are detected, it becomes more important to determine antibiotic sensitivities than to identify the bacteria themselves (Brumfitt & Hamillton-Miller 1990).

Urethral syndrome

Irritative symptoms within the lower urinary tract in women are common. However, in many the absence of any obvious pathology or infection makes treatment difficult. The definition of urethral syndrome is poor and clinicians are not always working to the same definition. However, urethral syndrome would certainly include women who suffer from recurrent episodes of dysuria, possibly suprapubic pain, frequency and urgency. Stamm et al (1980) defined urethral syndrome as acute dysuria and frequency of micturition in women who present with sterile urine. Therefore, in women where no bacteriuria will be found, further investigations need to be employed, including culture for fastidious organisms, chlamydia, mycoplasma and ureaplasma. Other investigations may include urodynamic studies and cystourethroscopy to exclude voiding dysfunction, and cytology and bladder biopsy to exclude malignancy. Other hypotheses regarding the aetiology of urethral syndrome include urethral obstruction, hypo-oestrogenism and psychogenic causes.

Sensory urgency

Sensory urgency is a diagnosis made during cystometry. There is no formal definition, the condition is generally described as an early first sensation and a reduced bladder capacity in the absence of detrusor instability. Catheterization is characterized as painful.

In many cases no underlying pathology can be found but urine culture should be taken to exclude UTI, and cystoscopy with bladder biopsy needs to be performed to exclude interstitial cystitis, calculi and transitional cell carcinoma.

Women who have no apparent cause for their symptoms may benefit from anticholinergic therapy and bladder retraining, including a reduction in stimulants like caffeine, alcohol and smoking.

Interstitial cystitis

Interstitial cystitis is a proliferation of mast cells within the detrusor, and can therefore be diagnosed only by bladder biopsy. Its aetiology is poorly understood and consequently treatment is often ineffective. Up to one-third of women who suffer idiopathic sensory urgency may experience early signs of interstitial cystitis (Frazer et al 1990). This is particularly distressing for women and a survey presented as part of a National Institute of Health consensus found that 40% of women were unable to work, 58% were unable to have sexual intercourse and 55% had considered suicide.

Treatment is mainly in the form of drug therapy including anticholinergics, antihistamines, anti-inflammatories and immunosuppressants. Women need considerable reassurance, with general advice about which fluid and food types aggravate their symptoms.

SUMMARY OF THE NURSE'S ROLE

All cases of lower urinary tract dysfunction can be distressing and often grossly embarrassing. The nurse is in a unique position to recognize and assess urinary dysfunction. With a small amount of knowledge, the nurse can provide reassurance and, most importantly, can realize potential problems that can so often be easily avoided or managed quickly.

A cause for most urinary tract symptoms can be identified through proper assessment and appropriate investigation. Nurses are ideally placed for teaching patients (and their carers) to understand about their own health or disease, to initiate and carry out behavioural therapy (such as bladder retraining) and to ensure that women are not only given the right appliance, if appropriate, but that they are using it correctly. It is the nurse's own responsibility to keep up-to-date on current trends of investigation and treatment for different causes of lower urinary tract disorders.

GLOSSARY

Biofeedback: where the patient is able to see, hear, or sense their treatment progress
Bladder drill: the process used to retrain the bladder to a normal voiding pattern
Cystitis: inflammation of the bladder
De novo: newly acquired condition
Detrusor: the muscle that makes up the bladder
Detrusor instability: condition where the bladder contracts involuntarily causing urgency and possibly urge incontinence

Diverticulum: Sac/pouch created by high pressure either within the bladder or urethra
Dysuria: pain on passing urine
Frequency: the need to void more than seven times during the day
Genuine stress incontinence: condition where leakage occurs in the absence of any detrusor activity
Hesitancy: the inability to initiate a void without delay
Intravesical: within the bladder

Low compliance: an increase in pressure within the bladder as the bladder fills (demonstrated during cystometry). It occurs because the bladder is unable to expand properly, due to fibrosis or long-standing detrusor instability
Nocturia: the need to wake more than twice to pass urine
Nocturnal enuresis: leakage of urine during sleep (bed-wetting)
Pelvic floor: this is made up of layers of muscle, connective tissue and skin that forms the floor of the pelvis and supports the pelvic organs

Retention: the inability to pass urine (either acute or chronic)
Stress incontinence: the loss of urine during episodes of raised abdominal pressure
Trabeculation: ridged appearance of the bladder mucosa
Ureteric reflux: the retrograde (backwards) flow of urine from the bladder up the ureter
Urge incontinence: the loss of urine associated with an intense desire to void
Urodynamics: the collective name for investigations that assess the function of the lower urinary tract

REFERENCES

Abbott GD 1972 Neonatal bacteriuria: a prospective study in 1460 infants. British Medical Journal 1:267–269

Abrams P, Blaivas JG, Stanton SL, Anderson JT 1989 The standardisation of terminology of lower urinary tract function. Scandinavian Journal of Urology & Nephrology (suppl) 114:5–19

Barrett DM 1981 The effect of oral bethanechol chloride on voiding in female patients with excessive residual urine: a randomized double blind study. Journal of Urology, November 126(5):640–642

Bates CP, Loose H, Stanton SLR 1973 The objective study of incontinence after repair operations. Surgery for Gynaecology & Obstetrics 136:12–22

Bhatia NN, Bradley WE, Haldeman S, Johnson BK 1981 Continuous monitoring of bladder and urethral pressures: a new technique. Urology 18(2):207–210

Bonney V 1923 On diurnal incontinence of urine in women. Journal of Obstetrics and Gynaecology of the British Empire 30:358–365

Brocklehurst JC 1993 Urinary incontinence in the community, an analysis of a MORI poll. British Medical Journal 306:832–834

Brubaker L, Benson JT, Bent A, Clark A, Shott S 1997 Transvaginal electrical stimulation for female urinary incontinence. American Journal of Obstetrics & Gynecology September 177(3):536–540

Brumfitt W, Hamilton-Miller JMT 1990 Urinary tract infection in the 1990s: the state of the art. Infection 18(suppl. 2):S34–S39

Burch J 1961 Urethrovaginal fixation to Copper's ligament for correct of stress incontinence, cystocole and prolapse. American Journal of Obstetrics and Gynecology 81:281–290

Burton G 1997 A three-year prospective randomised urodynamic study comparing open and laparoscopic colposuspension. Neurourology & Urodynamics 16(5) September:353–354

Cardozo LD 1990 The role of oestrogen in the treatment of female urinary incontinence. Journal of the American Geriatric Society 38:326–328

Cardozo LD, Stanton SL 1980 Genuine stress incontinence and detrusor instability. Neurourology & Urodynamics 6:256–257

Cardozo LD, Stanton SL 1984 Biofeedback. A five-year review. British Journal of Urology 50:521–523

Cardozo LD, Abrams PD, Stanton SL et al. 1978 Biofeedback in the treatment of detrusor instability. British Journal of Urology 50:250–254

Carter P, Lewis P, Shepherd A 1991 Urodynamic morbidity and dysuria prophylaxis. British Journal of Urology 67:40–41

Castleden CM, Duffin HM 1981 Guidelines for controlling urinary incontinence without drugs or catheters. Age and Ageing 10:246–249

Castleden CM, Duffin HM 1985 Factors influencing outcome in elderly patients with urinary incontinence and detrusor instability. Age & Ageing 14:303

Coolsaet B 1985 Bladder compliance and detrusor activity during the collection phase. Neurourology & Urodynamics 4:263–273

Creighton S, Stanton S 1990 Caffeine: does it affect your bladder? British Journal of Urology 66:613–614

Davila GW, Kondo A 1997 Introl™ bladder neck support prosthesis: international experience. International Urogynaecology Journal 8:301–306

Duffin H 1992 Assessment of urinary incontinence. In: Roe B (ed.) Clinical nursing practice. The promotion and management of continence. Prentice Hall, London, ch 3

Enhorning G 1961 Simultaneous recordings of the intravesical and intrurethral pressure. Acta Chirurgica Scandinavia (suppl.) 276:1–68

Fantl JA, Bump RC, Robinson D, McClish DK, Wyman JF 1996 Efficacy of estrogen supplementation in the treatment of urinary incontinence. The Continence Program for Women Research Group. Obstetrics & Gynecology November 88(5):745–749

Frazer ML, Haylen BT, Sissons M 1990 Do women with sensory urgency have early cystitis? British Journal of Urology 66:274–278

Freeman RM, Baxby K 1982 Hypnotherapy for incontinence caused by detrusor instability. British Medical Journal 284:1831–1832

Gallo ML, Hancock R, Davila GW 1997 Clinical experience with a balloon-tipped urethral insert for stress urinary incontinence. Journal of Wound & Ostomy Continence Nurse January 24(1):51–75

Glenning P 1985 Urinary voiding patterns of apparently normal women. Australian & New Zealand Journal of Obstetrics & Gynaecology. February 25(1):62–65

Haylen BT, Ashby D, Sutherst JR, Frazer MI, West CR 1989 Maximum and average flow rates in normal male and female populations – the Liverpool nomograms. British Journal of Urology 64:30–38

Hilton P 1988 Urinary incontinence during sexual intercourse, a common but rarely volunteered symptom. British Journal of Obstetrics & Gynaecology 95:377–381

Hilton P, Stanton SL 1982 The use of desmopressin (DDAVP) in nocturnal urine frequency in the female. British Journal of Urology 54:252–255

Hilton P, Tweedwell AL, Mayne L 1990 Oral and intravaginal oestrogens alone and in combination with alpha-adrenergic stimulation in genuine stress incontinence. International Urogynaecology Journal 1:80–86

International Continence Society 1990 The standardization of terminology of lower urinary tract function. British Journal of Obstetrics & Gynaecology 97(suppl. 6):1–16

Jarvis GJ 1981 A controlled trial of bladder drill and drug therapy in the management of detrusor instability. British Journal of Urology 53:252–256

Jarvis GJ 1994 Surgery for stress incontinence. British Journal of Obstetrics & Gynaecology 101:371–374

Jarvis GJ, Millar DR 1980 Controlled trial of bladder drill for detrusor instability. British Medical Journal 281:1322–1323

Kegal AH 1949 The physiologic treatment of poor tone and function of the genital muscles and of urinary stress incontinence. West. Journal of Surgical Obstetrics & Gynaecology 57:527–535

Kelleher CJ, Filshie J, Burton G, Khullar V, Cardozo LD 1994 Acupuncture and the treatment of irritative bladder symptoms.

Khullar V, Salvatore S, Cardozo LD, Hill S, Kelleher C 1994 Ultrasound of the bladder wall measurement – a non invasive test for detrusor instability. Neurourology & Urodynamics 13(4):461–462

Langer R, Golan A, Neuman M, Schneider D, Bukovsky I, Capsi E 1990 The effect of large uterine fibroids on urinary function and symptoms. American Journal of Obstetrics & Gynaecology 163:1139–1141

Lapides J, Dionko AC, Silber SJ, Lowe BS 1972 Clean intermittent catherization in the treatment of urinary tract disease. Journal of Urology 107:458–461

Larson JW, Swensen WM, Utz DC et al 1963 Psychogenic urinary retention in females. Journal of American Medical Association 184:697–700

Laycock J 1988 Interferential therapy in the treatment of incontinence. Physiotherapy 74:161–168

Lose G, Versi E 1992 Pad weighing tests in the diagnosis and quantification of incontinence. International Urogynaecology Journal 3:324–328

McLaren SM, McPherson FM, Sinclair F, Ballinger BR 1981 Prevalence and severity of incontinence among hospital and female psychogeriatric patients. Health Bulletin 39:157–161

Margolis GJ 1965 A review of literature on psychogenic urinary retention. Journal of Urology 94:257–258

Marsh F, Heldreth AJ, Hasan ST 1998 Evaluation of temporary neuromodulation and a permanent implantable neuroprosthesis in idiopathic detrusor instability. Proceedings of 5th Annual Meeting of International Continence Society (UK), Cambridge

Moore K 1995 Intermittent self catherization. Research-based practice. British Journal of Nursing 4(18):1057–1062

Mosso A, Pellacani P 1882 Sur les functions de la vessie. Methode de recherché. Archives Italiennes Biologie 1:97–128

Murray KHA, Feneley RCL 1982 Endorphins – a role in lower urinary tract function? The effect of opioid blockade on the detrusor and urethral mechanisms. British Journal of Urology 54:638–640

Norton PA, MacDonald LD, Sedgwick PM, Stanton SL 1988 Distress and delay associated with urinary frequency and urgency in women. British Medical Journal 297:1187–1189

Pengally AW, Booth CM 1980 A prospective trial of bladder training as treatment for detrusor instability. British Journal of Urology 52:463–466

Petros P, Ulmsten U 1995 Intravaginal slingplasty. An ambulatory surgical procedure for treatment of female urinary stress incontinence. Scand J Urol Nephrol 29:75–82

Philp T, Shah PJR, Worth PHL 1988 Acupuncture in the treatment of detrusor instability. British Journal of Urology 61:409–493

Plevnik S, Holmes DM 1985 Urethral conductance (UEC) – a new parameter for the evaluation of urethral and bladder function: methodology of the assessment of its clinical potential. In: Proceedings of the 15th International Continence Society Meeting, London: 90–91

Plevnik S 1985 New method for testing and strengthening of pelvic floor muscles. In: Proceedings of the 15th International Continence Society Meeting, London: 267–268

Plevnik S, Janez J, Vrtacnik P, Trasinar B, Vodusek DB 1986 Short term electrical stimulation: home treatment for urinary incontinence. World Journal of Urology 4:24–62

Sandford JP 1975 Urinary tract infection. Annual Review Medicine 26:485–905

Smith ARB, Hosker GL, Warrell DW 1989 The role of pudendal nerve damage in the aetiology of genuine stress incontinence in women. British Journal of Obstetrics & Gynaecology 96:29–32

Stamm WE, Wagner KF, Amsel R et al 1980 Causes of the acute urethral syndrome in women. New England Journal of Medicine 303:409–415

Stanton SL (ed) 1984 Clinical gynaecologic urology. Mosby, London

Stanton SL, Cardozo LD, Kerr-Wilson R 1979 Treatment of delayed onset of spontaneous voiding after surgery for incontinence. Urology 13:494–496

Stanton SL, Ozsoy C, Hilton P 1983 Voiding difficulties in the female: prevalence, clinical and urodynamic review. Obstetrics & Gynaecology 61:144

Stapleton A, Lathan RH, Johnson C, Stamm WE 1990 Postcoital antimicrobial prophylaxis for recurrent urinary tract infection. A randomised, double blind controlled trial. Journal of American Medical Association 264:703–706

Sutherst J, Brown M, Shawler M 1981 Assessing the severity of urinary incontinence in women by weighing perineal pads. Lancet 1:1128–1130

Thomas TM, Plymat KR, Blannin J, Meade TW 1980 Prevalence of urinary incontinence. British Medical Journal 281:1243–1245

Toozs-Hobson P, Khullar V, Cardozo L, Boos K 1998 Predicting incontinence six months after childbirth. Does urethral sphincter volume help? Neurourology & Urodynamics 17(4):369–370

Turner-Warwick R 1979 The evaluation of urodynamic function. Urology Clinics of North America 1(6):51–54

UKCC 1992 The Scope of Professional Practice. UKCC Guidelines, London

Ulmsten U, Johnson P, Rezapour M 1999 A three year follow up of TVT for surgical treatment of female stress incontinence. Br J Obstet Gynecol 106:345–350

Van Waalwijk van Doorn, Ernst, Anders K et al 2000 Standardization of ambulatory monitoring: report of the standardization sub-committee of neurology and urodynamics 19(2):113–125

von Garretts B 1956 Analysis of micturition: a new method of recording the voiding of the bladder. Acta Chirurgia Scandinavia 112:326–340

Walter S, Kielgaard B, Lose G et al 1990 Stress urinary incontinence in postmenopausal women treated with oestrogen (estriol) and an alpha-adrenoceptor-stimulating agent (phenylpropanolamine). A randomised double blind placebo controlled study. International Urogynaecology Journal 1:74–79

Webb RJ, Ramsden PD, Neal DE 1991 Ambulatory monitoring and electronic measurement of urinary leakage in the diagnosis of detrusor instability and incontinence. British Journal of Urology 68(2):148–152

Wheeler JS, Culkin DJ, Walter JS, Flanagan RC 1990 Female urinary retention. Urology 35(5):428–432

Wilson D, Herbison P 1995 Conservative management of incontinence. Current Opinion of Obstetrics & Gynaecology 7:386–392

Wolin LH 1969 Stress incontinence in young healthy nulliparous female subjects. Journal of Urology 101:545–549

FURTHER READING

Cardozo L 1997 Urogynaecology. The King's approach. Churchill Livingstone, London

Cardozo L, Cutner A, Wise B 1993 Basic urogynaecology. Oxford University Press, Oxford.

Mundy AR, Stephenson TP, Wein AJ 1994 Urodynamics: principles, practice and application, 2nd edn. Churchill Livingstone, Edinburgh

Norton C 1996 Nursing for continence, 2nd edn. Beaconsfield Publishers Ltd, Beaconsfield

Roe B 1992 Clinical nursing practice. The promotion and management of continence. Prentice Hall, London

Smith ARB 1995 Urogynaecology. The investigation and management of urinary incontinence in women. RCOG Press, London

Stanton SL 1984 Clinical gynecological urology. CV Mosby Company, St Louis

Stanton SL, Monga A 1998 Clinical urogynecology, 2nd edn. Churchill Livingstone, London

Stanton SL, Tanagho EA 1980 Surgery of female incontinence. Springer Verlag, Berlin

USEFUL ADDRESSES

The Continence Foundation
307 Hatton Square, 16 Baldwins Gardens, London EC1N 7RJ
Tel: 020 7404 6875
Incontinence Helpline (Mon–Fri, 9 a.m.–6 p.m.) 020 7831 9831

The Association for Continence Advice (ACA)
The Basement, 2 Doughty Street, London WC1N 2PH
Tel: 020 7820 8113

The Enuresis Resource and Information Centre (ERIC)
34 The Old Schoolhouse, Brittania Road, Kingswood, Bristol BS15 2DB
Tel: 0117 960 3060

Incontact (National Action on Incontinence)
Freepost, London NW1 1YU

International Continence Society (ICS) UK
C/o G Hosker, Honorary Secretary, Department of Urogynaecology, St Mary's Hospital, Whitworth Park, Manchester M13 0JH
Tel: 0161 276 6332

Royal College of Nursing (RCN) Continence Forum
Royal College of Nursing, 20 Cavendish Square, London W1M 0AB
Tel: 020 7409 3333

Interstitial Cystitis Support Group (ICSG)
76 High Street, Stony Stratford, Buckinghamshire MK11 1AM

Help the Aged
16–18 St James Walk, London EC1R 0BE
Tel: 020 7253 0253

Promocon
Disabled Living, St Chad's Street, Manchester M8 8QA
Tel: 0161 832 3678

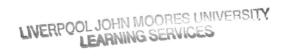

19

The climacteric

Janet Brockie

The **climacteric** is common to all ageing women regardless of race, education, religion or wealth. The word is derived from the Greek 'klima' (the ladder) and can be defined as occurring around the time menstruation ceases when ovarian function declines and women may experience menopausal symptoms. This period in a woman's life is often incorrectly termed the **menopause**, which is also derived from the Greek and literally means the last menstrual period. A woman is **postmenopausal** after a year from her last spontaneous menses.

The average age of the menopause is around 51 years and this has remained relatively unchanged since Aristotle wrote of the menopause in the third century BC. The age of the menopause is similar worldwide today (Payer 1991) but there are cultural differences in the menopause experience.

Over the twentieth century, female life expectancy increased dramatically in the Western world so that women can expect to live between one-third and one-half of their lives following the menopause, making the long-term consequences of the menopause much more significant (Whitehead & Godfree 1992).

PHYSIOLOGY OF THE CLIMACTERIC

The number of ova in the ovaries of the female fetus peaks at about 20 weeks gestation (when several million ova are present) and declines rapidly thereafter, so that at the menarche only about 300 000 remain. This number continues to decline during the reproductive years so that by the climacteric few remain and those that do become increasingly resistant to the **gonadotrophins**, **follicle stimulating hormone** (FSH) and **luteinizing hormone** (LH) (Burger 1996). Follicular development becomes spasmodic and increasingly infrequent and the ovaries produce less **oestrogen**, which in turn reduces the negative feedback on the anterior pituitary gland, causing FSH levels to rise. The overall gradual decline in oestrogen levels can result in troublesome menopause symptoms and the eventual low ostrogen levels result in the long-term metabolic consequences of the menopause. As the climacteric progresses, an increasing number of cycles are anovulatory, due to luteal deficiency and resulting in the production of unopposed oestrogen and dysfunctional uterine bleeding. Although some irregular bleeding in the climacteric is common, any very erratic or heavy vaginal bleeding should be reported and investigated.

As follicles mature irregularly during the climacteric, the serum FSH levels fluctuate dramatically, almost on a daily basis, between pre- and postmenopausal levels, thus limiting its diagnostic value of the menopause. Although the diagnosis of ovarian failure can be made as result of a single raised FSH level, it cannot be excluded as a result of a single low measurement, often a series of FSH measurements is required at regular intervals, i.e. 2-weekly, to confirm a diagnosis. LH levels also rise significantly after an increase in FSH levels. The gonadotrophins remain high for a number of years following ovarian failure and then fall gradually to premenopausal levels over the next decade or two. In most women it is unnecessary to check gonadotrophin levels to confirm diagnosis of the menopause because the patient is of menopausal age and her symptoms are strongly suggestive of the menopause. Usually, diagnosis needs only to be confirmed in case of a **premature menopause**, particularly after hysterectomy and the absence of menses or if there are inconclusive menopausal symptoms.

Following the menopause, the amount of the oestrogen, oestradiol, produced by the ovary is minimal. Androstenedione production is also reduced, although the ovary continues to produce small amounts of **testosterone**. However, the adrenal glands also produce androstenedione and this production is unchanged after the menopause. Androstenedione is converted in adipose tissue to oestrone. Premenopausally, oestradiol is the main predominant oestrogen but this changes in the postmenopause to oestrone, which is a weaker oestrogen. However, oestrone levels in obese women are higher than in women of normal weight due to more peripheral conversion, and may offer protection against the menopausal syndrome, although these women are more at risk of endometrial hyperplasia and endometrial carcinoma. The third naturally occurring oestrogen is oestriol, which is also biochemically weaker than oestradiol (Watson 1995).

TYPES OF MENOPAUSE

Most women will experience troublesome, self-limiting symptoms and irregular menstruation during the climacteric before finally having their last menstrual period, which is only known in retrospect. Ovarian failure occurs before the age of 40 in 1% of women and these women are considered to have a premature menopause; 0.1% will experience spontaneous ovarian failure before 30 years of age (Barlow 1996). Women with a premature menopause are at particular risk of the long-term consequences of oestrogen deficiency. They have different needs from the older menopausal woman because of fear of premature ageing, loss of fertility or concern about taking long-term treatment. These women often need counselling and careful follow-up.

However, other women will undergo a **surgical menopause** with the removal of functioning ovaries. These women also have special needs as they often experience more severe and prolonged menopausal symptoms (Spector 1989). For women who have had a hysterectomy but have ovarian conservation, the climacteric may be difficult to recognize without the presence of menstruation. However, hysterectomized women are likely to undergo ovarian failure on average 4 years earlier than women who have kept their uterus (Siddle et al 1987).

Increasing numbers of young women are surviving successful treatment of early malignancies and, like those women with a natural premature menopause, they will need close long-term support and supervision of treatment in the form of **hormone replacement therapy** (HRT).

A rare and poorly understood condition – **resistant ovarian syndrome** – occurs when the ovaries fail to respond to the gonadotrophins although ova are still present. Gonadotrophin levels rise and oestrogen levels drop, as in the menopause, and the only way of making a differential diagnosis is by ovarian biopsy. This is not usually done as treatment is the same as for menopausal symptoms. In some women the condition is reversed, either spontaneously or following hormonal treatments, and some women have achieved pregnancies (Kreiner et al 1988).

Short-term effects of the menopause

Eighty per cent of women will experience troublesome symptoms of oestrogen deficiency. The symptoms that each woman suffers are varied and acute menopausal symptoms fall into two groups, the **vasomotor symptoms** and the **psychological symptoms** (Box 19.1).

Vasomotor symptoms

Hot flushes and night sweats are the most common symptom, experienced by about 75% of women

---

Box 19.1 Acute menopausal symptoms

- **Vasomotor**:
  - hot flushes
  - night sweats
  - palpitations
  - headaches
  - giddiness
  - insomnia.
- **Psychological**:
  - depression
  - irritability
  - poor memory
  - difficulty in concentrating
  - tiredness
  - loss of libido.

(Thompson et al 1973). Some women will experience only an occasional flush but 25% of women will have persistent flushes for more than 5 years. A hot flush is described as a feeling of overwhelming heat starting in the body and moving up the neck and head. It lasts only for a minute or two but can leave a woman feeling cold and drained. The aetiology of the hot flush is unknown but it is thought to be due to a dysfunction in the thermoregulatory centre in the hypothalamus. The intense feeling of heat experienced by women during a hot flush is caused by inappropriate vasodilation of the superficial blood vessels causing the body core temperature to drop by as much as 1°C (Brockie et al 1991). Some women look very hot and red during a hot flush, others may sweat, both reactions can cause embarrassment. Vasomotor symptoms that occur at night are often associated with sweating and are termed night sweats. Severe night sweats may lead to disrupted nights, tiredness, depression and reduced libido with its additional implications.

Vasomotor symptoms tend to be more severe in women who experience rapid oestrogen withdrawal after oophorectomy and peak in severity before the menopause in climacteric women, suggesting that flushes are caused by changing levels of oestrogen rather than low levels.

Hot flushes can also occur in the premenstrual phase of the menstrual cycle and during pregnancy. Other causes of hot flushes include thyrotoxicosis, phaeochromocytoma and carcinoid syndrome and these conditions may need to be excluded if there is a lack of response to treatment.

Psychological symptoms

There is some debate about whether psychological symptoms such as depression, irritability and poor concentration can be attributed to the menopause. Some studies have shown a peak in psychological symptoms prior to the menopause and in many cases these symptoms are improved by HRT (Campbell & Whitehead 1977, Montgomery & Studd 1991). There are oestrogen receptors in the brain, suggesting a neurological basis for psychological menopausal symptoms. Sex steroids have a modulatory role on brain monoamine receptors, which may explain their effect on mood and memory. Sleep patterns are altered after the menopause and insomnia can still be a problem in the absence of vasomotor symptoms. Oestrogen seems to have a direct effect on the central nervous system and studies have shown that HRT does improve psychological symptoms in the absence of vasomotor symptoms (Ditkoff et al 1991). However, it is important to consider other life factors that may be occurring at the same time, such as ageing parents, ill health or bereavement, children leaving home, relationship problems, stressful work or vasomotor symptoms resulting in insomnia.

There are cultural differences in attitudes towards the menopause. In some Asian and African cultures, the cessation of menstruation offers liberation from taboos, more freedom and respect and removal of the threat of pregnancy. In our Western, youth-oriented society some women will perceive the menopause to be associated with old age and loss of attractiveness.

Long-term consequences of the menopause

Many women remain ignorant of the long-term consequence of the menopause (Hope & Rees 1995). Metabolic changes occur silently and they have a major impact on the health of older women, and also on the health and welfare provision of the ageing postmenopausal population.

Urogenital atrophy

The vagina and the distal urethra arise from the same embryonic origin and both contain oestrogen-dependent tissues that are affected by the menopausal hormonal changes. The low levels of oestrogen result in the thinning of the vaginal epithelium and the loss of the vaginal rugae. The vagina becomes shorter and less elastic, the walls becoming thinner and transparent due to the loss of vascularity. With the epithelial changes there is reduction in the glycogen content and reduced vaginal lactobacilli and a raised pH. These changes result in more susceptibility to infection, vaginal dryness and dysparunia.

Similarly, the low postmenopausal oestrogen levels cause thinning of the urethral epithelium leading to the urethral syndrome, which is characterized by urinary urgency, frequency, incontinence and, again, by an increased risk of infection.

Connective tissue atrophy

Oestrogens play a role in maintaining the dermis of the body and at the menopause there are changes in hair, skin and nails. Ageing women experience skin changes, their skin becoming dry, thin, wrinkled due to the loss of elasticity and more easily bruised. The loss of thickness in the skin is related to the menopause and the reduction in collagen levels rather than the ageing process (Brincat & Studd 1988).

Other atrophic changes caused by the low oestrogen levels include breast atrophy, hair loss, brittle nails and aching joints. All these respond to HRT.

Osteoporosis

Osteoporosis has been described as an epidemic of the 1990s. One in two women by the age of 80 years will have sustained as least one osteoporotic fracture. In the UK this results in approximately 60 000 hip fractures annually, at the cost of £750 million.

Osteoporosis can be defined in the reduction in bone mass and microarchitectural deterioration so that fractures are likely to occur with the minimum of trauma. Bone mass changes throughout life. The mass rises throughout childhood and in early adulthood until it peaks during the middle 30s. Then, in both sexes, there is a gradual ageing-related reduction in mass. However, there is an accelerated loss in the first few years after the menopause. Men generally have a greater peak adult bone mass and they develop osteoporosis some 20 years later than women. Bone is a living tissue that is constantly turning over, with bone being resorbed by the osteoclasts and renewed by the osteoblast cells. This is essential for the maintainance of a healthy skeleton. A number of hormones balance these two processes, including oestrogen, parathyroid hormone and calcitonin. However, the low oestrogen levels at the menopause result in a more rapid bone turnover, bone resorption rises but bone formation fails to keep up so that that there is a gradual loss in bone mass. Trabecular bone is at particular risk and fractures are most likely to occur in the vertebrae, wrist and neck of femur. Osteoporosis is likely to affect the spine first and vertebral crush fractures result in loss of height, bending of the spine and chronic backache,

which can severely reduce quality of life without making a great impact on the health services. Colles' fractures mostly cause only temporary pain and increased dependence, but hip fractures are associated with a considerable mortality; 20% of women die within 6 months of a fractured femur, mainly due to medical complications, and many other women lose their independence and need extensive long-term support. This problem is compounded by the falling birth rate and the increase in life expectancy so that the proportion of elderly in our population is becoming greater. This has a significant impact both economically and demographically. Our society is becoming more nuclear so that more elderly women live on their own without family support.

The development of osteoporosis is determined by two factors, the peak adult bone mass and the rate at which bone mass is lost. Ideally, women should have their bone density measured in the climacteric to assess bone mass and then again in the postmenopause to determine the rate of postmenopausal bone loss and thereby predict those women most at risk. However, bone densiometry facilities are limited in the NHS and it is important to predict those women at particular risk of developing osteoporosis by other means (Box 19.2). Unfortunately, once bone has been lost, it cannot be replaced to any significant degree and bone loss needs to be prevented in women at greatest risk. In many cases osteoporosis is only diagnosed when a woman presents with a fracture.

Cardiovascular disease

Coronary heart disease (CHD) is traditionally associated with stressed, middle-aged men. Up until the menopause, CHD remains five times more common in

---

Box 19.2 Osteoporosis risk factors

- Age
- Premature menopause or prolonged amenorrhoea
- Family history of osteoporosis
- Thin/petite
- Caucasian or oriental
- Sedentary lifestyle
- Smoking
- Prolonged use of steroids
- Previous osteoporotic fracture
- Nulliparous
- Low calcium or vitamin D intake or malabsorption disorders
- Excessive alcohol intake

Box 19.3 Risk factors for cardiovascular disease

- Premature menopause
- High cholesterol or triglyceride levels
- Hypertension
- Smoking
- Family history of cardiovascular disease
- Diabetes
- Obesity
- Sedentary lifestyle
- Poor diet

men than women. Following the menopause, there is a sharp increase in the incidence of CHD amongst women so that it becomes the major cause of death in postmenopausal women. First heart attacks in women are more likely to occur without warning and are more likely to be fatal than in men (Rehnquist 1993).

Many factors are recognized to increase the risk of CHD (Box 19.3). Most factors that affect risk in men do also in women, although in varying degrees of importance. Hypertension and diabetes are greater risk factors for women than men. Women have one unique factor over men and this is oestrogen withdrawal. Epidemiological data has shown the increasing risk of CHD in women but it has been hard to clarify the association with the low menopausal oestrogen levels and increasing age. Studies have found that oophorectomized women who had not received oestrogen replacement therapy had twice the risk of a myocardial infarction than those women who did receive treatment (Stampfer et al 1991).

The mechanisms that increase the risk following the menopause are not fully understood and involve several different areas, such as changes in serum lipoproteins, arterial blood flow, insulin resistance, body fat distribution and coagulation (Read 1997).

Changes in plasma lipids and lipoproteins. The changes that occur in the serum lipoproteins after the menopause are consistent with a greater CHD risk. The lipid profile changes with age, total serum cholesterol, low density lipoproteins (LDL) and triglyceride levels all increase but more rapidly after the menopause. Serum high density lipoproteins that are protective against cardiovascular disease change little, although the particles become smaller, which is consistent with a greater CHD risk.

Arterial blood flow. Oestrogens seem to have a direct effect on blood flow and arterial tone because of the presence of oestrogen receptors in the muscles of the arterial blood vessels that cause vasodilatation. Low

levels will reduce the blood supply in the coronary arteries, increasing risk of myocardial infarction.

Insulin resistance and carbohydrate metabolism. Disturbances in carbohydrate metabolism that are not sufficient to cause diabetes mellitus can cause an increase in risk of CHD. Insulin resistance increases with age and low oestrogen levels at the menopause appear to result in reduced insulin secretion, increased insulin half-life and progressive effects on insulin resistance.

Body fat distribution. There is a tendency for women to put on weight after the menopause and with the reduction in oestrogen there is a change in fat distribution from the female gynoid to a more android distribution, with more weight around the ribs, which is associated with an increased risk of CHD.

Coagulation factors. The formation of fibrin deposits within arteries and their degradation are key factors in the formation of artherogenic plaques. The menopause is associated with an increase in atherosclerosis, with the low postmenopausal oestrogen levels leading to a reduction in fibrinolytic activity, i.e. the degradation of atheroma.

Alzheimer's disease

This is the most common form of dementia. The prevalance alters with age but there is a dramatic increase in incidence after the age of 70 years. Several studies indicate that women are more at risk than men and, with the increase in life expectancy, the numbers of people at risk of Alzheimer's disease (AD) is rising. In AD the brain becomes smaller than in normal ageing, most prominently the hippocampus, which is the vital part of the brain for memory function. Decline in brain size is accelerated at about the age of 50 – around the time of the menopause. There are multiple risk factors, genetic mutations account for only a small number of cases. In addition in the reduction in brain size, there are also structural and chemical changes and a reliable diagnosis can be made on CT scan.

TREATMENT OF THE MENOPAUSE

There are opposing opinions regarding the management of the menopause. Some would argue that the menopause is a natural event in a woman's life and should be left untreated while others would argue that women were never intended to become menopausal, that it is a feature of the increased life expectancy and so should be treated.

Public awareness of the menopause and its effects are much more widely discussed than in previous generations – in women's magazines, on the radio, television and between women themselves. Telephone information lines are available, self-help books and various organizations offer help and information.

Despite this, many women still require more information and numerous studies have highlighted this, even amongst those already on therapy (Draper & Roland 1990). Ideally, every woman should have the opportunity to receive enough information about the menopause, HRT and alternative treatments to be able to make an informed decision whether to accept treatment or not.

HORMONE REPLACEMENT THERAPY

Oestrogens

Oestrogen deficiency is considered to be the most significant contributing cause of the troublesome acute self-limiting menopausal symptoms and the long-term consequences of the menopause. Therefore HRT is usually the first line of treatment and it aims to replace the oestrogen that the ovaries are no longer producing.

Many people believe that HRT is a relatively recent development, however, the use of ovarian extracts date back to 1919. The first synthetic oestrogens were first produced in the late 1930s followed by conjugated oestrogens that were better tolerated in the 1940s. Since the 1960s, treatment has been much more widely available using natural oestrogens and there have been many improvements in therapy. Now there are many different preparations involving different doses, combinations, treatment regimes and routes of administration. Despite these advances, the debate of how the menopause should or should not be treated is still ongoing.

Unlike the combined oral contraceptive pill, the oestrogens used in HRT are natural, not potent synthetic oestrogens. They are largely derived from plant sources, mainly yams, soya and cacti, and are chemically the same as the naturally occurring premenopausal oestrogens. The exception is the conjugated equine oestrogen present in some HRT preparations. This contains about 50% equine oestrogens that are derived from pregnant mares, urine. However, because it is a naturally occurring animal oestrogen it is still considered to be part of the same natural category. Synthetic oestrogens should not be used in HRT because of their metabolic impact.

Oestrogens in modern HRT regimes are given continuously and many different preparations are available, using different routes of administration, including oral, transdermal, percutaneous, subcuta-neous and vaginal. Each route has its indications and advantages.

Progestogens

In women with an intact uterus, a **progestogen** is added to the oestrogen to protect the uterine endometrium. Oestrogens stimulate the endometrium, causing it to proliferate. In the normal menstrual cycle, **progesterone** induces secretory differentiation, a process that induces enzymes involved in the breakdown of oestradiol and in turn causes menstruation as the endometrium is shed. Progesterone withdrawal at the end of the secretory phase of the menstrual cycle results in menstruation. In HRT the two hormones have a similar effect on the endometrium. The oestrogen alone causes similar proliferation and, if it was not opposed by a progestogen, there would be a high risk of simple endometrial hyperplasia developing. This risk may be as high as 50% depending on the dose and duration of therapy. There is probably about a 5% incidence of endometrial hyperplasia amongst women not on HRT. In some women, continued use of unopposed oestrogens may cause the hyperplasia to progress to complex hyperplasia, even with atypia, which is associated with an increased risk of endometrial cancer. Use of unopposed oestrogens at any stage increases this risk in the long term. Only women who have had a hysterectomy can use oestrogen-only HRT.

Unlike the natural oestrogens used in HRT, the progestogens most commonly used are synthetic, as oral progesterone is metabolized by the liver too rapidly to be effective. Progestogens are structurally different from progesterone and are divided into two groups:

- 17-hydroxyprogesterone derivatives such as dydrogesterone and medroxyprogesterone acetate
- 19-nortestosterone derivatives such as norgestrel and norethisterone.

The progesterone derivatives are not androgenic and do not have an adverse effect on blood lipids, while the testosterone derivatives are androgenic and can potentially negate some of the beneficial effects of the oestrogen in HRT, although studies have shown this is minimal in the usual doses used in HRT.

The future will probably include the introduction of a new generation of progestogens in HRT, which are well tolerated and lipid friendly (Barlow 1995).

The routes of administration for progestogens are oral and transdermal (combined with oestrogen in a patch). Progesterone, although not routinely given, is available for cyclical therapies as a vaginal gel and vaginal suppositories.

The levenorgestrel-releasing intrauterine system has yet to gain a product licence for use with HRT but it has been used successfully in perimenopausal women who are experiencing menstrual problems and provides contraception at a time when other methods are no longer an option. Releasing the progestogen continuously directly to the endometrium, systemic absorption of the levenorgestrol is minimal and it offers good endometrial protection and **amenorrhoea**. Oestrogen can then be added when menopausal symptoms appear (Andersson et al 1992)

Tibolone

This is a synthetic molecule that is not strictly an HRT preparation. It has oestrogenic, androgenic and progestogenic properties and it needs to be reserved for the postmenopausal woman with an atrophic endometrium to produce an amenorrhoeic regime. It provides an alternative therapy for the relief of acute menopausal symptoms, reducing vasomotor symptoms and enhancing mood and libido. Tibolone appears to offer long-term protection to the bones but the cardiovascular effects still need to be clarified. Studies on the long-term effect of Tibolone on breast tissue are underway, it does not have the oestrogenic effect on breast tissue and it may potentially be the treatment of choice in women with breast cancer, or in those at risk of breast cancer (Ginsburg & Prelevic 1995).

Treatment regimes

The type of HRT prescribed to a patient is first determined by whether a woman has had a hysterectomy. In the hysterectomized woman continuous oestrogen alone is given. There is no evidence that progestogens have any other benefit than protecting the endometrium. In the non-hysterectomized woman the progestogens can be given in a variety of ways, which are dictated by whether she is perimenopausal or postmenopausal.

In perimenopausal women the progestogen is usually given for 10–14 days each 28-day cycle, combined with an oestrogen that is given continuously. This regime usually results in a cyclical withdrawal bleed. About 5% of women do not bleed on these cyclical regimes and in most women this is completely satisfactory and is because the levels of the hormones

Case study: Jean

Jean, aged 49 years, works part-time in a local supermarket stocking shelves at night. At the age of 35 years she had a hysterectomy with ovarian conservation for menorrhagia. Four years later, she presented to her GP complaining of irritability, tiredness and generally feeling low. Her doctor prescribed antidepressants, which Jean never took feeling sure that her symptoms were cyclical and not due to depression. Then, aged 41 years she started experiencing hot flushes and night sweats. However, she did not see her GP as her mother, aged 61 years had just been diagnosed with breast cancer and Jean thought that she would be unable to take HRT with a family history of breast cancer. When she did see her GP again, at 49 years, her marriage had failed and she had a new partner. She presented complaining of dyspareunia and was found, on examination, to have atrophic vaginitis.

This case history highlights problems that many women experience following a hysterectomy. The hysterectomy solves one problem only to leave another – undiagnosed premature ovarian failure. Following hysterectomy, many women are not followed-up in general practice on a regular basis because they are no longer recalled for regular smears. Together with the absence of menstruation as an indicator, ovarian failure is missed.

Typically, Jean initially experienced psychological symptoms and many women do experience worsening of premenstrual symptoms in the years prior to ovarian failure. Psychological symptoms are common for many reasons other than the menopause but always need to be considered in young hysterectomized women. Women themselves need to be warned about the increased risk of early ovarian failure following a hysterectomy.

Many women get information about the menopause from the media and from friends and family rather than health professionals. This information is often incomplete or inaccurate, as in Jean's case. A family history of postmenopausal breast cancer is not a contraindication to HRT.

Jean's GP referred Jean to the practice nurse to discuss HRT fully. Jean has declined systemic HRT for the time being because of concern over breast cancer, although she understands that her risks from cardiovascular disease and osteoporosis are greater than her risk of breast cancer. She was supported in her decision. A bone scan is being arranged and if this is very poor she will reconsider her decision. However, in the meantime she is using a vaginal oestriol cream, which is not absorbed systemically to any significant degree. She has also received advice about diet, to increase her calcium intake and also to reduce her weight and to include regular exercise several times each week to protect her heart and bones are not sufficient to cause endometrial hyperplasia. If the woman is on other medication, such as phenytoin, phenobarbitone or carbimazole, this medication may be affecting the liver enzymes and there may be insufficient circulating oestrogens. As well as not stimulating the endometrium, the low levels of oestrogen may not be providing any long term protection to the cardiovascular system and bones. In these cases a transdermal therapy is preferred.

If a woman is late perimenopausal, with menstruation becoming less frequent, then a 3-monthly cyclic regime is an option, with 14 days of progestogen every 13 weeks giving only four withdrawal bleeds a year.

In postmenopausal women the progestogen can be given continuously with the oestrogen in order to achieve an amenorrhoea regime, although amenorrhoea may only be achieved after some months of irregular unpredictable bleeding until the endometrium becomes atrophic. Newer lower dose continuous combined preparations offer amenorrhea regimes aimed at older women. They have good bleeding control and fewer side-effects.

Following a subtotal hysterectomy, there is a small chance that some endometrium remains with the cervix and these women are usually given a cyclical therapy for 3 months. If there is no withdrawal bleed it is assumed that there is no endometrium present and the woman can continue with an oestrogen-only preparation.

If there is a possibility of endometrial deposits remaining in women who have undergone hysterectomy because of endometrosis then continuous progestogen or a continuous combined preparation are the regimes of choice initially.

Route of administration

Women tend not to be given a choice of HRT product or the route of administration (Hope & Rees 1995). This study showed that in 70% of cases, even if the doctor had discussed treatment options with the patient, the final decision was made by the doctor. Other studies have shown very poor long-term compliance in women with HRT (Coope & Marsh 1992) and this may be improved in some women if they are prescribed the treatment of their choice.

Oral

In most cases oral therapy is the first-line treatment and it is also the cheapest. It is easy to start and easy to stop. Alongside this, the majority of studies on the long-term benefits and safety have been done on oral therapies. Other preparations produce similar plasma levels and have the same therapeutic effects and are likely to have similar benefits and risks.

Oral administration of oestrogen means that the oestrogen is absorbed from the gut into the portal system, which passes through the liver where the oestrogen is largely metabolized to oestrone, which is less biochemically active, before entering the systemic circulation. Oral therapies contain higher doses of oestrogen to counteract this effect. Any woman with a history of liver disease should avoid oral therapies. However, oral therapies have the greatest benefits on blood lipid levels not only in suppressing the total- and LDL-cholesterol levels but also in producing beneficial effects on HDL-cholesterol levels, thus contributing to the cardiovascular benefits of HRT. Conversely, oral therapies cause a rise in triglyceride levels and, although their role in women is uncertain, triglycerides are associated with an increased risk of ischaemic heart disease in men (Crook 1995). Transdermal oestrogens are advised in women with hypertriglycierdaemia. High doses of equine oestrogens increase the production of a renin substrate, not the type usually associated with hypertension, and HRT has not been shown to increase blood pressure. Nevertheless, oral oestrogens should be avoided in women with a labile blood pressure.

Transdermal

There are two types of transdermal HRT skin patches. The older style reservoir patch contains the oestrogen in an alcohol-based reservoir in the centre of the patch. This patch has been superseded by the matrix patch, which holds the oestradiol in the adhesive. Some women do develop a skin allergy to the patches and this inhibits absorption of the hormones through the skin. Skin allergies are more frequently a problem with the reservoir patch but about 3% of women are allergic to the matrix patch. A number of different matrix patches are available, each contains a different combination of adhesives so a woman may be allergic to one patch but not another. An alternative route must then be found. Patches are easy to administer and are changed once or twice a week.

Transdermal therapies are advised in women with hypertriglyceridaemia and hypertension, and for those women with chronic gastrointestinal problems. Oestradiol is lipid soluble and can penetrate the skin, being absorbed into fat from where it is released into the peripheral bloodstream giving fairly constant levels of oestrogen. It bypasses the first-pass liver metabolism and so doses are much lower than in oral therapies. However, all oestrogens are eventually metabolized by the liver.

Percutaneous skin gel

This is a colourless, odourless oestradiol skin gel in an alcohol base. A measured amount is rubbed into the skin on a daily basis.

Skin gels have similar benefits and indications to transdermal therapies. They offer flexibility in dosage, minimizing any initial side-effects and, most importantly, provide an alternative for women who cannot tolerate a transdermal oestradiol patch.

Implants

Oestradiol implants are pellets of crystalline oestradiol that are inserted subcutaneously through a tiny incision under local anaesthetic. The oestradiol is released over many months, depending on the dosage. Implants remain active for 3–4 years – long after symptoms have returned to normal and they continue to stimulate the endometrium, which is significant for women who have not had a hysterectomy. Another concern with implants is tachyphylaxis. In a number of women, symptoms return despite adequate levels of oestrogen and women request repeated implants with increasing frequency, leading to supraphysiological levels of oestradiol. The long-term effects of these high levels, particularly on breast tissue, are uncertain (Garnett et al 1990).

Testosterone implants are sometimes used with HRT. Testosterone levels fall after the menopause and although its effects are controversial, it may be involved in improving libido and energy levels. The testosterone implants need replacing at 6–12 month intervals and although serum testosterone levels are elevated above premenopausal levels, androgenic side-effects are rare.

Vaginal oestrogens

These are useful in women with symptoms of urogenital atrophy and are available as creams, pessaries and tablets. Preparations containing natural oestrogens should be used. The oestriol preparations and low-dose oestradiol preparations are not absorbed systemically to any significant degree and do not appear to affect the endometrium. They can be given to women with a contraindication to HRT. All other preparations

---

> **Box 19.4** Absolute contraindications to HRT
>
> - Endometrial cancer
> - Breast cancer
> - Suspected pregnancy
> - Undiagnosed vaginal bleeding
> - Undiagnosed breast lump
> - Severe liver disease

are absorbed systemically and need to be monitored closely because of the potential deleterious effect of unopposed oestrogen.

Contraindications to HRT

Few conditions or indications contraindicate HRT use. For ease, these can be divided into absolute and relative contraindications.

Absolute contraindications (Box 19.4)

The main and most common contraindication to HRT is a history of an oestrogen-dependent malignancy, such as breast or endometrial carcinoma. Both these malignancies are responsive to oestrogens and some progestogens. These women are usually strongly discouraged from taking HRT although there is a lack of data to support this (Howell 1995). With the increased early diagnosis of breast carcinoma the long-term prognosis for many women is very good. Unfortunately, the use of chemotherapy in the treatment of the carcinoma leaves many women with a premature menopause and, together with the use of tamoxifen (which enduces vasomotor symptoms), many women are left with a poor quality of life and at greater risk long-term. Some small studies have not shown any adverse effects in women on HRT with a previous breast malignancy, but more data is needed. Endometrial adenocarcinoma is extremely oestrogen dependent. Following treatment by hysterectomy and bilateral salpingo-oophorectomy, HRT is usually considered only in women with an early stage disease.

Oestrogens are metabolized by the liver so that in women with severe active liver disease the increased burden on an already vunerable liver may be too great.

Relative contraindications (Box 19.5)

Although HRT can be prescribed with these conditions, investigations may be required first and then

---

Box 19.5 Relative contraindications to HRT

- Uncontrolled hypertension
- Past history of venous thromboembolic event
- Gall stones
- Fibroids
- Endometriosis
- Endometrial hyperplasia

---

the treatment tailormade to the individual patient. Relative contraindications include suspected pregnancy, undiagnosed irregular vaginal bleeding and an undiagnosed breast lump. In women with uncontrolled hypertension, this should be treated first and HRT should not be denied because these women are at increased risk of cardiovascular disease and are likely to benefit from the cardioprotection.

Recent studies have shown a small increased risk of venous thromboembolism (VTE) particularly associated with recent HRT introduction (Daly et al 1996, Grodstein et al 1996, Gutthann et al 1997, Jick et al 1996). Women with a history of VTE are always at increased risk of another event regardless of whether there is a known clotting abnormality or the event was associated with a predisposing risk factor. Advice from a haematologist should be sought before commencing HRT.

Transdermal oestrogens are favoured in women with a history of quiescent liver disease or a disturbance in liver function, and liver function is checked at intervals. Oral oestrogens change bile composition, which may in turn increase the risk of gallbladder disease and so, in women with established disease, HRT needs to be used with caution.

As previously described, HRT alters carbohydrate metabolism and therefore diabetic control needs to be more closely monitored during the first few months of therapy. Fibroids are oestrogen dependent and may enlarge during HRT use. In most women they remain asymptomatic but fibroid size should be monitored annually. If fibroids become problematic HRT should be discontinued or hysterectomy considered.

There are a number of conditions that, historically, have been thought to be contraindications to HRT, such as previous or current benign breast disease. There is no evidence that HRT has any increased risk on top of a woman's own inherent risk of breast cancer. Regular surveillance for any breast changes should be carefully established and maintained.

Although melanomas may be stimulated by the high levels of oestrogens during pregnancy there is no data to show any detrimental effect of HRT in patients with a history of melanoma.

Otosclerosis, which is a rare condition leading to a progressive irreversible hearing loss, is worsened by pregnancy but, again, there is no evidence that HRT has any adverse effect on the progress of this disease.

Short-term benefits of HRT

Most women seek HRT for the control of short-term, troublesome menopausal symptoms, and few for the long-term benefits. Oestrogen replacement is the most effective treatment for the control of all the menopausal oestrogen deficiency symptoms.

Vasomotor symptoms are usually the first to improve, usually significantly within the first month of treatment, with maximum improvement after 3 months (Coope et al 1975).

There is some controversy over the cause of psychological symptoms at the menopause, although some studies have demonstrated an improvement in these symptoms using HRT (Campbell & Whitehead 1977). Sometimes the psychological symptoms are compounded by other menopausal symptoms, such as night sweats and resulting insomnia, although it has been shown that oestrogen enhances mood in women irrespective of other symptoms. Although vasomotor symptoms are controlled quite rapidly, higher doses of HRT in the longer term are required to alleviate psychological symptoms. One study (unpublished) showed that psychological symptoms were only significantly improved after 12 cycles of HRT. The atrophic changes in the urogenital tract can be reversed or changed with the use of systemic or local oestrogens. Alleviation of the atrophic symptoms may take 3 months of therapy, with maximum improvement by 6 months.

Long-term benefits

With the increase in longivity, most clinicians are concerned with the long-term benefits of HRT, although few women present requesting HRT for cardiovascular, bone or Alzheimer disease protection.

Reduction in cardiovascular disease

It is important to stress that cardiovascular disease is multifactorial and that low postmenopausal oestrogen levels are just one of many factors that affect cardiovascular risk. It is currently believed that oestrogen provides a significant protection against CHD by nearly 50%, and little or no protection against strokes (Pederson et al 1997, Sullivan & Fowlkes 1996). This is based on a number of large epidemiological studies, case-controlled studies and from studies of angiographically defined disease. However, there have not been any large, randomized, controlled studies to prove the benefit but work is ongoing. The results of the Heart Estrogen/Progestin Replacement Study (HERS) was disappointing, it concluded that HRT did not offer protection in women with established coronary heart disease (Hulley et al 1998).

The importance of the effects of HRT on lipids is not fully understood. Oestrogen reduces LDL- and total-cholesterol levels, while raising HDL-cholesterol levels, thus reversing the atheromogenic lipid profile associated with the menopause. Transdermal therapies have less of an effect than oral oestrogens. Oral oestrogen raises triglyceride levels, which have a detrimental effect on CHD in men, but the importance of triglyceride levels in women in still being debated. There has been concern that adding a progestogen to HRT would partially or totally negate the beneficial effects of the oestrogens. The PEPI study showed that unopposed oestrogen had the most beneficial effect but that all hormone treatments were still significantly better than the placebo (PEPI 1995). In general the 17-hydroxyprogesterone derivatives have no adverse effect on lipids, unlike the 19-nortestosterone derivatives, which are androgenic. One study of women on continuous combined regimes showed that these regimes had more of an effect than sequential regimes in reducing LDL- and total-cholesterol but no studies have yet shown that continuous combined regimes reduce overall CVD risk. Another risk factor known to affect cardiovascular disease risk is lipoprotein (a), high levels of which are associated with atheroma formation. Oestrogens do not alter levels of lipoprotein (a), whereas the androgenic progestogens such as norethisterone cause a reduction in its concentrations. However, its significance is still to be demonstrated. The other non-lipid effects of oestrogen include a relaxant effect on the arterial system, which increases the blood flow through the coronary arteries, a reduction in peripheral resistance and an increase in the thickness in the left ventricular wall, increasing cardiac output.

Insulin resistance increases with age and this is important in the development of CHD. Transdermal oestrogen increases insulin production by the pancreas and increases its clearance, but how relevant this is, is still to be clarified.

Overall, there are good reasons to encourage oestrogen use in women as a primary prevention of CHD. Any benefits to the cardiovascular system from HRT seem to be lost within 2 years of discontinuing therapy and long-term treatment will need to be considered, although many cardiologists will be convinced of this only after large-scale, randomized, controlled studies looking specifically at cardiovascular disease. Some clinicians believe that HRT should routinely be give to women following a myocardial infarction to prevent reoccurrence.

Osteoporosis

HRT prevents bone loss at all recognized risk sites – the neck of femur, the vertebrae and the wrist – and studies have shown that its use is also associated with a reduction in fracture risk (Stevenson et al 1990). Most studies have focused on oral therapy, although a number of transdermal therapies have also obtained a licence for osteoporosis prevention. The doses of oestrogen that are known to be bone protective are shown in (Box 19.6).

Oestrogen has several roles in the prevention of bone loss. Its main effect is the reduction of the amount of bone that is absorbed by the osteoclasts. It also controls the body's calcium balance.

Bone loss is prevented only for as long as HRT is continued. When treatment is withdrawn then bone turnover increases again, and this leads to a fall in bone density.

Women have a rapid period of bone loss immediately after the menopause. HRT can prevent this if it is started during the perimenopause. However, when HRT is discontinued this accelerated period of bone loss will then occur. So if a woman is known to have a severe risk of osteoporosis then HRT should be continued in the long term. Some earlier studies have show that 5 years of HRT reduced fracture risk by half but it now seems doubtful that 5 years of HRT in a woman in her 50s will have any lasting protection for her in her 80s, when falls and resulting osteoporotic fractures are increasingly likely to occur. Just as there is concern

---

Box 19.6 Doses of oestrogen for osteoporosis prevention

Oral oestradiol	1–2 mg
Oestradiol transdermal patch	50 µg
Conjugated equine oestrogens	0.625 mg

over the long-term use of HRT, so there is a debate as to whether HRT should be commenced in an older woman whose bone density is known to be low, preventing it dropping any further and thus reducing fracture rates without increasing breast cancer risks.

Alzheimer's disease

Oestrogen has an effect on normal memory. HRT increases memory function in women following oophorectomy and modulates memory function through the normal menstrual cycle. It affects brain development in both sexes and has multiple actions; men convert testosterone to oestrogen in the brain. There is evidence to suggest that HRT can prevent or delay the onset of AD, and also that it can ameliorate the effects of AD, although it may have a greater action in preventing the disease rather than treating it. Small studies show readily detectable small improvements in cognitive function, but these may be only relatively short term. The duration and dose of treatment is significant. Long-term treatment is necessary for the protection against AD, probably starting early, as there is a long-term disease process that is thought to start in the third or fourth decade (Henderson 1997, Paganini & Henderson 1994). Progestogens also influence the brain but there is a lack of studies comparing the effects of combined HRT preparations with those of oestrogen-only regimes.

Risks of HRT

As with all drug therapies, there are risks associated with HRT use and these have to be weighed against the substantial benefits. Most of the concern with HRT is with the risk of breast cancer.

HRT and breast cancer

Breast cancer is possibly the disease that women fear most. Treatments are often disfiguring and seen as an assault on their femininity.

There are hormonal influences on breast cancer risk, shown by the increased incidence of breast cancer in women with an early menarche, late menopause, obesity in the postmenopausal women and the use of combined oral contraceptive pill before the first pregnancy. Oestrogen exposure is related to breast epithelial cell proliferation, perhaps making the breasts more sensitive to carcinogens or by stimulating early malignancies that may have laid dormant or even regressed after oestrogen withdrawal at the natural menopause.

There are two issues related to breast cancer and HRT use. First, the effects of HRT on the risks of developing breast cancer and on breast cancer reoccurrence. Second, the effect of HRT on the mortality from breast cancer associated with HRT use.

Many studies have been carried out looking at the risk, both case-controlled and cohort studies, and the results have not been consistent. As any effect of oestrogens on breast cancer risk is likely to be small, meta-analyses have been carried out to make sense of the data. The most recent analysis carried out contained data on 160 000 women. This analysis showed an increased risk of breast cancer with HRT use and suggested that the risk rises exponentially with HRT exposure (Beral et al 1997) However, it must be remembered that while breast cancer affects one in 12 women in their lifetime, cardiovascular disease kills one in two women and osteoporosis affects one in two women by the age of 70 years, with a high associated

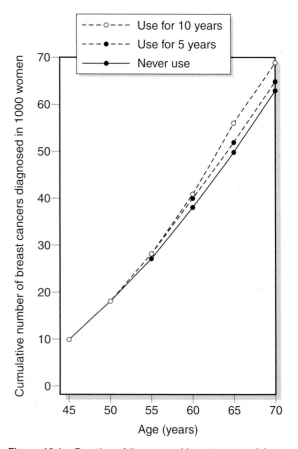

Figure 19.1 Duration of therapy and breast cancer risk. From Beral 1997, with permission.

mortality. Some women on long-term HRT who, would have died from cardiovascular disease without the HRT, will go on to develop breast cancer instead (Fig. 19.1).

Prognosis in women who develop a breast tumour on treatment appears to be better than in women not on HRT. Women who have taken HRT within 1 year of the diagnosis of breast cancer have a greater survival than other women (Willis et al 1996). There are two reasons for this. First, women taking HRT may well be more breast conscious and surveillance may be better, so the tumour is diagnosed earlier. Second, studies have indicated that women taking HRT develop a better grade of tumour, which can be treated more successfully. Mortality from breast cancer is 16% lower in women on HRT than in women not on HRT, even though the risk of developing the disease increases with HRT exposure. For women at increased risk of breast cancer because of a family history or the presence of benign breast disease, the use of HRT is not contraindicated. As with all areas of HRT use and breast cancer, more data would be welcomed but, at the moment, these women do not seem to be at an additional risk if they use HRT.

Little data exists for women with a history of breast cancer (Eden et al 1997). With the national breast screening programme, many women are being diagnosed with small tumours and long-term survival is good. Young women who have been rendered menopausal as a result of chemotherapy for the treatment for their breast cancer, or who are suffering menopausal symptoms as result of tamoxifen, would have a significant increase in their quality of life and the consequences of the premature menopause with HRT. However, there is obviously concern that HRT use will stimulate the proliferation of distant metastases. Although the small studies done to date have been encouraging, more data is required.

Endometrial cancer

Historically, unopposed oestrogen therapy was given to non-hysterectomized women and there was a significant rise in the incidence of endometrial adenocarcinoma. Modern treatment regimes contain between 10–14 days of progestogens per cycle, in sequential regimes or continuous progestogen, thus reducing the risk of endometrial hyperplasia and endometrial carcinoma to that of untreated women in the population (Voigt et al 1991).

> **Box 19.7** Side-effects of HRT
>
> - **Oestrogenic:**
>   - breast tenderness
>   - bloating
>   - leg cramps
>   - headaches
>   - nausea/dyspepsia
>   - nipple sensitivity.
> - **Progestogenic:**
>   - mood changes
>   - headaches
>   - fluid retention
>   - breast tenderness
>   - acne
>   - premenstrual symptoms.

Side-effects of HRT

The side effects of HRT can generally be divided into oestrogenic and progestogenic effects, although many of the symptoms overlap (Box 19.7). All women need to be warned about possible side-effects before starting treatment, as this will reduce their anxiety and encourage them to persist with treatment.

Many of the symptoms, particularly the oestrogenic symptoms, will improve over the first few months of therapy and it is essential that treatment is continued so that the symptoms have a chance to settle. One exception to this would be very severe oestrogenic side-effects, such as breast tenderness, which can be a problem in the postmenopausal women. Such severe symptoms can result in a woman abandoning therapy, in these cases it is much better to start on low-dose oestrogen and to increase the dose gradually to a bone sparing level if necessary. Careful questioning about side-effects is essential to establish whether they occur during the oestrogen-only phase of the cycle or during the addition of progestogen. Treatment options for oestrogenic side-effects are to reduce the dose, wait and encourage the patient to continue or change the route of administration. Progestogenic side-effects tend to be more problematic, particularly in cyclical regimes, and can be treated by changing the route of the progestogen, the type of progestogen and the frequency, i.e. a 3-monthly cyclical regime or continuous regime.

Care of the patient on HRT

Women on HRT need to be monitored to ensure that they are maximizing the benefits of treatment by early

---

Case study: Maureen

Maureen is aged 51 years and she works full-time as a legal secretary. She is well known to her GP because of multiple treatment failures with her HRT. She started experiencing menopausal symptoms at the age of 47 years when she was still menstruating regularly. These manifested as an increase in migraine headaches, inability to cope and vasomotor symptoms. She has a history of depression in her twenties following a failed engagement. She never married. After an initial consultation with her GP she started HRT in the form of continuous oral oestradiol and cyclical norethisterone. The GP offered Maureen counselling as her mood was low and work was very demanding. Maureen declined.

Maureen returned after 3 months with worsening of her premenstrual migraines, although the vasomotor symptoms were improved. The progestogen in the HRT was changed to a 17-hydroxyprogesterone derivative but the oestrogen was left unaltered. Two months later she returned, still with premenstrual migraine. Next the GP prescribed a combined oestrogen/progestogen reservoir patch but Maureen rapidly developed a skin allergy. Then she was prescribed a 3-monthly sequential regime, trying to reduce the frequency of the withdrawal bleeds and also the migraines. Maureen returned after 3 months complaining of irregular mid-cycle bleeding but a small reduction in the number of migraines. She was reassured that the irregular bleeding would settle in time. However, after a year on the 3-monthly regime she was still experiencing irregular bleeding and there was now no pattern to the migraines. This she found very difficult and she asked to return to a sequential regime. She then tried a sequential transdermal regime in the form of a matrix patch. This she was not allergic to and, with a review of her migraine medication, Maureen felt better. Her migraines were less severe, she had regular withdrawal bleeds, the vasomotor symptoms were well controlled and her mood after several months of therapy lifted. After a while on this therapy, she then flew to Australia to visit relatives and, during the 24-h flight, her left leg and ankle became swollen and painful. She was admitted into hospital soon after arrival with a suspected DVT. This was not proven on Doppler and she was not given anticoagulants although her HRT was discontinued. On her return home her GP undertook a clotting screen and the advice of the local haematologist was sought. The clotting screen was normal and the haematologist felt that is was unlikely that she had had a venous thromboembolic event and that she could restart her HRT.

This case history highlights the problems that some women face with side-effects, particularly progestogenic. Migraine can be a particular problem. The management of progestogen side-effects includes:
- changing the progestogen
- reducing the frequency
- changing the route of administration
- changing the treatment regime.

It is also important to review treatment in the light of recent research and to check whether the woman experiences other health problems. If Maureen had had a DVT she may well have been advised to discontinue therapy completely. Migraines tend to be better controlled with transdermal therapies.

---

recognition of problems and by minimizing any side-effects. There is no national agreement on the monitoring and management of women on HRT, although suggested guidelines do exist (Rees & Purdie 1999). A recent survey indicated that current levels of monitoring are very variable between practices (Tannu & Pitkin 1997). Monitoring needs to begin before a woman starts treatment to ensure she is suitable, to provide her with information so that she can participate in the choice of treatment and to give her realistic expectations (Hope & Rees 1995).

Provision of information

Uptake of HRT is low despite its recognized benefits and continuation is poor; many women discontinue therapy within the first 6 months, mainly due to side-effects.

Many women already taking HRT want more information (Roberts 1991). Media reports often cause anxiety and women need access to up-to-date, reliable, unbiased information. Although books, videos, leaflets and group meetings are helpful in providing information to women, individual counselling is essential. Time with either the nurse or doctor can help reinforce information, making it relevant to the patient and her history.

The climacteric is an emotive time of life, questioning and listening to a patient can help separate menopausal problems, which will respond to HRT, and other life problems that will need alternative approaches. Counselling can give women realistic expectations of HRT and provides an opportunity to build-up a rapport with a member of the menopause team. Many women discontinue therapy without returning to their doctor to discuss problems (Hope & Rees 1995). Such a rapport, together with easy access to a known clinician, may help with continuance on HRT.

Ideally, all women should have the opportunity to make an informed decision of whether to take HRT or not. Information using a variety of resources can be made available to all women in a practice through well women clinics, smear clinics and by targeting women who have had a hysterectomy.

Initial assessment

The aim of the initial assessment is to establish whether a woman will benefit from HRT because of menopausal symptoms or postmenopausal risk factors, while highlighting any possible contraindications. Some information can be accessed easily from records in general practice. The initial assessment gathers together information about menopausal status, gynaecological, obstetric, medical, surgical and family history, together with a general health assessment.

Menopausal and menstrual status. The patient is questioned about the presence of menopausal symptoms, their longivity and severity. The date of the last menstrual period should be noted to ascertain whether a women is peri- or postmenopausal. Questions about menstrual history will reveal any heavy or irregular bleeding, which may need investigating. Age, type of menopause (e.g. natural or other) may influence dose, route and duration of treatment. Previous experience with HRT is significant and detailed questioning about any problems in relation to the treatment cycle will establish whether they are oestrogenic or progestogenic in origin.

The patient needs to be asked if there are any nonmedical factors, personal and family stresses that may be contributing to the menopause scenario.

Gynaecological and obstetric history. Questioning should include parity, current use of contraception, cervical smear history, recent history of vaginal discharge, problems with intercourse and previous gynaecological surgery or problems.

Medical and surgical history. Of particular interest is a history of thromboembolic disease and liver disease, or a previous history of carcinoma, particularly that of the breast or endometrium. Specialist advice should be sought if there is a history of these problems. A history of any significant medical or surgical problems, together with bowel and urinary problems, should be noted. The patient should be up-to-date with mammography under the national screening programme.

Family history. The history of grandparents as well as parents, uncles, aunts and siblings should be considered when asking about family history of disease and the following diseases included: breast cancer, osteoporosis, heart disease, stroke, hypertension, dementia, thromboembolism and any other that the patient mentions. Between 5 and 20% of women have a family history of breast cancer but about 5% of breast cancers are due to a dominant breast cancer mutation (BRCA1 and BRCA2). Counselling of women with strong family histories of breast or ovarian cancers should be undertaken in specialist centres.

General health assessment. The following should be included: height, weight, blood pressure, allergies, smoking and alcohol consumption. A breast and pelvic examination are necessary to exclude obvious breast or pelvic pathology.

Special investigations. These may need to be carried out, for example, FSH levels to confirm the diagnosis in young or hysterectomized women. Other tests may include thyroid function (some menopausal symptoms can be confused with thyroid malfunction) and liver function. In women with a high risk of cardiovascular disease, fasting serum cholesterol and triglyceride levels will determine the route of therapy. Endometrial biopsy is performed to exclude uterine and pelvic pathology in women reporting menorrhagia and/or irregular vaginal bleeding.

If available, a bone mineral density measurement can be helpful when the decision to take HRT is not straightforward and, in the young woman, to confirm that HRT is conserving her bone mass.

The patient's own preferences need to be taken into account before prescribing HRT as this will improve continuance on therapy. Oral therapy remains the first-line treatment because of cost.

Bleeding patterns. Typical bleeding patterns need to be discussed. On cyclical regimes most women should expect a withdrawal bleed towards the end of the progestogen phase or within the first week of the oestrogen-only phase. Withdrawal bleeds during the first few treatment cycles tend to be heavier (Rees & Barlow 1991). Women should be warned and encouraged to continue. Withdrawal bleeds on monthly sequential regimes are of similar duration and flow to spontaneous menses. About 5% of women will not have a withdrawal bleed. Mid-cycle bleeding may occur initially on 3-monthly cyclic regimes but this settles with use.

Follow-up on therapy

A follow-up appointment should be made for about 3 months after the start of therapy but the patient should be encouraged to contact the surgery if problems arise. If therapy is modified, another 3-month appointment is made. Once a women is happily established on therapy, subsequent visits are at 6 month intervals, alternating between the doctor and nurse. The following assessments should be made:

- adequate symptom control
- side-effects of therapy (see p. 329)
- timing and acceptability of withdrawal bleeds
- weight and blood pressure changes
- patient's questions and concerns.

Adequate symptom control. Hot flushes are usually the first symptom to respond to therapy and should show significant improvement after 1 month and maximum improvement by 3 months. Urogenital symptoms should show some improvement by 3 months and maximum improvement by 6 months. Psychological symptoms take longer to respond and may not show significant improvement for 1 year. If symptomatology is still severe, establish that therapy is being taken correctly or if there are any problems, such as skin reaction with a transdermal patch, that will hinder oestrogen absorption. A change in therapy may be appropriate with poor symptom control either by increasing the dose of oestrogen or route.

Withdrawal bleeds. It is helpful at this visit if the patient has kept a record of the timing of her withdrawal bleeds in relation to the cycle day. Although there are monthly variations, the bleeds on a cyclical regime should be regular, relatively pain free and similar in length and flow to normal menstruation.

Bleeding problems may respond to a change in therapy. With severe dysmenorrhoea, the preparation needs to be changed. If bleeding problems persist, mid-cycle bleeding or menorrhagia, then endometrial pathology, needs to be excluded. If bleeding problems still continue than a hysteroscopy will exclude other pathology, such as an endometrial polyp.

On 3-monthly cyclic regimes, mid-cycle bleeding may occur but this settles with use. The data to show the level of mid-cycle bleeding after 1 year is not yet available.

With continuous combined preparations, initial irregular and unpredictable bleeding is very common. The amount can vary from nothing to weeks of bleeding on and off for months. After 3 months of therapy this bleeding should be reducing and should continue to lessen over the first 6 months. Sixty per cent of women are bleed-free by 6 months and 95% by 1 year (Christiansen & Riis 1991). An increase in the progestogen dose will help to control the loss but this can only be used as a temporary measure as it may cause unpleasant side-effects and some progestogens negate the beneficial effects of the oestrogens. Bleeding after 6 months on a continuous combined regime, or unexpected bleeding after a long period of amenorrhoea, should be treated as a postmenopausal bleed.

Weight and blood pressure changes. HRT is often blamed for weight increase although there is no scientific evidence to support this (Espeland et al 1997). Women do experience an age-related weight gain. Bloating and breast enlargement of atrophied breasts may cause discomfort and be confused with weight gain. Regular monitoring of weight, together with counselling about diet and exercise, can help women control their weight. HRT has not been shown to have an adverse effect on blood pressure.

Patient's questions. At each visit patients should be asked if there are any questions or anxieties about treatment in order to prevent any early discontinuation of therapy.

NON-HORMONAL TREATMENTS

Many women have concerns about HRT while others have contraindications and, if a woman declines HRT, alternative treatments should be investigated. There are possible alternative treatments for all the menopausal symptoms and consequences of the menopause. Alternatives fall into three categories: pharmological alternatives, lifestyle and dietary changes and complementary therapies.

Pharmacological alternatives

The antihypertensive drug clonidine, 50–75 µg twice daily, is helpful in reducing flush symptomatology in about 30% of women, about the same effect as a placebo. There is some evidence that it would be effective in higher doses but these are associated with side-effects. Propranolol is little used to control vasomotor symptoms now as studies have produced conflicting results of its effect. Progestogens have been used for some time for the control of menopausal hot flushes. Recent work has focused on megestrol acetate, which has not shown any oestrogenic effect and is sometimes used in the treatment of breast cancer. At a dose of 40 mg daily, flushes have been found to be significantly reduced after 1 month of treatment. Even though progestogens are effective in controlling hot flushes, their effect long term on the at risk breast is not known.

Bioadhesive vaginal moisturizer is helpful for the symptomatic relief of atrophic vaginitis. This is a slightly acidic gel containing water and a polycarbophil, which adheres to the dehydrated vaginal epithelium and encourages water back into the tissues, while restoring the protective pH of the vagina. Each application lasts for 3 days, so it is long-lasting compared to other simple vaginal moisturizers and in trials it compared well with vaginal oestrogen preparations (Nachtigall 1994). As it is not available on prescription, some women may find it prohibitively expensive.

Vaginal oestriol preparations remain an option for women who have contraindication to oestrogen as they are not absorbed systemically to any significant degree and are useful in treating all urogenital atrophic symptoms.

Etridronate, a bisphosphonate, is licensed to treat postmenopausal osteoporosis and is relatively free from side-effects (which are mainly gastrointestinal due to the calcium component of the treatment). It is a useful alternative in older women who find the side-effects of oestrogen intolerable and in which compliance is therefore poor. Patients need careful counselling about taking the therapy so as not to hinder its absorption. More long-term data is required to show long-term reduction in fracture rate, and second and third generation bisphosphonates are now being developed.

Alendronate, an aminobisphosphonate, also stops bone loss and reduces fracture risk at all clinically significant sites. Patients need to have a good calcium intake with therapy, often needing supplementation. Alendronate has been linked to gastric ulcers and patients need to adhere strictly to the instructions of its use.

A selective oestrogen receptor modulator (SERM), raloxifene, has now received its product licence for postmenopausal women at risk of non-traumatic vertebral osteoporotic fractures. Data remains limited but has shown a reduction in vertebral fracture risk. Side-effects include hot flushes and leg cramps. Raloxifene was shown to increase thromboembolic risk three-fold, so that a history of venous thromboembolism is a contraindication. Raloxifene has been shown to have a beneficial effect on lipids and a reduction in risk of invasive breast cancer. However, more studies are needed to confirm these findings and to show whether raloxifene offers protection against Alzheimer's disease or vaginal atrophy (Ettinger et al 1999).

Dietary and lifestyle modification

Cross-cultural experiences of the menopause vary enormously and the menopause is associated with fewer and less severe symptoms in Asian women. Diet and exercise may be important in reducing both vasomotor symptoms and depression (Payer 1991) and protecting against cardiovascular disease and osteoporosis (Clunie 1994, Pyoraia et al 1994).

Many foods contain phytoestrogens, which are potential oestrogen analogues, and in some cultures the diet is composed of many foods rich in these compounds, such as seed oils and soya. Phytoestrogens may reduce the severity of menopausal symptoms (Wilcox et al 1990) and, together with genetic and other lifestyle differences, affect the incidence of disease in different cultures (Ingram et al 1997). It is difficult to assess the absolute importance of dietary and behaviour factors in reducing the risk of osteoporosis. An active, healthy childhood with adequate calcium will help achieve the maximum peak adult bone mass. In older women, a daily intake of calcium of 1000–1500 mg will have a positive effect on bone turnover. Other lifestyle changes may be needed, such as a reduction in smoking and in alcohol, caffeine, salt and animal protein intake to minimize calcium loss and maximize calcium absorption. A significant number of elderly women are deficient in calcium and vitamin D, supplementation in this population has been shown to reduce fracture risk (Chapuy et al 1992).

A multitude of factors affect cardiovascular disease but there is evidence that modification of lifestyle will reduce the incidence of CHD. Nurses may need to help women identify areas of their lives that need modifying.

Exercise

There is some evidence to show that regular exercise can reduce vasomotor symptoms and depression (Payer 1991). Exercise in the young should be encouraged to maximize bone mass potential. Weight-bearing and muscle-strengthening exercises appear to play a role in maintaining and perhaps increasing bone mass, but will only have an effect for as long as the exercise is continued. The level of exercise needs to be modified to each woman and should be undertaken several times a week.

Complementary therapies

There is no scientific evidence that any complementary therapy improves menopausal symptoms, nevertheless many women do use and continue to use them. The choice of therapies is confusing but they have been reported to improve vasomotor, psychological, menstrual and urogenital symptoms, as well as helping in lifestyle changes. Any woman considering complementary therapy needs to find a therapy that she is happy with and to choose a therapist with care. Therapies that have been reported to be helpful include massage, aromatherapy, reflexology, homeopathy, acupuncture and herbalism (with caution in women with a contraindication to oestrogen).

CONTRACEPTION IN THE PERIMENOPAUSE

Many women welcome the menopause because it removes the threat of pregnancy. Fertility declines with age as the menopause approaches but pregnancy remains a risk until ovulation has finally ceased, and it is difficult to predict when this has happened. Pregnancy in the older woman carries significantly higher maternal and perinatal mortality, together with the ever-increasing risk of chromosomal abnormalities, most notably Down syndrome.

Although pregnancy in the older woman can be welcomed, some result in emotional and social hardship and 45% of pregnancies in women over 40 years are terminated (Office of Population Censuses and Surveys 1984), with all the resulting psychological effects. So women are advised to continue with contraception for 2 years following their last spontaneous mensus if it is before the age of 50 years or for 1 year if

menstruation ceases after 50 years. However, a problem arises in women who start HRT before menstruation ceases and the date of the menopause is unknown. HRT is not a method of contraception.

Generally, methods of contraception that are not effective enough in younger women, such as barrier methods, become extremely effective in older women with reduced fertility. Methods of contraception for use in the perimenopause are shown in Table 19.1.

THE NURSE'S ROLE IN THE CARE OF THE PERI- AND POSTMENOPAUSAL WOMAN

Nurses are in a unique position in caring for these women. In a recent survey nurses were shown to be under-used in the care of the menopausal woman and were more involved in monitoring than in initiation of treatment, that is, they covered the same parameters as the GP but with a different emphasis (Tannu & Pitkin 1997). Roberts (1995) showed that women preferred a clinic environment led by a female GP/practice nurse and did not like to be made aware of time constraints.

As with any specialist area, a good up-to-date knowledge is essential, together with clinical experience. Knowledge about the menopause in the general population is generally poor and the major role of the

Table 19.1 Methods of contraception

	Sterilization	Barrier methods	Coitus interruptus	Natural family planning	Spermicides	IUCD	IUS	POP	Injectables	COC
Effective	✓	✓	✓	✓	✓	✓	✓	✓	✓	✓
Unrelated to coitus	✓			(✓)		✓	✓	✓	✓	✓
Menopause not masked	✓	✓	✓	✓	✓	✓	✓			
No side-effects	✓	✓	✓	✓	✓					
Control of cycle										✓
Protection against infection		✓			(✓)		✓	(✓)	(✓)	(✓)
Protection against gynaecological pathology							✓			✓
Protection against symptoms of climacteric										✓
Protection against osteoporosis and other ageing effects of oestrogen deficiency										✓
May be used alongside hormone replacement therapy	✓	✓	✓		✓	✓	✓			

COC, combined oral contraceptive; IUCD, intrauterine contraceptive device; IUS intrauterine system; POP, progestogen-only pill nurse must be in the provision of information. This can be achieved in a number of different ways, from the provision of leaflets, videos and books, group meetings and discussion groups, to individual counselling. Individual counselling is the key to improve uptake of therapy amongst menopausal women and for greater long-term continuance. Spending time with a woman before she starts HRT has a number of different purposes:

- reinforcing information to build on a woman's basic understanding
- personalizing information and making the risks and benefits relevant to the woman and her history
- listening and disentangling life problems that are not related to the menopause and which require other treatments or therapies
- creating realistic expectations so that each woman understands likely effects of HRT in controlling her symptoms, the time course of symptom improvement and the possible side-effects
- establishing a rapport so that the woman is encouraged to contact the nurse if she encounters problems on therapy. Thirty-eight percent of women discontinue HRT without consultation.

Together with all the information-giving, nurses play a vital role in the information-gathering from a woman before she starts on treatment, and this continues when the nurse monitors the woman for the duration of her treatment.

There are some women at particular long-term risk of the metabolic consequences of the menopause, one such group being hysterectomized women, even those with ovarian conservation. The absence of menstruation makes the diagnosis more difficult. As these women miss out on the regular cervical screening, this is one group that nurses should target for regular general health check.

CONCLUSION

Enormous advances have been made in recent years in knowledge about effects of the menopause, together with a vast growth in the preparations available for treating menopausal women. Nurses face an increasing challenge to keep the menopausal population informed and to optimize their care.

GLOSSARY

Amenorrhoea: the cessation of menstruation
Climacteric: the time in a woman's life when menstruation ceases and she may experience menopausal symptoms
Follicle stimulating hormone (FSH): a hormone secreted by the pituitary gland. It can be used to diagnose ovarian failure, as levels rise with the decline in ovarian function
Gonadotrophins: the collective term for FSH and LH
Hormone replacement therapy: a main treatment for menopause syndrome, either oestrogen alone or oestrogen and progestogen
Luteinizing hormone (LH): this hormone is produced by the pituitary gland, levels rise at the menopause, but after the rise in FSH levels
Menopause: the last natural menstrual period
Oestrogen: this hormone is produced by the ovary during the menstrual cycle. Low postmenopausal levels of oestrogen lead to the menopause syndrome

Osteoporosis: reduction in bone mass so that fractures are likely to occur with a minimum of trauma
Postmenopausal: at least 1 year after the last spontaneous menstrual period
Premature menopause: a menopause before the age of 40
Progestogen: synthetic alternative to the naturally occurring progesterone
Progesterone: the naturally occurring hormone produced by the ovary during the menstrual cycle
Resistant ovarian syndrome: a poorly understood condition when the ovaries fail to respond to rising FSH levels although ova remain in the ovary
Surgical menopause: the surgical removal of functioning ovaries
Testosterone: male hormone, which occurs in women in low levels
Vasomotor symptoms: the most common menopause symptoms, include hot flushes and night sweats

REFERENCES

Andersson K, Mattson LA, Rybp G, Stadberg E 1992 Intrauterine release of levenorgestrel – a new way of adding progestogen in hormone replacement therapy. Obstetrics and Gynecology 79:963–967
Barlow DH 1996 Premature ovarian failure. The menopause: key issues. Baillière Tindal, London, pp. 361–384

Barlow DH 1995 Future developments and conclusion. Rees CMP (ed.) Menopause update. Reed Healthcare Communications, Sutton, pp. 57–59
Beral V 1997 Breast cancer and hormone replacement therapy: collaborative reanalysis of data from 51 epidemiological studies of 52,705 women with breast

cancer and 108,411 women without breast cancer. The Lancet 350:1047–1059

Brincat M, Studd JWW 1988 Skin and the menopause. In: Studd JWW and Whitehead MI (eds) The menopause. Blackwell Scientific, Oxford, pp. 85–101

Brockie JA, Barlow DH, Rees CMP 1991 Menopausal flush symptomatology and sustained reflex vasoconstriction. Human Reproduction 6:471–474

Burger HG 1996 The menopausal transition. In: Barlow DH (ed.) The menopause: key issues. Baillière Tindal, London, pp. 347–359

Campbell S, Whitehead MI 1977 Oestrogen therapy and the menopausal syndrome. In: Greenblatt RG and Studd JWW (eds) Clinics in obstetrics and gynecology. Saunders, London, pp. 31–48

Chapuy MC, Arlot ME, Duboeuf F, et al 1992 Vitamin D3 and calcium to prevent hip fractures in elderly women. New England Journal of Medicine 327:1637–1642

Christiansen C, Riis BJ 1991 Five years of continuous combined oestrogen/progestogen therapy. Effects on calcium metabolism, lipoproteins and bleeding pattern. British Journal of Obstetrics and Gynaecology 97(21):1087–1092

Clunie G 1994 Osteoporosis prevention. British Journal of Hospital Medicine 52:79–85

Coope J, Marsh J 1992 Can we improve compliance with long term HRT? Maturitas 15:151–158

Coope J, Thompson JM, Poller L 1975 Effect of 'natural oestrogen' replacement therapy on menopausal symptoms and blood clotting. British Medical Journal 4:139–143

Crook D 1995 Postmenopausal HRT, serum lipoproteins and cardiovascular disease. In: Rees CMP (ed.) Menopause update. Reed Healthcare Communications, Sutton, pp. 16–18

Daly E, Vessey MP, Hawkins MM, et al 1996 Risk of venous thromboembolism in users of hormone replacement therapy. The Lancet 348:977–980

Ditkiff EC, Crary WG, Cristo M, et al 1991 Estrogen improves psychological function in asymptomatic postmenopausal women. Obstetrics and Gynecology 78:991

Draper J, Roland M 1990 Perimenopausal women's views on taking hormone replacement therapy to prevent osteoporosis. British Medical Journal 300:786–788

Eden JA, Wren BG 1996 Hormone replacement therapy after breast cancer: a review. Cancer Treatment Reviews 22(5):335–343

Espeland MA, Stefanick ML, Kritz-Silverstein D, et al 1997 Effect of postmenopausal hormone replacement therapy on body weight and waist and hip girths. Journal of Clinical Endocrinology and Metabolism 82(5):1549–1556

Ettinger B, Black DM, Mitlak BH, et al 1999 Reduction of vertebral fracture risk in postmenopausal women with osteoporosis treated with raloxifene. The Journal of The American Medical Association 282:637–645

Garnett T, Studd JWW, Henderson A, et al 1990 Hormone implants and tachyphylaxis. British Journal of Clinical Investigations 97:917–921

Ginsberg J, Prelevic GM 1995 Tibolone in postmenopausal women with a history of breast cancer. Journal of British Menopause Society 1:24–25

Grodstein F, Stampfer MJ, Goldhaber SZ, et al 1996 Prospective study of exogenous hormones and risk of pulmonary embolism in women. The Lancet 348:983–987

Gutthann SP, Garcia-Rodriquez LA, Castellsague J, Oliart AD 1997 Hormone replacement therapy and risk of venous thromboembolism: population-based case-control study. British Medical Journal 314:796–800

Henderson VW 1997 The epidemiology of estrogen replacement therapy and Alzheimer's disease. Neurology 48(5 suppl 7):27–35

Hope S, Rees CMP 1995 Why do British women start and stop hormone replacement therapy? Journal of the British Menopause Society 1:26–28

Howell A, Baildam A, Bundred N, et al 1995 'Should I Take HRT, Doctor?' Hormone replacement therapy in women at increased risk of breast cancer and in survivors of the disease. Journal of British Menopause Society 1:9–17

Hulley S, Grady D, Bush T et al 1998 Randomised trials of estrogen plus progestin for secondary prevention of coronary heart disease in postmenopausal women. Journal of the American Medical Association 280:605–613

Ingram D, Sanders K, Kolybaba M, Lopez D 1997 Case-controlled study of phyto-oestrogens and breast cancer. The Lancet 350:990–994

Jick H, Derby LE, Myers MW, et al 1996 Risk of hospital admission for idiopathic venous thromboembolism among users of postmenopausal oestrogens. The Lancet 348:981–983

Kriener D, Droesch K, Navot D, et al 1988 Spontaneous and pharmacologically induced remissions in patients with premature ovarian failure. Obstetrics and Gynecology 72:926–928

Montgomery JC, Studd JWW 1991 Psychological and sexual aspects of the menopause. British Journal of Hospital Medicine 45:300–302

Nachtigall LE 1994 Comparative study: Replens versus local oestrogen in menopausal women. Fertility and Sterility 61:78–80

Office of Population Censuses and Surveys 1984 Statistics for fertility and mortality 1981 & 1982. HMSO, London

Paganini-Hill A, Henderson VW 1994 Estrogen deficiency and risk of Alzheimer's disease in women. American Journal of Epidemiology 140(3):256–261

Payer L 1991 The menopause in various cultures. In: Burger H, Boulet M (eds) A portrait of the menopause. Parthenon Publishing Group, Lancashire, pp. 3–22

PEPI Trial 1995 Effects of estrogen or estrogen/progestin regimes on heart disease risk factors in postmenopausal women. Journal of American Medical Association 273:199–208

Pyoraia K, De Backer G, Grahm P, et al 1994 Prevention of coronary heart disease in clinical practice. European Heart Journal 52:1300–1331

Pederson AT, Lidegaard O, Kreiner S, Ottesen B 1997 Hormone replacement therapy and risk of non-fatal stroke. The Lancet 350:1277–1283

Read C 1997 Cardiovascular system. In: Barlow DH, Collin P (eds) Managing the menopause. Fusion Communication and Publishing Ltd, London, pp. 32–55

Rees CMP, Barlow DH 1991 Quantitation of hormone replacement induced withdrawal bleeds. British Journal of Obstetrics and Gynaecology 98:106–107

Rees M, Purdie W 1999 Management of the menopause. BMS Publications Ltd, Marlow, Bucks

Rehnquist N 1993 Heart disease in women. Realties of mid life in women. Proceedings of the Novo Nordisk International Symposium, Copenhagen.

Roberts PJ 1991 The menopause and hormone replacement therapy: views of women in general practice receiving hormone replacement therapy. British Journal of General Practice 41:421–424

Roberts PJ 1995 Reported satisfaction among women receiving hormone replacement therapy in a dedicated general practice clinic and a normal consultation. British Journal of General Practice 45:79–81

Siddle N, Sarrell P, Whitehead ML 1987 The effect of hysterectomy on the age of ovarian failure: identification of a subgroup of women with premature loss of ovarian function. Fertility and Sterility 47:94–100

Spector TD 1989 Use of oestrogen replacement therapy in high risk groups in the United Kingdom. British Medical Journal 299:1434–1435

Stampfer MJ, Colditz GA, Willet WC, et al 1991 Postmenopausal estrogen therapy and cardiovascular disease. New England Journal of Medicine 325:756–762

Stevenson JC, Cust MP, Ganger KF, et al 1990 Effects of transdermal oral hormone replacement therapy on bone density in spine and proximal femur in postmenopausal women. The Lancet 335:265–269

Sullivan JM, Fowlkes LP 1996 Estrogens, menopause and coronary artery disease. Cardiology Clinics 14(1):105–116

Tannu NK, Pitkin J 1997 Monitoring patients on HRT within the primary care setting. Journal of the British Menopause Society 3(3):11–15

Thompson B, Hart SA, Durna D 1973 Menopausal age and symptomatology in general practice. Journal of Biosocial Science 5:71–82

Voigt LF, Weiss NS, Chu J, et al 1991 Progestogen supplementation of exogenous oestrogens and risk of endometrial cancer. The Lancet 338:274–277

Watson N 1995 Pathophysiology of the menopause. In: Rees CMP (ed.) Menopause update. Read Healthcare Communications, Sutton, pp. 9–11

Whitehead M, Godfree V 1992 Hormone replacement therapy: your questions answered. Churchill Livingstone, Edinburgh, pp. 1–6

Wilcox G, Wahlquist ML, Burger HG et al 1990 Oestrogenic effects of plant foods in post menopausal women. British Medical Journal 301:905–906

Willis DB, Calle EE, Miracle-McMahill HL, Heath CW 1996 Estrogen replacement therapy and risk of fatal breast cancer in a prospective cohort of postmenopausal women in the United States. Cancer Causes and Control 7:449–457

FURTHER READING

Abernethy K 1997 The menopause and HRT. Baillière Tindall, London

Hope S, Rees M, Brockie J 1999 Hormone replacement therapy. Oxford University Press, Oxford

McPherson A, Waller D 1997 Women's health. Oxford University Press, Oxford

Rees M, Purdie OW 1999 Management of the menopause. BMS Publications Ltd, Marlow, Bucks

Strategies for managing the menopause Dr Jean Coope Publishing Initiative Books Beckenham, Kent 1997

USEFUL ADDRESSES

British Menopause Society
36 West Street, Marlow, Bucks SL7 2NB
Tel: 01628 890199
(Information available to members only)

The Amarant Trust
11–13 Charterhouse Buildings, London EC1M 7AM
Tel: 02074013855
Helpline: 01293 413000

National Osteoporosis Society
PO Box 10, Radstock, Bath BA3 3YB

Tel: 01761 471771
Helpline: 01761 472 721

Institute of Psychological Medicine
11 Chandos Street, London W1M 9DE
Tel: 020 7580 0631 Women's Health Concern
PO Box 1629, London W8 6AU
Tel: 020 7938 3932

N.B. Your nearest menopause clinic and menopause nurse specialist will probably be happy to offer advice.

20

Gynaecological surgery

Jacky Cotton

The majority of gynaecological surgery is undertaken as elective planned admissions. This provides nurses with the opportunity to prepare women both physically and psychologically for the intended surgery prior to their admission to hospital.

With the advances in both medical techniques and technology, many procedures previously carried out on women as inpatients are now carried out as day cases or even in outpatient departments. Those procedures that do still require inpatient admission are performed with much shorter convalescent periods and women are being discharged earlier back to their home and family. This increases the speed of the recovery and reduces the incidence of postoperative complications (Taylor et al 1993).

PREOPERATIVE ASSESSMENT

It is important to ensure that the woman is physically fit to undergo surgery and a general anaesthetic. A preoperative assessment provides the nurse with the opportunity to assess the woman's knowledge and understanding of the planned surgery, explaining associated risks and benefits. It is well known that thorough psychological preparation of the woman will reduce anxiety and aid recovery (Wilson-Barnett 1979).

Preoperative assessment usually occurs prior to the woman being admitted for surgery, although in some units it may still be done on the day of admission. This allows time to detect any abnormalities in the woman's health that may be affected by a general anaesthetic and also gives the nurse the opportunity to provide the woman with the information she requires before coming into hospital. In many cases, it reduces the need for the woman to be admitted the day before her planned major surgery and increases the number of procedures that can be carried out as a day patient.

Nurse-led preoperative assessment clinics are now well developed in many units. It has been recognized that nurses have the skills and expertise to assess the differing needs of women and are usually the most appropriate healthcare professional to advise women in these circumstances (Dulaney et al 1990). Physical examination of women, especially those undergoing minor surgery, can be performed by nurses. Clinical guidelines provide a framework within which nurses can work, recommending occasions when medical staff need to review a patient.

A nurse is capable of assessing the woman holistically to take into account the different aspects of the woman's life that will be affected by her planned surgery. These can be divided into physical, psychological, social and spiritual needs.

Physical assessment

The woman must be assessed as being physically fit to undergo both surgery and a general anaesthetic. It is common for this assessment to be undertaken using a questionnaire, which can be completed by the nurse with the patient. This questionnaire must be agreed with medical staff within the unit to ensure that appropriate information is collected. The underlying principle of any assessment is to identify deficits in the woman's health that may be compromised by the stress of surgery. Details of the woman's presenting history may also be recorded, although it would be expected that these details would have been recorded at the initial outpatient attendance.

It is important to record any previous surgical history, noting any problems encountered with general anaesthetics. Any underlying medical conditions must be noted, especially heart or lung problems such as angina or asthma, or hormonal conditions such as diabetes or thyroid disorders. The nurse must also be alert for undiagnosed conditions such as cardiac failure or hypertension. The woman should be asked about how she copes with exercise such as climbing stairs, identifying breathlessness, swelling of ankles or chest pain.

Any medication the woman is taking must be noted as these may affect her anaesthetic. Particularly important is any recent steroid intake. Any hormone preparations must also be noted.

Known drug allergies must be highlighted within the case notes to ensure these preparations are avoided.

The first day of the last menstrual cycle must be recorded to prevent surgery being performed on a woman in the early stages of a pregnancy. If there is any doubt about this information, a urinary pregnancy test should be performed to eliminate the risk of an unknown pregnancy.

Lifestyle issues that may also affect the woman's health status, such as smoking or alcohol intake, should be noted. Excessive indulgence may be affected by an anaesthetic and the nurse can take this opportunity to discuss health education around these topics.

Diagnostic investigations are carried out to provide a baseline for comparison both intraoperatively and postoperatively. The current trend is to perform tests only when there is a clinical indication, so reducing the costs of many unnecessary diagnostic tests. Individual units will have clinical guidelines as to which tests should be performed routinely. Table 20.1 lists the tests that are routinely undertaken; other tests may be indicated, depending on the woman's history. If the woman requires auscultation of the heart and lungs, this should be performed by a doctor or a nurse who has undergone appropriate training (UKCC 1992). Any deviations from the expected norm should be reported to medical staff for further assessment.

Written informed consent must be obtained prior to surgery and this can be done at the preoperative assessment. Increasingly, this is now being obtained by nurses who have undergone further education to work at specialist level (UKCC 1992). However, it is important nurses are aware of their accountability and responsibility in this area and ensure that they are supported legally by their Trust through vicarious liability. There is much debate currently about the nurse's role in obtaining written consent. Although a nurse is often the most appropriate person to do this because they will explain all aspects of the risks and benefits and

Table 20.1 Preoperative investigative tests

Test	Rationale
Full-blood count	Identify haemoglobin, white cell count and platelets within normal levels
Group and save serum	Identify blood group and save serum in laboratory in case emergency cross-match is needed
Cross-match	Units of blood cross-matched and assigned to patient prior to surgery
Biochemical profile	Confirm urea and electrolytes are within normal levels
Chest X-ray	Identify any lung and chest abnormalities
ECG	Identify any irregularities of heart beat

what the procedure entails, the Clinical Negligence Scheme for Trusts (CNST) now advises that the person who obtains the written consent should be capable of performing that procedure. However, CNST does accept that nurses who have undergone appropriate training programmes may be more suitable to obtain informed written consent than inexperienced junior doctors.

Social assessment

During the preoperative interview, the nurse can determine the social background of the woman. The rapport she builds at this time enables her to discover about the woman's family, friends and work background. This provides the woman with the opportunity to discuss any fears about how her family will function during her hospital stay. Often the woman is the unofficial head of the family, organizing the other members and ensuring their lives operate smoothly. She may prepare all the meals and perform all the household duties. This may have occurred for many years and she may be concerned that the family will not be able to function without her. The woman may also have young children and be worried about the mutual separation. Advice about visiting hours, length of stay and the support needed on discharge may help allay some of these fears.

Women in employment may be concerned about the time needed away from work to recover and their job security. Advice about the expected recovery period will enable her to inform her employers about the expected length of absence.

The preoperative assessment is the ideal opportunity for the nurse to start discharge planning. Any deficits in support or circumstances at home can be identified and the involvement of outside agencies such as Social Services can be initiated before admission. This will not only reassure the woman but can also reduce the length of stay postoperatively.

Psychological assessment

Admission to hospital for surgery is worrying for any patient. Combined with the perceived assault on a woman's femininity, gynaecological surgery can be a particularly anxious experience. A nurse's experience and skills can be used to support the woman by imparting the information she requires. Each patient must be assessed individually as not all women have the same information requirements. Indeed, some women want to know only the minimum about their

impending surgery and it may be psychologically damaging to be given a full and frank explanation about the procedure. The skill of the nurse is to be able to identify how much the woman really wants to know.

Details about what will happen to the woman whilst she is in hospital preoperatively, intraoperatively and postoperatively can do much to reduce anxiety. Many women are very anxious about having a general anaesthetic administered. An informed explanation by the nurse combined with a visit from a member of the theatre staff can do much to allay these fears (Martin 1996).

Another area of concern is postoperative pain. An explanation should be given by the nurse about the type of analgesia and how it will be administered. Hayward's (1975) study demonstrated how people who were given appropriate information experienced fewer pain control problems postoperatively. Many units now use patient-controlled analgesia (PCA) for gynaecological patients and an explanation and demonstration of the equipment will be useful. It is important that the woman understands that, with current techniques and drugs, pain relief will be possible.

Details of recovery time and progress can also help the woman to plan her convalescent period to include appropriate support once home. It will allow her to plan with her partner and family what her expected needs will be once she is discharged home (Raleigh et al 1990). This explanation should also include an estimated discharge date. Some gynaecology units now operate an early discharge scheme, whereby patients who fulfil certain predetermined criteria can be discharged 2–3 days after major surgery (Taylor et al 1993). They are supported at home by their family and by visits from a nurse linked to the gynaecology ward. Plans for inclusion in such a scheme should be initiated at this visit.

Written information should also be given to support the verbal discussion that has taken place between the nurse and the woman. This will enable reinforcement of the information as the woman can read the literature once home.

Spiritual assessment

Gynaecological surgery, especially removal of parts of the female genital tract, can be most upsetting for many women. It should be remembered that, for some women, a **hysterectomy** is a bereavement process and they need to mourn the loss of their uterus. Support and time should be given to allow the woman to express any fears and visits by spiritual advisors from their home environment should be encouraged.

GYNAECOLOGICAL SURGICAL PROCEDURES

Minor surgery

Most minor gynaecological surgical procedures are now performed on a day case basis. Many of them are also carried out in the outpatient department without the need for general anaesthetic, thus reducing the risks to the woman.

Details of the most common **minor procedures**, including pre- and postoperative care, are listed in Table 20.2.

Intermediate surgery

Laparoscopy

Laparoscopy may be used as either a diagnostic or a therapeutic procedure. It may be used to diagnose unexplained pelvic pain, endometriosis, infertility or ectopic pregnancy. Therapeutic uses include sterilization, division of pelvic adhesions, treatment of ectopic

Table 20.2 Minor gynaecological procedures

Procedure	Indication	Surgical procedure	Preoperative care	Postoperative care	Comments
Hysteroscopy	Menorrhagia Irregular bleeding Postmenopausal bleeding	Hysteroscope introduced via cervix to view endometrial cavity either under direct view or connected via camera to television screen	Full blood count Preoperative check	Monitor pulse, blood pressure, per vaginal loss	Difficult to get good view if woman menstruating
Dilatation & curettage (D&C)	Menorrhagia Irregular bleeding Postmenopausal bleeding	Cervix dilated using metal dilators. Curette introduced into endometrial cavity and endometrium shaved off	Full blood count Preoperative check	Monitor pulse, blood pressure, per vaginal loss	Only performed in conjunction with hysteroscopy to obtain endometrial biopsy. Can be performed in outpatient department using smaller equipment
Polypectomy	Menorrhagia Irregular bleeding Postmenopausal bleeding	Endometrial polyps removed during curettage	Full blood count Preoperative check	Monitor pulse, blood pressure, per vaginal loss	Performed to remove endometrial polyps that cannot be removed at outpatient hysteroscopy.
Diathermy loop excision of cervix	Usually performed as outpatient in colposcopy clinic. Performed under general anaesthesia for very tense, anxious women	Wire heated by electric current removes and cauterizes affected area of cervix	Full blood count Preoperative check	Monitor pulse, blood pressure, per vaginal loss	Allow cervix to heal – no sex or tampons for 6 weeks. Advise regarding per vaginal loss
Insertion of Mirena IUD	Menorrhagia Irregular bleeding	Device coated with levonorgestrol inserted into uterine cavity. Bleeding reduced by slow release of progesterone	Full blood count Preoperative check. Ultrasound scan shows regular uterine cavity	Monitor pulse blood pressure, per vaginal loss	Can be done as outpatient. Done under general anaesthetic in conjunction with hysteroscopy and D&C. Advise that bleeding pattern may take 3–6 months to settle

pregnancy and laser ablation of sacral nerve and laparoscopically assisted hysterectomies, which will be dealt with later.

Procedure. Whilst under general anaesthetic, a trocar is introduced into the abdominal cavity through the skin beneath the umbilicus. This part of the operation is performed blind, so there is a possiblity of perforation of abdominal organs at this time. The laparoscope is then inserted through this incision. The abdominal wall is inflated to enhance the view of the pelvis. This is achieved by introducing carbon dioxide into the pelvic cavity. The laparoscope can be used by the operator under direct vision or a camera can be attached to the eyepiece and the view transmitted to a television screen.

Further incisions will be made in the lower quadrants close to the pubic hair line to enable other instruments to be inserted to grasp or move pelvic organs to enable a close examination of all areas of the pelvis.

An instrument known as Currie's uterine manipulator is inserted via the cervix into the endometrial cavity and the assistant uses this to antevert the uterus. This enables a good view of the fundus, posterior wall of the uterus (see Plate 36), tubes and ligaments.

At the end of the procedure, as the instruments are withdrawn, most of the carbon dioxide also escapes via the portals. The incisions may be sutured, depending on surgeon preference. During laparoscopy, there is a risk that excessive bleeding or damage to other pelvic organs may occur. In this case, a laparotomy may be required.

Indications. *Pelvic pain* Laparoscopy can be a useful diagnostic tool in unexplained pelvic pain. Endometriosis or pelvic adhesions may be noted and endometriotic spots may be diathermied. Ablation of the uterosacral nerve can also be achieved via the laparoscope. This is thought to assist women who have had long-standing pelvic pain, but further research is required to evaluate its efficacy.

Infertility In addition to laparoscopy and inspection of the pelvis, dye can be introduced through a cannula via the cervix. Laparoscopic observation of the dye spilling from the fallopian tubes indicates patency of the tubes. However, this cannot guarantee the state of the lining of the tubes. Although the tubes may be patent, the cilia may have been destroyed by a previous infection.

Adhesions between pelvic organs (see Plate 37) may prevent the required elements for successful conception from making contact. These adhesions can be divided via the laparoscope, commonly using the neodymium:yttrium–aluminium–garnet (Nd–YAG) laser.

Ectopic pregnancy Laparoscopy has both a diagnostic and therapeutic role for ectopic pregnancy. Laparoscopy as described in Chapter 5 may be the only method of providing a definitive diagnosis in many cases of ectopic pregnancy. Once diagnosed, the surgeon can then assess how best to treat. It is possible to perform salpingectomy via the laparoscope but the Nd–YAG laser can be used to open the tube and destroy the trophoblast (Keckstein et al 1990). Excessive bleeding due to a ruptured ectopic pregnancy may need to controlled by performing a laparotomy.

Sterilization is one of the most common procedures performed via the laparoscope. Filshie clips can be applied to the fallopian tubes via an applicator introduced through the lower portals. The woman must be thoroughly counselled before this procedure on the following points:

- the operation is permanent and irreversible
- there is a small failure rate: approximately 2 in 1000 operations
- if the woman does become fertile, there is a high risk of an ectopic pregnancy developing
- if the procedure is difficult, if the patient is grossly obese or if excessive bleeding occurs there is a risk that a laparotomy may have to be performed at the time of surgery
- male sterilization is a simpler procedure, carrying fewer risks because it can be carried out under local anaesthetic.

Preoperative care. Routine preoperative checks should be made in preparation for theatre. Shaving is not indicated unless there is gross hair growth around the umbilicus.

Explanation should be given to the woman about the effects she will experience postoperatively. These include the possibility of shoulder tip pain. Carbon dioxide introduced during the procedure to inflate the abdominal wall can collect under the diaphragm. This irritation causes referred pain via the phrenic nerve and the woman may experience shoulder, upper back or chest discomfort. She should be reassured this will subside as the excess carbon dioxide is absorbed into the bloodstream and, after gaseous exchange in the alveoli, is then exhaled through the lungs.

The woman should also be warned that she may have some slight loss per vagina (p.v.). This is due to the introduction of the obturator into the uterine cavity.

Postoperative care. Routine observations should be performed to detect early signs of haemorrhage. In addition, the laparoscopy sites on the abdomen should be closely observed for bleeding. Paracetamol usually provides adequate pain relief both for abdominal discomfort and shoulder pain.

Endometrial ablation

This technique is performed as an alternative to hysterectomy for women suffering with menstrual disorders. It can be carried out as a day case with much less inconvenience to the woman than undergoing major surgery. It is estimated that nearly 80% of procedures requiring laparotomy can now be achieved by minimally invasive surgery (Sutton 1993). However, this figure may not be as high in actual practice as there are several disadvantages of such procedures to the gynaecological unit. The procedures often take longer in the operating theatre, require expensive new technology and both nursing and medical staff have to gain new skills in the procedures and care. The cost implications of these factors may have contributed to minimally invasive techniques not replacing more traditional forms of surgery. The procedure involves removing the endometrial lining of the uterine cavity by destroying the cells with heat. There are several different techniques of endometrial ablation depending on the source of the heat destruction. These are summarized in Table 20.3.

Preoperative preparation. In order to perform this procedure safely, the endometrial cavity should be smooth, without the presence of submucous fibroids. The woman should have a **hysteroscopy** to assess this before planning ablation, as discussed in Chapter 6.

Postoperative care. Routine postoperative care should be given, with particular attention paid to any signs indicating fluid overload, such as oedema or respiratory difficulties. Uterine perforation should also be observed for.

Complications. Some complications have been identified, mainly due to inexperienced operators (Macdonald 1993). Closer supervision and higher training standards for gynaecologists have now reduced the incidence. The most serious complications include:

- uterine perforation
- fluid overload
- perforation of other pelvic organs (bladder, ureter, major blood vessels)
- haemorrhage
- infection (endomyometritis, pyrexia).

Postoperative success. Published information on the long-term effects of this treatment has only recently started to become available on a wide basis. In addition, the amount of blood loss prior to the procedure is not measured scientifically, so results are somewhat subjective. Patient satisfaction can be judged on whether further treatment was required. A study undertaken at the Royal Northern Hospital, London (Macdonald 1993) of 187 patients who underwent endometrial ablation showed that following the procedure, 54% had amenorrhoea, 25% had light loss and 9% had moderate loss; 32 (17%) patients required repeat ablation and 18 (10%) required hysterectomy. Endometrial ablation is widely used as an alternative to hysterectomy and the incidence of serious complications is reducing with the introduction of strict training guidelines for surgeons.

Table 20.3 Methods of endometrial ablation

Technique	Surgical procedure	Comments
Laser ablation	Uterine cavity distended with fluid via hysteroscope. Endometrium is exposed to Nd–Yag laser light. Light is scattered and absorbed by endometrium. Laser energy converted to heat, destroying cells	Risk of absorption of fluid distension media. Risk of uterine perforation
Transcervical resection of endometrium (TCRE)	Rollerball electrode used to destroy endometrium on contact, or loop electrode used to cut away endometrium	Risk of absorption of fluid distension media. Risk of uterine perforation
Radiofrequency-induced ablation	Probe introduced to uterine cavity. Radiofrequency electromagnetic energy conducted via probe to destroy tissue	No distension media used. Simpler and cheaper procedure Not frequently used than hysteroscopic methods
Balloon ablation	Probe introduced to uterine cavity Balloon around probe tip contains heated water, which destroys endometrium	No distension media used

Major surgery

Major gynaecological surgery can be performed via an abdominal or vaginal route. Surgery is usually performed to remove organs of the upper genital tract, although it may be used to correct displacements of organs. These operations are known as **repairs**. Complex surgery is usually carried out for the treatment of gynaecological cancers and has been described in Chapters 13, 14 and 15.

Abdominal surgery

The most common procedures performed abdominally to correct gynaecological disorders are summarized in Table 20.4.

Total abdominal hysterectomy

This operation is usually performed for menstrual disorders that have failed to respond to the woman's satisfaction using other forms of treatment. It is important that the woman is not persuaded to undergo this surgery unless she feels mentally prepared to accept it. It can mark a major life event for the woman; the end of her ability to reproduce. The woman may have already decided that she did not want any more children but the finality of this not being possible can have a profound effect on some women's feelings of sexuality. The ovaries may also be removed (bilateral salpingo-oophorectomy) or the cervix left (subtotal hysterectomy). The nursing care will be similar in all these cases.

Preoperative care. A full preoperative assessment should be carried out to determine that the woman is fit to undergo major surgery and a general anaesthetic, as detailed on p. 340. If the woman is suffering from menorrhagia, particular attention should be paid to the haemoglobin level, which may be lowered due to the heavy menstrual loss. Treatment of low haemoglobin in these circumstances will depend on the clinical need of the woman. Surgery may be deferred and the woman treated with iron supplements such as ferrous sulphate 200 mg three times daily. This is not always appropriate as the woman's haemoglobin levels may continue to fall because she will still be experiencing heavy periods. In some cases, iron therapy may be prescribed in conjunction with a drug that will cause cessation of periods, such as Zoladex. Stopping menstruation allows the body to restore haemoglobin levels prior to surgery. This therapy can take 2–3 months. In individuals where the haemoglobin levels are extremely low, such as below 6 g/l, it may be necessary to offer a blood transfusion.

Table 20.4 Common gynaecological abdominal operations

Operation	Indications	Comments
Total abdominal hysterectomy (TAH)	Dysfunctional uterine bleeding Menorrhagia Endometrial hyperplasia	May be suprapubic or midline incision depending on indications and size of uterus. Uterus including cervix removed. Vagina oversewn to form vault
Subtotal hysterectomy	As above, especially if woman wishes to retain her cervix. Not appropriate if high risk of cervical cancer	As above but only body of uterus removed leaving cervix. Will need to continue to have cervical smears
Bilateral salpingo-oophorectomy (BSO)	Performed in conjunction with TAH if woman is perimenopausal or menopausal	Removal of fallopian tubes and ovaries. Hormone replacement therapy (HRT) will be necessary if woman perimenopausal prior to surgery
Wertheim's hysterectomy	Cervical cancer	Complex operation including TAH and BSO and removal of pelvic lymph nodes and upper third of vagina
Ovarian cystectomy	Ovarian cyst	Simple fluid-filled cysts may be aspirated laparoscopically. Larger or more complex cysts as diagnosed on ultrasound scan may require laparotomy. Midline or suprapubic incision depending on size of cyst. Ovarian function maintained by shelling out cyst
Burch colposuspension	Stress incontinence Failure of previous vaginal surgery	Anterior vaginal wall elevated with urethra via suprapubic incision. Paravaginal fascia sutured on each side to inguinopectineal ligaments

This may be done 2–3 weeks before surgery. It is not advisable to do this transfusion immediately prior to or during surgery as this increases the risk of the development of venous thromboses. On arrival, the normal admission procedure of the unit should be carried out by a nurse assigned to the woman for her period of stay. This will enable a close relationship to develop that will help to reduce any fears and anxieties the woman may have. Discharge planning, if not initiated at the preoperative assessment clinic, should be started now to ensure support arrangements for the woman on discharge are in place. Other preoperative care may include:

- Pubic shave – this may be necessary if the incision is going to be along the suprapubic hairline. A depilatory cream may be used as this reduces the risk of infection but if a shave has to be performed it should be done on the day of surgery to reduce the colonization of the skin by commensal organisms. The woman must be allowed to perform this herself if she wishes but the nurse may need to supervise the procedure.
- Bowel preparation – this is not now considered to be necessary by many surgeons. However, it is important that the woman is not grossly constipated at the time of surgery as normal bowel function will be affected postoperatively. Women often complain of painful wind and constipation following surgery and this can be difficult to treat if already constipated. In this case, glycerin suppositories the evening before surgery may be helpful.
- Fasting – the woman should fast for at least 5 h prior to surgery, although this will depend on the policy of the unit.
- Bath/shower – this should be taken prior to surgery. It will enable the woman to feel clean and refreshed and will also reduce the number of commensal organisms on the skin.
- Preoperative preparation – this will include routine checks that must be undertaken prior to the woman leaving the ward area for operating theatre. Dentures should be removed and a note made of any loose or crowned teeth. Any prostheses should also be removed. The woman should be wearing a wristband with her name and hospital registration number. This must be checked against the notes and the request slip from the theatre assistant who collects her. The woman should have a good understanding of what the operation entails and the consent form should have been signed. It is not good practice for this to be done after premedication has been given as the

woman is likely to suffer from a reduction in mental accuity.
- Premedication – this may include prophylactic antibiotic therapy such as cefuroxime and metronidazole and thromboembolic prophylaxis such as subcutaneous heparin. A mild hypnotic such as temazepam 10 mg may be given to relax the woman.

Postoperative care. *On return from surgery* to the ward, the nurse should make careful observations of certain vital signs. These can then be used as a baseline to compare future observations, enabling the nurse to closely monitor the woman's progress. Regular recordings of pulse and blood pressure should be instigated to monitor any signs of primary haemorrhage. The wound site and sanitary pad should also be checked for abnormal amounts of bleeding. An intravenous infusion will be in situ to prevent dehydration. The rate and type of infusion fluid should be checked with the prescribed rota. The intravenous infusion site should have been fixed with clear adhesive to allow inspection, and should be checked for any signs of inflammation. An indwelling catheter may have been inserted during surgery. This will allow urine to drain from the bladder, preventing retention of urine and undue pressure on the surgical site by an overfull bladder. The catheter and drainage bag should be checked for any kinks to allow free drainage and prevent any stasis or backflow. The colour and amount of urine should be checked. Small amounts of dark, concentrated urine may indicate dehydration. Haematuria may indicate damage to the bladder or ureters during surgery and should be closely monitored. If the woman is not catheterized, all self-voided urine must be noted to monitor the presence of urinary retention.

A vacuum drain may be in place to prevent a haematoma forming in the pelvis postoperatively. The amount and type of exudate drained should be noted. Strong analgesia such as morphine will be administered intravenously either by a continuous syringe driver whose rate can be altered by an experienced nurse to meet the woman's requirements or by a pump that can be controlled by the woman herself. Patient-controlled analgesia systems have a button on handset, which the woman can press to deliver analgesia as she requires it, enabling her to be in control of her medication. There is a safety lockout device to prevent the woman from operating the system continuously.

It is important that relatives have been made aware previously of all the equipment that will be attached to the woman during the immediate postoperative period. Nurses must be aware that, although this is normal routine postoperative care, it can be very alarming for visitors to see their loved ones with so many tubes attached.

Day 1. Recovery after total abdominal hysterectomy is now encouraged to be a rapid process, which starts on the first postoperative day. The woman should be encouraged to mobilize to reduce the risk of deep vein thrombosis and should sit out of bed for short periods. She should be helped to maintain her personal hygiene and may take a shower or have a bedbath. Attention should be paid to mouthcare and general appearance. Analgesic requirements may now be reducing and the level of analgesia can be altered. Morphine and derivatives can make the woman very sleepy and nauseous, so discontinuation of the intravenous therapy, when the woman can tolerate it, will often make her feel much improved. Oral analgesia such as co-dydramol should be prescribed but should not be administered until the woman can tolerate oral fluids. The nurse has an important role in assessing when the woman can tolerate oral therapy instead of intravenous. The presence of bowel sounds will assist in this assessment, indicating the absence of paralytic ileus. The intravenous infusion can be discontinued as soon as the woman is tolerating oral fluids and a light diet can be commenced that day. The food should be attractively presented as the woman may not feel like eating, but she should be encouraged to take some nutrition orally to regain normal bowel function as quickly as possible. The urinary catheter will usually be in situ for only 24 h and will be removed according to the unit policy. In many units now, catheters are removed late evening. This allows the woman to sleep during the night and then micturate on waking; a normal physiological function. If a catheter is not used, careful note must be made of the amount of urine being voided.

The vacuum drain will remain until no further exudate appears to be draining. The nurse should check that the vacuum is maintained within the system.

Day 2. Progress continues and any remaining attachments are usually removed on the second day. It is important to note that the woman voids urine after the removal of the catheter and a fluid balance chart should be maintained to record all output. Occasionally a woman experiences difficulty in voiding urine and a urinary catheter may need to be reinserted.

The woman should now be encouraged to eat more, although a light diet may be all she can tolerate, and to mobilize more around the unit and for longer periods. A common but very painful problem experienced by women around day 2–3 is wind. The woman may complain of a feeling of trapped wind that she cannot pass as flatus or by belching. The discomfort may be relieved by 10 ml peppermint water mixed with warm water, or by 10 ml of gripe water. She will still experience tiredness and should rest in between mobilization. Assistance may be needed to maintain personal hygiene and a shower or bath should be taken. The wound may now be left exposed unless there are any signs of exudate oozing. It should be checked daily for any signs of inflammation, which may indicate the development of an underlying infection.

Day 3. The woman should be encouraged to self-care and return to a normal diet. She may experience the 'postop blues' on the third day and feel very weepy. The nurse should reassure her that this is a normal reaction, although the reason for it is not fully understood. It is important that bowel function is noted as constipation can become a painful problem that may take several days to resolve. Lactulose 10 ml at night should help produce a soft stool that can be passed without too much discomfort. Glycerine suppositories may be required for more stubborn cases.

Many women are now discharged home on day 3, as long as she has appropriate family support at home, has no complications and feels able to cope at home.

Day 4–5. Most women will have been discharged by now. An outpatient appointment is arranged for 6 weeks, although some women may attend their GP for this review. Advice should be given about the convalescent period. The woman should be encouraged to remain active on discharge, taking regular walks. Heavy housework and exercise should be avoided. The woman may drive when she feels able to perform an emergency stop. She should be advised to sit in a stationary car and rehearse the procedure to ensure it is not too painful.

Sexual intercourse should be avoided until the vaginal vault is fully healed. This may take up to 6 weeks. The woman should not return to work until she feels able to perform her role completely. This may take 6–8 weeks or longer in some cases.

Postoperative review. In many units this consultation is now carried out by a nurse. At this review, progress should be discussed and any remaining queries addressed. The wound should be inspected and a speculum examination performed to ensure healing of the vaginal vault. Issues such as hormone replacement therapy can be discussed at length. A nurse is the most appropriate professional to take this opportunity to discuss and promote healthy lifestyles.

Ovarian cystectomy

The nursing care for patients undergoing these operations is similar to that for total abdominal hysterectomy, although recovery may be quicker and discharge home earlier in women undergoing ovarian cystectomy, especially if they are young and fit prior to surgery. For further information, see Chapter 9.

Wertheim's hysterectomy

Due to the more extensive nature of the surgery involved in this operation, recovery may be longer and care more intensive than for an abdominal hysterectomy. High-dependency care may be needed for the immediate postoperative period, depending on the preoperative fitness of the woman and the extent of surgery. In addition to an intravenous infusion and urinary catheter, the woman may have a nasogastric tube. This will be dependent on the extent of micro-invasive disease, and consequently the extent of the surgery. Increased handling of the bowel will obviously increase the risk of a paralytic ileus developing postoperatively. The nasogastric tube should remain on free drainage although aspiration may be needed if the woman complains of nausea. All drainage and aspirate should be recorded on a fluid balance chart to accurately monitor fluid input and output. The nasogastric tube may need to remain in situ for several days postoperatively until bowel sounds can be detected. Oral fluids should be introduced, starting with small amounts of water and increased gradually as tolerated. Once the woman can tolerate free fluids and a light diet, the intravenous infusion can be discontinued. To prevent a pelvic haematoma forming, two vacuum drains may be inserted during the operation; one in the pelvis and one in the lymphatic system if lymphadenectomy has been carried out. These should remain until no further drainage is noted and the drain within the lymphatic system may continue to drain for longer and so will need to stay in longer.

Postoperative recovery is likely to be longer than for abdominal hysterectomy owing to the extent of the surgery, even though many women may be in a younger age group. Mobilization should be encouraged as soon as possible and thromboembolic prophylaxis should be continued until the woman is fully mobile.

In addition to physical care, the woman will require psychological support from the nurse caring for her. She will not only have to cope with the realization of undergoing major surgery for cancer but also that she will be unable to have any more children. Due to the young age range of many women who have to undergo this radical surgery, they may not even have had the opportunity to have a child and this may be a constant reminder to her about her disease. Histology results should be discussed with the woman and her close family as soon as they are available. Any further treatment options should also be explored to reassure her. Regular follow-up will be needed to reassure the woman that treatment has been successful

Burch colposuspension

This abdominal operation is performed to treat genuine stress incontinence. The woman will have an abdominal wound and postoperative care will be similar to that for a woman undergoing abdominal hysterectomy. There is a need to monitor urinary output very closely and to assess the woman's ability to self-void urine. Postoperatively, a suprapubic catheter will be used to monitor urinary output. The catheter should be allowed to drain freely for the first few days. Once the woman is mobile and recovery is established, the suprapubic catheter should be clamped and the woman encouraged to self-void urine per urethra. After each episode of micturition, the catheter should be unclamped and any residual urine draining from the bladder measured. If the woman has problems self-voiding, the catheter can be unclamped and the bladder drained. This procedure can continue until the woman can pass urine per urethra. It is usual for the woman to experience difficulties in self-voiding immediately postoperatively due to the new supportive position of the bladder. She must be reassured that this is normal and that, given time, the bladder function will return to normal. In some cases, the woman may be discharged home with the catheter still in situ or trained to perform intermittent self-catheterization (ISC). If this is the case, the woman must be given much reassurance and psychological support by the nurse to prepare her for discharge. Patients often expect to leave hospital 'cured' and still having a catheter in the bladder or needing to perform ISC is often perceived by the woman as failure of her treatment. She should be taught to care for the catheter aseptically and how to check residual amounts of urine left in the bladder after voiding urine per urethra. Once the residuals are below 50 ml, the catheter can be removed.

It may take several weeks for normal bladder function to return following surgery and the woman may need psychological support to cope with this.

Vaginal surgery

Due to the access to the lower genital tract, many conditions can be treated surgically via the vagina. This

Table 20.5 Common gynaecological vaginal operations

Operation	Indications	Comments
Vaginal hysterectomy	Stress incontinence due to uterine prolapse Menorrhagia	Uterus pulled down vagina and surgery undertaken at introitus. Oophorectomy may be performed if ovaries not too high in pelvis. Cervix oversewn to create vaginal vault. Vaginal approach not used if any suspicion of cancer. Ring pessary should be removed at least 2 weeks prior to surgery and postmenopausal women should have local oestrogen applied to ensure tissues less friable and aid healing
Anterior colporrhaphy (anterior repair)	Cystocele – prolapse of bladder through anterior vaginal wall	Incision made in anterior wall of vagina. Bladder supported with buttress sutures. Redundant vaginal tissue may be removed to make support more effective. Must be aware if still sexually active so that vagina is not rendered too narrow for sexual intercourse. May be performed in conjunction with vaginal hysterectomy. Removal of ring pessary and local oestrogen as for vaginal hysterectomy
Posterior colpoperineorrhaphy (posterior repair)	Rectocele – prolapse of rectum through posterior vaginal wall	Incision made in posterior wall of vagina. Rectum supported to prevent further prolapse. May be performed in conjunction with vaginal hysterectomy and/or anterior repair if vaginal walls very weak
Laparoscopic assisted vaginal hysterectomy (LAVH)	Menorrhagia Benign pathology that would normally require abdominal approach, e.g. endometriosis, fibroids	Uterine vessels ligated via laparoscope then uterus removed vaginally. Procedure may take longer time in theatre than vaginal hysterectomy Average length of stay in hospital less than total abdominal hysterectomy – up to 2 days. Recovery more rapid – may be back at work after 2 weeks. Reduced risk of wound infection. Increased risk of pelvic haematoma

reduces the need for abdominal incisions and recovery is consequently much quicker. In the past, vaginal surgery tended to be carried out solely for uterine or vaginal prolapses. Commonly, the women were postmenopausal and being treated for urinary symptoms such as stress incontinence due to prolapse. However, with advances in surgical expertise, vaginal surgery is now performed for women with menorrhagia, providing the uterus is not grossly enlarged with fibroids and there is some uterine descent. This is not always possible in nulliparous women. Advances in minimal access surgery has led to the development of laparoscopic assisted vaginal hysterectomy. Common vaginal operations are described in Table 20.5.

Vaginal hysterectomy

This approach to hysterectomy often results in a quicker recovery than the abdominal approach due to the lack of an abdominal incision. It can be performed for uterine displacement or for menorrhagia. Psychological support is important for women undergoing vaginal hysterectomy as they may also be affected by the loss of their ability to have children.

Preoperative care. This will be similar as the care for a woman undergoing an abdominal hysterectomy. Preoperative assessment must be carried out to ensure the woman is fit to undergo surgery. On the day of admission, the nurse responsible for the woman's care during her hospital stay should inform her of the procedures and events the woman can expect over the next few days. Discharge planning must be commenced at this stage if it has not already been started, especially if the woman is elderly. Support from Social Services may be needed postoperatively and prompt attention to this will prevent a delay in discharge arrangements. In some units a pubic shave is no longer thought necessary although a perineal shave may be necessary to aid access to the surgical site.

Routine preoperative assessment should be undertaken prior to the women transferring from the ward to theatre.

Postoperative care. On return from theatre, the nurse must undertake recordings of vital signs to monitor potential haemorrhage. An intravenous infusion will be established to prevent dehydration. A vaginal gauze pack may be in situ to exert pressure on the sutures in the vagina. To prevent it becoming uncomfortable and difficult to remove when dry, the ribbon gauze is soaked in a cream prior to insertion. If the woman is premenopausal this may be glycerine; if the woman is postmenopausal, it is an oestrogen cream. Per vaginal bleeding through the pack should be monitored closely and excessive bleeding reported promptly to medical staff. It is likely that a urinary catheter will also be in situ. Pressure on the bladder and urethra from the vaginal pack often makes it difficult for the woman to self-void urine. In many instances, if a vaginal pack is not used neither is a urinary catheter. Postoperative pain will be controlled by methods used for abdominal hysterectomy although the vaginal approach often causes less discomfort.

Day 1. The vaginal pack is removed and it is recommended that the woman remains in bed for a short while after this procedure in case it has precipitated vaginal bleeding. The nurse will decide when it is appropriate to discontinue the intravenous infusion once it is clear there is no active bleeding. The woman may mobilize later in the day and may decide to take an assisted bath to meet her hygiene needs. The urinary catheter if used may be removed that night.

Day 2. Postoperative recovery continues and any remaining 'attachments' are removed. The woman should be encouraged to mobilize and commence normal diet and fluid intake. Urinary output should be noted to alert staff to urinary retention developing following removal of the catheter. Some women with good support at home, or who are participants in an early discharge scheme, may be discharged on day 2.

Day 3. Attention and advice should be given regarding bowel movements. A common minor postoperative complication is constipation, which can be extremely uncomfortable for the woman. It is not advisable for the woman to be straining at stool following this surgery. Lactulose solution 10 ml is often useful in these circumstances.

There is a tendency for a vault haematoma to develop following this surgery, and this might become infected. Signs to indicate this might have occurred include a general feeling of malaise, unexplained pyrexia and a dark bloodstained discharge with an offensive smell. The haematoma may start to drain spontaneously or may be encouraged by a digital vaginal examination. Broad spectrum antibiotics should be prescribed and the woman reassured that the loss will subside. An infected vault haematoma will resolve once it has drained and been treated appropriately and will not cause any residual problems.

Anterior repair (colporrhaphy)

An anterior repair may be carried out in isolation or in conjunction with a vaginal hysterectomy. Care for women undergoing this surgery is similar to that for vaginal hysterectomy. Preoperatively, it must be ascertained whether the woman is still sexually active. This will determine the extent of surgery performed on the anterior vaginal wall. If too much tissue is excised, it may result in narrowing of the vagina, making intercourse difficult in the future.

Increases in abdominal pressure can cause stress on the suture line while healing is progressing. Conditions that cause an increase in abdominal pressure, such as vomiting or coughing, should be treated to reduce this stress. Chronic chest conditions should be treated and the woman advised against smoking. Postoperative vomiting should be controlled with appropriate antiemetics.

It is important that, if a urinary catheter is used, it remains draining the bladder for 24–48 h to allow immediate postoperative surgical oedema to subside. Special attention must be paid to monitoring urinary output as this may be affected by the surgery.

If an anterior repair is the only surgical procedure carried out, recovery is usually fairly rapid with the woman fit for discharge after 48 h providing she is self-voiding urine in satisfactory amounts.

Prior to discharge, a digital vaginal examination may be carried out by the doctor to prevent vaginal adhesions forming between the vaginal walls, which may cause difficulties with sexual intercourse in the future.

Posterior repair (colpoperineorrhaphy)

This may be performed in isolation or in conjunction with an anterior repair and/or vaginal hysterectomy. Care is similar to that for vaginal hysterectomy or anterior repair. Sexual activity should be established to determine the extent of vaginal tissue that can be removed from the posterior wall of the vagina.

Postoperatively, attention should be paid to the perineal area as sutures may extend from the vaginal wall to the perineum. There is a risk of infection developing in the warm, moist environment around the suture line. The woman should be advised about the need for maintaining the hygiene of this area and of ensuring gentle though thorough drying following bathing.

Because of the close proximity of the suture line to the rectum, it is especially important that the woman does not become constipated, as straining at stool may cause extreme discomfort and strain on the sutures.

As with anterior repairs, vaginal examination may be required prior to discharge to prevent the formation of vaginal adhesions.

Laparoscopic assisted vaginal hysterectomy

Laparoscopic assisted vaginal hysterectomy (LAVH) has not been developed to replace vaginal hysterectomy but to increase the number of hysterectomies carried out by the vaginal approach that traditionally would have been performed abdominally. The avoidance of an abdominal incision reduces the length of stay in hospital and postoperative convalescence period and reduces the risk of wound infection.

During the procedure the uterine vessels are ligated via a laparoscopic approach and then the uterus is removed vaginally (Kovac et al 1990).

Preoperative care. Prior to admission, the woman may be treated with gonadotrophin releasing hormone (GnRH) analogues for up to 3 months to reduce the size of uterine fibroids. Shrinking any fibroids in the myometrium should make the vaginal removal of the uterus easier. Routine preoperative preparation is similar for abdominal hysterectomy. Because of the risk of increased bleeding during LAVH, some centres cross-match two units of blood prior to surgery.

The operative time for this operation is generally considerably longer than for traditional abdominal or vaginal hysterectomy. This must be taken into account when the woman is assessed for general anaesthetic and planning theatre lists and may have a cost implication for the organization (Kohli et al 1997).

Postoperative care. On return from theatre, the nurse should undertake regular monitoring of vital signs. Special attention should be paid to the amount of vaginal loss in case of bleeding around the vaginal vault. An intravenous infusion may be in situ but this will be necessary for only a short period. Initial analgesia may be via PCA or intravenous pump, or the woman may require only oral analgesia. Mobilization should be encouraged as soon as the woman feels able. Normal diet and fluids may be recommenced when tolerated. This is often earlier than with other major surgery, especially if morphine is not required for analgesia, as there will not be the side-effects of nausea.

Average length of stay is often as little as two days (Miekle et al 1997), although vault haematoma and subsequent infection must be observed for closely during this time. The cost to the organization of the lengthy theatre time used is often offset by the early discharge of the woman. The woman and her family

should be psychologically prepared by the nurse for this early discharge and recuperation. Women often have the expectation that a hysterectomy, regardless of how it has been performed, is a major operation that will render her incapable of functioning normally within her social system for many weeks. The reassurance given by the informed advice and support from the nurse preoperatively has been shown to help patients cope physically with postoperative outcomes positively (Gammon & Mulholland 1996).

Postoperative complications

Complications can occur in gynaecological surgery that can severely compromise the wellbeing of the woman. Their occurrence is fortunately the exception rather than the norm. However, the gynaecology nurse must be aware of the signs and symptoms that may be apparent in order to facilitate early intervention and treatment.

The complications may be due to undergoing a general anaesthetic, undergoing pelvic surgery or may result as a combination of the two. The most common complications are described below.

Primary haemorrhage

This can occur after any surgery due to incomplete haemostasis. Regular observations must be carried out postoperatively to detect any signs of surgical shock. Table 20.6 lists these observations and deviations from the expected norm.

Medical staff must be alerted to such changes in the woman's condition. Fluid intake must be increased. An intravenous infusion should be initiated if not already in place.

Uterine perforation

This may occur whenever a uterine sound or other instrumentation is introduced into the endometrial cavity. The operator may push the instrument through the fundus of the uterus, causing a perforation. Particularly at risk are women undergoing an evacuation of retained products of conception as the pregnant uterus is softer and more prone to perforation. If this is noted at the time it occurs, a laparoscopy may be performed to assess the extent of the perforation. Frequent observations of pulse, blood pressure and abdominal discomfort must be carried out postoperatively. An increase in pulse rate, decrease in blood pressure, increase in abdominal discomfort and, in the

Table 20.6 Signs of primary haemorrhage

Observations	Indication of haemorrhage	Rationale
Pulse rate	Increased, thready	Increased heart rate to maintain supply of oxygenated blood to major organs
Blood pressure	Decreased	
Loss per vagina	Heavy, clots, bright red – fresh	
Level of abdominal pain	Excessive, not relieved by analgesia	Irritation to peritoneum due to increased abdominal pressure due to bleeding into abdominal cavity
Level of consciousness	Restless	
Colour	Pallor, may be clammy	
Urinary output	Decreased	Fluid retained by body in effort to maintain haemodilution

later stages, an increase in abdominal girth, will indicate excessive bleeding into the abdominal cavity. If the perforation is not noted during the procedure, any of the above signs occurring during the normal observations undertaken should be reported to medical staff.

Uterine perforations usually resolve spontaneously and it is unlikely that a laparotomy will have to be performed unless the perforation is a large one and the woman's condition deteriorates. Prophylactic antibiotics are likely to be prescribed.

Bowel perforation

This can occur due to the close proximity of the pelvic organs including the bladder, bowel and uterus. It may occur either during open abdominal surgery or during laparoscopy. A large perforation can cause leaking of faecal matter into the pelvic cavity resulting in peritonitis. Signs of this may not present until 24–48 h postoperatively. These include pyrexia, tachycardia and increase in abdominal pain with guarding. Urgent treatment must be initiated as this is potentially a life threatening complication. Intravenous antibiotics will be prescribed to resolve the peritonitis. Laparotomy may be indicated to repair the bowel followed by nursing care related to specialist bowel surgery.

Bladder perforation

This is most likely to occur during abdominal surgery owing to the close anatomical relationship of the urinary tract to the upper genital tract. Pelvic adhesions can make the bladder adherent to the uterus and so at risk during surgery to the uterus.

Signs include reduced urinary output, frank haematuria, increased abdominal discomfort and an increase in abdominal girth. If a redivac drain is in the pelvic cavity, straw-coloured fluid resembling urine may drain into it.

Treatment includes antibiotic therapy and close observation of symptoms. If a urinary catheter is not already in situ, it may be necessary to insert one. This should then be left on free drainage for up to 5 days. The perforation may resolve spontaneously or may require surgical repair.

Urinary retention

Urinary retention is a common postoperative complication following gynaecological surgery. Oedema, sutures and handling of the organs can all contribute to dysfunction of the bladder. It should be noted if a woman has not passed urine at least 8 h after surgery. If she is left for any longer than this, she will experience considerable discomfort from the full bladder exerting pressure on the surgical site. If the woman is unable to self-void urine, it may be necessary to pass a urinary catheter. The woman may have been catheterized during surgery and may experience problems in emptying her bladder once the catheter is removed. If this occurs, she may need to be recatheterized. In this instance, the insertion of a suprapubic catheter is recommended. This will prevent the woman having numerous urethral catheters passed, which can be uncomfortable and increases the risk of introducing infection to the urinary tract. A suprapubic catheter can then be clamped and the woman allowed to void urine per urethra. If she still experiences problems, the urine can be drained by releasing the clamp on the suprapubic catheter. This procedure can be continued until the woman is able to self-void urine. Once this is happening satisfactorily, the suprapubic catheter can be removed.

Urinary tract infection

Many gynaecological procedures involve bladder catheterization, which increases the risk of urinary tract infections. Reduced mobility and surgery to other pelvic organs in close proximity to the bladder can contribute to difficulty in emptying the bladder fully. Urinary stasis and retention provides a medium for potential infection. Signs include dysuria, frequency, burning and stinging on micturition, difficulty initiating micturition and incomplete emptying of the bladder. A midstream specimen of urine should be sent for microscopic examination and culture to confirm the presence of infection. Antibiotics specific to the bacteria cultured should be prescribed.

Chest infection

This is more likely to occur after major surgery where the woman has been under general anaesthetic for a prolonged time. Women more at risk are those with underlying chest conditions such as chronic bronchitis or asthma. Smoking is known to be the most important predisposing factor. Women should ideally give up smoking before undergoing major surgery but, if this is not possible, they must be advised to reduce the number of cigarettes they smoke daily. In addition, the increase in abdominal pressure caused by coughing postoperatively can be detrimental to any vaginal repair surgery.

Reduced mobility and shallow breathing due to abdominal pain can contribute towards the development of a chest infection. Preventative measures can be taken, including a preoperative explanation of the need to breathe deeply. Adequate analgesia will encourage deep breathing postoperatively and early mobilization will also reduce the risk. If the woman does develop a chest infection, deep breathing and coughing can be encouraged by nurses after ensuring adequate analgesia has been administered. Fluid intake must be increased to allow expectoration of any sputum. If sputum appears infected, a sample should be sent to the bacteriology laboratory for culture and sensitivity. A broad spectrum antibiotic may be prescribed and early mobilization should be encouraged.

Wound infection

This may occur at any surgical site. Signs to look for include inflammation, redness, swelling, and pain, and exudate may be apparent at the site. A swab should be taken of any exudate present and the area kept clean and dry. Lower abdominal wounds just above the pubic hair line may be particularly susceptible if the woman is obese. The overhanging abdominal skin provides a moist, warm environment around a surgical incision ideal for bacterial colonization. This area should be dried thoroughly after bathing. The incision may be kept uncovered or have a small dry gauze dressing applied for comfort. Large bulky dressings should be avoided as these add to the warmth of the environment. Specific antibiotics should be prescribed and the wound checked daily. If the wound dehisces and the suture line becomes separated, the nurse must assess the most appropriate wound dressing.

Deep vein thrombosis and pulmonary embolism

Women undergoing abdominal and pelvic surgery are at an increased risk of formation of deep vein thrombosis (DVT), which may develop into a pulmonary embolism, a condition that can be life threatening. The risks should be minimized by using preoperative precautions such as antithromboembolic stockings or subcutaneous heparin. Guidelines produced by the Royal College of Obstetricians and Gynaecologists (RCOG) for thromboembolic prophylaxis assist in identifying risk factors and appropriate treatment (RCOG 1995). Unfortunately, thrombosis can still occur despite these measures.

Signs to observe for a deep vein thrombosis include pain, inflammation and redness in the calf. Medical staff must be informed and should instigate investigations such as ultrasound, to confirm the diagnosis. An ultrasound beam detects movement of red blood cells within the vein. Lack of reflection from moving red blood cells indicates the presence of an occlusion. If this is the case, the ultrasound contact gel should not be removed from the skin by massaging the leg as this may dislodge an embolus.

Treatment includes intravenous heparin. Daily blood clotting profiles should be taken and advice sought from a haematologist. Oral warfarin will be prescribed on the haematologist's recommendation. It is usually taken at the same time as the heparin, which

Case study: Deborah

Deborah is a 52-year-old married woman with one son who was admitted electively from the waiting list for a total abdominal hysterectomy. The decision to perform a hysterectomy was reached in consultation with Deborah after several diagnostic investigations.

Deborah had originally been referred to the consultant gynaecologist by her GP with a history of irregular bleeding whilst on hormone replacement therapy (HRT). She had been on HRT since she was 39 and originally started taking it for mood swings. Deborah had been taking Premique for 18 months and had no bleeding until February 1998, when she experienced continuous spotting for 3 weeks.

It was decided that it would be appropriate to see Deborah for her first consultation at the outpatient hysteroscopy clinic. Here, a detailed history was taken to determine any other relevant problems. She had been depressed and had recently started antidepressant medication – sertraline 50 mg daily. During the last few months she had been experiencing troublesome hot flushes and was not sure if these symptoms were due to her antidepressant treatment or the menopause.

Following the history taking, Deborah was given a thorough explanation of the procedures that were to follow and was then invited to a screened area of the clinic for examination. Physical assessment of the female genital tract followed a systematic review to ensure signs and symptoms were not overlooked. A bimanual pelvic examination was performed to assess the size and position of the uterus and detect any adnexal masses. It is important to know the position of the uterus before introducing the hysteroscope into the cervical canal. If the uterus is retroverted, the cervical canal follows a different direction so techniques must be adapted to compensate.

Although a vaginal ultrasound scan is usually performed at this stage to assess the pelvis and the thickness of the endometrium, because Deborah had already been referred by her GP for an ultrasound scan, which showed no ovarian masses but did not comment on the thickness of the endometrium, it was decided not to repeat the investigation at this stage.

After pelvic examination, a speculum examination was performed to assess Deborah's vulva, vagina and cervix. All appeared normal and healthy. A recent cervical smear, taken within the last year, was normal. Sterile lignocaine gel was introduced into the cervical canal. This acts as a lubricant, a local anaesthetic and assists in dilating the canal. The amount used is important as too much will transfer into the endometrial cavity and obscure the view. The gel was left in situ for a short time, during which Deborah was reassured by the nursing staff assisting in the clinic. Sodium chloride was used as the irrigating fluid and was attached to the flushing channel of the hysteroscope via a giving set. A light source cable was attached to a light source and another chamber of the hysteroscope. Once the equipment had been assembled, the hysteroscope was gently introduced into Deborah's cervical cavity. A camera was attached to the eyepiece and the image was viewed by Deborah and the staff onto a television scheme. Although initially unsure about

seeing the image, Deborah, like many other women, was overcome by curiosity and was quite amazed by the television picture of inside her uterus. The hysteroscope was introduced gently with no problems through the cervical canal. This can be a difficult time in the procedure as there are many blind crypts within the cervix and perforation or trauma can occur. Deborah did not find the procedure painful but experienced slight discomfort similar to mild period pain. As the hysteroscope passed into the endometrial cavity, the irrigating fluid was introduced under slight pressure to distend the cavity. Three polyps were seen, two arising from the fundus and one long one, which filled the cavity. The endometrium was apparently healthy with no abnormal appearances (see Plate 38).

The hysteroscope and saline were withdrawn and a biopsy of endometrium was taken using a pipelle. This is a thin, plastic, straw-like instrument that has an inner stilette, which, when withdrawn, creates a small vacuum within the instrument. Once the vacuum had been created, the end of the pipelle was pulled gently against Deborah's endometrial lining to obtain a sample. The sample was placed in formulin for preservation and sent for histological performance.

Deborah experienced most discomfort during the pipelle biopsy but this soon settled and she refused any analgesia. Following her appointment, she spent a short time resting in a waiting area before going home. The appointment had taken only 20 min in total. An appointment was made for her to see the consultant when the results of the biopsy was available and discuss her further treatment.

At her next outpatient appointment, Deborah was able to discuss with the consultant all the results of her investigations. The endometrial biopsy showed inactive endometrium. It was felt that the irregular bleeding she had been experiencing was due to the endometrial polyps, which would need to be removed surgically. However, due to the large size of one of them, it was not felt that this would be a simple procedure. Deborah wanted a definitive surgical procedure, which would guarantee a solution to the irregular bleeding. After discussing the risks and benefits of major surgery, Deborah elected to have a hysterectomy. Due to her age, and the fact that she was postmenopausal, her ovaries were now inactive and it was decided to perform a bilateral salpingo-oophorectomy at the same time.

Deborah was placed on the waiting list and was admitted for her operation 2 months later. She was seen in the preadmission clinic by the nurse practitioner for preoperative assessment. Here a summary of her gynaecological history was noted, including information about previous contraception and details of cervical cytology. This information all helped to ensure appropriate advice was given about her planned treatment. In addition, details were recorded about previous medical and surgical history. Deborah had no systemic medical illnesses but had already had three operations via abdominal incisions. These included an emergency lower segment caesarian section, a left ovarian cystectomy and

Case study: Deborah (*contd*)

an appendicectomy. Adhesions may have formed following these operations, which may have made surgery more difficult than expected. She had not experienced any problems following general anaesthetics except for sickness after undergoing tonsillectomy.

Examination of her cardiovascular and respiratory systems by auscultation of the heart and lungs revealed no abnormalities. Previous operation scars were noted on abdominal examination. Blood samples were taken to check full blood count and the blood group.

Deborah mentioned that she had experienced problems coping with the stress of her job as a teacher and had started antidepressant therapy 9 months previously. The expected length and progress of the recovery period were discussed because, although Deborah's husband and son were very supportive, she was concerned about being fit enough to return to her teaching post for the start of the new academic year. After a full discussion about the proposed surgery, including risks of major gynaecological surgery, Deborah gave her written informed consent and left the clinic feeling reassured and less anxious.

On admission to the ward on the morning of her planned surgery, Deborah was slightly nervous but refused any premedication. She received a prophylactic dose of heparin 1 hour before being transferred to theatre. During her surgery, the left ovary was absent, having been removed during previous surgery so a total abdominal hysterectomy, right salpingo-oophorectomy and left salpingectomy were performed. On return to the ward, an intravenous infusion was in progress to prevent dehydration, a urinary catheter was in the bladder and an intravenous infusion via a pump was in progress administering morphine as analgesia. Deborah's nurse undertook regular monitoring of her vital signs to detect early signs of haemorrhage.

On the first postoperative day, Deborah felt extremely well with only slight nausea. Pain experienced was minimal and, in view of the nausea and drowsiness being caused by the morphine, Deborah requested the pump to be discontinued. She felt able to take oral fluids so was prescribed oral analgesia and the intravenous infusion was discontinued. She was assisted with a wash at her bedside as she did not feel up to a shower. By the evening, she was mobilizing gently around her bed area and tolerating light diet. Her husband was delighted to see the progress she was making. Before settling for the night, the urinary catheter was removed.

On the second postoperative day, Deborah continued to progress and was now able to undertake much of her care herself with support from nursing staff. She self-voided urine with no obvious problems and was able to increase mobilization and dietary intake. The dressing was removed from her abdominal scar and the wound was noted to be healing well with slight bruising over the upper aspect. The wound was left exposed and, as the skin suture used was a continuous one that would dissolve, no further treatment was required.

By the third postoperative day, Deborah was anxious to go home to complete her recovery at home with her family. It was felt that this would be appropriate as Deborah was self-caring now in most aspects. However, concern was expressed by nursing staff because Deborah's bowel function had not returned to normal. Preoperatively, Deborah suffered from irritable bowel syndrome with alternating bouts of constipation and diarrhoea. Although she had suffered with wind, a common occurrence following this type of surgery, she had not yet had her bowels open. Deborah did not feel it would be a problem and after discussions about how to manage any constipation that may occur, she was discharged home with a supply of lactulose. In addition, both verbal and written advice were given about the progress of her recovery with guidelines about increasing her activity levels. Her hormone replacement therapy was altered as she now required an oestrogen only preparation.

Deborah was reviewed 6 weeks after her discharge by the nurse practitioner. In some units this review is carried out by medical staff and in others by the woman's GP. In this unit, the nurse practitioner had the opportunity not only to exam Deborah to assess her physical recovery but also to discuss any problems encountered and plans for the future. It is an ideal situation in which to promote healthy lifestyles and practices.

Deborah had continued to make a full and relatively uneventful recovery since discharge. The two biggest problems she encountered were constipation and tiredness. Unfortunately, she did not have her bowels open naturally postoperatively, despite taking regular lactulose orally. After 6 postoperative days, she was feeling very uncomfortable but did not feel able to strain at stool. The situation was resolved by a visit from her GP and the administration of two glycerine suppositories. Deborah then ensured, through her diet and fluid intake, that she did not become constipated again. Tiredness is usual after such major surgery and although this had been explained to Deborah preoperatively and on discharge, she admitted that she hadn't realized just what an impact this would have on her.

A physical examination was performed, which included inspection and palpation of the abdominal scar and speculum examination of the vaginal vault. Both areas were healing well so Deborah was reassured that physically everything was healing well and that the tiredness would recede. This was the area causing Deborah most concern due to her job. She was a teacher at a junior school and the new academic year was due to start in 2 weeks' time. After a long discussion, she decided to meet with her head teacher early the following week in order to assess whether she then felt able to begin the new school term. Despite this concern, Deborah was pleased that she had had the surgery, as the irregular bleeding she had originally suffered with had now ceased. She also expressed her surprise at how relatively quickly she had returned to her previous lifestyle.

can be discontinued after about 4 days. The length of therapy depends on the severity of the DVT but should extend for at least 1 week after the disappearance of all symptoms. Regular checks must be made of the woman's blood clotting time whilst on warfarin therapy.

Pulmonary embolism may present as chest pain or the woman may collapse, often suffering a cardiac arrest. Complaints of chest pain, especially postoperatively, must be investigated thoroughly. A perfusion scan may be recommended to check the blood supply to the lungs. The treatment is similar to that for a deep vein thrombosis.

If the patient collapses, emergency resuscitation must be carried out and the woman's condition stabilized before treatment is commenced.

Anaemia

Postoperative anaemia can occur following blood loss during or immediately after surgery. The woman will be at greater risk if her haemoglobin was low preoperatively. Blood should be taken for a full blood count. Iron therapy is recommended, especially if the woman has undergone a hysterectomy. In this case, she will no longer be losing menstrual blood and her body will be able to restore haemoglobin levels during convalescence. The woman should be advised about this outcome.

A blood transfusion may be indicated if the haemoglobin level is excessively low but this decision should be made in conjunction with the woman. Patients are often anxious about receiving blood transfusions because of the associated risks of blood-borne infections, and this decision should be based on individual circumstances.

Secondary haemorrhage

This can occur 10–14 days postoperatively due to infection of a surgical site. Haemostasis may be required if haemorrhage is excessive. Investigations for infection, such as swabs from the affected site, may be taken and a broad spectrum antibiotic such as metronidazole or augmentin prescribed.

CONCLUSION

The elective nature of the majority of gynaecological surgery enables the nurse to plan care for the woman and her family both prior to and during her hospital stay. Psychological support is paramount to enable the woman to cope with the stress of undergoing surgery. Current research has shown the importance of providing appropriate, timely information. It is important that the nurse is well informed to advise the woman about planned treatments and procedures. This will help reduce anxiety and enable the woman to make an informed choice about her treatment.

GLOSSARY

Dilatation and curettage: minor surgical procedure, often referred to as 'a scrape', to obtain a sample of the endometrium. The cervix is dilated using metal dilators then a curette is introduced to endometrial cavity
Colposuspension: major surgical procedure via abdominal route to support bladder. Used to treat cases of stress incontinence or failed previous vaginal surgery
Hysterectomy: surgical removal of uterus. This may be performed via an abdominal or vaginal route
Hysteroscopy: examination of uterine cavity using endoscopic techniques

Laparoscopy: examination of the pelvis or abdominal cavity using endoscopic techniques
Minor procedure: term used to describe a small surgical procedure. These procedures are usually performed as day cases or in outpatient settings. Operations of this type include hysteroscopy and dilatation and curettage
Repair: term used to describe a vaginal operation performed to repair vaginal prolapse. May be prefixed by anterior or posterior, depending on the area of vaginal wall where surgery is performed

REFERENCES

Dulaney PE, Crawford VC, Turner G 1990 A comprehensive education and support program for women experiencing hysterectomies. Journal of Obstetric, Gynaecologic and Neonatal Nursing 19(4):319–324

Gammon J, Mulholland CW 1996 Effect of preparatory information prior to elective total hip replacement on post-operative physical coping outcomes. International Journal of Nursing Studies 33(6):589–604

Hayward J 1975 A prescription against pain. Royal College of Nursing, London

Keckstein J, Hepp S, Schneider V 1990 A new technique for conservation of the Fallopian tube in unruptured ectopic pregnancy. British Journal of Obstetrics and Gynaecology 97:352–354

Kohli N, Jacobs P, Sze E, Roat T, Karram M 1997 Open compared with laparoscopic approach to Burch colposuspension. Obstetrics and Gynecology 90(3):411–415

Kovac SR, Cruikshank SH, Retto HF 1990 Laparoscopy-assisted vaginal hysterectomy. Journal of Gynaecologic Surgery 6:185–189

Macdonald R 1993 Audit applied to endometrial ablation. In: Sutton CJG (ed) New surgical techniques in gynaecology. Parthenon Publishing Group, Carnforth, Lancashire

Martin D 1996 Pre-operative visits to reduce patient anxiety: a study. Nursing Standard 10(23):33–38

Meikle S, Weston Nugent E, Orleans M 1997 Complications and recovery from laparoscopy-assisted vaginal hysterectomy compared with abdominal and vaginal hysterectomy. Obstetrics and Gynaecology 89(2):304–310

Raleigh EH, Lepczyc M, Rowley C 1990 Significant others benefit from preoperative information. Journal of Advanced Nursing 15:941–945

Royal College of Obstetricians & Gynaecologists (RCOG) 1995 Report of RCOG Working Party on Prophylaxis Against Thromboembolism. In: Gynaecology and obstetrics. Chameleon, London

Sutton CJG 1993 New surgical techniques in gynaecology. Parthenon Publishing Group, Carnforth, Lancashire

Taylor J, Goodman M, Luesley D 1993 Is home best? Nursing Times 89(37):31–33

United Kingdom Central Council (UKCC) 1992 The scope of professional practice. UKCC, London

Wilson-Barnett J 1979 Stress in hospital. Churchill Livingstone, Edinburgh

FURTHER READING

Forrest APM, Carter DC, Macleod IB 1994 Principles of practice of surgery, 2nd edn. Churchill Livingstone, Edinburgh

Govan ADT, McKay Hart D, Callander R 1993 Gynaecology illustrated, 4th edn. Churchill Livingstone, Edinburgh

Llewellyn-Jones D 1990 Fundamentals of obstetrics and gynaecology, vol 2: Gynaecology, 5th edn. Faber & Faber, London

Sutton CJG 1993 New surgical techniques in gynaecology. Parthenon Publishing Group, Carnforth, Lancashire

USEFUL ADDRESSES

Women's Health

52 Featherstone Street, London EC1Y 8RT
Helpline: 020 7251 6850 Admin: 020 7251 6580
Fax: 020 7608 0928
Produce wide range of leaflets giving advice on women's health issues. Will provide further contacts for women requiring support following hysterectomy.

NHS Health Information Service

Tel: 0800 665444
Provides information for public and professionals on medical conditions, treatments, medical procedures, where to get treatment, hospital waiting times and self-help groups.

Patient's Association

8 Guildford Street, London
Represent patient interests to government and professional bodies. Offers support and advice to patients by telephone or correspondence.

Well Being

27 Sussex Place, Regent's Park, London NW1 4SP
Research charity of RCOG. Funds research into women's health. Educates and informs women. Provides written advice.

Index

Page numbers in **bold** type refer to illustrations and tables.